Kimberley Bush Medicine

Kimberley Bush Medicine

MEDICINAL PLANTS OF THE KIMBERLEY REGION OF WESTERN AUSTRALIA

MADISON KING AND
JOHN HORSFALL

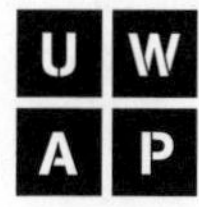

First published in 2023 by
UWA Publishing
Crawley, Western Australia 6009
www.uwap.uwa.edu.au
UWAP is an imprint of UWA Publishing,
a division of The University of Western Australia.

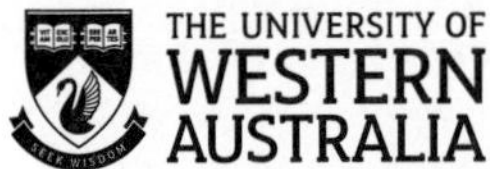

Front cover photo: Sam Fraser-Smith
Back cover photos: Ian Sutton, Mark Marathon and Craig Nieminski

ISBN: 9781760802196

Design by Upside Creative
Printed by Imago in China

Contents

DISCLAIMER

This book has been written for educational purposes based on information accumulated by the authors from personal knowledge and third parties, including books, websites, records, documents that other parties have prepared, and from Indigenous elders with traditional food and healing knowledge. While the authors have made their best efforts to produce an accurate account of plants used for food by the Indigenous people of the Kimberley region of Western Australia, they do not warrant or make any claim as to the accuracy or otherwise of the information and accept no responsibility whatsoever in the event of any inaccurate information contained in the book. It is the authors' recommendation that people wishing to collect or cultivate the plants described in this book and use them for culinary purposes for themselves, family or their friends, should consult with elders who have knowledge of the plants in their area before doing so.

All native plants on Crown land are protected in Western Australia by law. Section 171 of the Biodiversity Conservation Act 2016 states that you need a licence to take part or all of any native plant on Crown land or permission from the owners if the flora is on privately owned land. In Western Australia, the penalties are severe if people disregard the law related to flora and fauna.

Section 182 of the *Biodiversity Conservation Act 2016* includes a defence if the person taking the flora and fauna is of Australian Aboriginal descent and they are taking the flora and fauna for Aboriginal customary purposes, that is for ceremonial, food or medicinal purposes, providing that they comply with parts of the Act that relate to the taking of flora, and providing they can prove they are of Aboriginal descent. Aboriginal persons are advised to read Section 182 of the Act relating to Aboriginal people. A copy of the Act can be viewed at: www5.austlii.edu.au/au/legis/wa/num_act/bca201624o2016355/

The authors of this book wish to acknowledge and pay their respects to the traditional owners and elders, past and present, of the Kimberley region of Western Australia, the owners of the knowledge contained in this book.

Acknowledgements

The authors wish to acknowledge the following people for allowing us to use their beautiful photographs of plants: Craig Nieminski, Russell Cumming, Bill and Mark Bell, Harry Rose, Arthur Chapman, John Tann, Jean and Fred Hort, Steve and Alison Pearson, Ria Tan, Forest and Kim Starr, and the many others who generously make their images available through Creative Commons for projects such as ours.

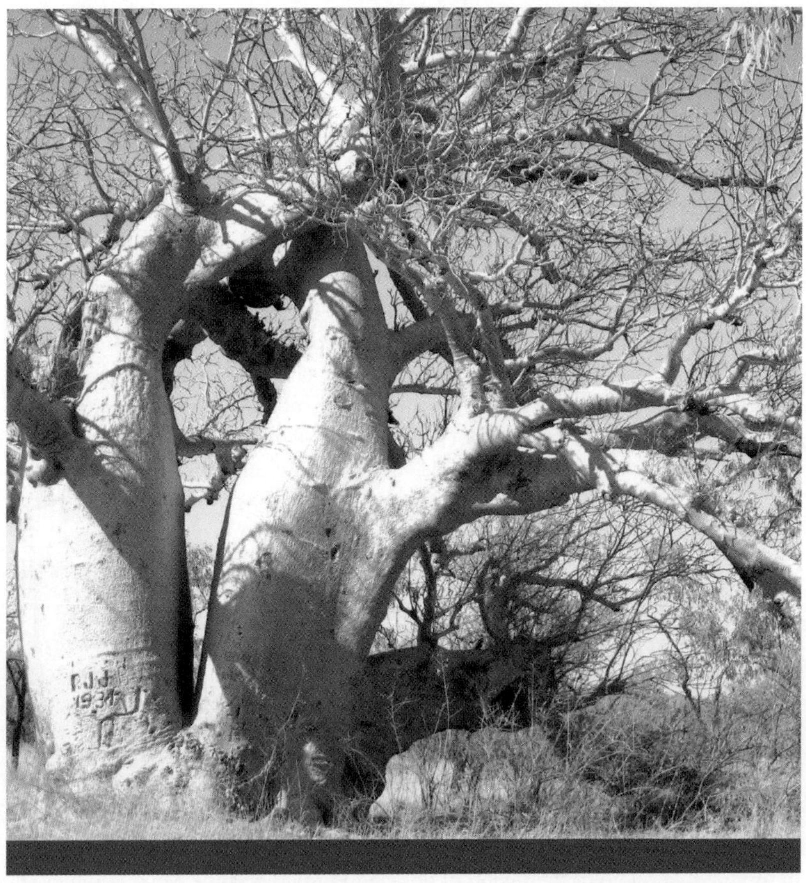

About the Authors

Madison's Story

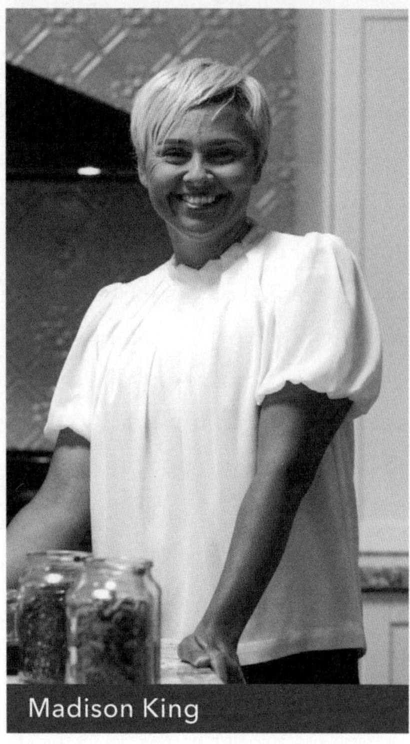
Madison King

From the bustling city of Perth to the remote landscapes of the East Kimberley, Madison King's journey as an Aboriginal woman has been a rich tapestry of cultural heritage, education, and entrepreneurial spirit. Hailing from five traditional groups across the Kimberley region, including Oombulgurri, Broome, Bidyadanga, Derby, Fitzroy, and Wyndham, Madison was instilled with a deep passion for foraging bush foods at an early age. It was here, among the stunning scenery and abundant wildlife of the East Kimberley, where she developed a deep appreciation for the traditional bush foods of her people.

Growing up, Madison fished, hunted, and tracked alongside her great-grandmother, Doris Morgan, grandmother, La La Gwen and other community members of Oombulgurri where learning about the seasons, food sources, and medicines of the land through quiet observation began. Learning the skill of sitting in silence allowed Madison and other members of her family and community members a deeper understanding of their immediate environment through the observation of weather patterns, temperature, and vegetation changes. Flowers in bloom, such as the Boab tree, kapok, and waterlily, played a crucial role in determining when and where to find food. The blooming kapok flower, for example, signalled the time to pick and collect crocodiles' and turtles' eggs, but also served as a reminder to be wary of territorial crocodiles when fishing. While the waterlily is another food source during the cooler wet season, it too, was a valuable survival tool for underwater activities such as snorkelling.

Madison went on to attend high school at St Brigid's College Perth and then earned a double degree in Psychology, Criminology, and Justice while pursuing a law degree. Her passion for creativity and taking on challenges led her to launch Kimberley Bush Superfoods, which will soon be available to a select group of chefs and businesses across Australia and, eventually, online. With her sights set on farming bush foods in the Kimberley region, Madison hopes to bring more job opportunities to the region and continue the tradition of bush food for future generations.

As Madison says, "Food is a connection to land, and land is a connection to memories." Join her in this exciting endeavour to preserve the rich culinary heritage of the Kimberley and to pass on this legacy to future generations.

John's Story

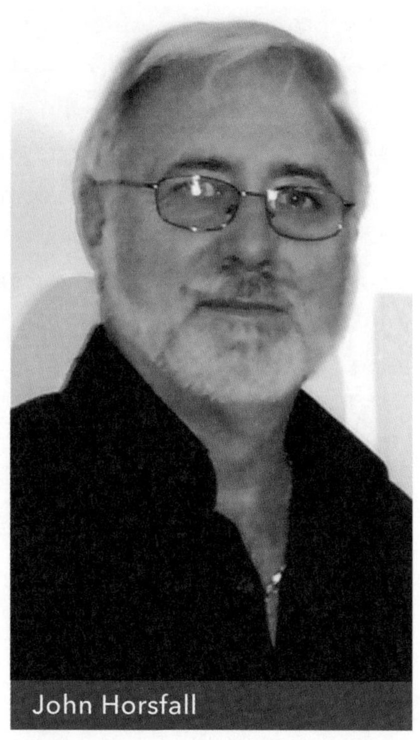
John Horsfall

John Horsfall was born in Melbourne, Victoria, and completed his schooling there. After finishing school, he worked for two years on Groote Eylandt in the Northern Territory, where he had their first contact with an Australian Aboriginal community, the Warnindilyakwa people. John was employed by BHP and later Groote Eylandt Mining Company, and spent his days off hunting and fishing with the Aboriginal men of the island. While on the island, John noticed how fit and healthy the Warnindilyakwa people were, as they often spent long periods away from the missions hunting, fishing, crabbing and gathering bush tucker and bush medicine, and getting plenty of exercise doing so.

After commencing his nursing career in Perth in 1967, John became interested in alternative medicine and completed a diploma in naturopathy and herbal medicine. He lectured at the Western Australian School of Nursing for some years before going into staff development at Graylands Hospital. In 2007, John was appointed to the position of associate lecturer at the Centre for Aboriginal Studies at Curtin University to teach in the Indigenous Community Health Degree course. It was there that he came into contact with Aboriginal Australians from all over Australia and learnt a great deal more about Aboriginal culture, lore and protocols.

While researching session notes on bush medicine, John noticed that there was little coverage of the full range of wild medicinal and edible plants used by Western Australian Aboriginal groups. While working at Curtin University, he met Vivienne Hansen, a Wadjuk Ballardong Noongar elder, who had traditional bush food and bush medicine knowledge passed down to her from her grandparents and parents. Vivienne has also completed a diploma in herbal medicine at Marr Mooditj. The two collaborated on two books: *Noongar Bush Medicine: Medicinal Plants of the Southwest of Western Australia* and *Noongar Bush Tucker: Bush Food Plants and Fungi of the South-west of Western Australia*.

John was fortunate to meet Madison, his co-author, while working at the Specialist Aboriginal Mental Health Service in his final position as a training coordinator before retirement.

Introduction

The Kimberley

The Kimberley region of Western Australia ranges from Broome in the south to Kununurra and the border with the Northern Territory in the north. It covers some 424,517 square kilometres. Characterised by its distinct wet and dry seasons, the Kimberley experiences a sub-tropical climate. The dry season extends from May to October and the wet season from November to April.

The estimated residential population of the Kimberley was 36,230 in 2017, with the Shire of Broome accounting for over 40% of the population. The region is culturally rich with approximately half the population comprising Aboriginal people who represent more than 30 traditional Aboriginal language groups.

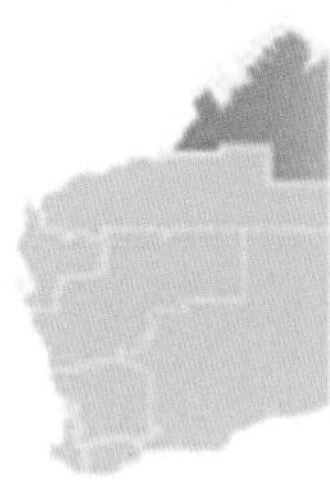

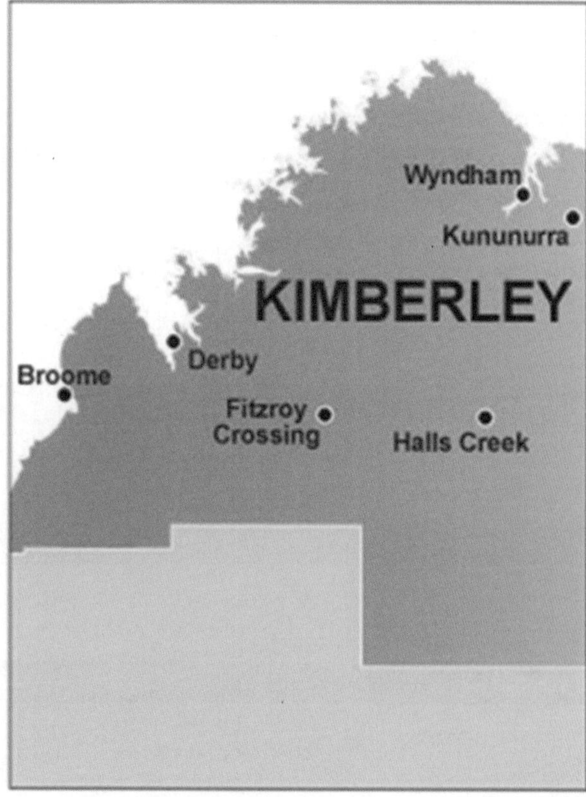

Source: Department of Primary Industries and Regional Development, Western Australia.

Kimberley Languages

Aboriginal people of the Kimberley region of Western Australia speak a variety of languages. Language groups include the following:

Bardi Type	This includes Warwar, Nimanburu, Ongarang and Djaul Djaui languages.
Garadjeri Type	As for Nyangamada type in the Murchison, this includes Garadjeri, Mangala, Yaoro, Djungun, Ngombal, Djaberadjabera and Nyul Nyul languages.
Ungarinyin Type	This includes Umedi, Wungemi, Worora and Wunumbul languages.

Kimberley Seasons

The calendar of the **Yawuru** and **Karajarri** people of the Kimberley has six seasons. The Yawuru are the native title holders of the town of Broome, including areas of land and sea in and around that area. The Karajarri people are the traditional owners of the land and waters along the south-west Kimberley coast.

Man-gala	
Summer - December to March	The wet season with strong winds - the monsoon.
Marrul	
Late summer - April	The hot season with very little wind and high tides.
Wirralburu	
Autumn - May	The dry season with no rain. The days are hot and the nights are cool.
Barrgana	
Winter - June to August	The cold season with some fog and dry winds.

Wirlburu	
Spring - September	The warming season with the days and nights getting hotter.
Laja	
Early summer - October and November	Building up to the hot season when the days and nights are getting hotter.

The **Miriwoong** calendar only has three major seasons broken down into eight sub-seasons, covering the hot, wet and cold times of year. The area around Kununurra in the Kimberley is the heart of Miriwoong and Gajirrabeng land.

Nyinggiyi-mageny	
Wet weather December to March	**Barrawoodang** December, January: Strong winds, thunder, lightning and big rain. **Jaloorr-mageny** February, March: Rain (coinciding with monsoonal downpours).
Warnka-mageny	
Cold weather April to August	**Genkaleng** April, May: South winds start, introducing cold weather. **Werlthang** June: Dew forms overnight and dries in the morning. **Manbilying** July and August: Irregular cold weather rain (doesn't occur yearly).
Barndenyirriny	
Hot weather September to November	**Boornbeng** September: Country starts warming up. **Dilboong** October: Country dries out and becomes brown and dusty. **Deroorr-mageny** November: Thunder, heat and humidity, introducing the wet season.

The **Gooniyandi** language group calendar from people of the Fitzroy Valley in the Kimberley has four seasons.

Barranga	
September to November	Very hot weather time.
Yidirla	
December to March	Wet season time when the rivers run.
Ngamari	
April and May	Female. Cold weather time.
Girlinggoowa	
June to August	Male. Cold weather time.

The **Walmajarri** people, who have migrated into the Fitzroy Valley area from southern desert locations, have three seasons on their calendar.

Parranga	
September to November	Hot weather time
Yitilal	
December to March	Raining time
Makurra	
April to August	Cold weather time

Adapted from the Bureau of Meteorology and the CSIRO websites.

The **Wunambal** and **Kwini** people of the Kalumburu area have seven seasons in their calendar.

Season	Time	Description
Yirma	May to August	Winter commences and the south-east winds blow steadily.
Yuwala	September to November	The hottest period of the year.
Djaward	Mid-November to late December	The approach of the wet season.
Wundju	January and early February	The wet season when heavy rains fall almost daily.
Maiaru	Late February and March	The rains ease and the leaves fall from some trees.
Bande Manya	April	The wet season has ended and the first of the new season's root crops are reaching maturity.
Goloruru	End of April	The south-east trade winds begin to blow and more root crops reach maturity.

Adapted from Crawford, 1982.

The **Gija** or **Kija** people of the eastern Kimberley have five seasons in their calendar.

Jadagen	
December to mid-March	The full wet season with heavy rain, thunder and lightning.
Lintharrg	
Mid-March to mid-May	The end of the wet season but still quite hot. The rivers and creeks begin to slow up.
Warnkan	
Mid-May to the end of July	The start of the cold weather when night temperatures can get down to zero.
Barnden	
August and September	The cool weather merges into hot weather. The ground begins to heat up and the waterholes begin to dry up.
Werrgalen	
October and November	This is the time of very hot weather. The waterholes are dry and there is very little water around.

Adapted from Purdie et al., 2018.

The **Bardi** people from Dampierland just north of Broome have six seasons in their calendar.

Mangal	
December and January	The wet season or monsoon season. Little fruit is available, though some roots are dug from the ground.
Ngalandany	
February to mid-March	The end of the wet. Temperatures and humidity are high. There is little or no wind.

Iralbu	
Mid-March and April	The period of king or big tides. Much fruit is available.
Bargana	
May to July	The cold season when people light night fires. Dugong hunting season.
Djallalayi	
August to mid-October	The warming up season. The west winds start. Dugong hunting ends. Low spring tides for reefing.
Lalin	
Mid-October to November	The build-up to the wet. Hot and humid. Winds shift to the north-west bringing the rain. Turtle hunting time.

Adapted from Smith & Kalotas, 1985.

The **Bunuba** people from north-west of Fitzroy Crossing follow four seasons on their calendar.

Maurri	
Mid-April to July	Winter rains arrive. Bush turkeys are the fattest. Fire management continues.
Barrangga	
August to mid-December	Gales start as heat builds up. Turtle eggs hatch with the first rains. Freshwater crocodiles lay their eggs.
Bullurru	
Mid-December to early February	The big rains arrive, flooding the rivers. Fire management of the country begins. Many fruits become available.

Girinybali	
Late February to mid-April	This is the most active time when the country is alive. The goannas are fat. Fishing is good. Barramundi (Balga) swim upstream. Mussels are collected.

Adapted from the Bunuba Seasonal Calendar, Bush Heritage Australia.

The **Nyikina** people, whose country encompasses the lower reaches of the Fitzroy River, describe six seasons in their calendar.

Wilakarra	
December to February	Wilakarra, around Christmas time, is the wet season.
Koolawa	
March to mid-May	'Knockem down rain' comes at the end of the wet season, before it goes into Koolawa time, the start of winter.
Jirrbal	
Mid-May to June	At this time, the Seven Sisters (stars) come out early in the morning. The bright pinpoint light of these stars warns that cold weather is on the way.
Wilbooroo	
June to August	At the end of July, when koolbarn (a type of Acacia) leaves turn green, the cold weather is coming to an end.
Barrkana	
September	The middle of the dry season when the Warimba flowers dry up, and Kardookardoo (whitewood) flowering begins. Kardookardoo flower is the main food for cockatoos while they're nesting.
Lalin	
October to December	This is the build-up to the rainy season. White gums and Coolibahs, Walarriy (white river gum) and Majala (freshwater mangrove) are all in flower.

Adapted from the West Kimberley Place Report

The **Jaru** or **Djaru** people, who live in the East Kimberley near Halls Creek, divide the annual cycle of weather patterns into four major seasons. Wightman (2003) advises that 'The timing of these seasons can vary a lot from year to year as the onset and duration of seasons can be significantly different each year.'

Malirri	
May to July	Cold weather time when the temperature gets very low at night. Temperatures during the day time are also lower and the air is very dry.
Barrangga	
August to November	The build-up time, when temperatures and the humidity build up. The Jaru term 'Barrangga' literally means the time of the sun, when the creeks and rivers have dried up and only big waterholes and springs contain water.
Ngababura	
December to March	This is the wet season, the time of monsoonal weather, with torrential rain, thunder and lightning. The rivers and creeks are flowing strongly again and often flood. The grasses are greening up.
Wurrgal	
April	This is the time of green grass. The rain has stopped. The ground has not yet dried out and the rivers and creeks are still flowing.

Adapted from Wightman, 2003.

Traditional Pharmacological Preparations, Healing Methods and Healers

Although plants were, and still are, an important part of medical treatment in the Kimberley, they are only one of the many forms of healing treatments available. Some of the others include the use of minerals, insect products, healing songs, the removal of 'foreign objects' by knowledgeable traditional healers and, of course, modern Western treatment by medical professionals in hospitals and Aboriginal community health centres.

Aboriginal people in the Kimberley had many traditional ways of preparing plant material for treating all types of ailments. To make infusions (teas), parts of plants, or sometimes the whole plant, were crushed and soaked in hot or cold water. Decoctions were made by boiling parts or whole plants in water. Water was traditionally heated by placing hot stones in rock pools or coolamons; nowadays, billies and metal cans are used to boil plant material. Infusions and decoctions were either taken internally or applied externally depending on the condition being treated and the level of toxicity of the plant.

Many plant preparations were only used externally. Infusions and decoctions, when used externally, were applied as antiseptic washes to cuts, sores and wounds to aid and quicken healing. Other decoctions and infusions were rubbed on painful parts of the body to treat headaches and rheumatic pain, or rubbed on the head and chest to treat the symptoms of cold and influenza. Sometimes sap from certain plants, such as Caustic Bush (*Cynanchum viminale* subsp. *australe*; p. 100), was applied to sores or rubbed on certain parts of the body to aid healing, or rubbed on the breasts of nursing mothers to promote lactation (the flow of milk). Tonics made from certain plants, such as Gadji (*Flagellaria indica*; p. 212) were taken to maintain good health.

The leaves of certain plants were heated whole or crushed and applied as poultices to wounds to aid healing or to painful areas of the body for pain relief. Certain vines, such as Snakevine (*Tinospora smilacina*; p. 510), were mashed and tied around the head to relieve a headache. Often plants were ground to a paste and mixed with animal fat, usually from reptiles or emus, and applied as salves to painful areas. Sometimes the ashes of some plants were more effective for treating sores and wounds than the fresh material. The gum or resin from some species, especially eucalypts, was ground and applied to sores and wounds as an antibiotic powder to aid healing.

Smoke from certain plants was another therapeutic tool and was thought to make people, especially babies, strong and healthy. Babies would be held over smoking leaves for a few seconds. People with colds and influenza would stand stooped over smouldering fires to inhale smoke from smoking aromatic leaves from plants with volatile oils, such as the Broad-leaved Paperbark (*Melaleuca leucadendra*; p. 70). Another treatment was crushing the leaves from certain plants, such as eucalypts or melaleucas, that were then held under the nose of people with colds and influenza so they could breathe in the vapours. Massage was another tool that was used to heal certain conditions, especially headaches and back pain (Clarke, 2008; Ens et al., 2017; Smith, 1991).

Some Aboriginal groups in Western Australia ate red earth for stomach conditions (Williams, 2013).

Aboriginal people all over Australia used emu oil, the fat or oil extracted from fatty deposits under the skin of emus (*Dromaius novaehollandiae*), externally as a liniment and anti-inflammatory to relieve minor arthritic aches and pains, to help wounds heal quicker and to protect the skin from the elements, including the sun (Bennett et al., 2015; Whitehouse, 1998). Sometimes emu oil was mixed with red clay and applied to wounds (Williams, 2013). Recent studies have shown that emu oil contains the anti-inflammatory substance vitamin E (Grossmann, n.d.). Goanna oil or fat from various *Varanus* species, such as the Argus Monitor (*Varanus panoptes*), either used by itself or mixed with other ingredients, was also smeared on wounds to aid healing (Mader, 2007).

Each Aboriginal group had their traditional healers or 'clever men or women' to whom knowledge of plant medicine and healing techniques were handed down from previous generations. Traditional healers knew what medicinal plants were available in certain areas and in what season. Healers were considered to have the ability to 'see' into the body of their patients and to diagnose what was ailing them. They dealt with mental health issues as well as physical ones. Clarke (2008) explains that:

> *In Aboriginal Australia, the healer's job is to diagnose problems, advise on remedies, suggest and perform ritualised healing procedures, explore the impact of community social and cultural issues upon the illness, and to reassure their patients that they can be cured.*

He goes on to say that:

> *The healer's set of special skills was considered fundamental for treatment in cases where sickness was blamed upon supernatural things, such as sorcery, contact with spirits and the breaking of taboos. When illness is diagnosed as being caused by foreign objects entering the body, the healers will treat the patient with singing, massage and sucking to 'remove' the offending article, which may be revealed as a fragment of wood, bone, shell, stone and since European colonisation even wire or glass.*

The Plants

The purpose of this book is to preserve the bush medicine plant knowledge for future generations of Aboriginal and non-Aboriginal people from the Kimberley region of Western Australia, and elsewhere, as information could be lost over time with the passing of elders and clever men and women.

Only plants that are endemic or native to the Kimberley region of Western Australia and were present before colonisation will be discussed in this book, with the exception of Mimosa Bush (*Vachellia farnesiana*; p. 334), Stinking Passionflower (*Passiflora foetida;* p. 528), and Tamarind *(Tamarindus indica;* p. 542). There are many other introduced plants that have medicinal properties that are covered elsewhere and will not be discussed in this book. The authors have tried to include most of the indigenous plants that grow in the Kimberley that have medicinal properties. We were unable to find written evidence for the use of some of the plants by Aboriginal groups, but we have included the plants anyway as they may have been used by Aboriginal people over the 60,000-plus years that they have occupied the land before colonisation.

The plants are listed and discussed on the following pages in the order of the most common name they are known by in Western Australia, or wider Australia if no common name is mentioned in the Western Australian Herbarium (FloraBase) database. The plants may be known by other common names elsewhere. Care has been taken to list as many English common names as possible for each plant where more than one common name is known. Some common names presented are also the Aboriginal names for the plants or an anglicised version of them.

Albayi

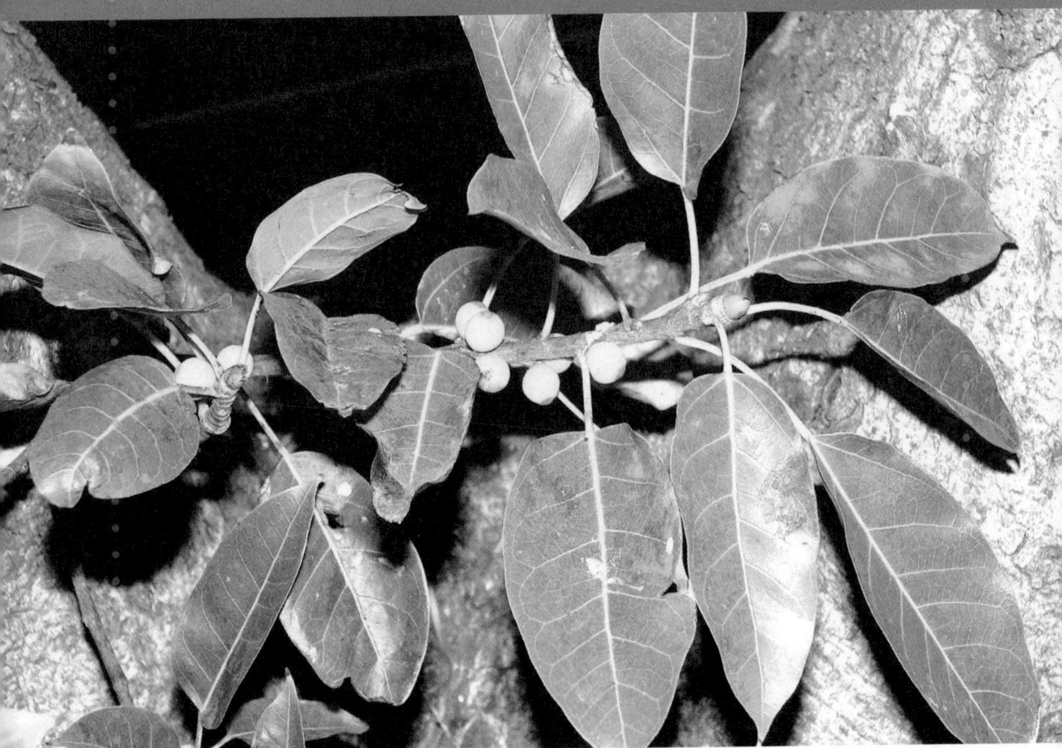

Scientific Name *Ficus virens* Aiton.

Common Names Albayi, Banyan, Mountain Fig, White Fig.

Aboriginal Names Yawurru (Wunambal, Gaambera) (Karadada et al., 2011), Albayi (Bardi) (Smith & Kalotas, 1985), Barlngel (Gija) (Purdie et al., 2018; Wightman, 2003).

Field Notes Albayi is a deciduous, monoecious tree that is found growing up to 30 m in height, at first an epiphytic strangler, but becoming a tree with aerial and prop roots with a canopy wider than the height of the tree. Its leaves are oblong-elliptic to ovate or lanceolate and up to 200 mm long and 60 mm wide. According to Fern (2022), 'these trees produce three types of flower: male, a long-styled female and a short-styled female flower'. The flowers are present between April and December. Its globose, pinkish brown to white fruit are up to 15 mm in diameter. Albayi prefers sand or alluvium over sandstone, limestone or basalt, and is found

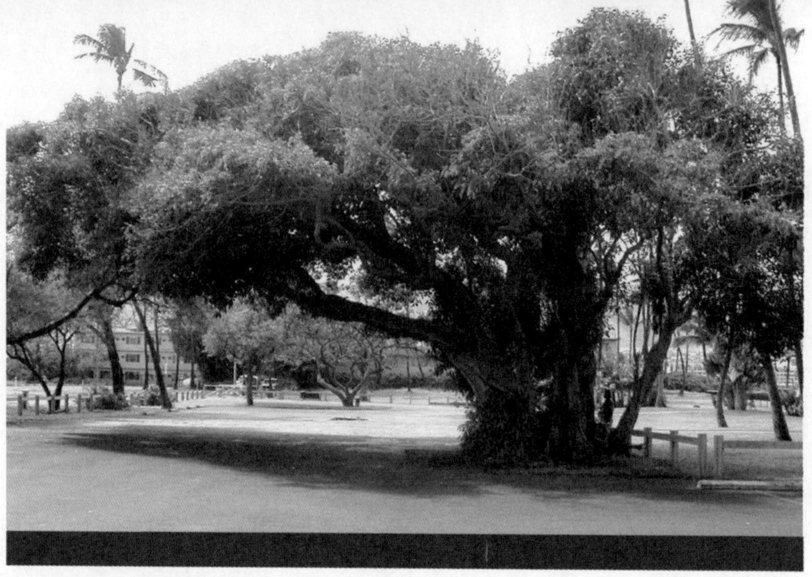

in a variety of habitats, frequently in vine thickets on sandstone. It occurs across the top end of Australia from the Pilbara and Kimberley regions of Western Australia through the Northern Territory and down the Queensland coast to the border with New South Wales. It also occurs in China, Japan, the Indian subcontinent, Sri Lanka, through tropical Asia to New Guinea and the Solomon Islands (ALA, 2022; Tree Logic, 2015; WAH, 2022).

Medicinal Uses In Far North Queensland, Aboriginal groups took decoctions of the leaves internally to treat an 'upset stomach'. Small aerial roots were chewed and tied around the head to relieve headaches and fever. Juice from aerial roots was used as an eyewash to treat conjunctivitis (Edwards, 2005). Parts of the tree are used in Ayurvedic medicine in India and Sri Lanka in the treatment of leucorrhoea. Decoctions of the bark were applied externally to treat leg ulcers and as a gargle for excessive salivation (Fern, 2021). In Pakistan, the leaves are used to treat diabetes (Khan et al., 2011)

Other Uses The fruit of the Albayi tree are edible when they are speckled whitish and ripe, which is usually from June to August. In some Asian countries, the young shoots and young leaves are eaten raw, cooked as a vegetable or added to curries (Fern, 2021; Fox & Garde, 2018; Low, 1991; Purdie et al., 2018; RFCA, 1993; Vigilante et al., 2013; Wightman, 2003).

Apple Bush

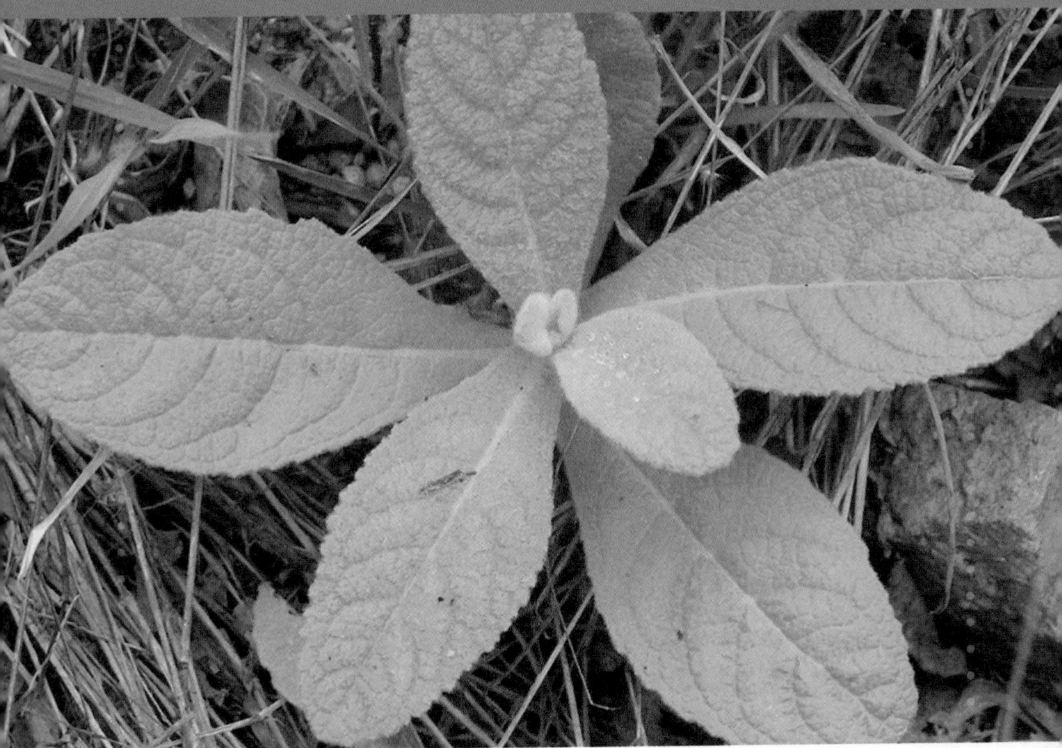

Family **Asteraceae** **Bercht. & J. Presl.**

Scientific Name *Pterocaulon sphacelatum* (Labill.) F.Muell.

Common Names Apple Bush, Fruit Salad Bush, Woolly Tobacco, Horehound.

Aboriginal Names Ngalil (Bardi) (Kenneally et al., 1996), Gooroongoony (Gija) (Purdie et al., 2018), Manyani (Ngardi) (Cataldi, 2004), Parntingunma-ngunma, Tjurrtjungurnu-ngurnu (Kukatja) (Valiquette, 1993), Ngurnungurnu (Jaru) (Wightman, 2003).

Field Notes Apple Bush is an erect or straggling perennial herb or shrub that grows up to 1.2 m in height. It has furry, oblanceolate leaves, and spherical, blue, purple, white or pink flowers that appear from April to October. It is found in a variety of habitats right across the top half of Australia from Carnarvon in the west to Brisbane in the east and as far south as Cooper Pedy in South Australia (ALA, 2022; PlantNET, 2020; WAH, 2022). It also occurs in Indonesia, New Guinea and New Caledonia (Kenneally et al., 1996).

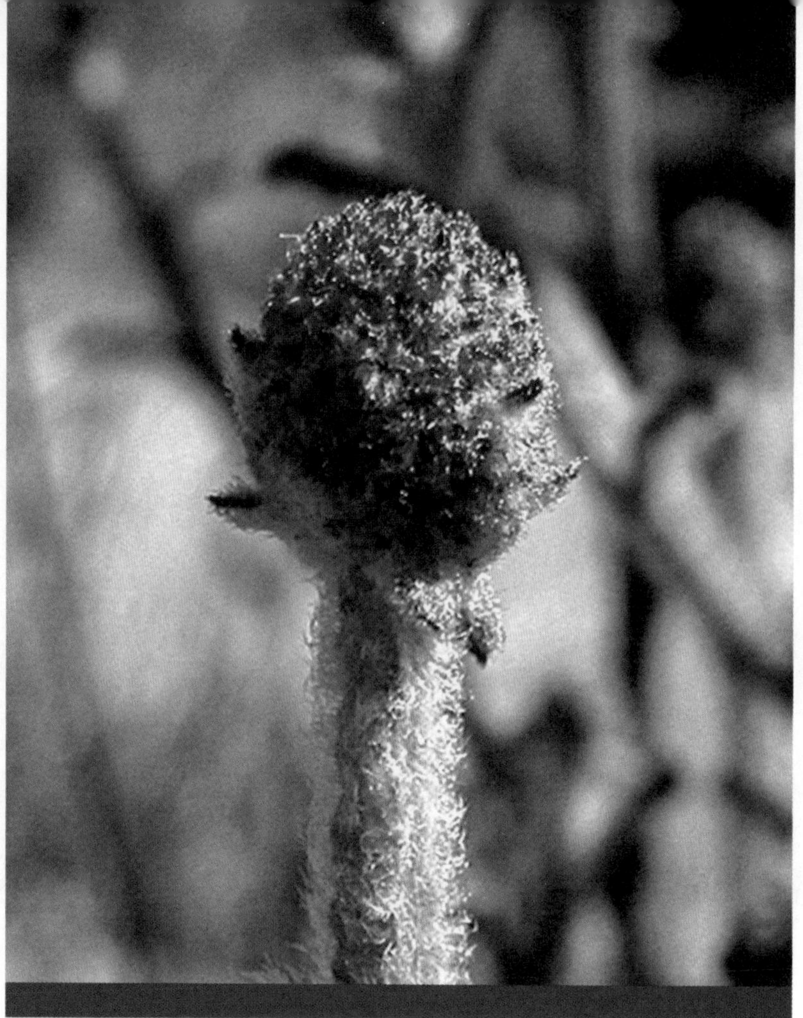

Medicinal Uses Decoctions of the leaves were taken internally to ease the symptoms of colds and influenza. Crushed leaves were inserted into the nose, wrapped as a pillow, or mixed with animal oil to make a massage ointment to relieve the symptoms of colds, such as a stuffy nose or chest congestion (Clarke, 2008; Cock, 2011; Low, 1990; Wightman, 2003; Williams, 2013). Decoctions of the leaves were used as an eyewash to treat conjunctivitis, as an antiseptic wash for sores of the skin and badly infected cuts (Cock, 2011; Devanesen, 2000; Smith, 1991; Williams, 2013) and rubbed on the chest to ease the symptoms of colds and influenza (Valiquette, 1993).

Other Uses The leaves of Apple Bush were sometimes used as chewing tobacco when other tobaccos were scarce (Clarke, 2007).

Arid Wattle

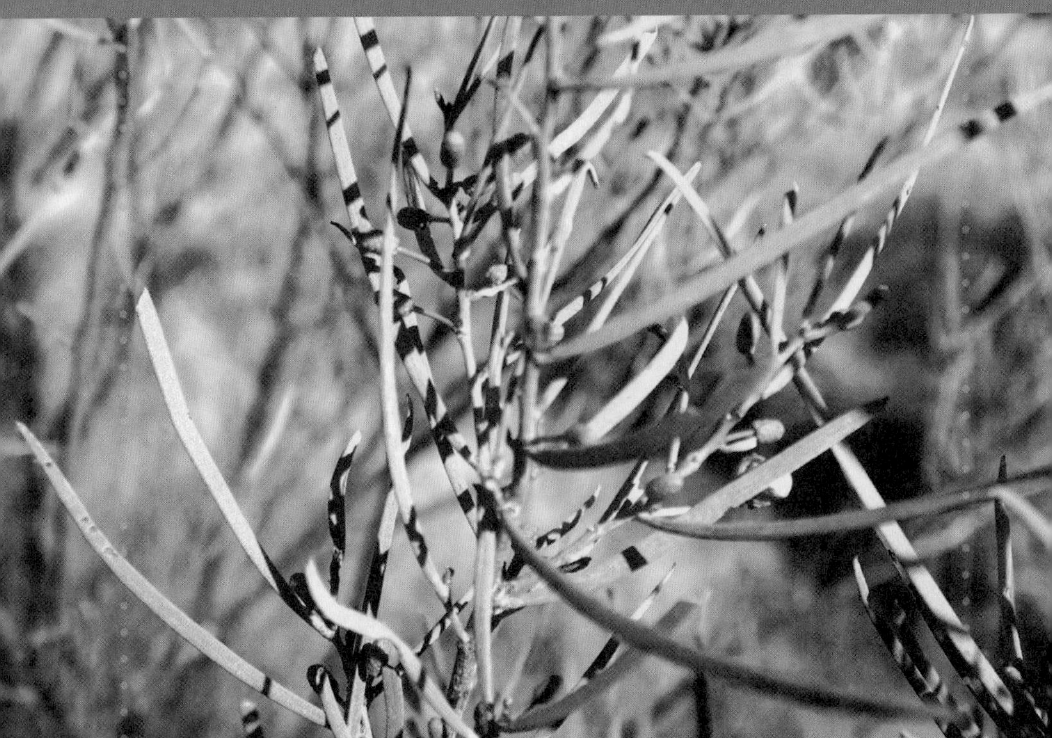

Scientific Name *Acacia arida* Benth., also known as *Acacia trachycarpa* E.Pritz.

Common Names Arid Wattle, False Melaleuca.

Field Notes There are some 1350 species of acacia worldwide and roughly 1000 of these are found in Australia. Acacias are commonly known as wattles. Acacias are the largest genus of vascular plants in Australia. Many acacias have edible seeds or gum, and many are used for their medicinal properties. Fern (2021) reports that, on analysis, 'Acacia seeds are highly nutritious and contain around 26% protein, 26% available carbohydrate, 32% fibre and 9% fat. The fat content is higher than most legumes with the aril providing the bulk of fatty acids present.'

Arid Wattle is a multi-stemmed shrub that grows to around 3 m in height. It has minni-ritchie, or curling red bark, and linear to narrowly oblong leaves, or more correctly phyllodes, that are up to

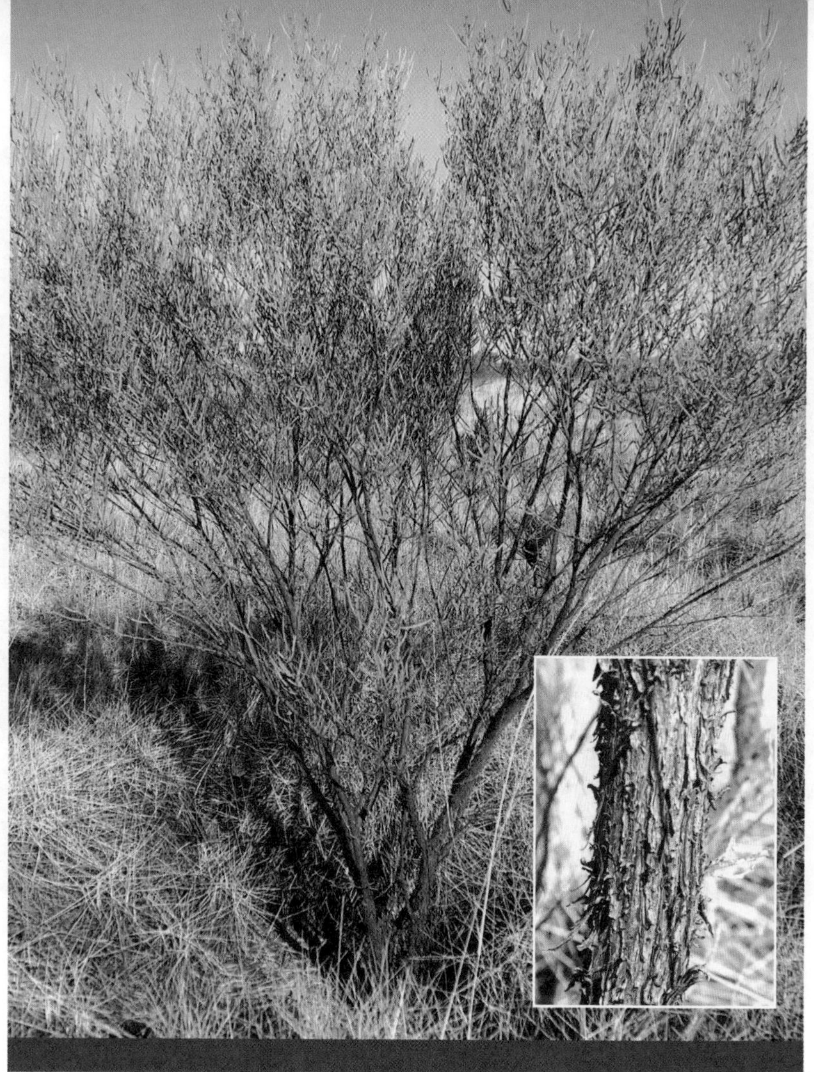

80 mm long and 6 mm wide. Its golden flower spikes are 24 mm long and appear from February to March or June to August. Its brownish-black seed pods are narrowly oblong-elliptic and up to 7 mm long. Arid Wattle is often found on red sandy and stony soils and is endemic to the Pilbara and Kimberley regions of Western Australia (ALA, 2022; Maslin et al., 2010; WAH, 2022).

Medicinal Uses Decoctions of the phyllodes of Arid Wattle were used as an eyewash to treat conjunctivitis (Young & Vitenbergs, 2007). Decoctions or infusions of the mashed phyllodes and twigs were used to bathe the head to ease headaches. Crushed phyllodes and twigs were rubbed on the body to treat swellings and internal pain (Williams, 2011).

Arrow-leaf Morning Glory

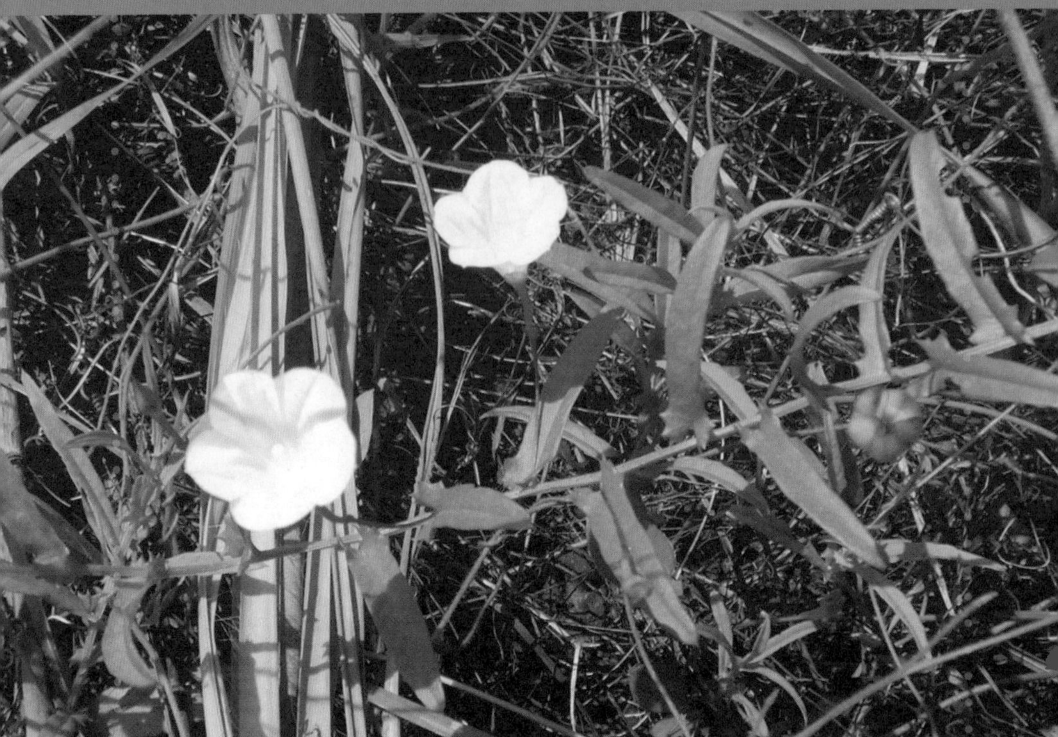

Scientific Name *Xenostegia tridentata* (L.) D.F.Austin & Staples, previously known as *Merremia tridentata* (L.) Hallier f.

Common Name Arrow-leaf Morning Glory.

Field Notes Arrow-leaf Morning Glory is a prostrate, scrambling or twining perennial herb or climber producing wiry stems up to 4 m long. Its lanceolate leaves are up to 100 mm long by 20 mm wide. Its white-cream, trumpet-like flowers are present from March to August in Western Australia. Its fruit are globose capsules that are up to 9 mm in diameter. The capsules usually contain four seeds. Arrow-leaf Morning Glory occurs in sandy soils, red gravel and skeletal soils over sandstone across the top end of Australia from the Kimberley region in Western Australia to northern Queensland (ALA, 2022; WAH, 2022). It also occurs in tropical and southern Africa through to tropical Asia (Fern, 2021).

Medicinal Uses In Australia, decoctions of the whole plant were used as an antiseptic wash to treat sores, cuts and other wounds (Cock, 2011). Arrow-leaf Morning Glory is also widely used in folk medicine in Africa and parts of Asia. The leaves are crushed and applied as poultices to the head to treat fever and snakebites. Decoctions of the whole plant or the roots are used for treating rheumatism and dysentery. Decoctions of the roots are used as a mouthwash or relieving toothache. Decoctions of the whole plant, or the roots, are used to treat haemorrhoids, swellings and urinary disorders. The roasted seeds are reported to have anthelmintic, diuretic and antibilious properties (Fern, 2021).

Asparagus Fern

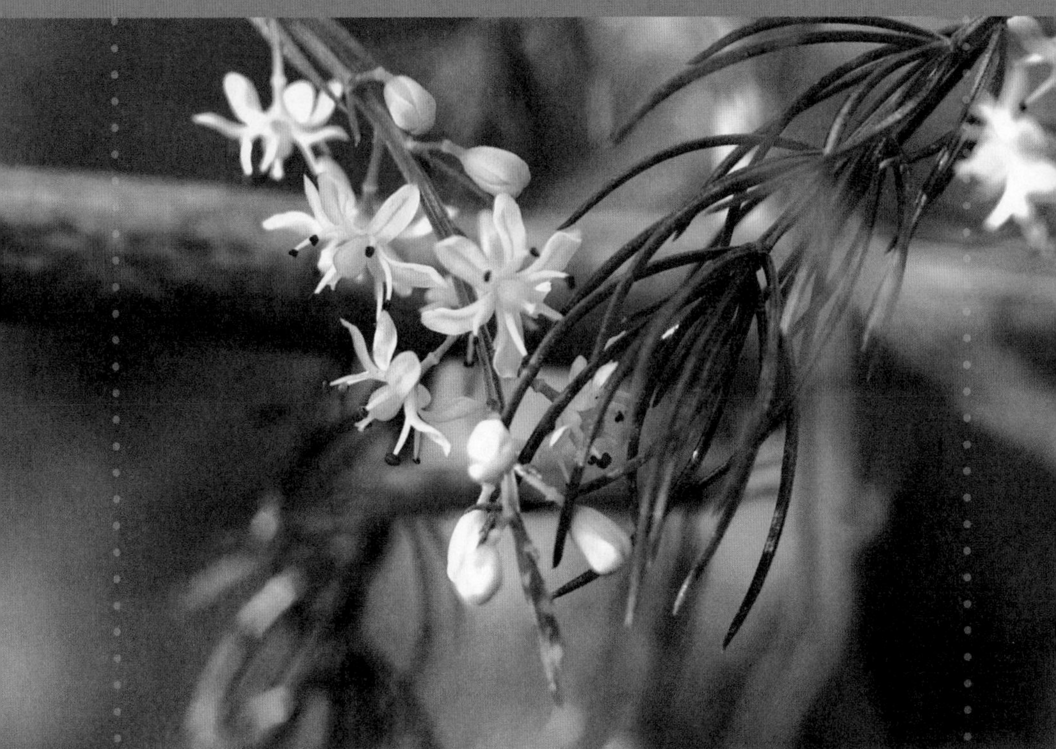

Scientific Name *Asparagus racemosus* Willd.

Common Names Asparagus Fern, Native Asparagus.

Aboriginal Name Leiwaleiwa manya (Kwini) (Cheinmora et al., 2017).

Field Notes Asparagus Fern is a rhizomatous and tuberous perennial herb and climber climbing sometimes to 5 m in height. It has small pine-needle-like phylloclades, and tiny cream-white, star-shaped flowers that are present in Australia between May and August. Its fruit are small green berries that turn brown later. Asparagus Fern is often found in coastal bush throughout tropical Africa, through Arabia and tropical Asia, including India and Sri Lanka. In Australia it is native to the coastal and near-coastal areas of the Kimberley region in Western Australia, the Northern Territory, the Cape York Peninsula and the east coast of Queensland, reaching as far south as the border with New South Wales (ALA, 2022; ATRP, 2020; Fern, 2021; WAH, 2022).

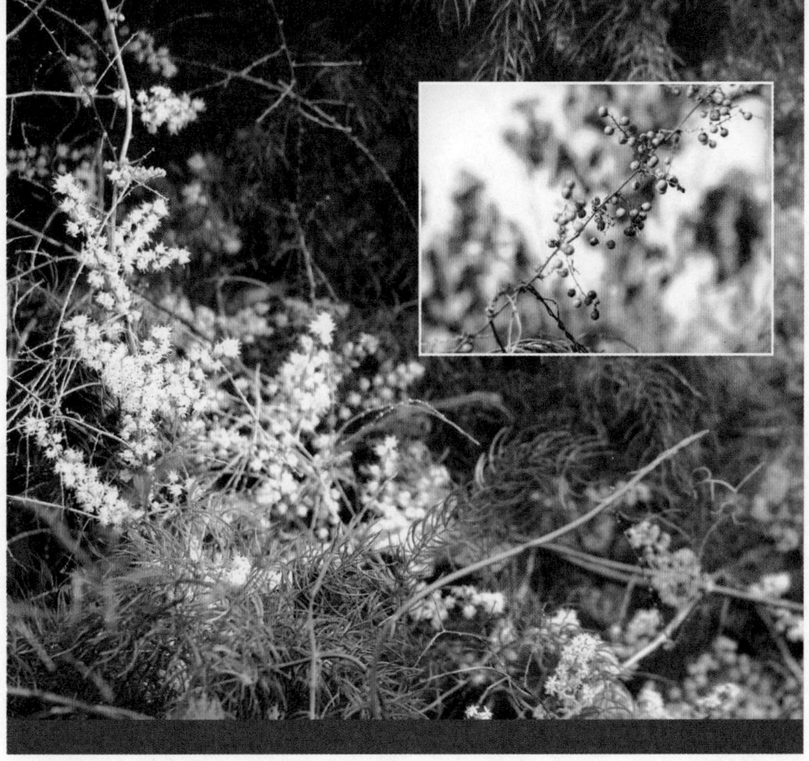

Medicinal Uses In Australia, decoctions of the crushed roots were applied directly to skin sores, especially leg ulcers on the ankles (Devanesen, 2000; Smith, 1991; Wightman, 2017). The tuberous roots were crushed and rubbed onto women's breasts to reduce swellings, take away lumps and to treat breast cancer (Smith, 1991). Decoctions of the fleshy lateral roots were used as a wash and taken internally to treat chest infections (Tiwi Land Council, 2001). Asparagus Fern is also used in traditional medicine in other countries, including Ayurvedic medicine in India and Sri Lanka. The rhizome is a tonic that acts on the circulatory, digestive, respiratory systems and female reproductive organs. It is taken internally for infertility, loss of libido, threatened miscarriage, menopausal problems, hyperacidity, stomach ulcers and bronchial infections. It is used externally in the treatment of stiffness in the joints, diarrhoea and dysentery (Fern, 2021).

Other Uses The tender young shoots can be cooked and eaten as a vegetable. In other countries the tubers are candied and eaten as a sweetmeat (Fern, 2021).

Baderi

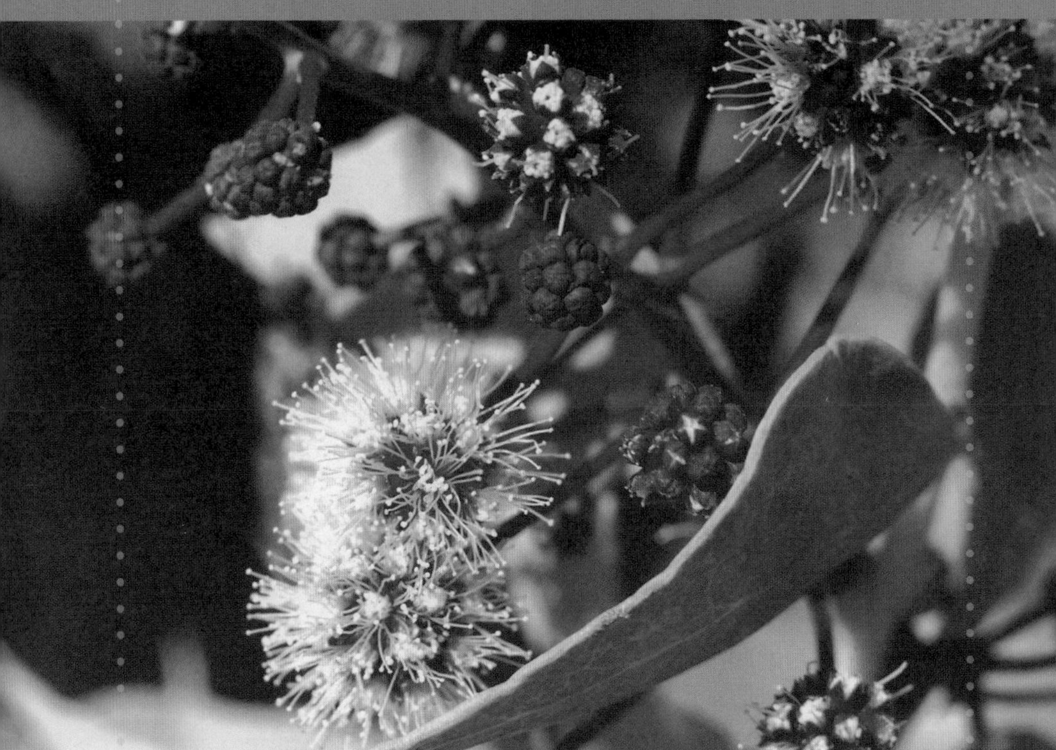

Scientific Name *Acacia inaequilatera* Domin.

Common Names Baderi, Camel Bush.

Aboriginal Name Janjilyngi (Ngardi, Warlpiri) (Cataldi, 2004).

Field Notes Baderi is a prickly shrub or tree that grows up to 8 m in height. Its bark is dark grey to black, rough, thick and corky. Its phyllodes are ovate to elliptic or obovate, and up to 70 mm long and 45 mm wide. Yellow flowers with red centres appear in spherical clusters from May to October. Its seed pods are flat and curved and up to 100 mm long and 10 mm wide. Baderi occurs in sandy and loamy, occasionally stony, soils on plains, stony hillsides and rocky plateaus in the Pilbara and Kimberley regions of Western Australia and the western half of the Northern Territory (ALA, 2022; WAH, 2022; World Wide Wattle, 2022).

Medicinal Uses Decoctions of the inner bark of Baderi were used as a wash to bathe skin problems. The decoctions were also sipped

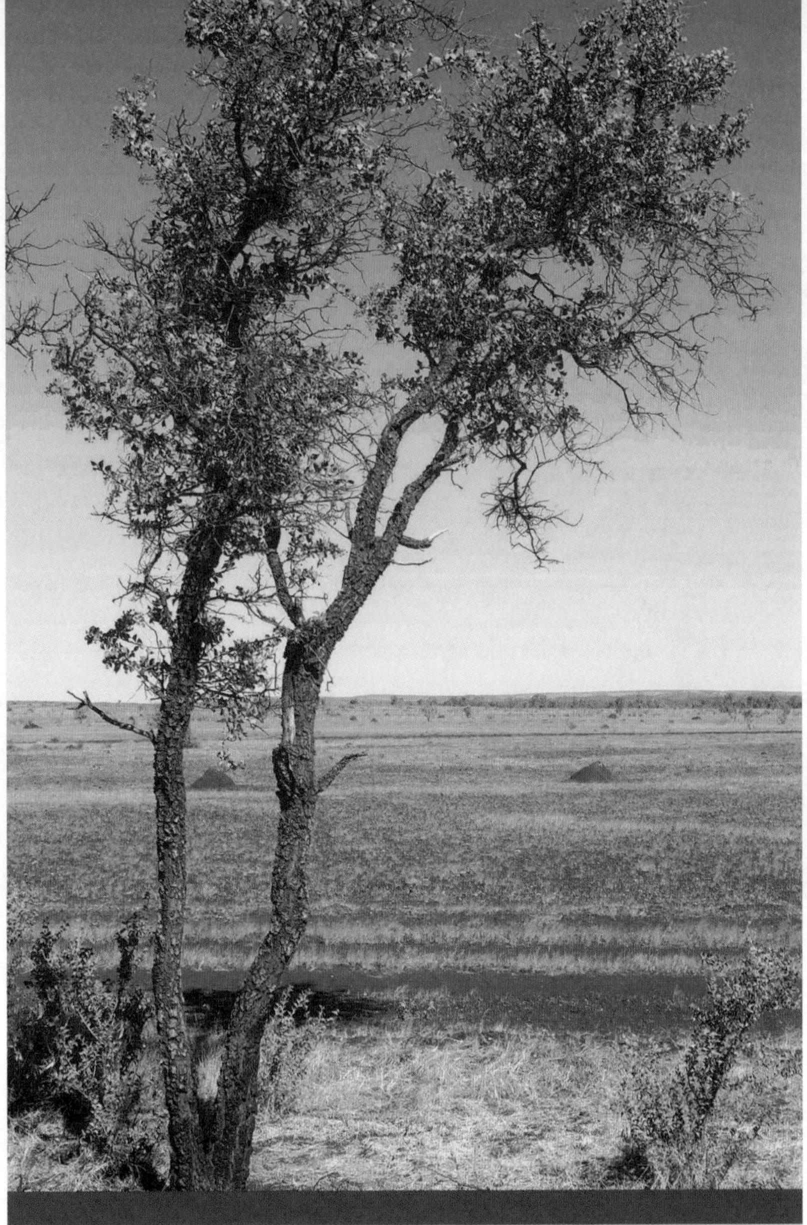

to treat cold and influenza symptoms. The bark was burnt and the ashes were rubbed over infants to heal sores, especially those due to chickenpox. This ritual is still practised today in parts of the Pilbara (Trails WA, n.d.).

Other Uses The seeds of Baderi are edible (Glasby, 2018).

Banyjood

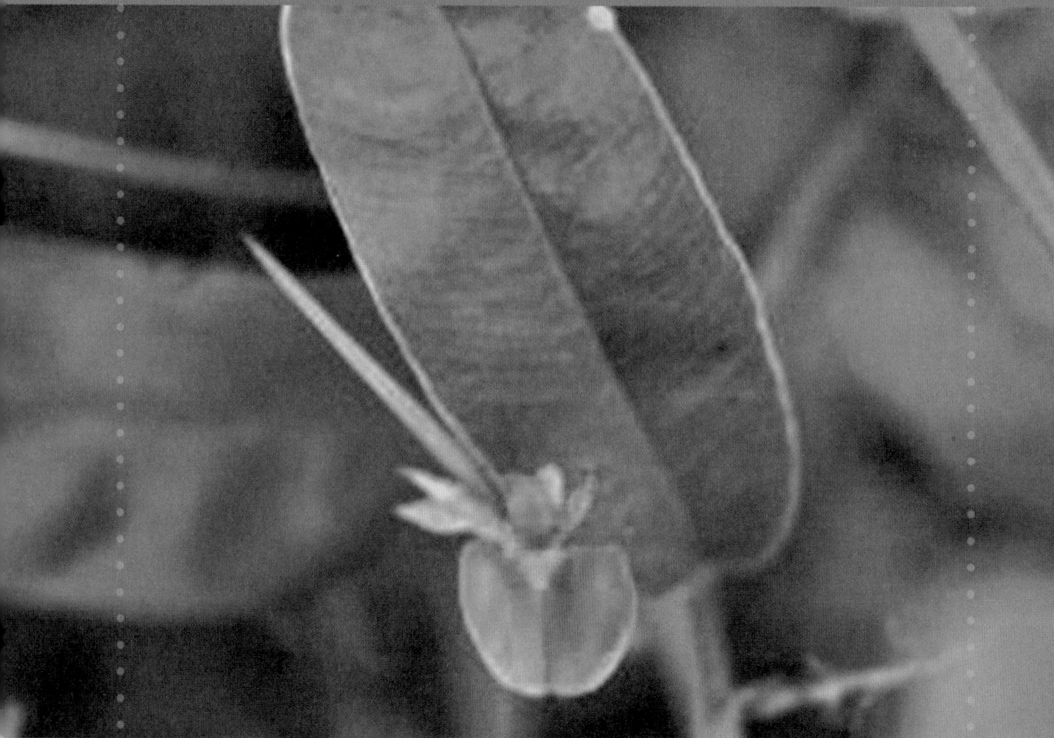

Scientific Name *Tephrosia crocea* Benth.

Common Name Banyjood.

Aboriginal Name Banyjoord (Bardi) (Kenneally et al., 1996; Paddy et al., 1993).

Field Notes Banyjoord is a prostrate to sprawling herb or shrub that grows to only around 500 mm in height. Its orange-red, pea-type flowers are present between January to April or during September. It prefers sandy soils and occurs along coastal regions from Dampier in the north-west of Western Australia into the Northern Territory (ALA, 2022; WAH, 2022; Young et al., 2012).

Medicinal Uses Decoctions of the leaves of Banyjoord were used as an eyewash to treat conjunctivitis (Young et al., 2012). The juice of the green roots was applied to bites and stings (Kenneally et al., 1996; Paddy et al., 1993; Smith & Kalotas, 1985). The small, young roots are reported to be the strongest (Kenneally et al., 1996).

Other Uses The ground-up roots of the Banyjoord were the most commonly used fish poison, which, when thrown in water, made the fish float to the top so they were easily collected (Smith & Kalotas, 1985).

Bardi Bush

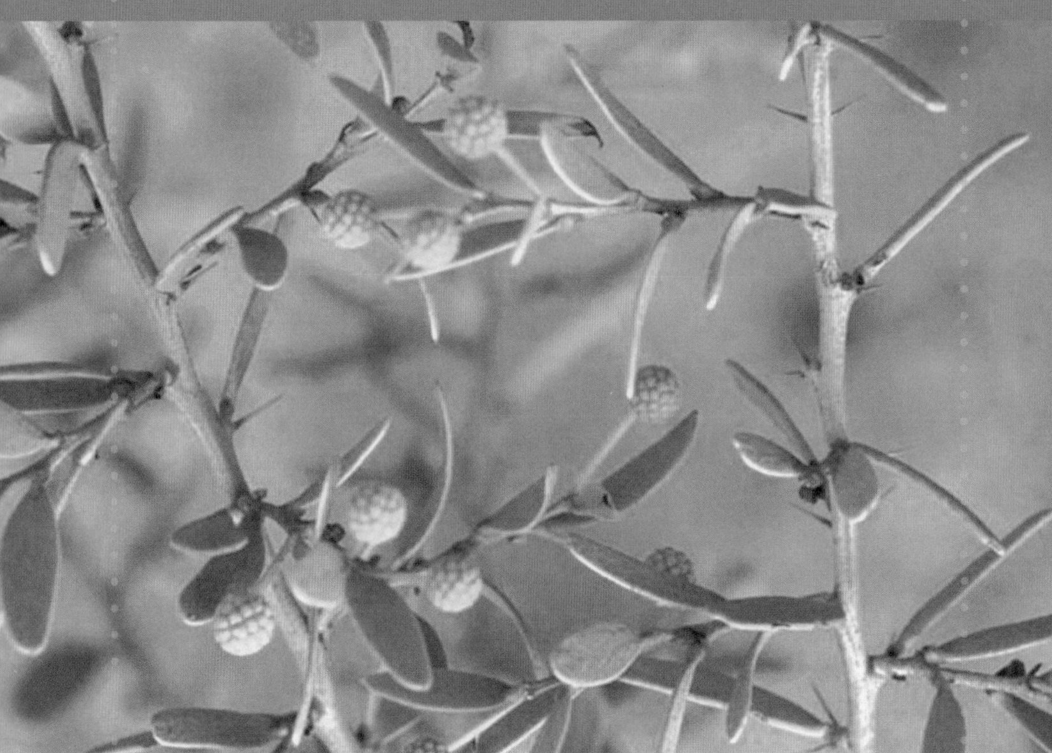

Scientific Name *Acacia synchronicia* Maslin.

Common Name Bardi Bush.

Aboriginal Name Bundalji (Jaru) (Deegan et al., 2010).

Field Notes Bardi Bush is a wattle that grows as a spreading shrub or tree up to 3 m in height. Its bark is grey and finely fissured at the base of the main stems, with smooth upper branches. Its phyllodes are mostly narrowly elliptic and up to 35 mm long. Its yellow, globose flower heads appear from August to December. Its seed pods are oblong. Bardi Bush is found in rocky sand, clay or loam over limestone or quartz, along drainage lines, alluvial flats, clay depressions and stony plains. It occurs in the Gascoyne, Mid-West, Kalgoorlie-Esperance, Pilbara and Kimberley regions of Western Australia, and in the western part of the Northern Territory (ALA, 2022; Maslin et al., 2010; WAH, 2022).

Medicinal Uses Decoctions of the bark were taken internally for the treatment of diarrhoea and dysentery. They were also applied externally as an antiseptic wash to treat wounds, other skin problems, some eye problems and as a mouth wash (Fern, 2021).

Other Uses The seeds of the Bardi Bush are edible and were usually ground into flour and mixed with water to make damper. The gum that exudes from wounds in the tree is also edible and was eaten like candy or mixed with water to make a sweet drink (Fern, 2021; Wheatstone Project, n.d.). Edible grubs can be found in the stems and roots of this Wattle (Deegan et al., 2010).

Barrier Saltbush

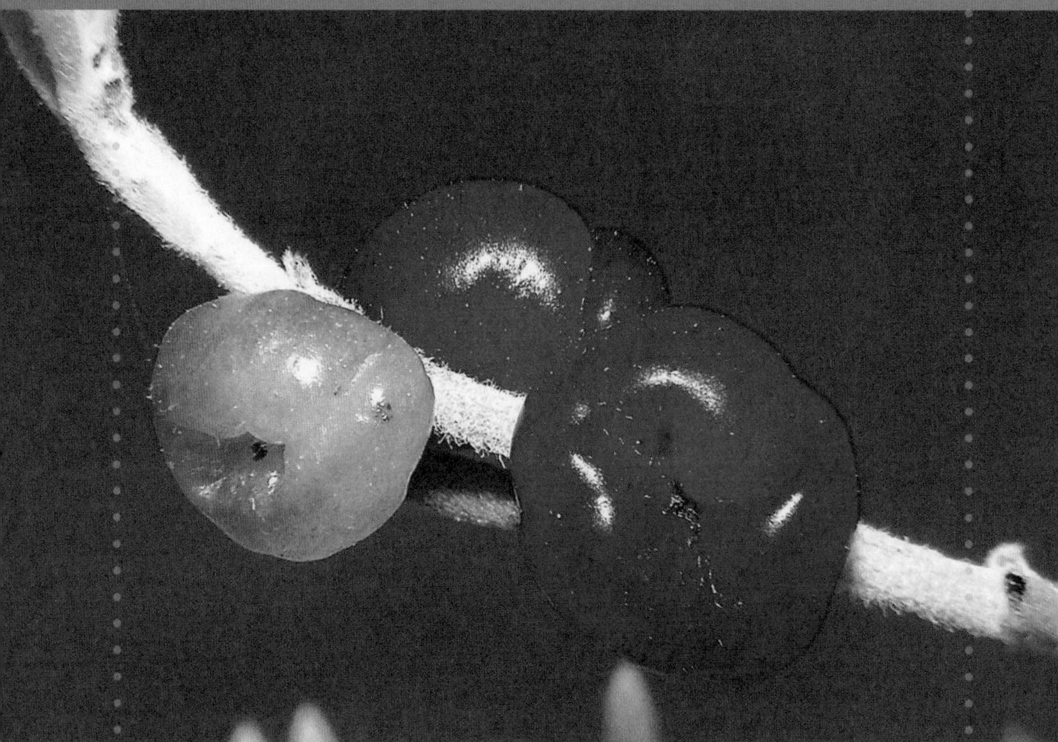

Scientific Name *Enchylaena tomentosa* R.Br.

Common Names Barrier Saltbush, Ruby Saltbush.

Aboriginal Names Tjilpi-tjilpi, Yili (Kukatja) (Valiquette, 1993).

Field Notes Barrier Saltbush grows as a prostrate or erect shrub to around 600 mm in height. Its cylindrical, semi-succulent leaves are up to 20 mm long. Both leaves and stems are covered in hairs. Its white, small and insignificant flowers appear from May to September. It bears edible, button-like fruit about 5 mm in diameter that are bright red when ripe. The berries are present throughout the year. The plant grows in a variety of soils both around the coast and inland (NACC, 2022; WAH, 2022). It occurs in all Australian states except Tasmania, in tropical, sub-tropical and more temperate regions (ANBG, 2022).

Medicinal Uses The fruit contain ascorbic acid (vitamin C) and would have helped to prevent scurvy in places where they were eaten (Fern, 2021).

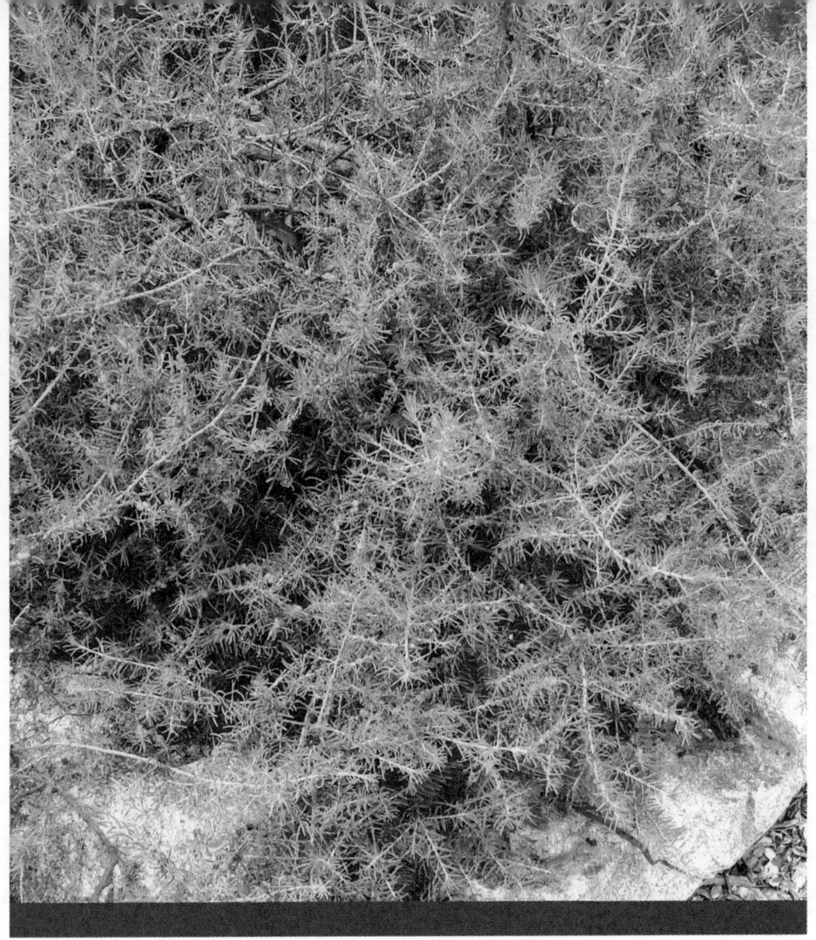

Other Uses The succulent, button-shaped berries are eaten fresh as a snack food or dried and soaked in water and reconstituted later (Cribb & Cribb, 1981; De Angeles, 2005; Gott, 2010; NACC, 2022). The fruit have a black seed inside that is also edible (ANBG, 2022). The leaves can be boiled or steamed and eaten as a vegetable but should only be eaten in small quantities due to their high oxalate content (Low, 1991; NACC, 2022).

Beach Cabbage

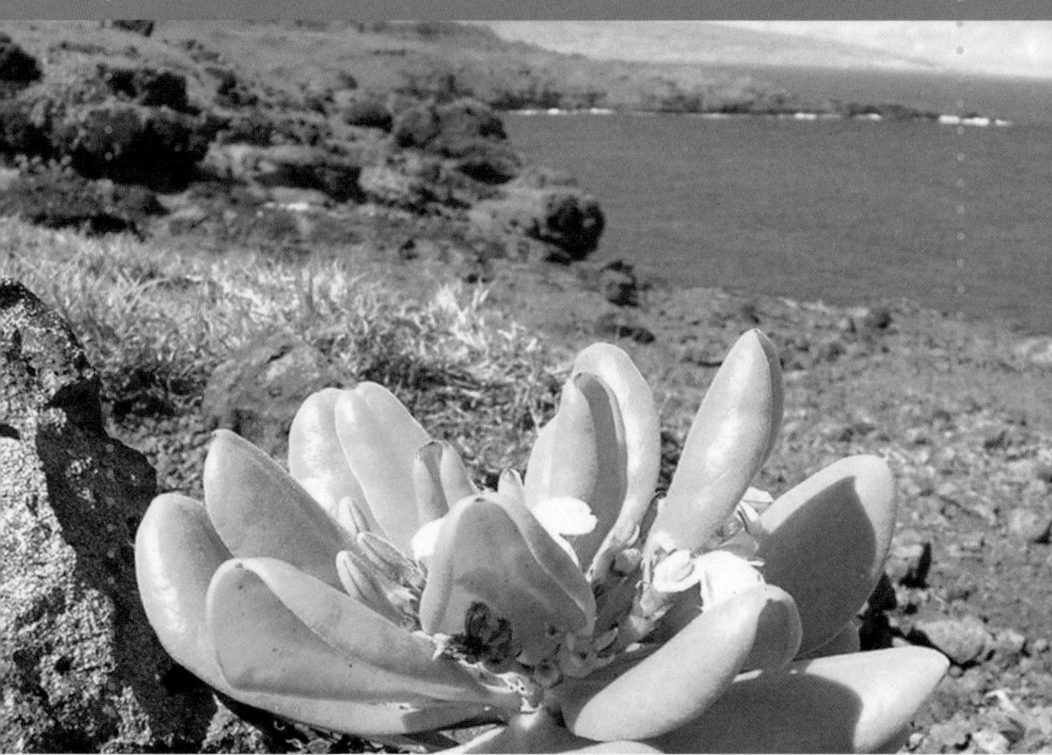

Scientific Name *Scaevola taccada* (Gaertn.) Roxb.

Common Names Beach Cabbage, Native Cabbage, Sea Lettuce, Sea Fanflower, Cardwell Cabbage.

Aboriginal Names Amanganan (Bardi) (Smith & Kalotas, 1985), Nulul (Pender Bay area) (Kenneally et al., 1996).

Field Notes Beach Cabbage is an erect, dense shrub that grows up to 2.5 m in height. It has large, thickish, ovate leaves and small white or blue, fan-shaped flowers that appear from March to October. Its fruit are white fleshy drupes up to 15 mm in diameter. Beach cabbage is a coastal plant that prefers sandy soils. In Australia, it occurs on coastal beaches and dunes around the top end from Broome in the north-west of Western Australia to Brisbane in Queensland (ALA, 2022; Fern, 2021; WAH, 2022). It also occurs in coastal locations in the tropical areas of the Arabian Sea, the tropical Indian Ocean and the tropical islands of the Pacific (Fern, 2021).

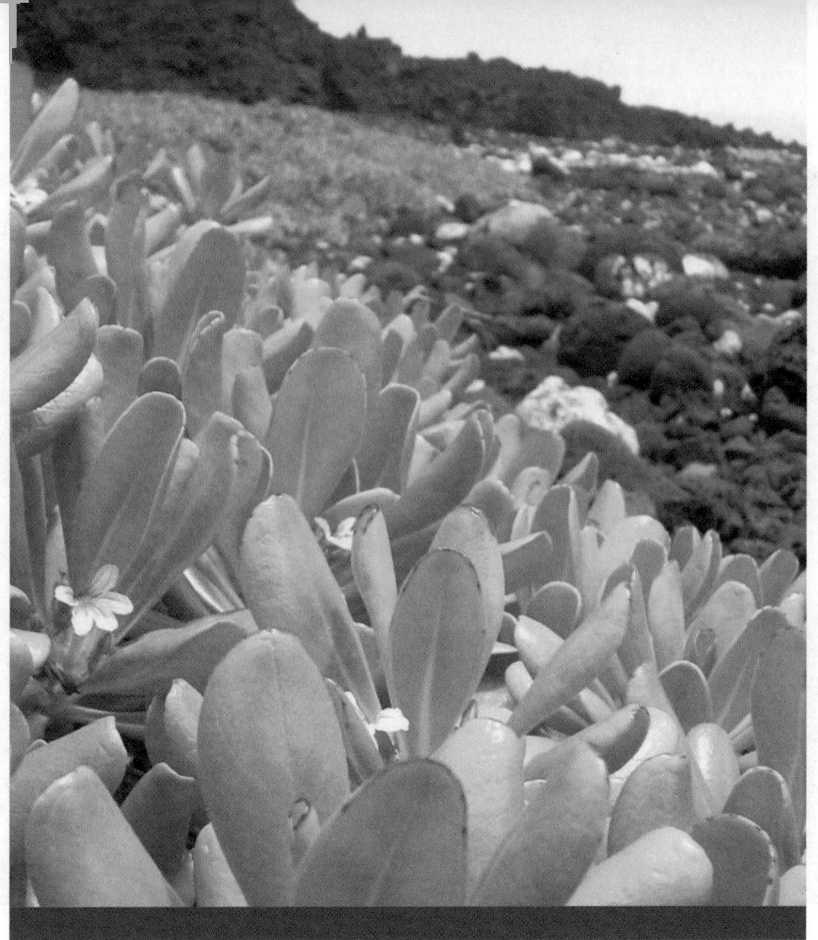

Medicinal Uses The fruit of Beach Cabbage have antifungal properties and were crushed and rubbed on parts of the body affected by dermatophytosis (tinea corporis or ringworm). The juice was also used to treat conjunctivitis, wounds and sores. Decoctions of the leaves and fruit pulp were used externally to treat wounds and skin sores (Cock, 2011; Edwards, 2005; Lassak & McCarthy, 2001; Low, 1990; SMIP, 2022). The fruit and young stems of Beach Cabbage were applied to stings to relieve pain and itching (Low, 1990; Smith, 1991). The leaves were heated over hot stones and draped over swollen joints to ease swelling and pain (Edwards, 2005; SMIP, 2022), and over the eyes to relieve the symptoms of conjunctivitis (Smith, 1991).

Other Uses The fruit of Beach Cabbage are edible. The young leaves are also edible and are usually cooked before they are eaten (Fern, 2021; Maiden, 1889).

Beach Moonflower

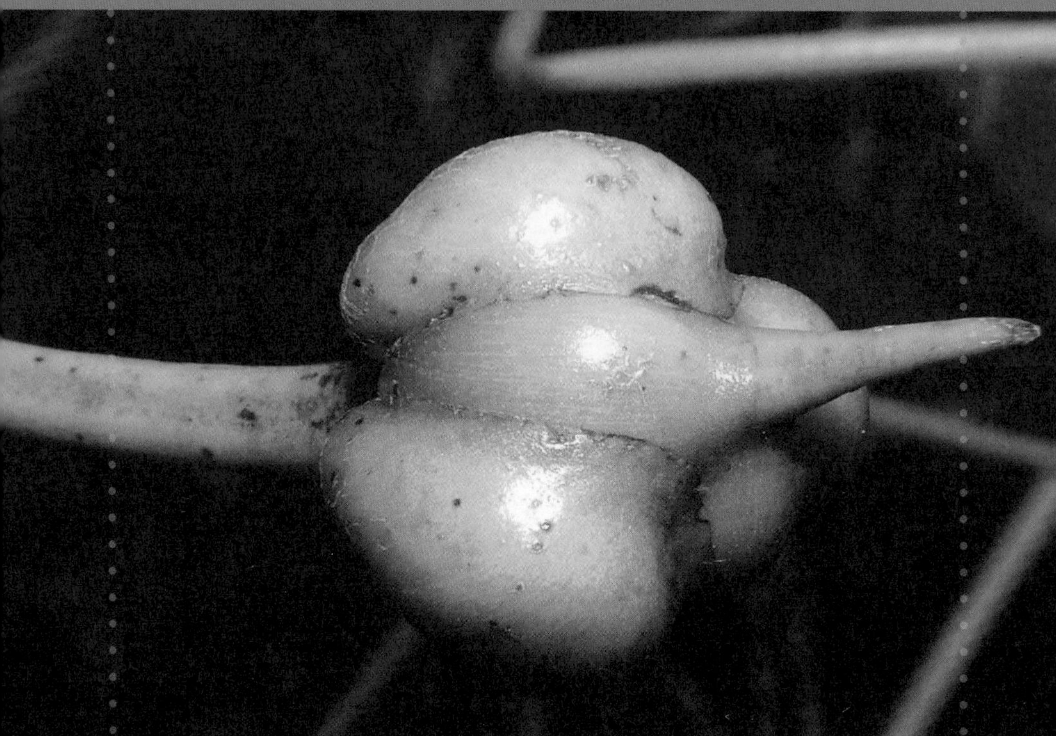

Scientific Name *Ipomoea macrantha* Roem. & Schult.

Common Names Beach Moonflower, Morning Glory, Beach Morning Glory.

Aboriginal Name Yingka winya (Kwini) (Cheinmora et al., 2017).

Field Notes Beach Moonflower is a prostrate, climbing or scrambling perennial plant growing up to 3 m in height. Its leaves are heart-shaped or roundish, and up to 140 mm long by 130 mm wide. Its white flowers, which occur singly or in small bunches, are trumpet-shaped and tube-shaped at their base, and up to 100 mm long. The flowers only open at night, hence the name Beach Moonflower. Flowering occurs between March and July. Its fruit are globular or capsicum-shaped capsules roughly 25 mm in diameter, containing four or more seeds. Beach Moonflower is found in beach sand, basalt or sandstone on rocks above high tide mark and amongst mangroves around the northern coast from the Kimberley

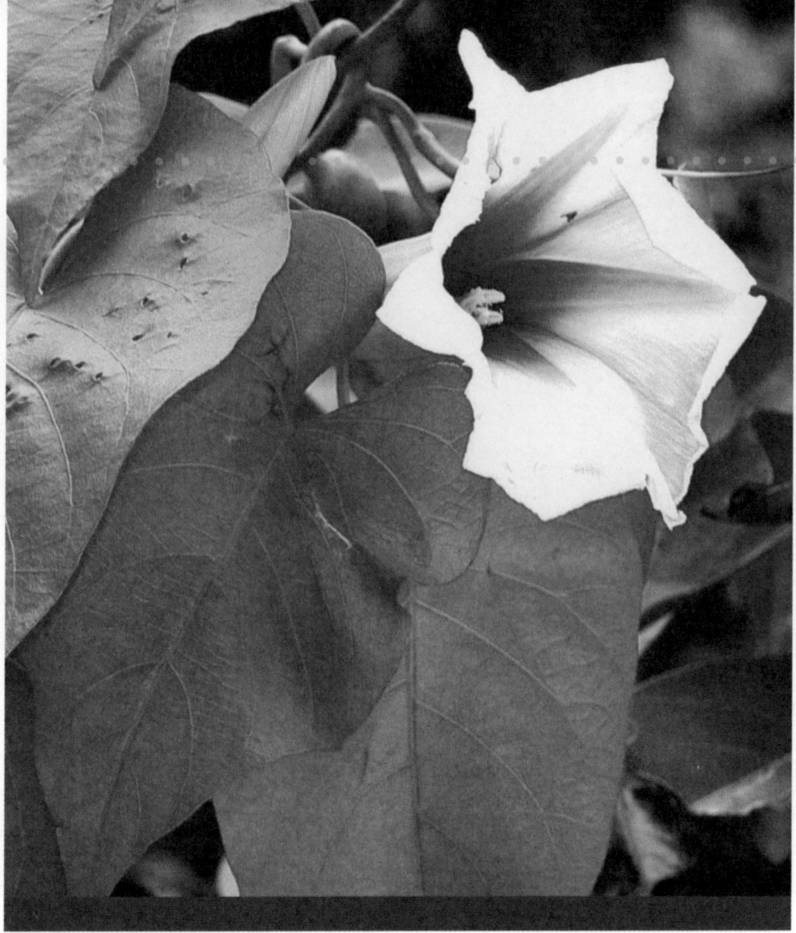

region in Western Australia to Townsville and Magnetic Island in Queensland. It also occurs in tropical America, tropical East Africa, Asia, Indonesia, Malaysia, New Guinea, the Philippines and on some Pacific islands (ALA, 2022; SMIP, 2022; WAH, 2022).

Medicinal Uses Decoctions of the leaves and juice from the fruit have been used as an antiseptic wash to treat burns (SMIP, 2022).

Other Uses Beach Moonflower is related to the Sweet Potato, so the roots are edible. Aboriginal groups roasted them in hot ashes before eating (Cheinmora et al., 2017; Vigilante et al., 2013).

Beach Morning-glory

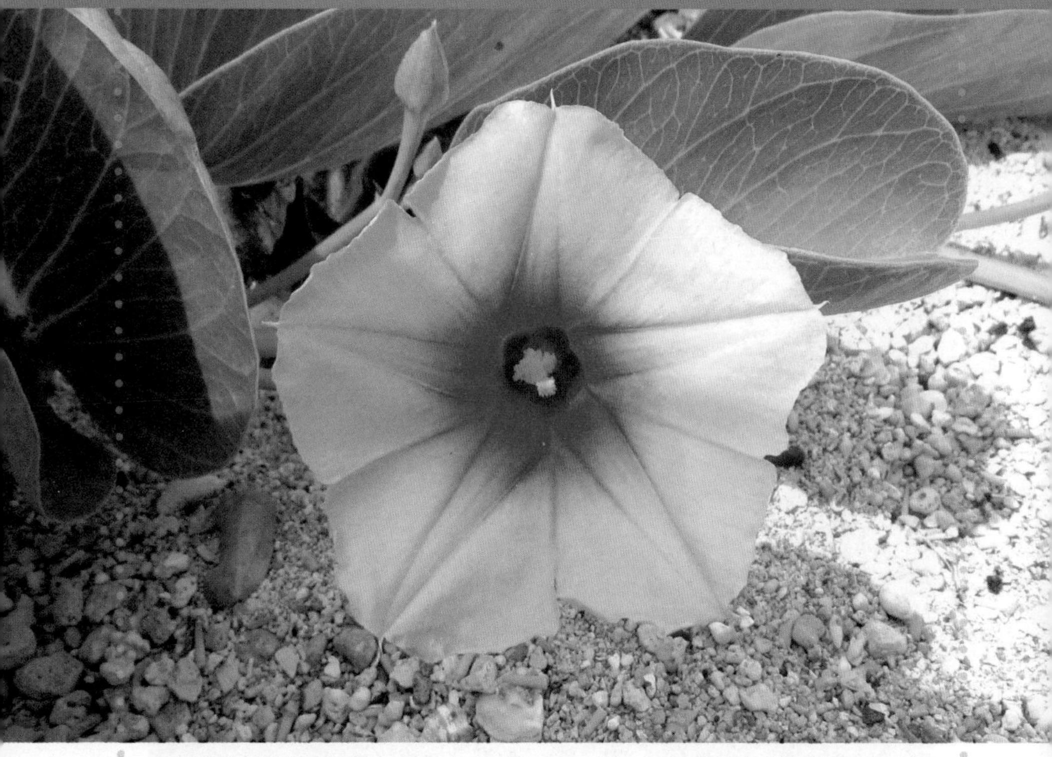

Scientific Name *Ipomoea pes-caprae* subsp. *brasiliensis* (L.) Ooststr.

Common Names Beach Morning-glory, Goat's Foot Convolvulus, Bay Hops, Convolvulus, Goat's Foot, Coast Morning Glory.

Aboriginal Names Gudayun (Bardi) (Smith & Kalotas, 1985), Yinga (Kwini) (Crawford, 1982), Waljuru (Nyangumarta), Waljaru (Karajarri) (Willing, 2014).

Field Notes Beach Morning-glory is a prostrate, creeping or trailing perennial herb. Trailing stems can be several metres long. The leaves are an unusual shape, and it is aptly named because of the shape of its leaf (*pes-caprae* is Latin for 'foot of a goat'). Its round, pink flowers are darker in the centre. In Australia they appear from January to August or October to November. Beach Morning-glory occurs in beach sand or clay loam in coastal or near-coastal areas around the top end of Australia from Carnarvon in the north-west

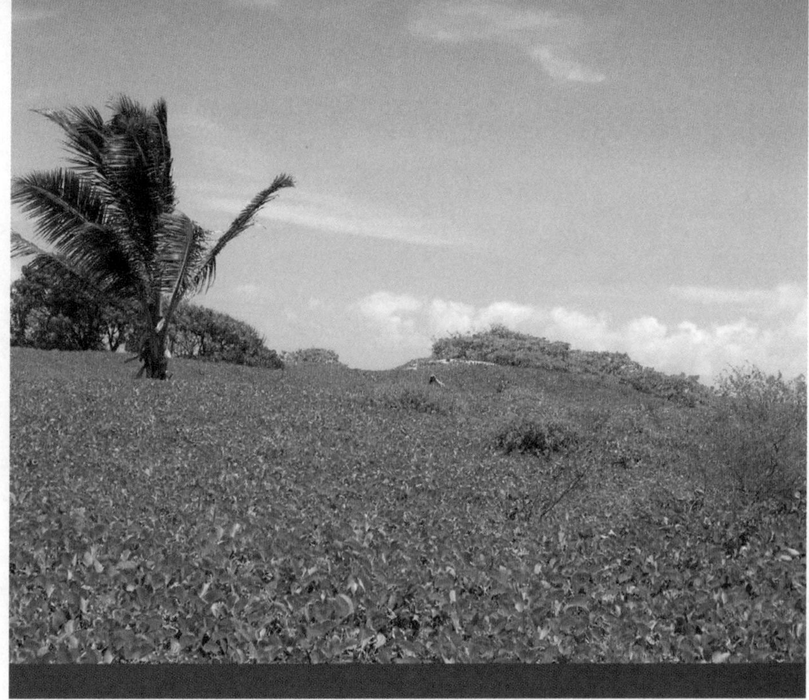

to the New South Wales border with Victoria. It also occurs in Africa, Asia and the Pacific islands (ATRP, 2020; WAH, 2022).

Medicinal Uses The juice of the Beach Morning-glory plant has diuretic properties. Decoctions of the crushed leaves were applied to sores to aid healing and used as a wash to treat aching joints and general malaise. Poultices of heated, crushed leaves were applied to boils and carbuncles to drain them and were placed on swollen joints and sore backs for the relief of rheumatic pain (Edwards, 2005; Lassak & McCarthy, 2001; Williams, 2012). Some Aboriginal communities applied heated leaves to the stings of stingrays, stonefish and green tree ants as well as to the head to ease headaches (Edwards, 2005; Low, 1990).

Other Uses Beach Morning-glory is closely related to the Sweet Potato so it has starchy, edible tubers, which were probably roasted before they were eaten. Because it is not very palatable, it was only eaten by Aboriginal and Torres Strait Islander people when other foods were scarce (Glasby, 2018; Isaacs, 1987; Low, 1991; Vigilante et al., 2013).

CAUTION: Glasby (2018) warns against eating excessive amounts of the tubers as they may be toxic in large quantities.

Beach Spinifex

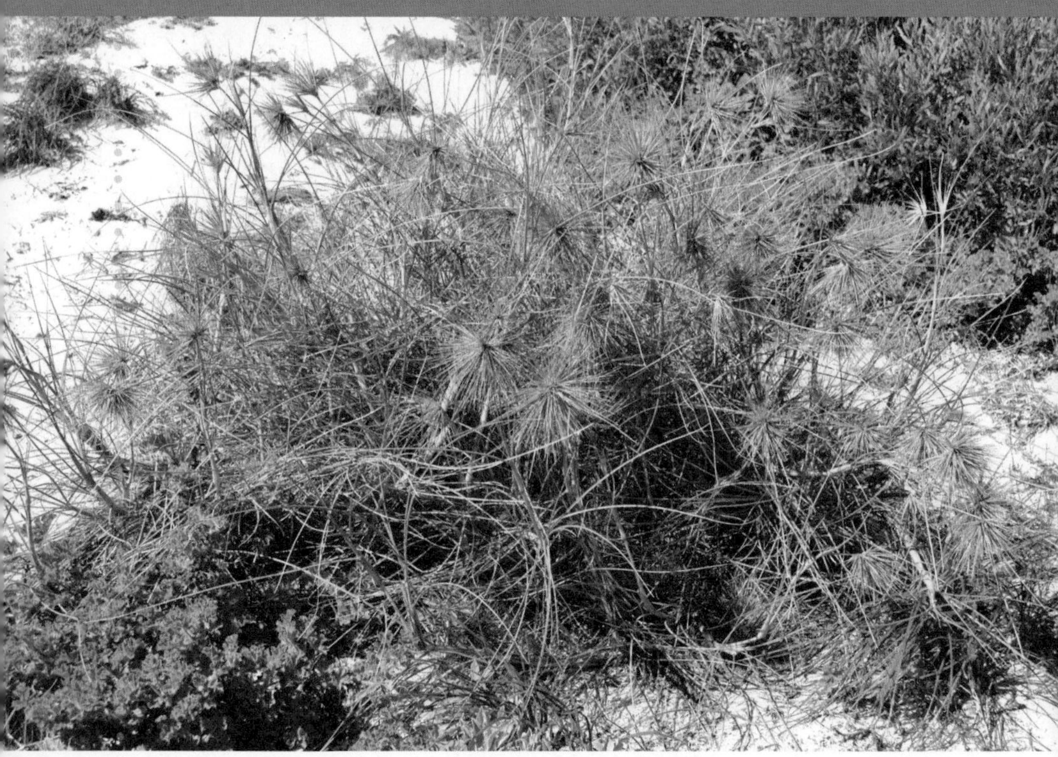

Scientific Name *Spinifex longifolius* R.Br.

Common Names Beach Spinifex, Long Leaved Spinifex.

Aboriginal Names Wurrngulungulu (Wunambal, Gaambera) (Karadada et al., 2011), Ural (Bardi) (Smith & Kalotas, 1985), Oorral (Bardi), Rrarrga Rrarrga (Yawuru) (Kenneally et al., 1996).

Field Notes Beach Spinifex is a coarse grass with long thin leaves that grow up to 300 mm in height. There are male and female plants. The rhizomatous roots spread through the sand forming the grass into large tussocks. The green-brown flower spikes, barely 10 mm long, appear from April to January. Beach Spinifex occurs in white sand on coastal sand dunes around the northern Australian coast from northern Queensland and the Northern Territory down along the west coast to Cape Leeuwin. It also occurs on Rottnest, Garden, Carnac, Seal and Penguin islands, and in New Guinea and Indonesia (ALA, 2022; Rippey & Rowland, 1995; WAH, 2022).

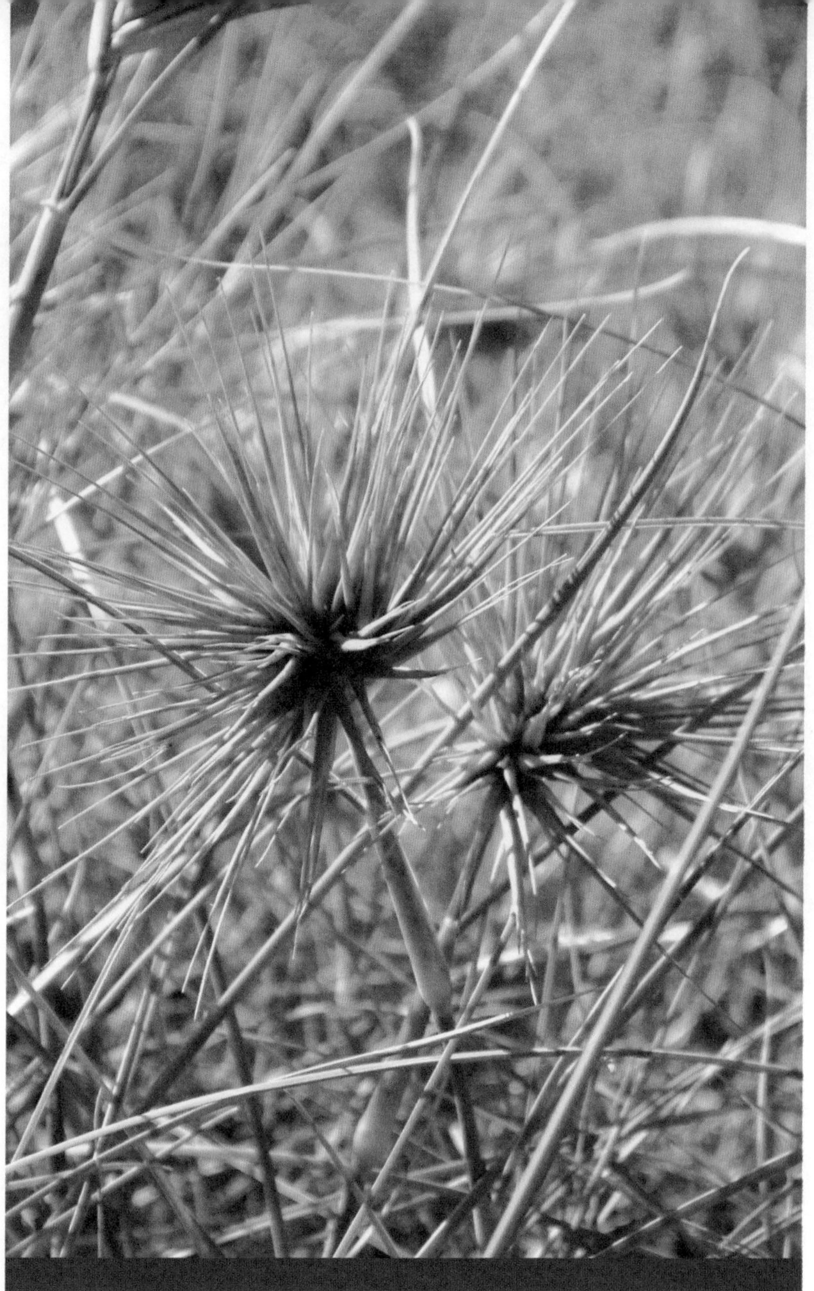

Medicinal Uses Juice from the young tips (obtained by squeezing them with fingers) was dripped into the eyes to treat conjunctivitis. Infusions of the crushed leaves were also used to bathe sore eyes and as a wash to treat wounds, burns and sores (Hansen & Horsfall, 2016; Lassak & McCarthy, 2001; Low, 1990; Smith, 1991). Decoctions of the young stems were drunk to relieve internal pain (Smith, 1991).

Beefwood

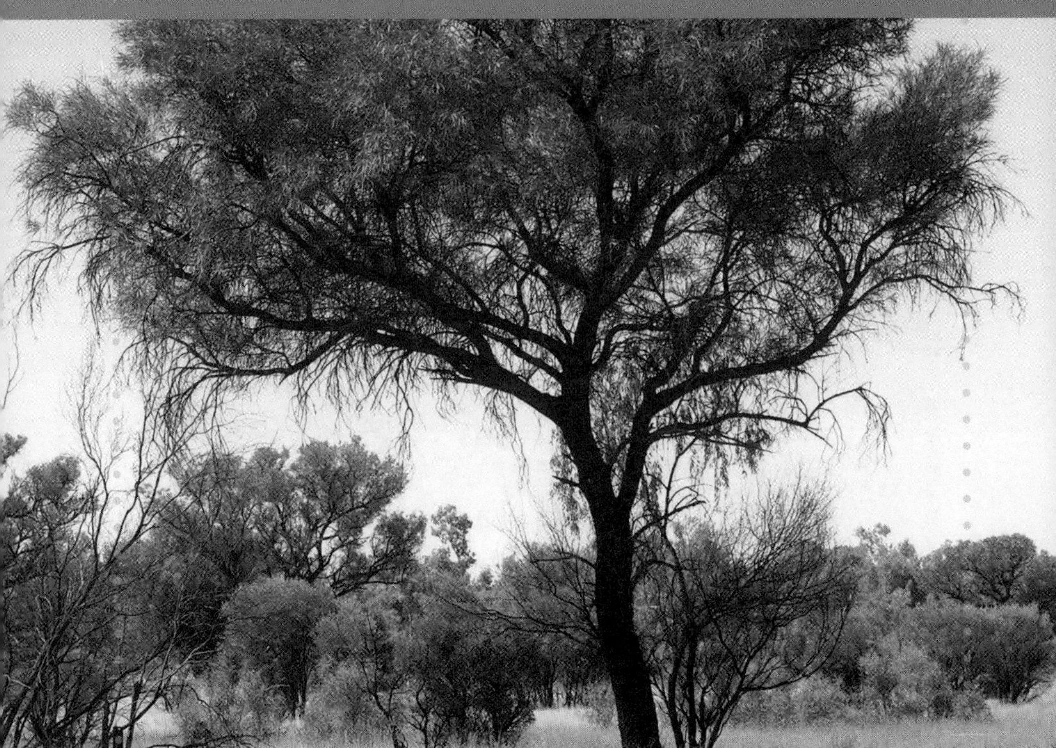

Scientific Name *Grevillea striata* R.Br.

Common Names Beefwood, Silvery Honeysuckle.

Aboriginal Names Derrending (Miriwoong) (Leonard et al., 2013), Jawilyiny (Gija) (Purdie et al., 2018), Jirrirnti, Jawalyi, Japilji (Ngardi) (Cataldi, 2004), Pantal-pantalpa, Yiltilpa, Yirltirlpa (Kukatja) (Valiquette, 1993), Jirrirndi, Jalwilyi (Jaru) (Wightman, 2003), Jarangkarr (Nyikina) (Smith & Smith, 2009).

Field Notes Beefwood grows as a tree or shrub up to 15 m in height. It has tessellated bark and long strap-like leaves. Its white-cream to yellow-green flowers hang in racemes. They can be present from July to December or January to March. Beefwood occurs in red sand, loam or clay near watercourses, and on plains in most areas across the top half of Australia from Carnarvon in Western Australia to the Sydney area in New South Wales (ALA, 2022; Fern, 2021; Lassak & McCarthy, 2001; WAH, 2022).

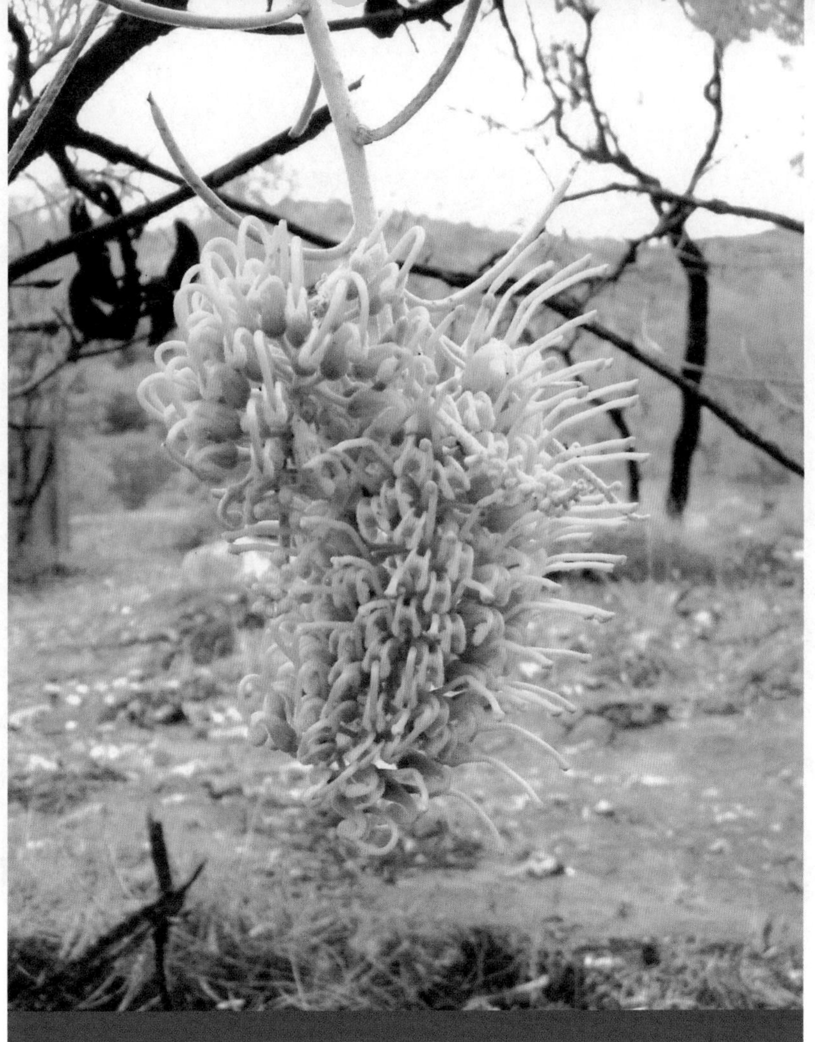

Medicinal Uses Ground-up charcoal from the Beefwood bush was applied to wounds and sores to aid healing. The resin from this bush has been used for preparing healing ointments (Eulo, n.d.; Lassak & McCarthy, 2001). A wash made from the powdered resin was used to facilitate the healing of sores and wounds. Decoctions of the leaves were used for the same purpose (Williams, 2010).

Other Uses The roots and nectar of Beefwood are edible (Eulo, n.d.). The nectar was either sucked directly from the flowers or the flowers were soaked in water to make a sweet drink. The seeds are also edible (Land for Wildlife, n.d.). Resin extracted from the roots of Beefwood made a good glue. The timber from Beefwood was used to make boomerangs and fighting sticks (Deegan et al., 2010; Eulo, n.d.; Purdie et al., 2018; Wightman, 2003).

Belalie

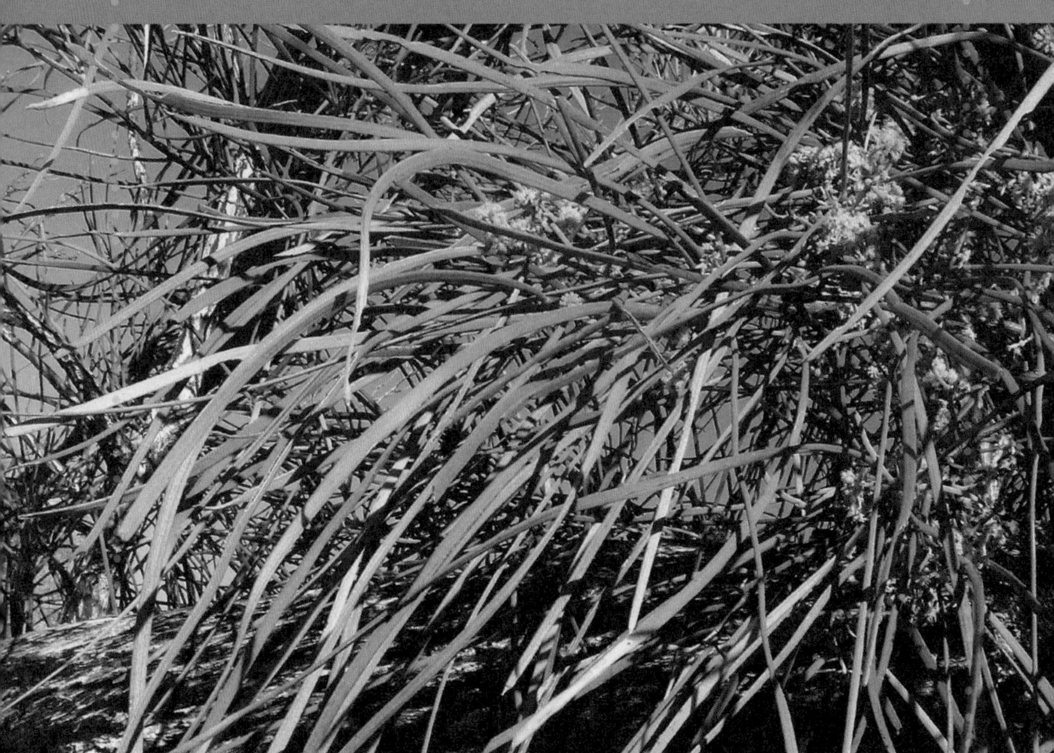

Scientific Name *Acacia stenophylla* Benth.

Common Names Belalie, Balkura, Black Wattle, Dalby Myall, Dalby Wattle, Dunthy, Eumong, Gooralee, Gurley, Ironwood, Munumula, Native Willow, River Cooba, River Myall.

Aboriginal Names Warrkila (Kukatja) (Valiquette, 1993), Burlwirri, Bugurlbirri (Jaru) (Wightman, 2003).

Field Notes Belalie is a wattle that grows as a straggly shrub or tree up to 20 m high in good conditions. Its bark is dark grey and fibrous. Its phyllodes are strap-like and up to 400 mm long and 7 mm wide. Its yellow, globular flower heads appear on short stems between March and June. Its woody seed pods are up to 260 mm long and 12 mm wide with large seeds up to 9 mm long. Belalie occurs in grey sand or clay soils on floodplains and along drainage lines in the Pilbara and Kimberley regions of Western Australia, and

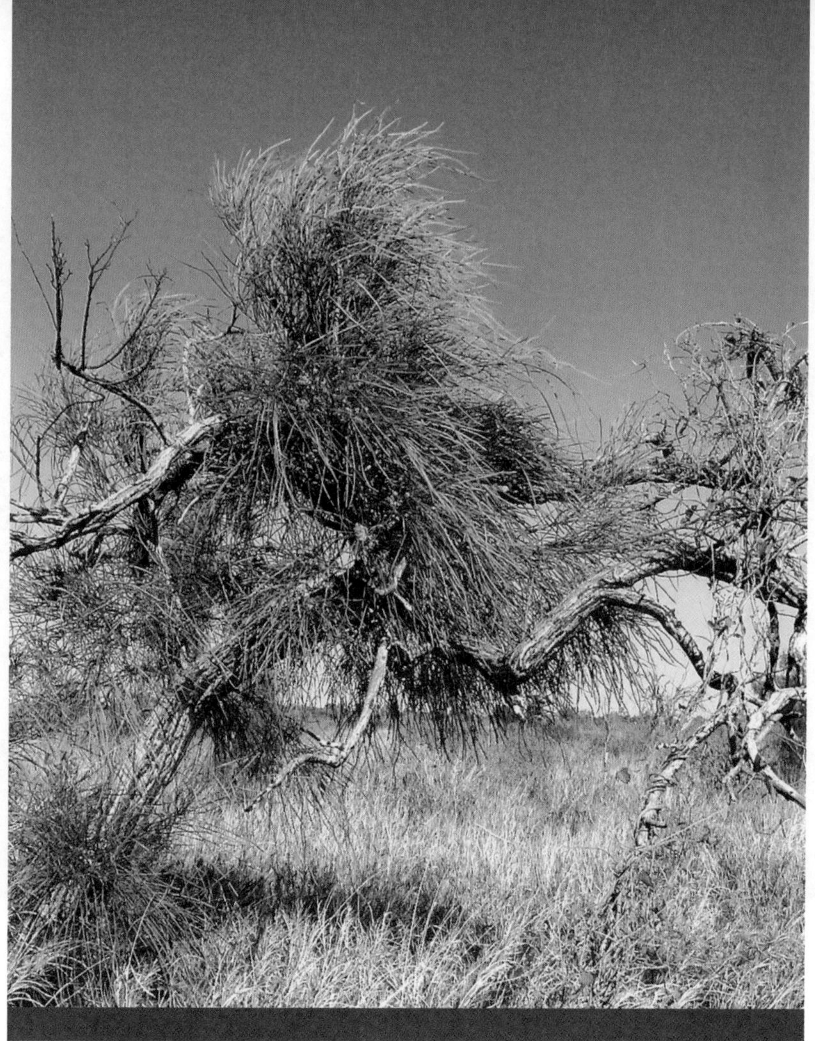

in all other mainland states and territories (ALA, 2022; Maslin et al., 2010; WAH, 2022).

Medicinal Uses Decoctions or infusions of the crushed leaves of Belalie are applied as an antiseptic wash to wounds and sores to aid the healing process. The leaves are also used by the Kukatja for 'medicinal smoke' (Valiquette, 1993).

Other Uses The seeds of Belalie are edible (Williams, 2011). The gum that oozes from wounds in the tree is also edible and is reported to have a salty taste (Deegan et al., 2010; Wightman, 2003; Williams, 2011). Edible grubs are found in the stems and the roots of this wattle (Deegan et al., 2010).

Bendee

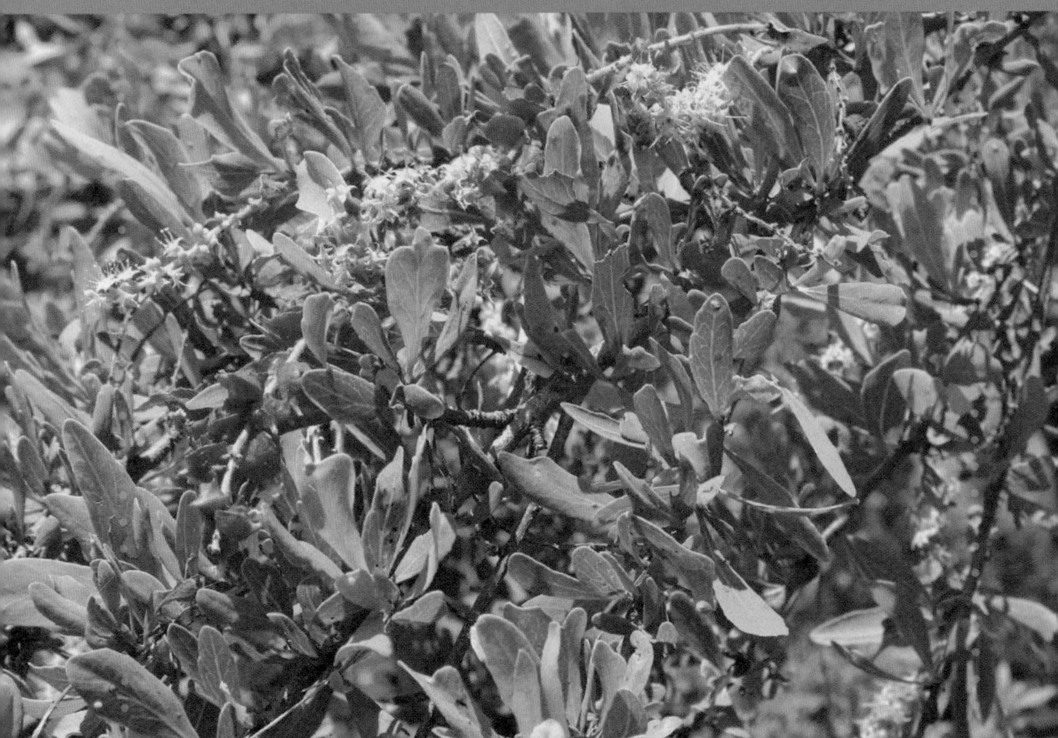

Scientific Name *Terminalia bursarina* F.Muell.

Common Names Bendee, River Gum Tree.

Aboriginal Names Biriwiri (Bunuba) (Oscar et al., 2019), Yirriru (Wunambal, Gaambera) (Karadada et al., 2011), Warraroony or Warraruny (Gija) (Purdie et al., 2018), Yirriyarri (Jaru) (Wightman, 2003), Yirrirru manya (Kwini) (Cheinmora, et al., 2017).

Field Notes Bendee is an erect, straggly tree that grows up to 8 m in height. Its bark is deeply fissured. It has ovate leaves that are tapered at the base and small, star-shaped, yellow-white flowers that are borne on racemes. Flowering is between June and September. Its fruit are red, ovate pods. Bendee occurs in stony sandy soil or sandstone in rock crevices and river beds in the Kimberley region of Western Australia, the Northern Territory and the north-west corner of Queensland (ALA, 2022; WAH, 2022).

Medicinal Uses The gum from Bendee is considered to be

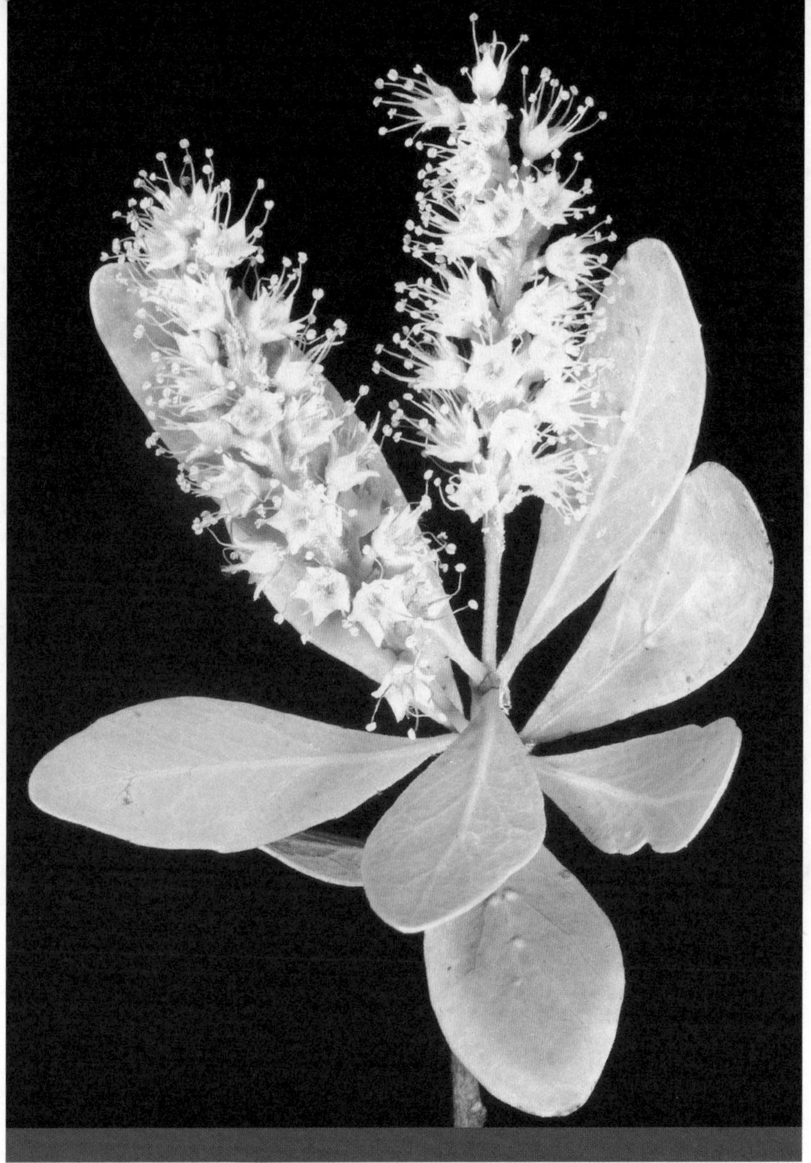

an excellent medicine by the Jaru, who use it as a detoxifying agent and as a treatment for certain cancers (efficacy unknown) (Wightman, 2003).

Other Uses The gum that oozes from wounds in the Bendee Tree is edible and can be heated in a fire to soften it if it has gone hard (Cheinmora, et al., 2017; Karadada et al., 2011; Oscar et al., 2019; Purdie et al., 2018; Wightman, 2003; Williams, 2011). Wightman (2003) reports that, 'The gum from the trees at Yirriyarri (Blue Hole) near Purnululu is considered by some Jaru people to be the sweetest and tastiest of all Yirriyarri trees.'

Berrigan

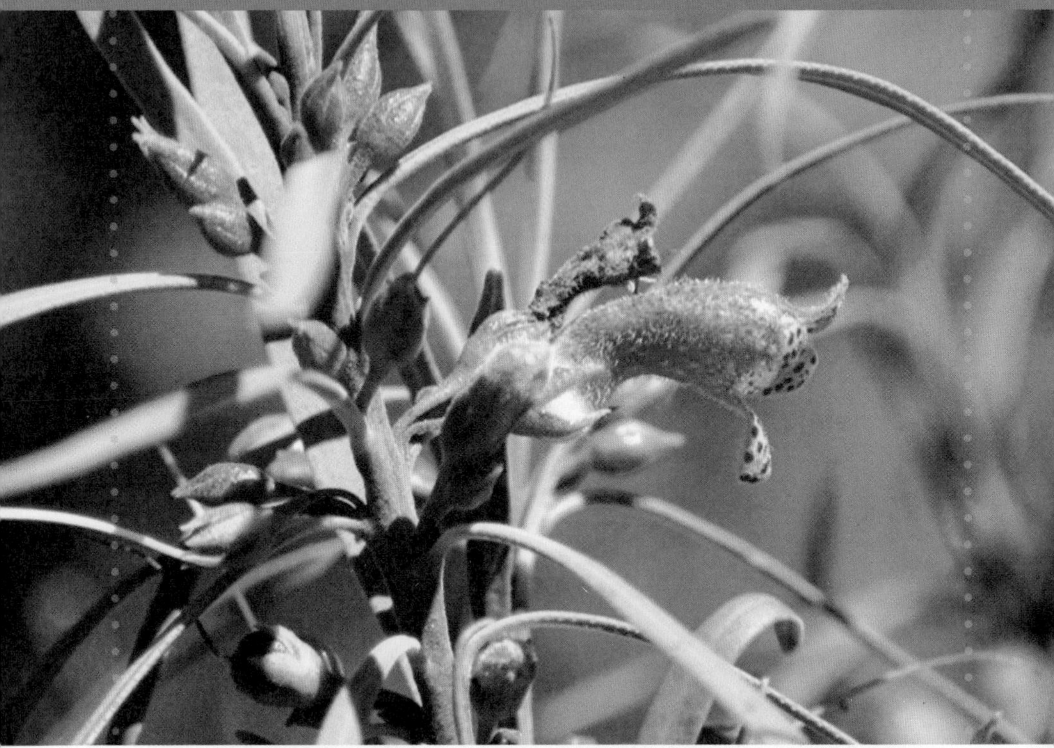

Scientific Name *Eremophila longifolia* (R.Br.) F.Muell.

Common Names Berrigan, Emu Bush, Emu Apple, Dogwood, Juniper Tree, Long-leaved Eremophila.

Aboriginal Names Kulaki (Ngardi) (Cataldi, 2004), Milyulyu, Ngularnpa, Tulykurrpa, Tjulypurrpa (Kukatja) (Valiquette, 1993).

Field Notes Eremophila is a large genus of 214 species, all endemic to Australia. Berrigan grows as an often-weeping shrub or tree up to 6 m in height. Its mature bark is dark grey with a rough surface and squarish segments. Its dull green, linear to lanceolate leaves have a bent or hooked tip and are up to 200 mm long and 7 mm wide. Its red to pink-red, tubular flowers appear on short stalks in leaf axils, either singly or in groups of two to three and sometimes up to five, between March and November. Its globular fruit are blackish-purple when ripe and are up to 11 mm in diameter. Berrigan is often found on stony, red sandy or clay

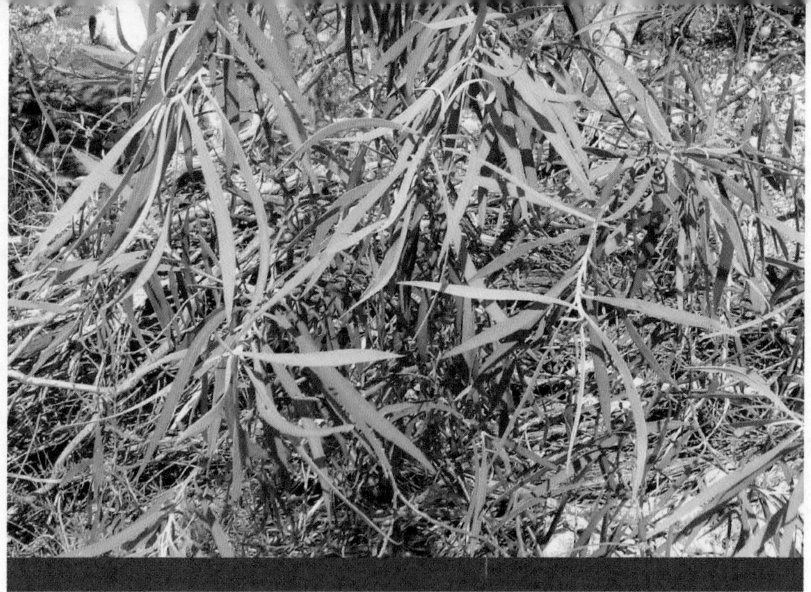

soils along watercourses, floodplains, stony rises and ridges in the drier regions of every mainland state including the southern part of the Kimberley region of Western Australia (ALA, 2022; Lassak & McCarthy, 2001; WAH, 2022).

Medicinal Uses Decoctions of the leaves were rubbed on the skin as a wash to treat scabies infestations, cuts and sores. Alternatively, the crushed leaves were mixed with animal fat, which was used as an ointment for the same purpose. Sometimes a small amount of the decoctions were drunk to relieve the symptoms of colds and influenza (Lassak & McCarthy, 2001; Smith, 1991; Webb, 1959; Williams, 2013). The Kukatja rubbed the decoctions on the head, neck and shoulders of women to relieve 'women's pains' and headaches (Valiquette, 1993). Poultices of the crushed leaves were used to draw out boils and carbuncles. Newborn babies and mothers were held over pits of burning Berrigan wood to inhale the fumes, which was thought to strengthen the baby as well as stop postpartum haemorrhage in the mother (Australian Plants Online, 2022; Williams, 2013). Smoke from this bush is reported to provide relief for headaches (Valiquette, 1993).

Other Uses The fruit is edible and is eaten fresh off the bush (Fern, 2021).

Billabong Tree

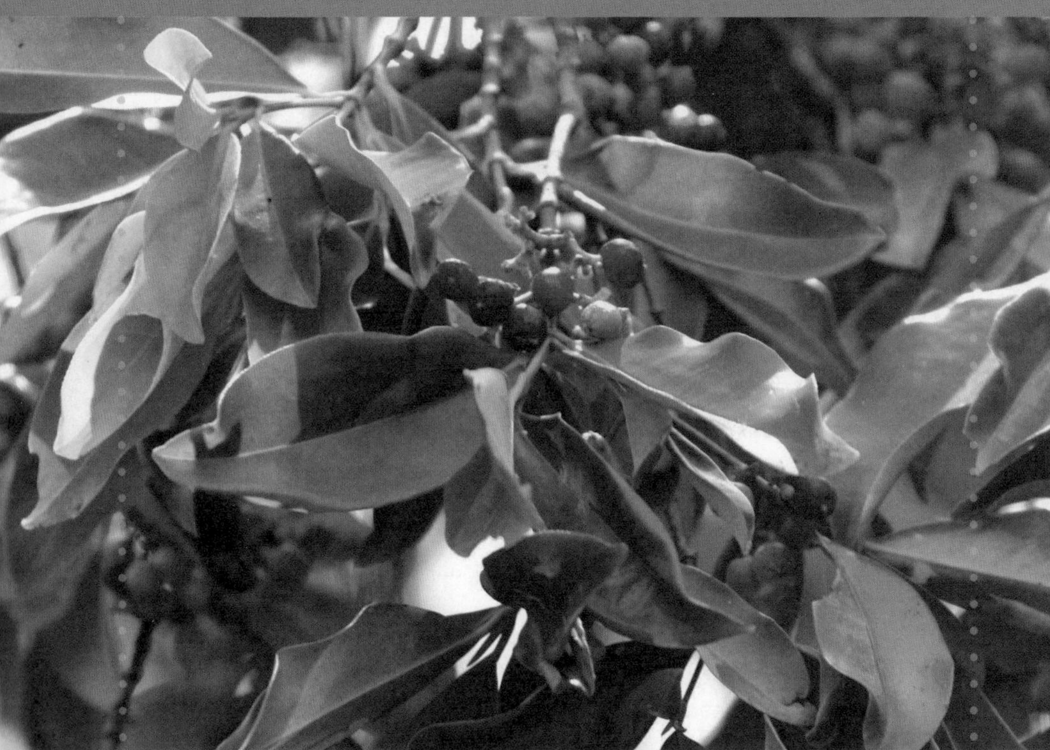

Scientific Name *Carallia brachiata* (Lour.) Merr.

Common Names Billabong Tree, Carallia, Bush Currant, Freshwater Mangrove, Palamkat, Shengali, Karalli, Caralla Wood, Andi, Maniawiga, Corkwood, Corky Bark.

Aboriginal Names Burrgungayi, Barnbii (Wunambal, Gaambera) (Karadada et al., 2011), Dumulinggu (Wunambal) (Vigilante et al., 2013), Joonjoonool or Junjunul (Gija) (Purdie et al., 2018; Wightman, 2003).

Field Notes Billabong Trees (occasionally buttressed) are found growing up to 20 m in height. They have ovate leaves that are pointed at the apex and measure up to 120 mm long and 70 mm wide, and small, white-cream-green flowers that form in clusters at the end of branchlets from June to September. Their fruit are globular or depressed globular drupes that are about 9 mm in diameter. Billabong trees occur in sand, peat or loam

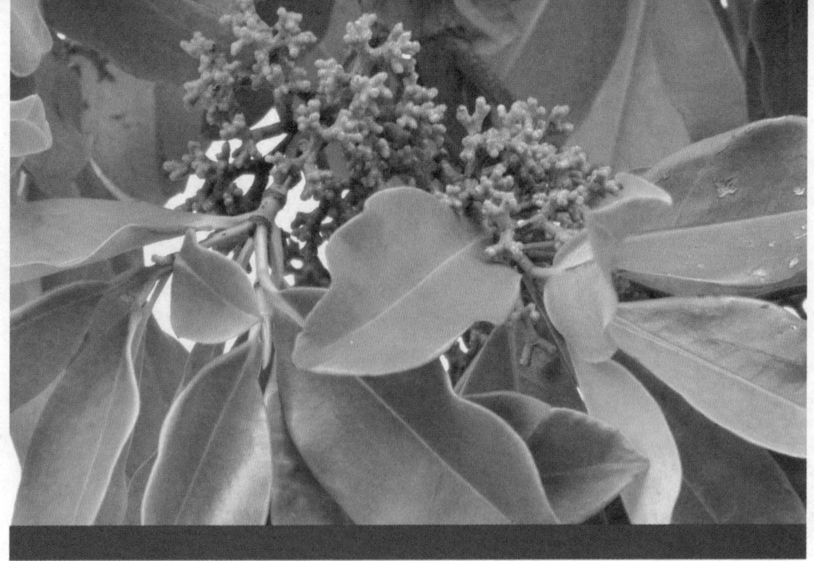

on the margins of streams and swamps across the top end of Australia and down the east coast as far as Townsville (ALA, 2022; ATRP, 2020; WAH, 2022). They also occur in Africa, East Asia, Madagascar, southern China, the Indian subcontinent, Myanmar, Thailand, through Indochina and South-east Asia to the Solomon Islands (ATRP, 2020).

Medicinal Uses Billabong Trees are used in folk medicine in Africa and some Asian countries. The juice extracted from the crushed leaves was used in the treatment of fevers. Pulverised bark was rubbed on the body to treat the rash of smallpox. The leaves and bark were crushed and used to treat blood poisoning (Septicaemia) and itchy skin (Fern, 2021). Some Aboriginal groups in Australia pounded then boiled the bark to make a poultice which was applied to the skin to ease skin irritations and itches (Hiddins, 2001). Aboriginal groups from the Kimberley rubbed fine black ash from burnt wood into wounds and cuts to aid the healing process (Karadada et al., 2011).

Other Uses The small fruit of Billabong Trees are edible and are eaten raw when red and ripe. Fruiting is between July and September (Edwards, 2005; Glasby, 2018; Fox & Garde, 2018; Hiddins, 2001; Karadada et al., 2011; Purdie et al., 2018; Vigilante et al., 2013). The Gija use the wood from young Billabong Trees to make the shafts of throwing sticks or woomeras (Wightman, 2003).

Black Bean

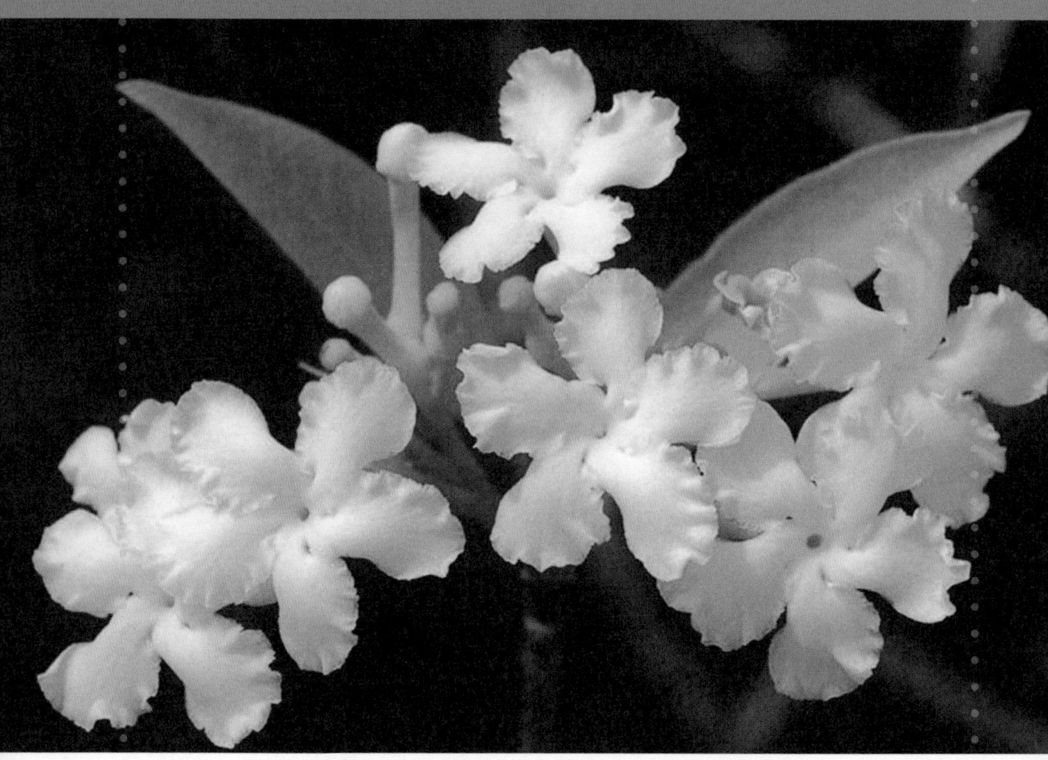

Scientific Name *Tabernaemontana orientalis* R.Br., previously known as *Ervatamia orientalis* (R.Br.) Domin.

Common Names Black Bean, Banana Bush, Eastern Gondola Bush, Rosebay, Bitter Bark, Iodine Plant.

Field Notes Black Bean is a small to medium-sized spreading shrub with milky sap that grows to around 3 m in height. Its light green, hairy leaves are an elongated oval shape, tapering to the base with a pointed tip and prominent veins. Its perfumed white, tubular flowers with petals in a rotating pattern appear from August to December. Its fruit are a yellow-orange colour, in a curved, three-sided banana shape and around 2 mm long. The fruit have reddish seeds. Black Bean is found along the banks of streams, on rainforest margins, in monsoon forests and vine thickets along and near the coast across the top half of Australia from Broome in the north-west to the Sunshine Coast north of Brisbane (ALA, 2022; Native

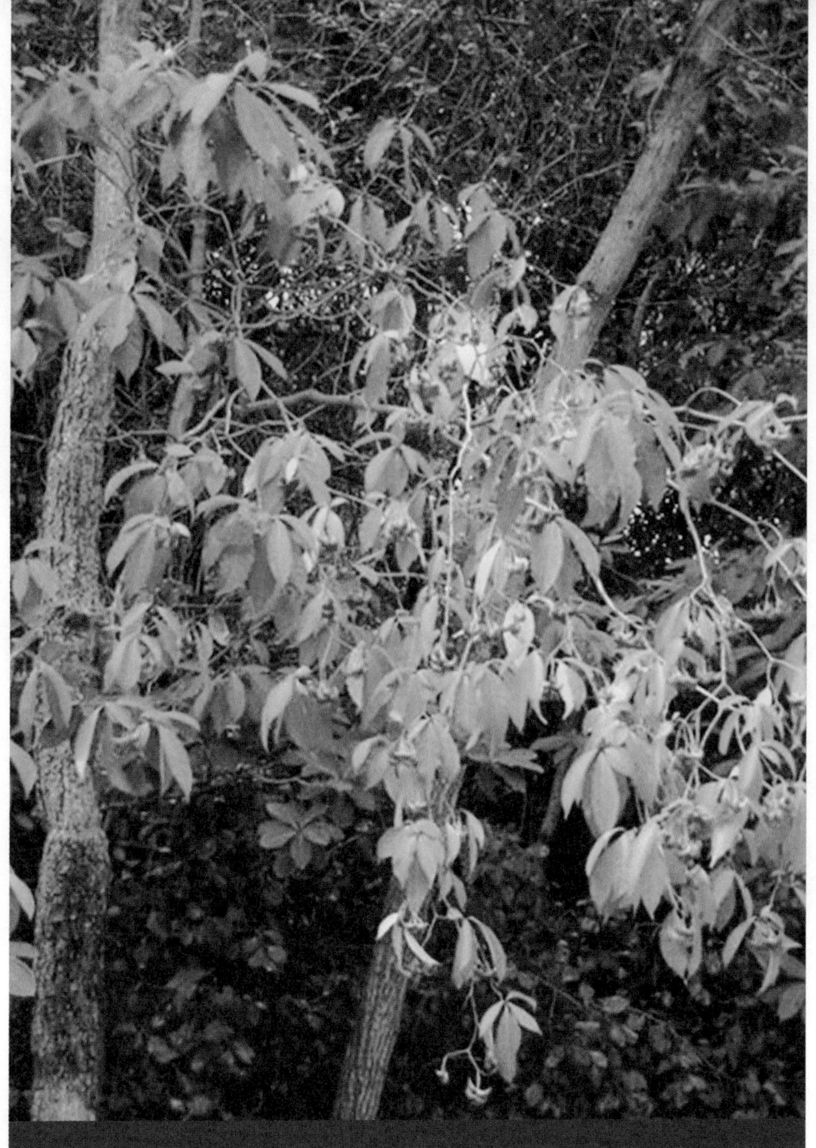

Plants Queensland, 2020; WAH, 2022). It is also found in Indonesia, Melanesia and Papua New Guinea (SMIP, 2022).

Medicinal Uses The sap of Black Bean was used like iodine to disinfect ulcers and sores. The fruit was crushed and rubbed on wounds and sores to aid healing, and as a treatment for tinea corporis (ringworm) (Cock, 2011; Fern, 2021; Lassak & McCarthy, 2001; Low, 1990).

Other Uses The fruit of the Black Bean shrub are edible (Fox & Garde, 2018; Territory Native Plants, 2022).

Black Orchid

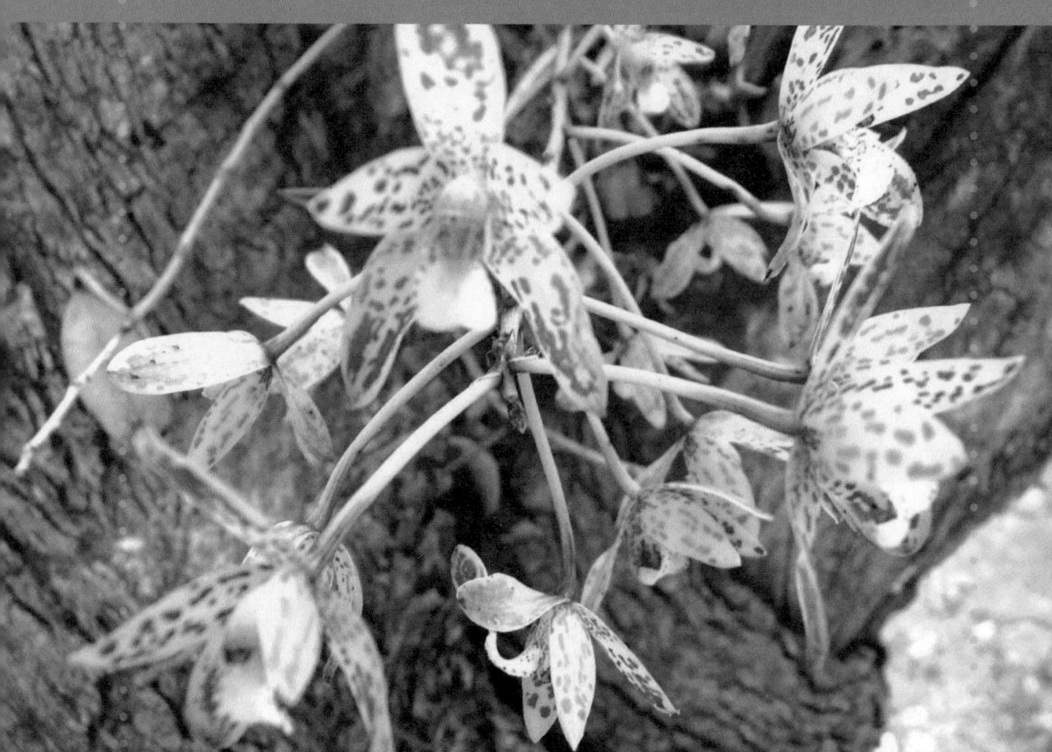

Scientific Name *Cymbidium canaliculatum* R.Br.

Common Names Black Orchid, Tiger Orchid, Banana Orchid, Queensland Black Orchid, Channel Leaf Orchid, Channelled Boat-Lip Orchid, Tiger Boat-Lip Orchid, Small Groove-leafed Cymbidium.

Aboriginal Names Dangilyangal (Wunambal, Gaambera) (Karadada et al., 2011), Banggaldjun (Bardi) (Smith & Kalotas, 1985), Pungulyon (Bardi) (Kenneally et al., 1996), Garloonggoony (Gija) (Purdie et al., 2018), Mirrinymirriny (Jaru) (Wightman, 2003).

Field Notes Black Orchid is an epiphytic (a plant that gets its moisture and nutrients from the air), clump-forming, perennial herb that grows on rotting wood in hollow trees. It has long thin leaves and greyish-green pseudobulbs. Its flowers are olive green, yellow, brown or purple, often with spots or blotches, and appear in November or February. Black Orchid is found in tropical and sub-tropical Australia from the northern parts of Western Australia,

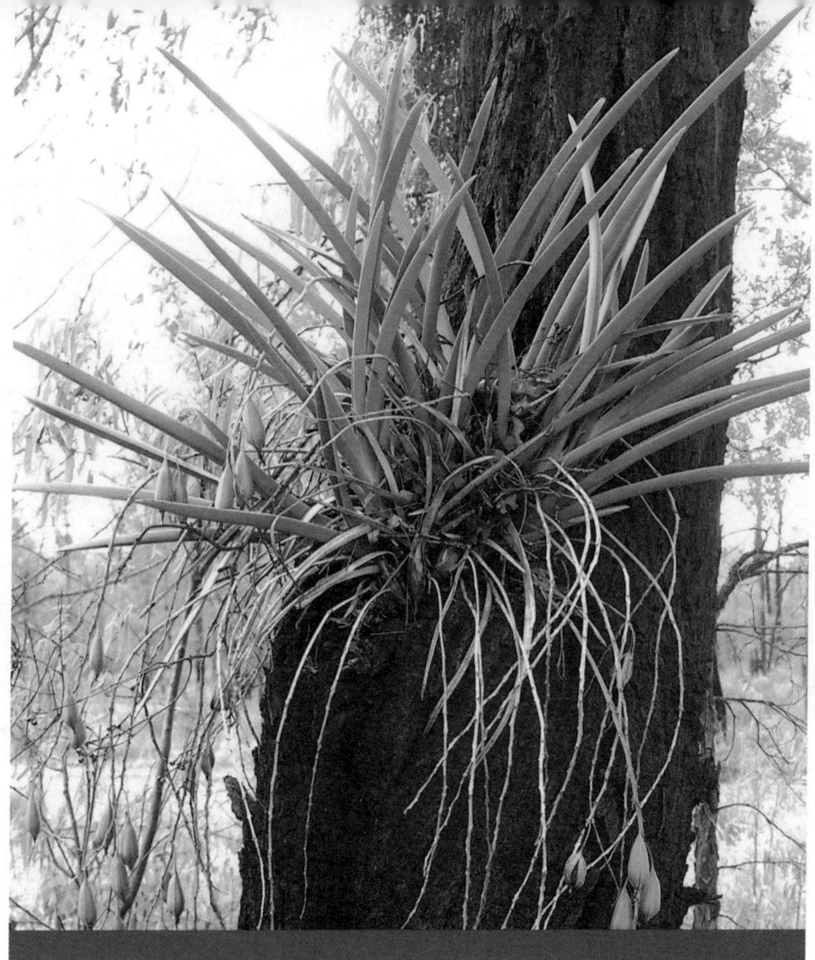

Northern Territory, Queensland (except the dry south-west) and north-east New South Wales (Oz Native Plants, 2022; WAH, 2022).

Medicinal Uses Some Aboriginal groups ate the base of the stems of tree orchids to relieve diarrhoea and dysentery (Cock, 2011; Low, 1990; Williams, 2010). The sap from the pseudobulbs was squeezed out directly onto sores and wounds to aid healing. It was also used to provide relief to itchy skin (Hiddins, 2001; Smith, 1991; Williams, 2011). The leaves were heated and the sap painted onto the skin to treat scabies infestations (Wiynjorrotj et al., 2005).

Other Uses The corms at the base of the leaves are edible and were eaten raw or roasted (Hiddins, 2001; Kenneally, et al., 1996; Smith & Kalotas, 1985). Edwards (2005) relates that, in Far North Queensland, Aboriginal 'Women ate the root part of the cluster of orchid stems as a contraceptive' (efficacy not recorded).

Blistering Ammannia

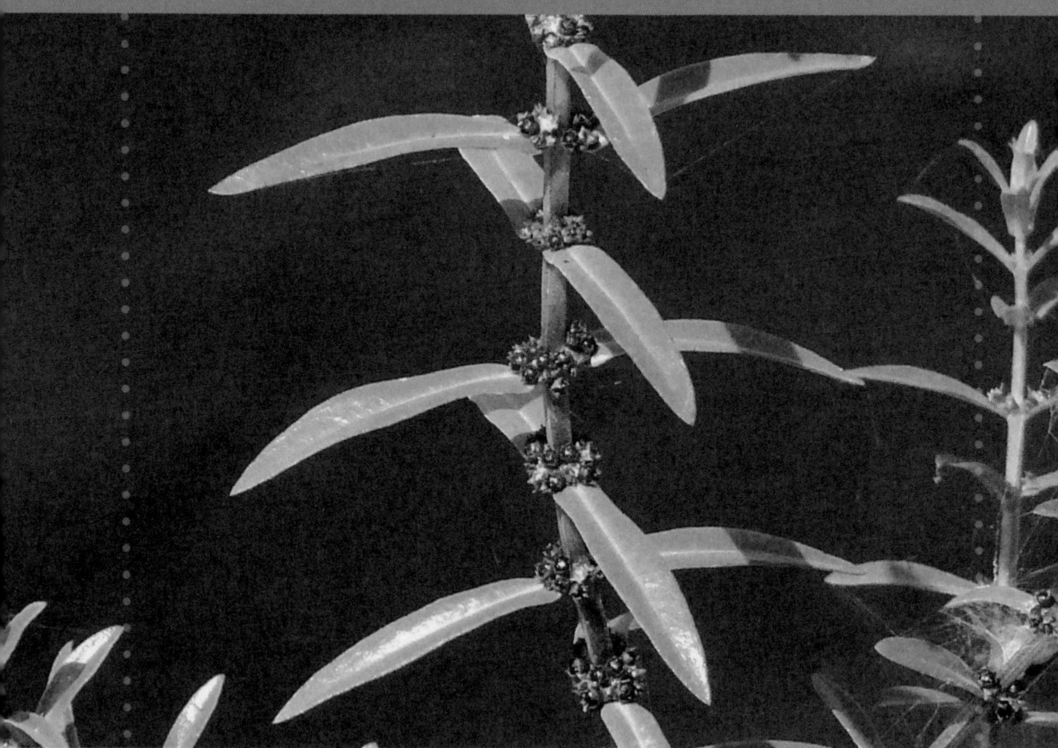

Scientific Name *Ammannia baccifera* L.

Common Names Blistering Ammannia, Acrid Weed, Monarch Redstem, Tooth Cup.

Field Notes Blistering Ammannia is an erect to spreading annual herb that grows to around 600 mm in height. Its leaves are glabrous, opposite, lanceolate to oblanceolate, and up to 70 mm long and 15 mm wide. Its small, red-brown flowers are present between May and September. Its tiny, red fruit are globose capsules only 2 mm in diameter and contain many seeds. Blistering Ammannia occurs in alluvium, sandy loam and clay on the edges of creeks and rivers in seasonally wet depressions and on mud flats in the Pilbara and Kimberley regions of Western Australia, the northern part of the Northern Territory and northern Queensland. It also occurs in tropical Africa, India, Pakistan, Thailand, Cambodia, Laos, Vietnam, Malaysia and the Philippines (ALA, 2022; WAH, 2022).

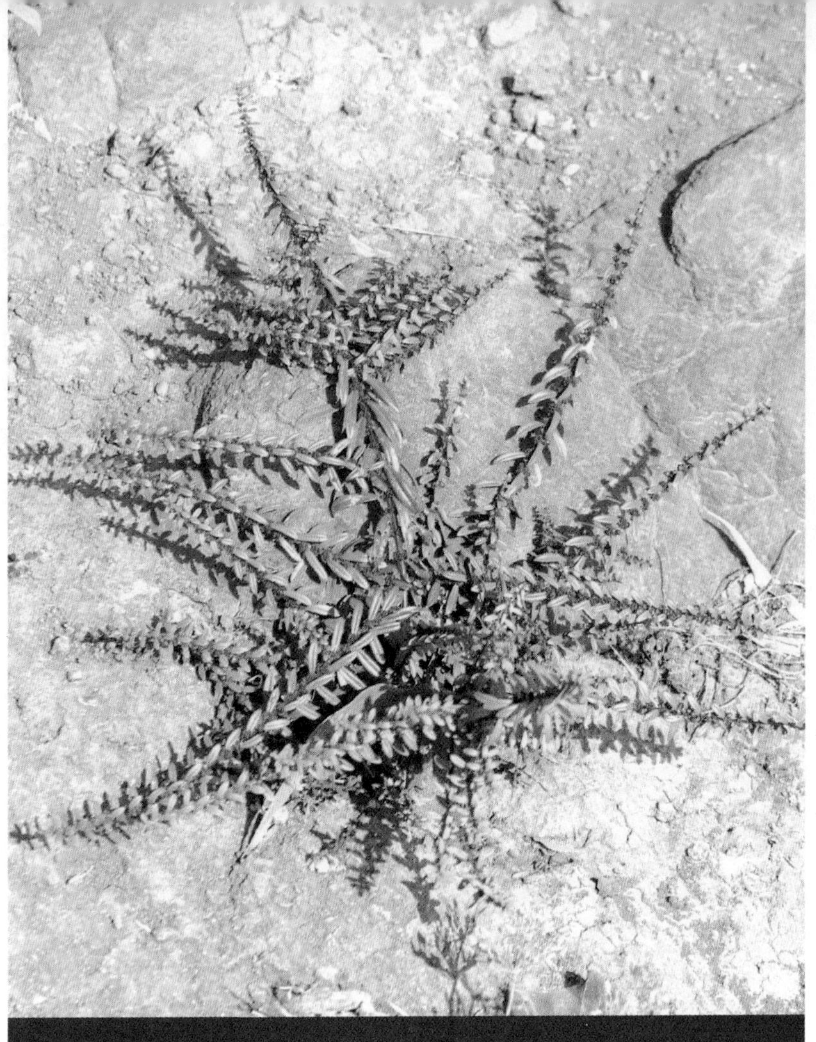

Medicinal Uses Blistering Ammannia is used in Ayurvedic folk medicine in India. Bruised fresh leaves are used for raising blisters to treat rheumatic pain and fever. The crushed leaves or the ashes of the plant are mixed with oil and applied to cure herpetic eruptions. The fresh, bruised leaves have been used in skin diseases as a rubefacient and as an external remedy for dermatophytosis (ringworm and tinea) (Fern, 2021; Flowers of India, 2022).

Blue Flax-lily

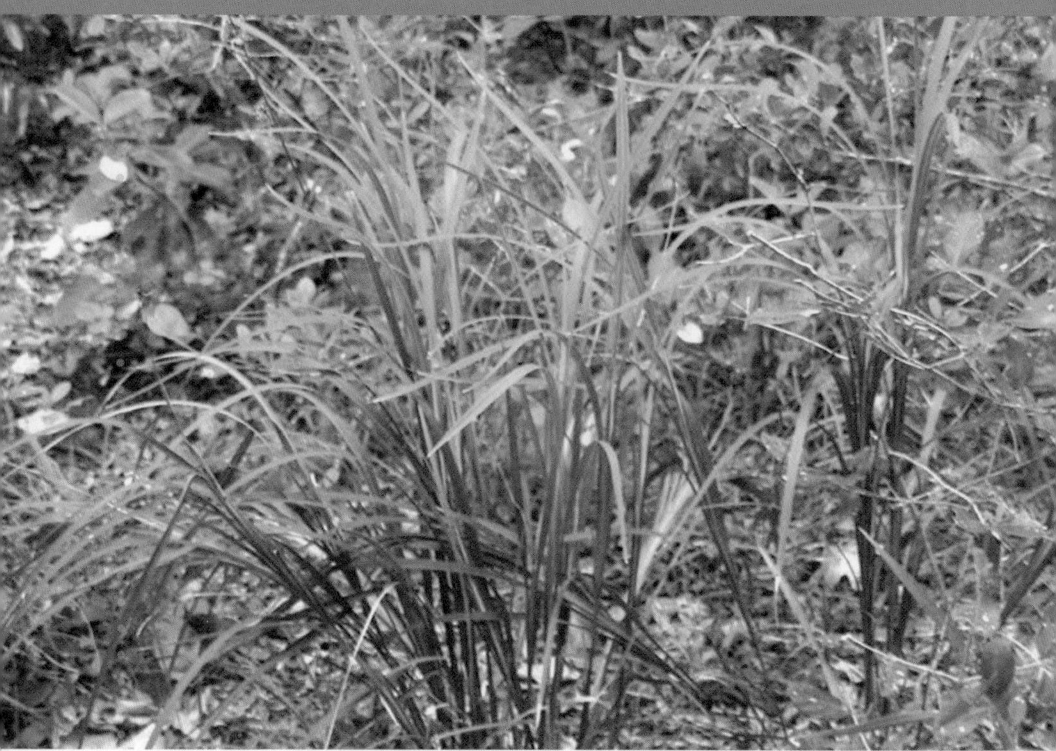

Scientific Name *Dianella longifolia* R.Br.

Common Names Blue Flax-lily, Spreading Flax Lily, Pale Flax Lily, Smooth Flax Lily, Smooth-leaved Flax Lily, Greater Blueberry Lily.

Field Notes Blue Flax-lily is a rhizomatous, tufted, perennial plant that grows up to 800 mm in height. Its leaves are up to 800 mm long and arise from the base of the plant. Its whitish to dark-blue or blue-green star-shaped flowers appear from January to March. The fruit is a fleshy berry that is up to 7 mm in diameter and contains about five seeds. The fruit turns purple when ripe. Blue Flax-lily is often found in lateritic loam in the Kimberley region of Western Australia, the top end of the Northern Territory, the Cape York Peninsula, and down the eastern side of Queensland, New South Wales, all over Victoria, parts of South Australia and Tasmania (ALA, 2022; PlantNET, 2022; WAH, 2022).

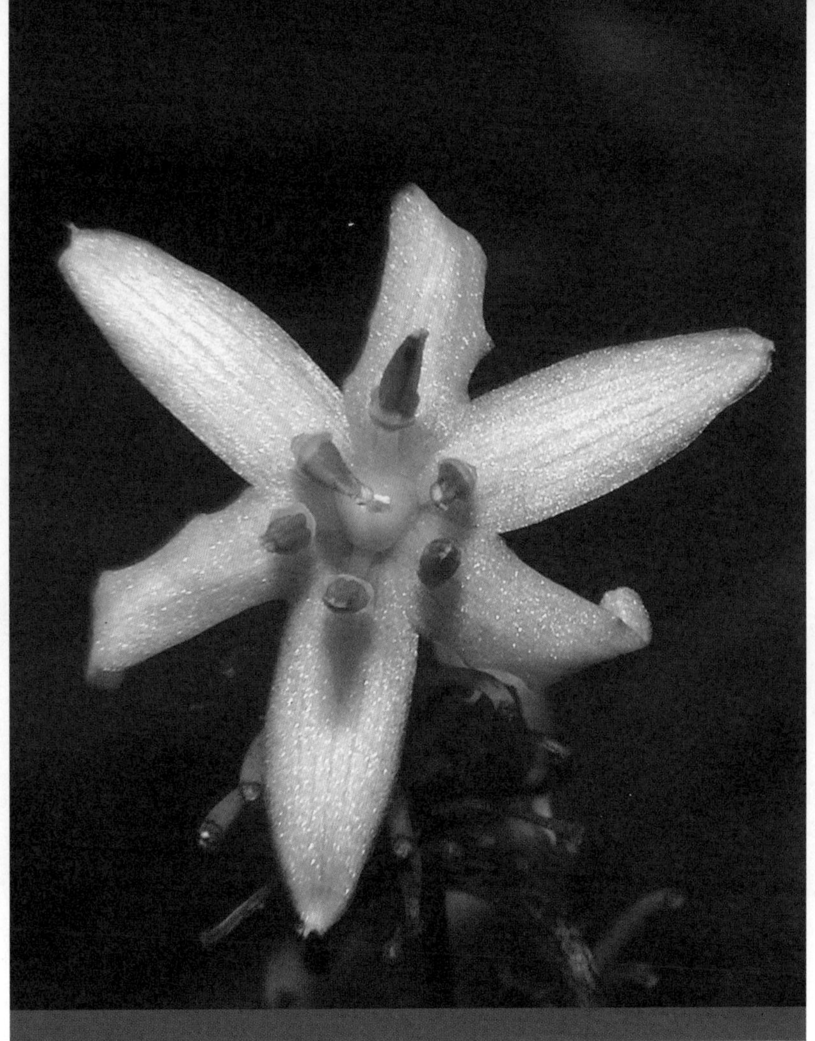

Medicinal Uses The Boandik people of the Mount Gambier region of South Australia and western Victoria took decoctions of the roots of Blue-Flax lily internally to treat the symptoms of colds and influenza (Clarke, 1987).

Other Uses The purple berries of the Blue Flax-lily are edible when ripe, from late October to January, and are reported to be sweet and tasty. Some Aboriginal groups used the tough leaves to weave dillies and baskets (Low, 1991; Sustainable Gardening Australia, 2020).

Blue Water Leaf

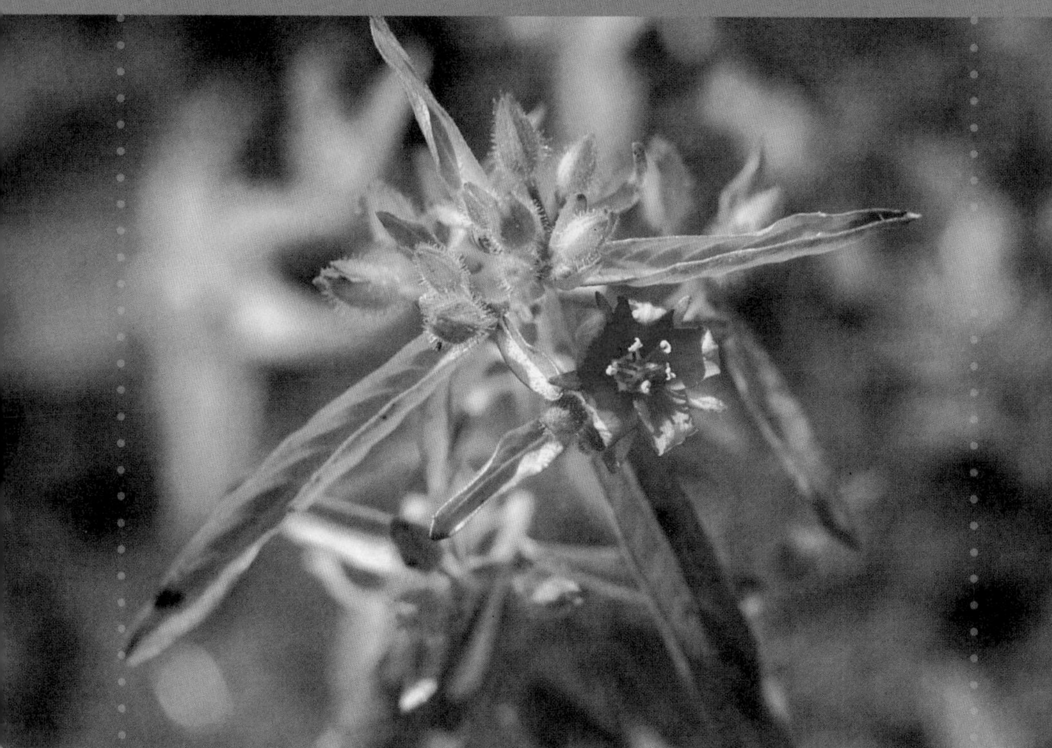

Scientific Name *Hydrolea zeylanica* (L.) Vahl.

Common Names Blue Water Leaf, Water Olive, Ceylon Hydrolea.

Field Notes Blue Water Leaf is an erect to prostrate herb, sometimes rooting from lower nodes, that grows up to 1 m in height. Its leaves are lanceolate to ovate, and up to 100 mm long and 25 mm wide. Its bright-blue flowers with five ovate petals form in terminal panicles. Its fruit or seed capsules are small and ovoid. Blue Water Leaf occurs on pond margins, beside streams, in open forests and in swampy or inundated soil in the Kimberley region of Western Australia, the northern half of the Northern Territory and northern Queensland. It also occurs in China, India, Sri Lanka, Myanmar, Thailand, Malaysia, Indonesia and the Philippines (ALA, 2022; WAH, 2022).

Medicinal Uses Blue Water Leaf was used by Aboriginal Australians and in Ayurvedic and folk medicine in Asian countries. The leaves

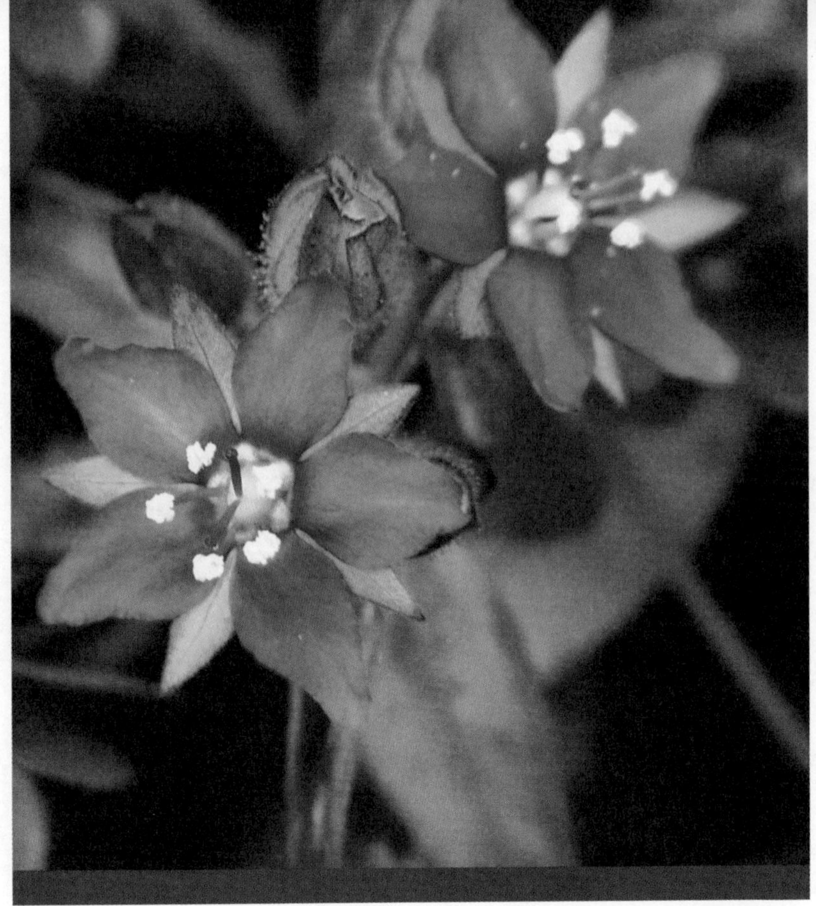

were beaten into a pulp then used as a poultice to aid the healing of neglected and callous leg ulcers. Decoctions of the leaves were also used for healing ulcers. Decoctions of the leaves and twigs were used in the treatment of diabetes and are thought to reduce blood sugar levels (Bailey, 1881; Philippine Medicinal Plants, 2020).

Other Uses The young leaves and shoots of Blue Water Leaf can be cooked and eaten as a vegetable. The leaf tips can be eaten raw in salads (Fern, 2021; Philippine Medicinal Plants, 2022).

Blush Plum

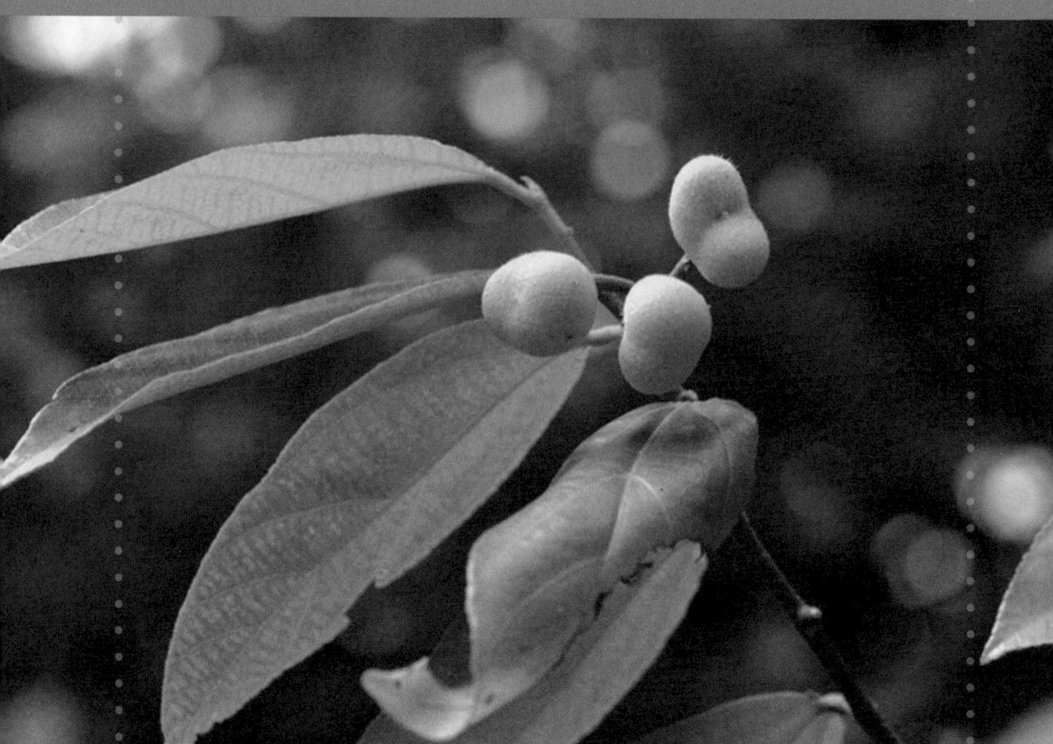

Scientific Name *Grewia oxyphylla* Burret.

Common Name Blush Plum.

Aboriginal Names Wuloy (Wunambal, Gaambera) (Karadada et al., 2011), Wilawa minya, Ngururr minya (Kwini) (Cheinmora et al., 2017).

Field Notes Blush Plum is a deciduous climber, shrub or tree that grows up to 8 m in height. Its bark is grey to brown and can be fibrous or smooth. Its leaves are usually ovate to elliptic and up to 130 mm long. Its beautiful green-white flowers have lanceolate to ovate petals that curl backwards and long stamens. They appear between January and May. Its fruit are drupes that are succulent and mucilaginous when ripe, and usually have three or four globular parts. They turn brown when ripe. Blush Plum is usually found in sand over sandstone in vine thickets close to the coast in the northern Kimberley region of Western Australia, the Northern

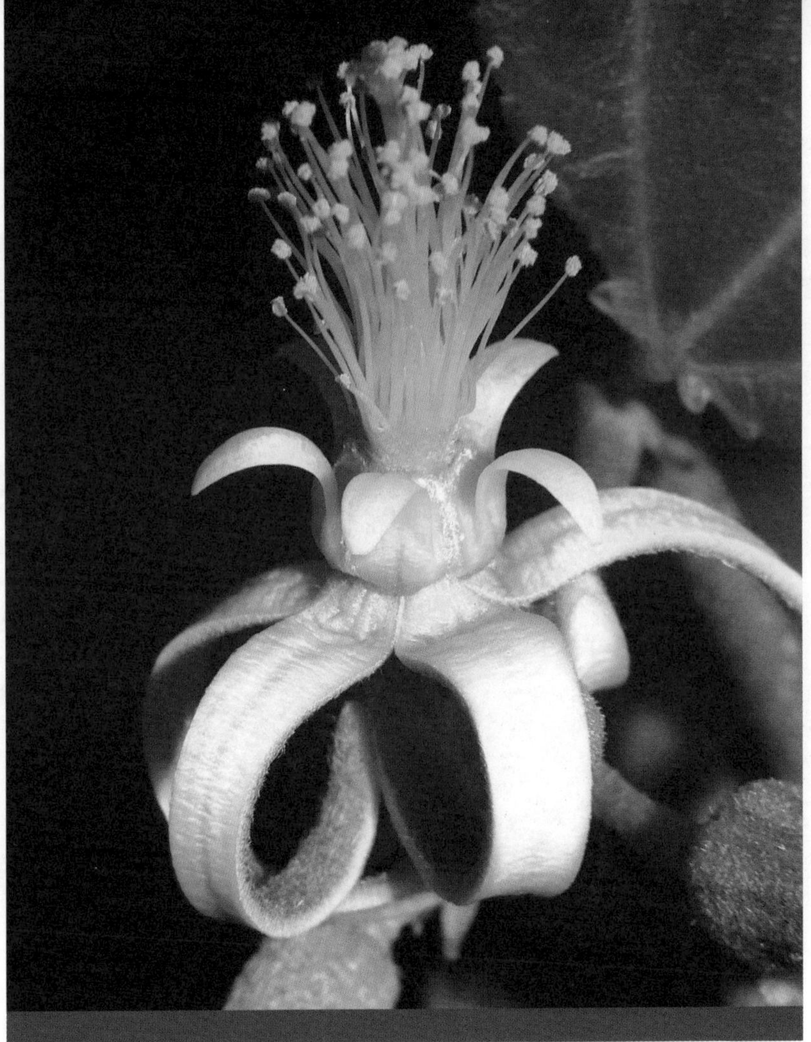

Territory and Queensland coasts as far south as Mackay (ALA, 2022; ATRP, 2020; FloraNT, 2022; WAH, 2022).

Medicinal Uses Decoctions of the inner bark from the base of the stems and roots of Blush Plum were used as a wash to treat boils, carbuncles, wounds, sores and cuts (Devanesen, 2000; Smith, 1991).

Other Uses The fruit of the Blush Plum are edible and were eaten raw when ripe. The fruit are available from the end of April through May (Cheinmora et al., 2017; Crawford, 1982; Karadada et al., 2011; Smith, 1991; Vigilante et al., 2013). The Kwini used the stems of larger Blush Plum to make spear shafts (Cheinmora et al., 2017).

Boab Tree

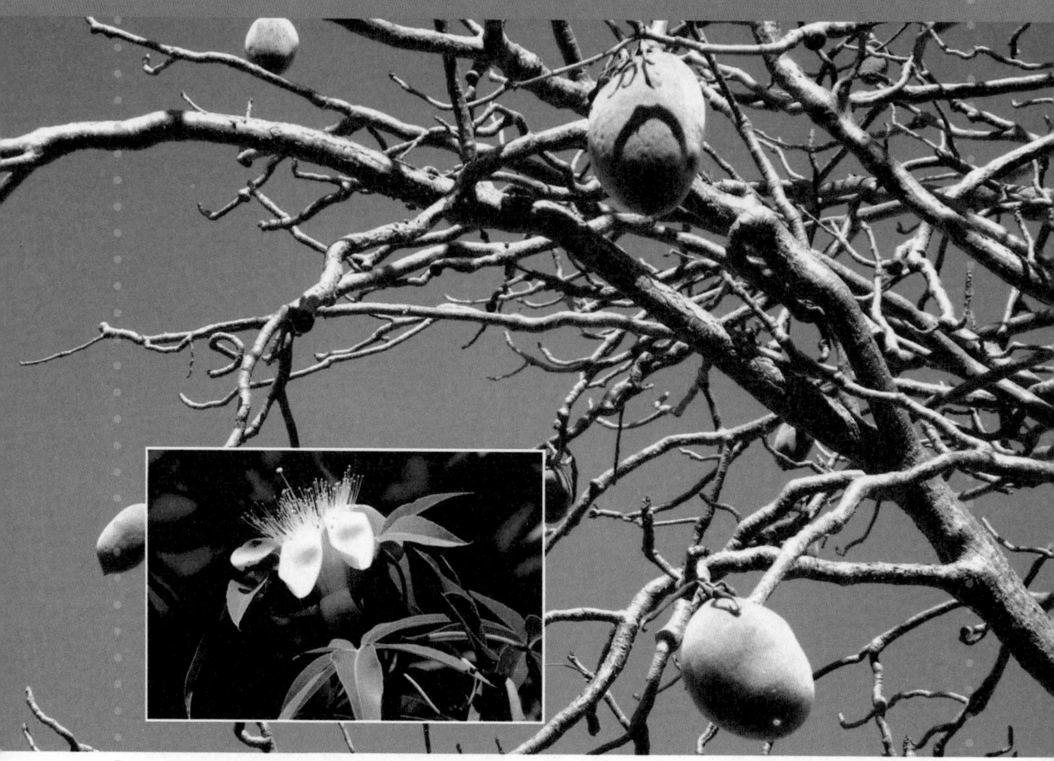

Scientific Name *Adansonia gregorii* F.Muell.

Common Names Boab Tree, Australian Baobab, Bottle Tree, Upside Down Tree, Dead Rat Tree, Gouty Stem Tree, Monkey Bread Tree, Cream of Tartar Tree, Gourd-gourd Tree, Sour Gourd.

Aboriginal Names Bodgurri (Wunambal, Gaambera) (Karadada et al., 2011), Potkurri, Junguri and Jarragan (northern Worrorran), Jumulu (southern Worrorran and Kwini), Kertewun or Gerdewoon (Gajirrabeng and Miriwoong), Jamula (Ngumpin) (McConvell et al., 2013), Largarda or Largirda (Bardi) (Smith & Kalotas, 1985), Larrkarti (Walmajarri) (Richards & Hudson, 2012), Joomooloony (Gija) (Purdie et al., 2018), Girdiwun (Miwa) (Kimberley Specialists, 2020), Larrgardi (Jaru) (Wightman, 2003), Jumulu manya, Jumuli manya, Junguri manya (Kwini) (Cheinmora et al., 2017; Crawford, 1982), Larrkardiy (Nyikina) (Milgin, 2009), Jungura inja, Jungurim mana (Worroorra) (Clendon et al., 2000), Larrgari (Bunuba) (Oscar et al., 2019), Larrkardiy (Nyikina) (Smith & Smith, 2009).

Field Notes The Boab Tree is a large, deciduous tree that can grow up to 15 m in height with a spread of around 12 m. Its trunk is bottle-shaped and is filled with soft fibrous wood that enables it to store water. It has thin, lanceolate leaves and large, fragrant, showy, cream-coloured flowers that appear from December to May. Its fruit are large, brown, oval-shaped, woody and hairy pods that are roughly 180 mm long. The Boab Tree is found in sandy and loamy soils across the Kimberley region of Western Australia and in the western part of the Northern Territory. (ALA, 2022; ANPSA, 2022; Kings Park Botanic Gardens, n.d.; McConvell et al., 2013; WAH, 2022).

Medicinal Uses Infusions of the leaves and roots of Boab Trees were used to treat digestive complaints and chest infections (Native Tastes of Australia, 2022). The fruit is high in ascorbic acid (vitamin C) and would have helped prevent people consuming them from getting scurvy (Fern, 2021; McConvell et al., 2013).

Other Use: The pith of the fruit and the seeds of Boab Trees are edible. The pith, soaked in water, makes a refreshing drink. Sometimes a drop of sugarbag is added for a bit more sweetness. The seeds were eaten raw or roasted. The fruit are at their best and are usually picked between late February and August. Unripe fruit were often buried for a while to ripen them (Cheinmora et al., 2017; Crawford, 1982; Karadada et al., 2011; Oscar et al., 2019; Wightman, 2003). The roots are also edible and were usually eaten raw (Cheinmora et al., 2017; Oscar et al., 2019; Vigilante et al., 2013). Some Aboriginal groups in the Kimberley ate the sap or soaked the sap in water to make a sweet drink (Crawford, 1982). Fibre from the bark and roots was used to make cordage. Water can be obtained from the porous trunk (Crawford, 1982; Karadada et al., 2011; McConvell et al., 2013).

Bootlace Oak

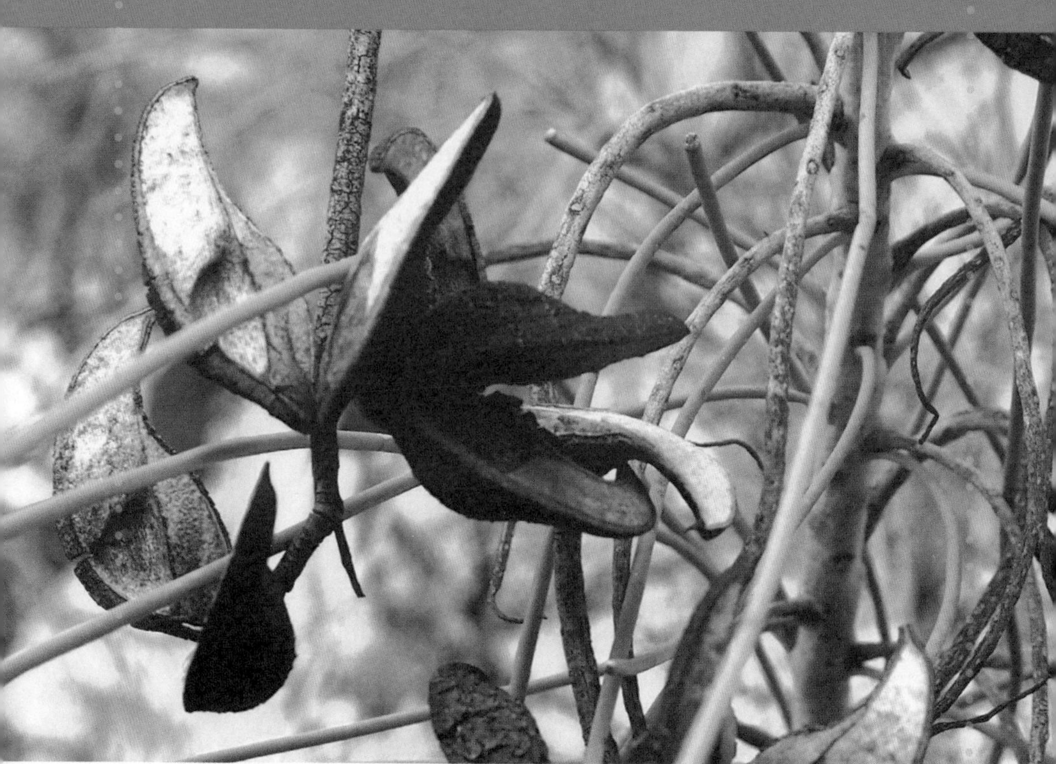

Scientific Name *Hakea chordophylla* F.Muell.

Common Names Bootlace Oak, Bootlace Tree, Corkwood, Bull Oak.

Aboriginal Names Jani, Janbij, Jarni, or Jaani (Jaru) (Wightman, 2003), Kumpalpa, Mililinti (Kukatja) (Valiquette, 1993), Wiyinti, Piriwa (Ngardi) (Cataldi, 2004).

Field Notes Bootlace Oak is a lignotuberous hakea that grows as a shrub or tree up to 5 m or more in height. Its leaves are terete (cylindrical or slightly tapering), usually simple, and up to 420 mm long and 2.9 mm in diameter. Its typical hakea-type, spidery, cream-yellow or red flowers are present between June and September. Its fruit or seed capsules are up to 40 mm long, with long obscure to prominent beaks. Bootlace Oak occurs in red or brown sand and rocky or stony soil on sandplains in the Pilbara and Kimberley regions of Western Australia, the Northern Territory and

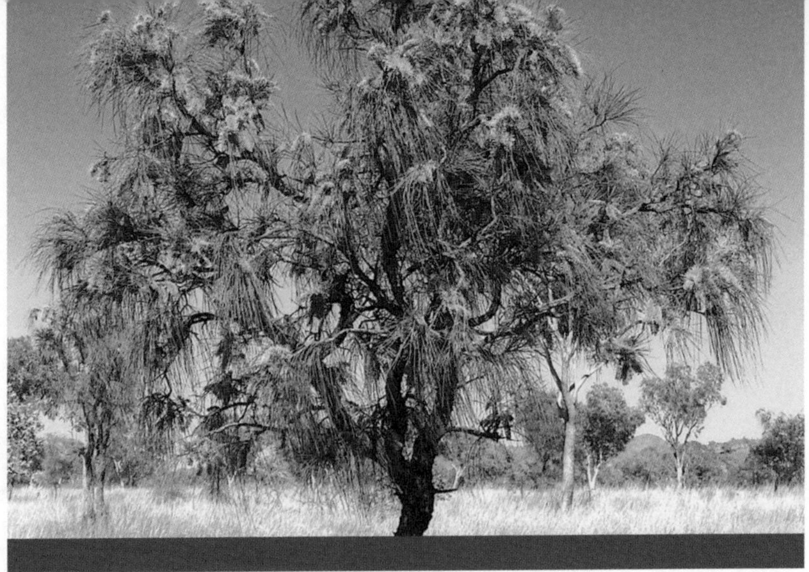

Queensland (ALA, 2022; eFlora.SA, 2022; WAH, 2022).

Medicinal Uses The bark of Bootlace Oak was burnt, mixed with goanna fat and applied as an antiseptic and healing salve to treat burns and skin conditions, such as eczema and psoriasis, scabies infestations and gum abscesses (Morse, 2005; Nyinkka Nyunyu Art and Culture Centre, n.d.). Decoctions of the bark were used as an antiseptic wash to treat sores, boils, carbuncles and skin rashes (Nyinkka Nyunyu Art and Culture Centre, n.d.). The Ngardi heat the bark from this tree and rub newborn babies with it to strengthen them. They also use infusions of the flowers, which are full of nectar, to treat 'cold sickness', the symptoms of colds and influenza (Cataldi, 2004).

Other Uses Bootlace Oak flowers are full of nectar, which was sucked directly from the flower. Alternatively, the flowers were soaked in water to make a sweet drink (Cataldi, 2004; Nyinkka Nyunyu Art and Culture Centre, n.d.; Wightman, 2003). The Jaru curled the leaves of Bootlace Oak into a circle and placed it on the head to make it easier to carry heavy coolamons. They placed a little soft grass in the middle to protect the top of their head. The wood can be used to make coolamons. The Jaru also soaked the leaves in ngarlu (bush honey), and then sucked the leaves to get more flavour from the honey (Wightman, 2003).

Broadleaf Paperbark

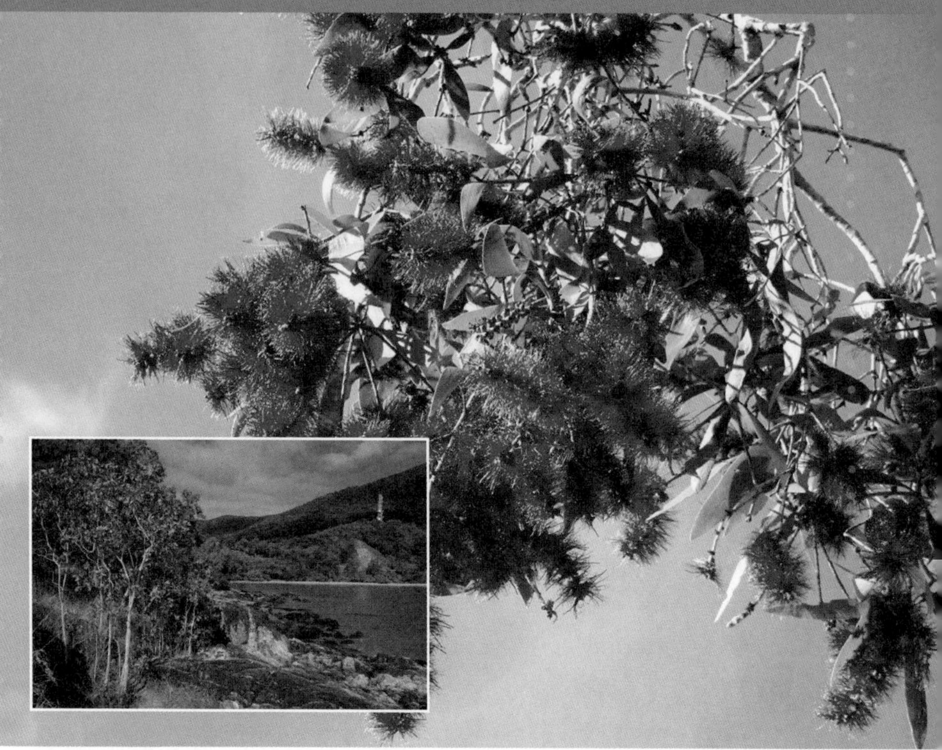

Scientific Name *Melaleuca viridiflora* Gaertn.

Common Names Broadleaf Paperbark, Broad-leaved Paperbark, Weeping Red Flowering Paperbark.

Aboriginal Names Walamanggar (Nyul Nyul) (Dobbs et al., 2015), Andamalal (Wunambal, Gaambera) (Karadada et al., 2011), Nimalgoon (Bardi) (Kenneally et al., 1996), or Nimalgan (Bardi) (Smith & Kalotas, 1985), Moonggoolji or Mungkulji (Gija) (Purdie et al., 2018; Wightman, 2003), Ngarli minya (Kwini) (Cheinmora et al., 2017).

Field Notes Broadleaf Paperbark grows as a shrub or tree up to 20 m in height. It has white, brownish or grey papery bark and wide, thick, broadly elliptic and aromatic leaves that can be up to 190 mm long. Its bottlebrush-type flowers can be cream but are more often red. They are present any time between January and August. Flowering is followed by the appearance of fruit, which are woody capsules up to 6 mm long. Broadleaf Paperbark is found in sand over sandstone, and sometimes clay, along watercourses, in swampy areas and seasonally damp sites all across the tropical north of Australia and down the east coast as far as the Queensland and New South Wales border (ALA, 2022; ANPSA, 2022; ATRP, 2020; WAH, 2022).

Medicinal Uses Fresh leaves of the Broadleaf Paperbark were crushed then held under the nose and the vapours inhaled to relieve sinusitis and the symptoms of colds and influenza. Decoctions of the fresh leaves were used as a body wash for the relief of headaches, fever, the symptoms of colds, influenza and the associated general body aches and pains. Decoctions of the fresh leaves were also used as an antiseptic wash for sores, cuts and other wounds (Edwards, 2005; Smith, 1991; Williams, 2011). Infusions of the crushed leaves were sipped as a cough suppressant (Williams, 2011). Some Aboriginal groups in Far North Queensland used the leaves as smoke medicine to smoke newborn babies to 'make them strong' (Williams, 2011). Well-filtered infusions of the inner bark were used as eye drops or an eyewash to treat sore eyes due to conjunctivitis (Williams, 2011).

Other Uses The flowers of Broadleaf Paperbark are usually full of nectar that can be sucked directly from the flowers. Alternatively, the flowers can be soaked in water to make a sweet drink. Water can usually be obtained from swellings that grow on the trunk. The swellings are chopped open to release the water (Fox & Garde, 2018). Sugarbag honey is often found in this tree (Williams, 2011). The bark of Broadleaf Paperbark was used to build shelters, for wrapping food, to make bark coolamons and as a body wrap for the deceased (Williams, 2011).

Broad-leaved Cherry

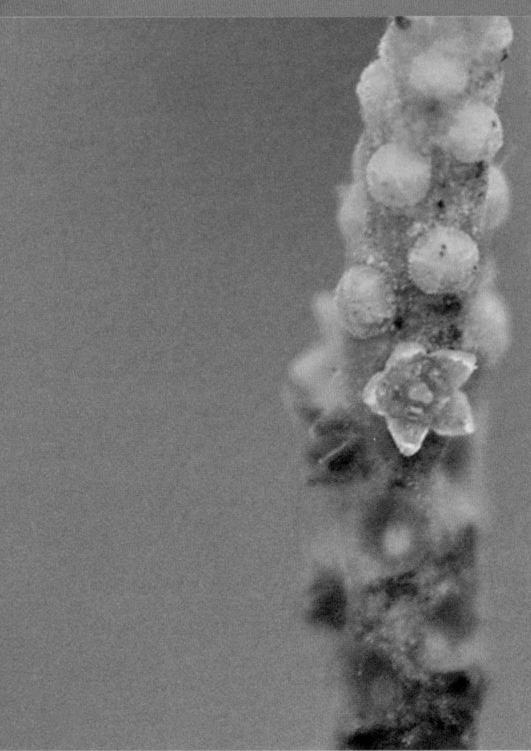

Scientific Name *Exocarpos latifolius* R.Br.

Common Names Broad-leaved Cherry, Broad-leaved Native Cherry, Mistletoe Tree, Broad-leaved Ballart.

Aboriginal Names Wundugu (Wunambal, Gaambera) (Karadada et al., 2011), Djamba-djamba (Bardi) (Smith & Kalotas, 1985), Jarnba (Bardi) (Kenneally et al., 1996).

Field Notes Broad-leaved Cherry grows as a small tree or shrub up to 10 m in height. It is hemiparasitic on the roots of other trees. The leathery leaves are ovate and up to 100 mm long. The small, green, cream-yellow or orange-brown flowers are produced in slender spikes approximately 10 mm long. They can be present any time between March and November. The fruit starts as a green drupe. As it matures and ripens, the stem behind the fruit swells and becomes fleshy. Broad-leaved Cherry occurs in sand or clay, in sandstone gullies, on sand dunes and riverbanks across the top

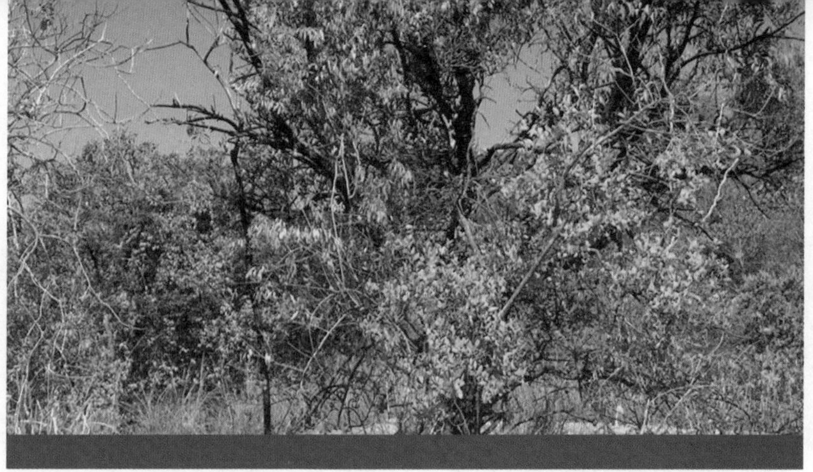

end of Australia from the Kimberley region in the north of Western Australia, through the Northern Territory and along the Queensland and New South Wales coasts as far south as Newcastle. It also occurs throughout South-east Asia and the Pacific Islands (ALA, 2022; Fern, 2021; Low, 1991; WAH, 2022).

Medicinal Uses Decoctions of the leaves of Broad-leaved Cherry were widely used as an antiseptic wash to treat cuts and sores. Decoctions of the inner bark were used as a wash for the head to ease the symptoms of colds and influenza. They were also taken internally in small amounts for the same purpose (Smith, 1991; Williams, 2010). Decoctions of crushed leaves were used as a compress and squeezed onto the head to treat headaches (Edwards, 2005). Infusions of the bark and the seeds were supposedly used as a contraceptive by some Aboriginal groups, but the efficacy of this method of contraception has not been proven (Fern, 2021). The leaves and wood were burnt in campfires to repel insects (Low, 1991; Williams, 2010). The foliage was often used to smoke babies 'to make them stronger' (Low, 1990; Smith, 1991). In tropical Queensland, poultices made from the rough bark and roots that were crushed and mixed with water were applied to boils and carbuncles to help draw them out (Williams, 2020).

Other Uses Aboriginal groups throughout the top end of Australia eat the sweet fruit of Broad-leaved Cherry. The fruit form after flowering finishes in December (Edwards, 2005; Low, 1991; Maiden, 1889; Smith, 1991; Vigilante et al., 2013).

Broad-leaved Paperbark

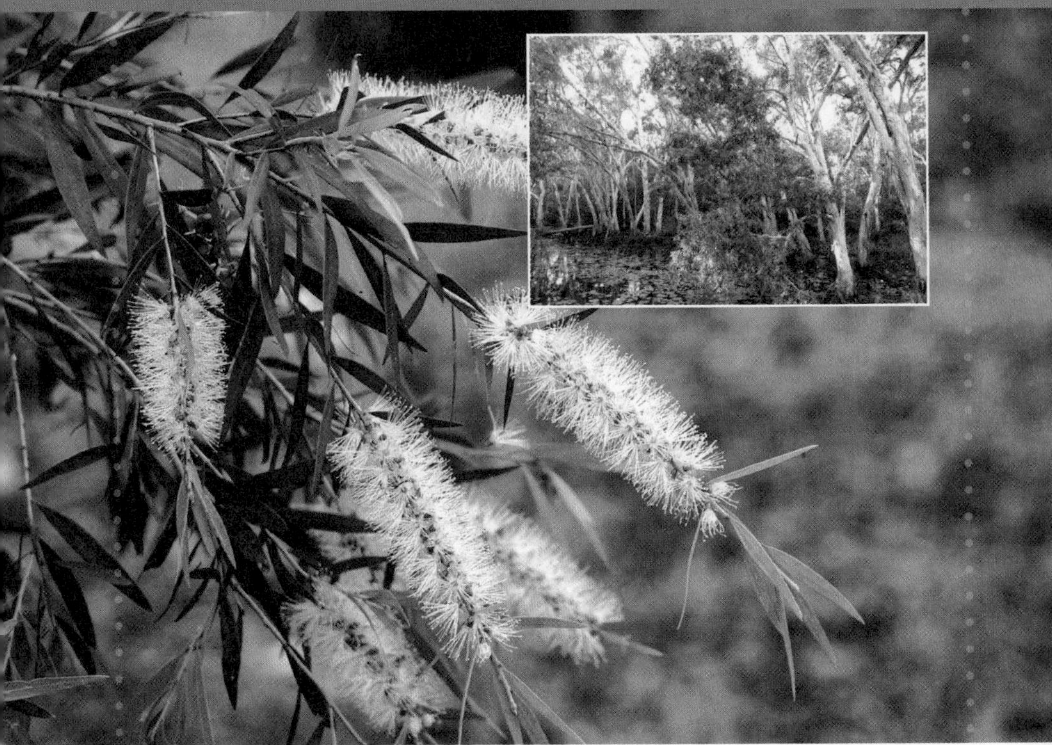

Scientific Name *Melaleuca leucadendra* (L.) L.

Common Names Broad-leaved Paperbark, Fresh-water Paperbark, Weeping Paperbark, River Cadjeput, Bandaran.

Aboriginal Names Wulu (Bunuba) (Oscar et al., 2019), Ngarli (Wunambal, Gaambera) (Karadada et al., 2011), Merndany or Merntany, Lamerntarlel (Gija) (Purdie et al., 2018), Warrapa (Karajarri) (Willing, 2014), Lambu (Jaru) (Wightman, 2003), Ngarli minya (Kwini) (Cheinmora et al., 2017).

Field Notes Broad-leaved Paperbark grows as a small or large tree to 30 m in height. Its trunk is covered with thick, white, papery bark and it has weeping thinner branches. Its leaves are alternate, wide, flat, ovate or lanceolate, tapering to a point and up to 270 mm long. Its green to cream or white, bottlebrush-type flowerheads appear on the ends of branchlets. They are present between March and October. Flowering is followed by fruit that are woody capsules up to 5 mm in diameter. Broad-leaved Paperbark occurs in sand or alluvium over sandstone along watercourses and around swamps across the tropical north of Australia from the Kimberley region in Western Australia to Far North Queensland. It also occurs in Indonesia and New Guinea (ALA, 2022; ATRP, 2020; WAH, 2022).

Medicinal Uses Decoctions of the papery bark were drunk to relieve bad headaches associated with colds and influenza, as a cough suppressant and to reduce fever. Alternatively, the decoctions were applied warm to the head, neck and ears to relieve a headache. Fresh leaves were crushed, held under the nose and the vapours inhaled to relieve the symptoms of sinusitis, colds and influenza. Alternatively, decoctions of the leaves were used as a body wash for the same purpose. Decoctions of the leaves were sometimes drunk to treat general malaise. Occasionally a person would sit near a fire on which some fresh leaves had been placed so they could inhale some of the smoke to help a cold, influenza or general malaise (Edwards, 2005; Hiddins, 2001; Lassak & McCarthy, 2001; Smith, 1991; Webb, 1959; Wightman, 2003; Williams, 2011).

Other Uses Like most melaleucas, the flowers are full of nectar which was sucked straight from the flower. Alternatively, the flowers were soaked in water to make a sweet drink (Calvert, 2018; Fox & Garde, 2018; Hiddins, 2001; Williams, 2010). Water can usually be obtained from swellings on the trunk by chopping open the lumps (Fox & Garde, 2018). Sugarbag is often found in the trunk of this tree (Oscar et al., 2019). The bark of Broad-leaved Paperbark is used as a mat to place food on when cooking and as a wrapping. The bark sheets are also used to wrap up meat to be cooked in ground ovens. The bark was also used as a covering for shelters and to make coolamons (Cheinmora et al., 2017; Hiddins, 2001; Karadada et al., 2011; Kenneally et al., 2018; Wightman, 2003). Dugout canoes were often made from the straight trunks of the larger trees (Cheinmora et al., 2017).

Broad-winged Hop Bush

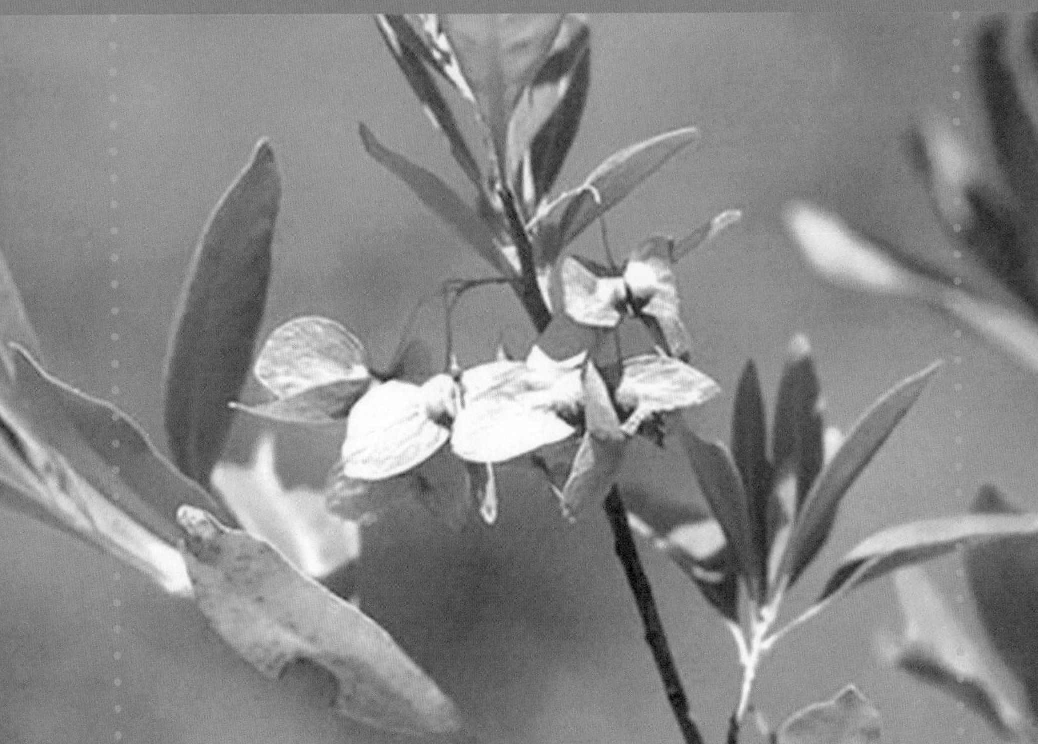

Scientific Name *Dodonaea platyptera* F.Muell.

Common Names Broad-winged Hop Bush, Hopbush.

Aboriginal Names Biindanjoon (Bardi) (Moss et al., 2021), Alarga (Bardi) (Smith & Kalotas, 1985), Alarrgarr (Bardi) (Kenneally et al., 1996).

Field Notes Broad-winged Hop Bush grows as an erect shrub or tree up to a height of 6 m in good conditions. Its ovate leaves are up to 100 mm long by 45 mm wide. Its small, white-green flowers are present between January and May. Its fruit are three or four-winged capsules up to 30 mm long by 13 mm in diameter. Broad-winged Hop Bush occurs in sandy, skeletal soils on coastal dunes and sandstone screes across the north of Australia from the Kimberley region of Western Australia through the top end of the Northern Territory and into Far North Queensland (ALA, 2022; ATRP, 2020; WAH, 2022).

Medicinal Uses Decoctions of the leaves were used as a body wash to treat general malaise and as a liniment to treat back pain. Crushed leaves were boiled and applied warm as a poultice to the back to treat back pain (Edwards, 2005).

Broom Wattle

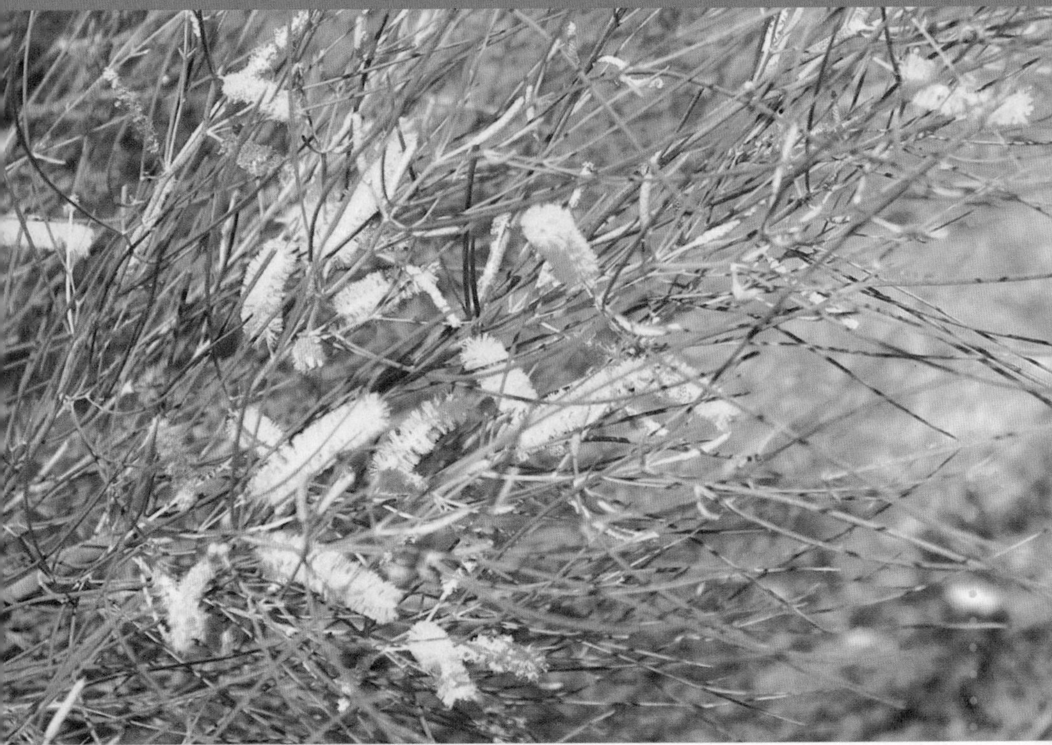

Scientific Name *Acacia tenuissima* F.Muell.

Common Names Broom Wattle, Narrow-leaved Wattle.

Aboriginal Names Minyinkura (Ngardi) (Cataldi, 2004), Minyina or Minyirna, Minyinkura, Mungilpa, Palykanypa (Kukatja) (Valiquette, 1993).

Field Notes Broom Wattle is a slender, erect shrub that grows up to 3 m in height. Its phyllodes are slender and up to 150 mm long. Its pale yellow to light-golden flowers appear on spikes up to 15 mm long between May and October. Its seed pods are up to 70 mm long and 3 mm wide. Broom Wattle occurs in stony clay, loam or red sand on rocky ironstone ranges, in gullies, on rocky clay flats and sandstone screes across the Pilbara and Kimberley regions of Western Australia through the Northern Territory and the top of South Australia, and into Queensland and north-west New South Wales (ALA, 2022; Maslin et al., 2010; WAH, 2022).

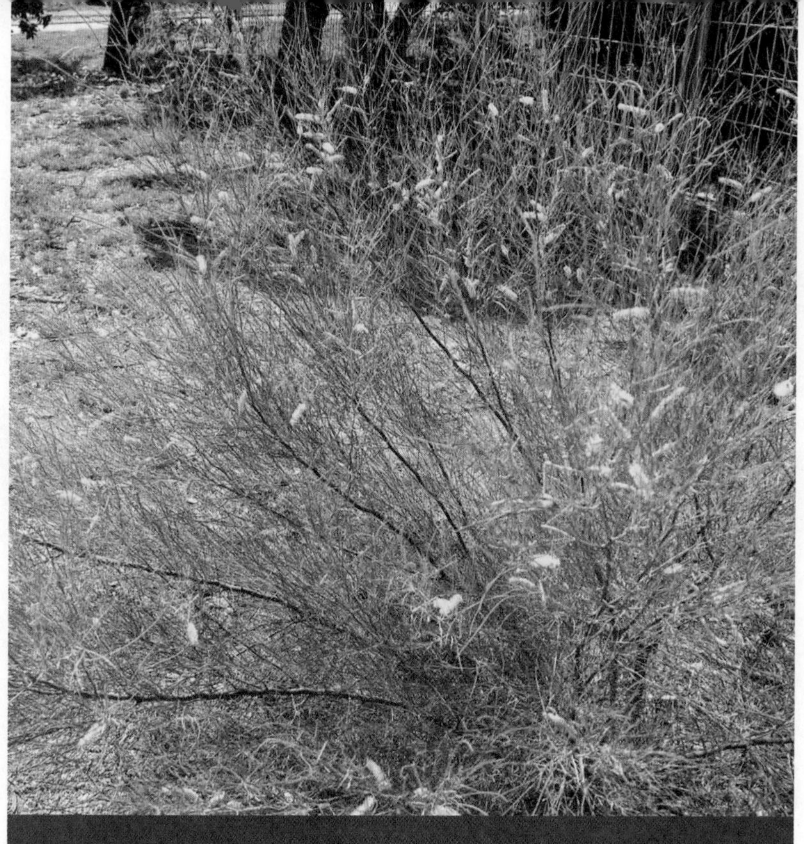

Medicinal Uses The phyllodes of Broome Wattle were crushed and mixed with fat for use as a medicinal ointment that was applied to wounds and sores. Alternatively, decoctions or infusions of the crushed phyllodes were used as an antiseptic wash for the same purpose (Kemarre, 2019; Valiquette, 1993; Williams, 2011).

Other Uses The seeds of the Broom Wattle are edible. Aboriginal groups ground them into flour to make damper or ate them raw. Mature seeds are available between September and November (Bindon, 2014; Brand-Miller & Holt, 1998; Fern, 2021; Maslin et al., 2010; Valiquette, 1993).

Broome Pindan Wattle

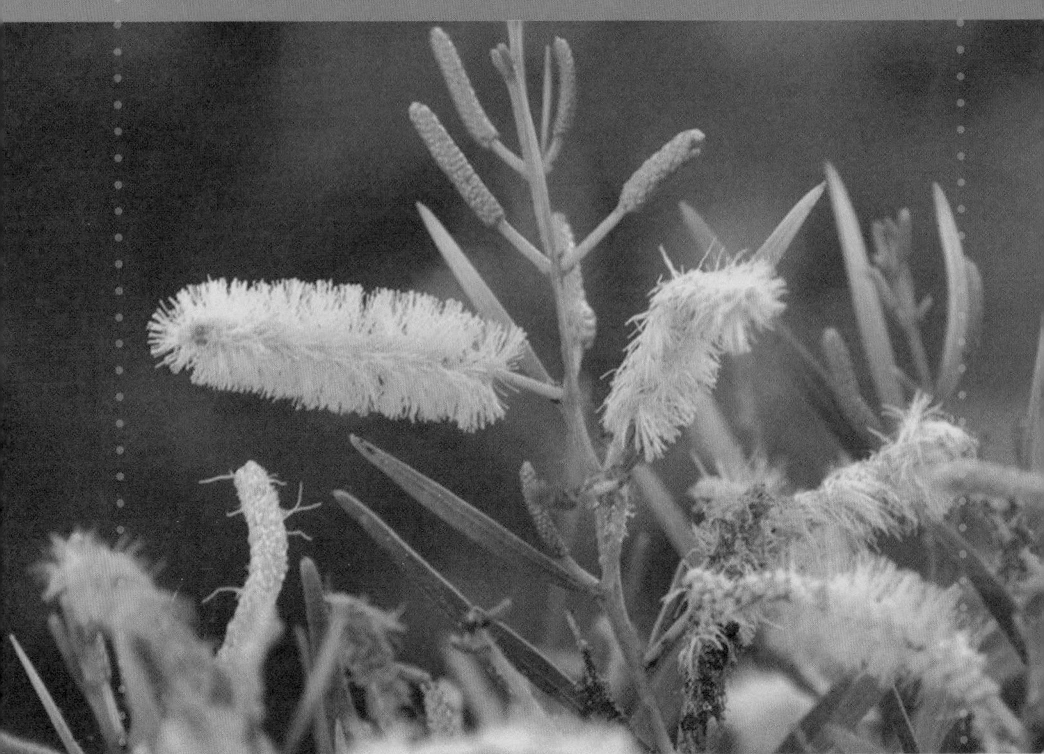

Scientific Name *Acacia eriopoda* Maiden & Blakely.

Common Names Broome Pindan Wattle, Narrow Leaf Pindan Wattle.

Aboriginal Names Irroogool or Irgul (Bardi) (Smith & Kalotas, 1985), Yirragulu (Yawuru) (Kenneally et al., 1996), Nyalyka (Walmajarri) (Richards & Hudson, 2012), Yirrakulu (Karajarri) (Willing, 2014), Yirrakooloo (Nyikina) (Smith & Smith, 2009).

Field Notes Broome Pindan Wattle is a shrub or tree that grows to around 6 m in height. It either has a single trunk or up to four trunks. Its bark is mid-grey to light grey and finely longitudinally fissured, becoming flaky with age. Its branchlets tend to be smooth. Its phyllodes are linear and up to 240 mm long and 5 mm wide. Its yellow flowers are peduncles on spikes up to 50 mm long. They are present between April and September. Its seed pods are droopy and up to 150 mm long or more. Broome Pindan Wattle occurs in

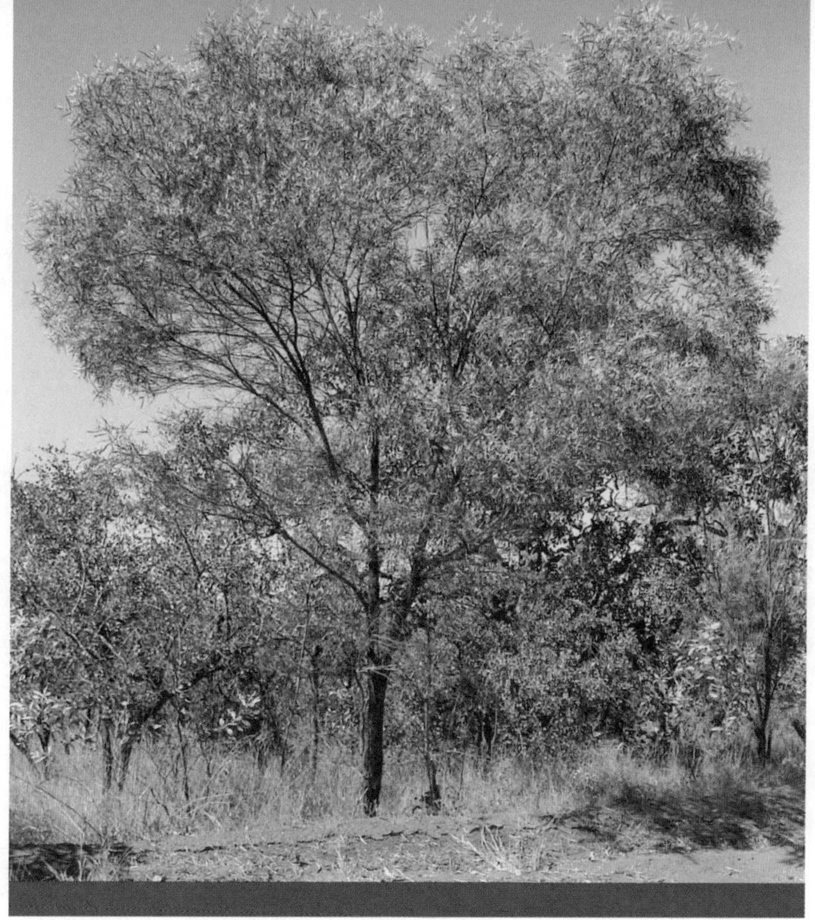

red sandy soils in the Pilbara and Kimberley regions of Western Australia (ALA, 2022; Maslin et al., 2010; WAH, 2022).

Medicinal Uses Decoctions of the bark of Broome Pindan Wattle were taken internally to treat diarrhoea, dysentery and internal bleeding. Decoctions of the bark were also used as a wash to treat wounds and other skin problems, haemorrhoids, perspiring feet, conjunctivitis and as a mouthwash. Infusions of the gum were taken internally to treat diarrhoea and haemorrhoids (Fern, 2021).

Other Uses The gum from the Broome Pindan Wattle is edible and is high in protein (47%). The insect larvae (commonly called Witchetty Grubs), found in the roots of the tree, are also edible and were eaten raw or slightly roasted (Fern, 2021; Kane, 2022). The seeds are edible and were ground to flour to make damper (Australian Bushfoods, 2022). Branches of Broome Pindan Wattle have been used to make spears (Kane, 2022).

Brown Beech

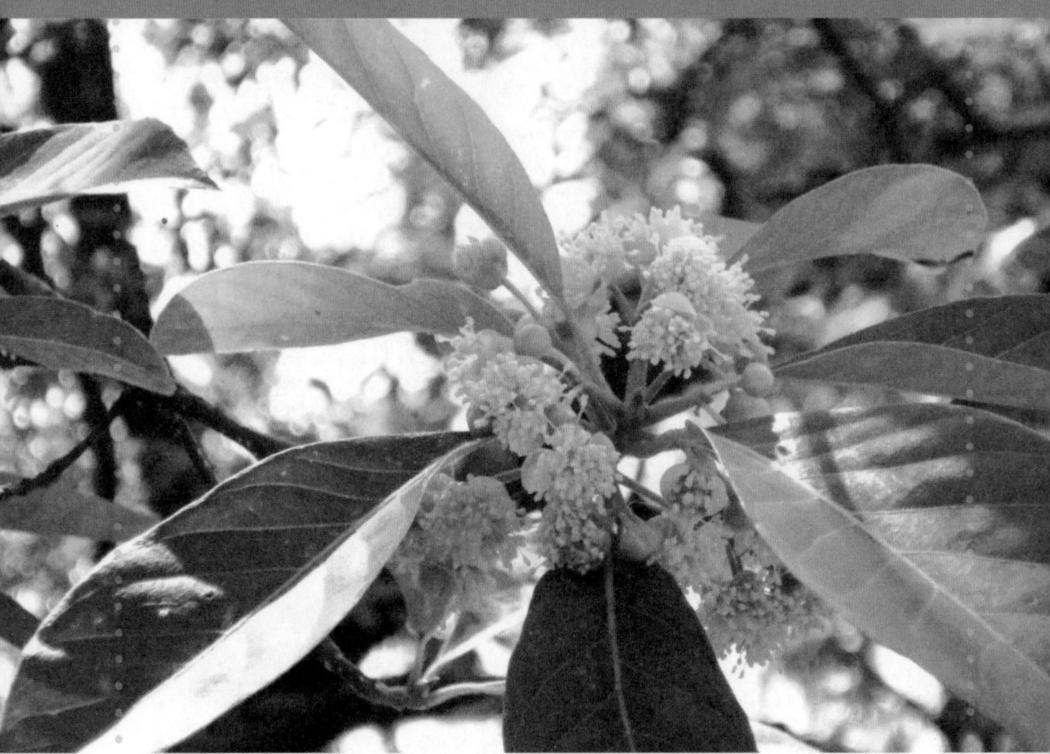

Scientific Name *Litsea glutinosa* (Lour.) C.B.Rob.

Common Names Brown Beech, Brown Bollywood, Beech Bolly, Bollywood, Bollygum, Soft Bollygum, Brown Bollygum, Bolly Beech, Indian Laurel.

Field Notes Brown Beech is a tree or shrub that grows to around 12 m in height in good conditions. It has large, hairy, lanceolate leaves that are up to 280 mm long by 185 mm wide. The flower heads that form in umbels from January to February contain many small, yellow flowers. Its purplish-black, globular fruit are approximately 8 mm or less in diameter. Brown Beech occurs in lateritic and basaltic soils in the Kimberley region of Western Australia and around the northern coast to Rockhampton in Queensland. It is also native to parts of South-east Asia, including the Indian subcontinent, Myanmar, Thailand, Cambodia, Laos, Vietnam, Malaysia, Indonesia, China and the Philippines (ALA, 2022; ATRP, 2020; Lassak & McCarthy, 2001; PFAF, 2022; WAH, 2022).

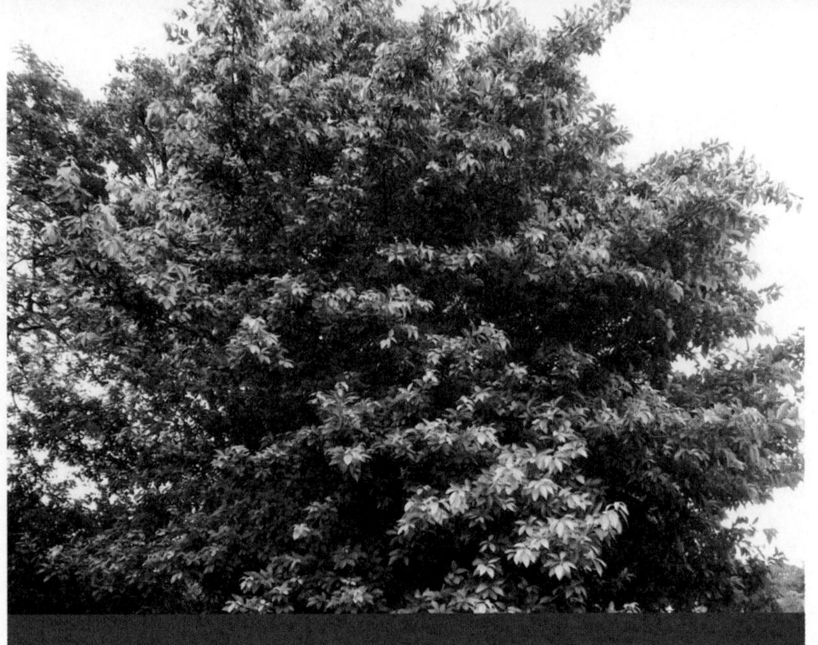

Medicinal Uses Decoctions of the bark were used externally to treat scabies infestations and were applied to cuts and sores to aid healing. Decoctions of the leaves and bark were used externally as a liniment for rheumatic pain. Leaves were crushed and the resulting juice was used to treat conjunctivitis (Cock, 2011; Fern, 2021; Lassak & McCarthy, 2001; Low, 1990; Webb, 1959). Decoctions of the leaves were drunk to relieve the feeling of nausea and to control vomiting (Smith, 1991). Decoctions of the root bark and leaves were used medicinally to reduce fever, reduce swelling and to treat diarrhoea (PFAF, 2022). Chewed leaves were applied as a poultice directly on skin infections, cuts and sores to aid healing (Webb, 1959). In Far North Queensland, Aboriginal groups boiled the leaves to make a jelly-like substance that was applied to the lower back for backache and as a body wash for headaches and general malaise (Edwards, 2005).

Other Uses The fruit of Brown Beech are edible when purplish-black and ripe and are reported to have a sweet, creamy pulp (Fern, 2021; PFAF, 2022; SMIP, 2022).

Bulrush

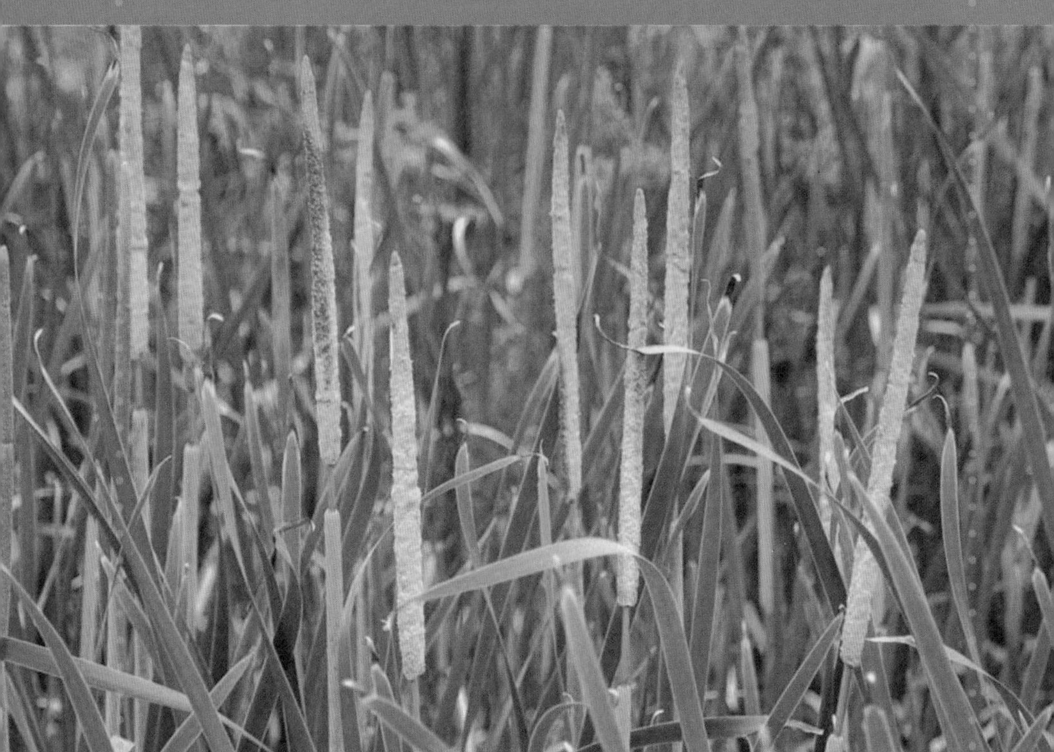

Scientific Name *Typha domingensis* Pers.

Common Names Bulrush, Reedmace, Narrow-leaved Cumbungi.

Aboriginal Names Tjinal-tjinalpa, Tjuna-tjuna (Kukatja) (Valiquetta, 1993), Thulmirri (Bunuba) (Oscar et al., 2019), Jankerriny, Beramarral or Peramarral (Gija) (Purdie et al., 2018; Wightman, 2003), Lirrimbi manya, Jabûrrenyee minya (Kwini) (Cheinmora et al., 2017; Crawford, 1982).

Field Notes Bulrush is a water-loving plant that lives for several years. It grows to 3 m in height. The rhizomes grow to 20 mm in diameter. The blade-like leaves are up to 2 m long and 20 mm wide. The flowers of both sexes grow on a single plant. Its brownish flowers grow on long stalks that are up to 400 mm long. Flowering is from May to September. Bulrushes occur in sand substrate soils beside freshwater swamps, creeks and rivers throughout Australia and in many other countries. Although they are endemic

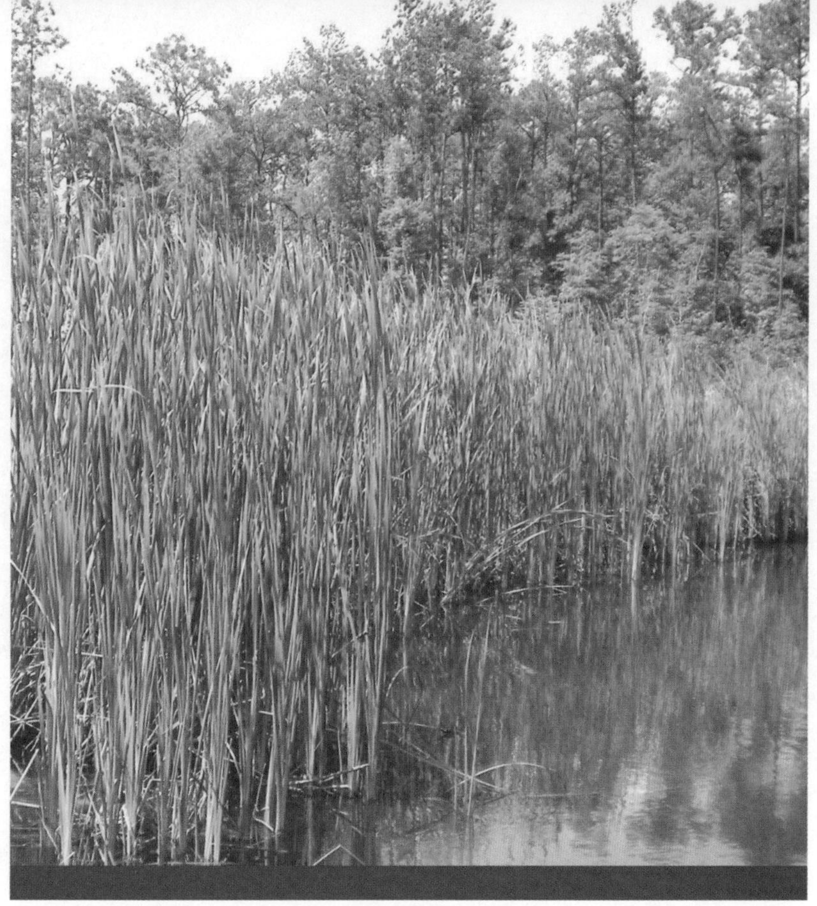

to the Kimberley region, they are more prolific in the south-west of Western Australia (ALA, 2022; Flora of Australia Online, 2022; WAH, 2022).

Medicinal Uses The crushed female flowers of the Bulrush had medicinal uses as an antiseptic to treat sores and wounds (Revoly, 2019). The seed down is haemostatic and was applied externally to cuts and wounds to halt bleeding (Fern, 2021).

Other Uses The tuberous roots of the Bulrush contain starch like that of sweet potatoes and were a good source of food for Aboriginal people who ate them raw or roasted. The young shoots are also edible as a vegetable, as are the base of mature stems. The leaves can be dried and woven into mats and baskets (Calvert, 2016; Fern, 2021).

Bunch Speargrass

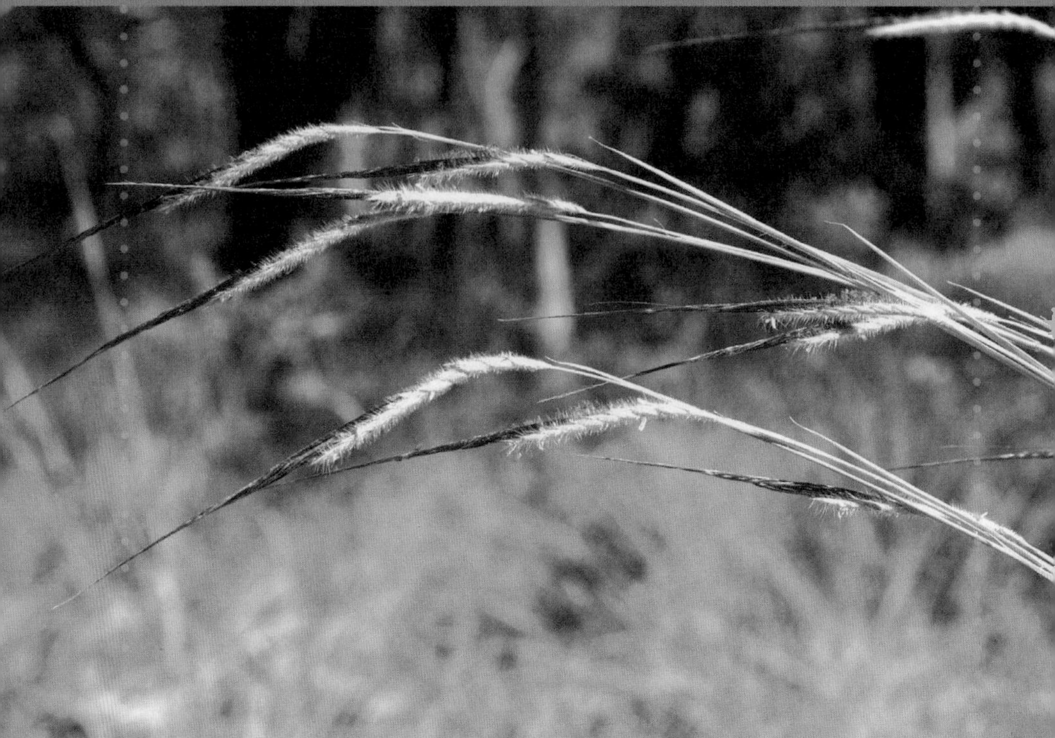

Scientific Name *Heteropogon contortus* (L.) Roem. & Schult.

Common Names Bunch Speargrass, Black Speargrass, Tanglehead Grass.

Aboriginal Names Ngalara (Nyikina), Marlil (Gija) (Wightman, 2003).

Field Notes Bunch Speargrass is a densely tufted, perennial grass that grows up to 1 m in height. It has green, glabrous leaves and culms. The leaf sheaths and blades are folded along the mid-rib. The leaves are up to 300 mm long. Its flowers are green florets that appear between January and August. Bunch Speargrass occurs in sandy, clay, red sand and lateritic soils around the top end of Australia from Broome in the Kimberley region of Western Australia to Newcastle in New South Wales (ALA, 2022; Department of Primary Industries, 2022; WAH, 2022). It also grows in other warm, temperate to tropical and sub-tropical areas of the world (ATRP, 2020).

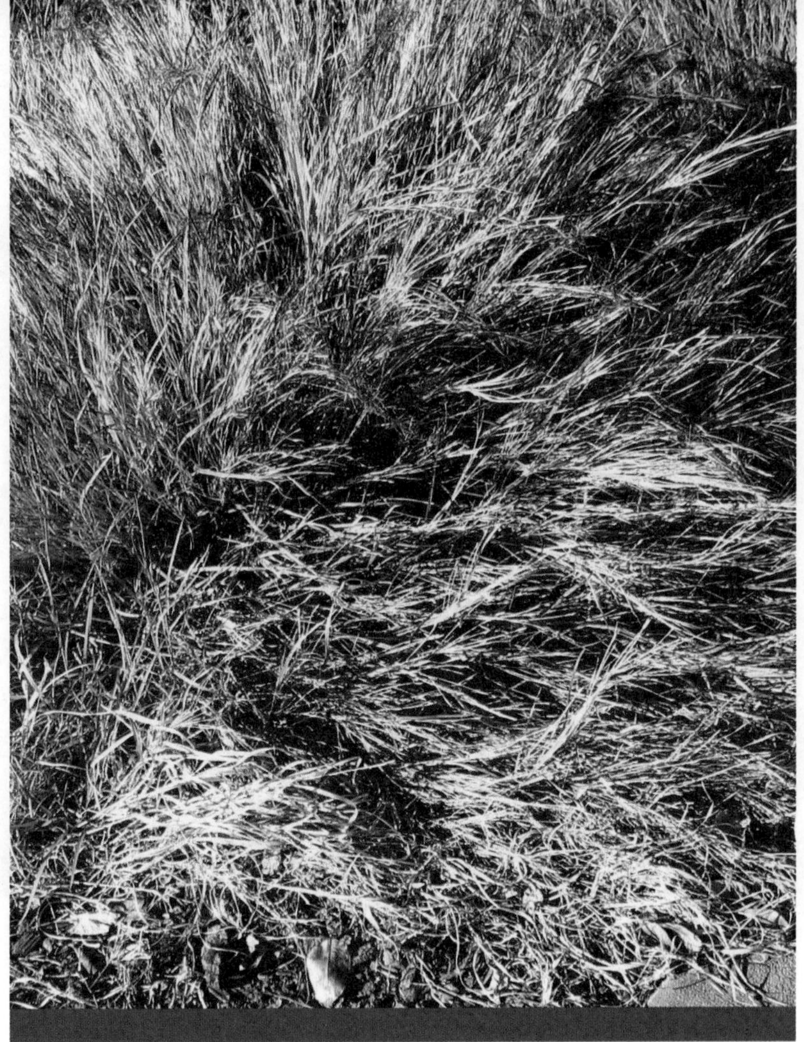

Medicinal Uses Cold or warm infusions of the mashed leaves were taken internally for coughs. Some Aboriginal groups chewed the leaves like tobacco (Lassak & McCarthy, 2001; Reid, 1986; Native Tastes of Australia, 2022; Webb, 1959). The Zulus of South Africa used the plant in the treatment of burns, wounds and rheumatic pain. The plant is reported to have diuretic properties (Pl@ntUse, 2022).

Bunu

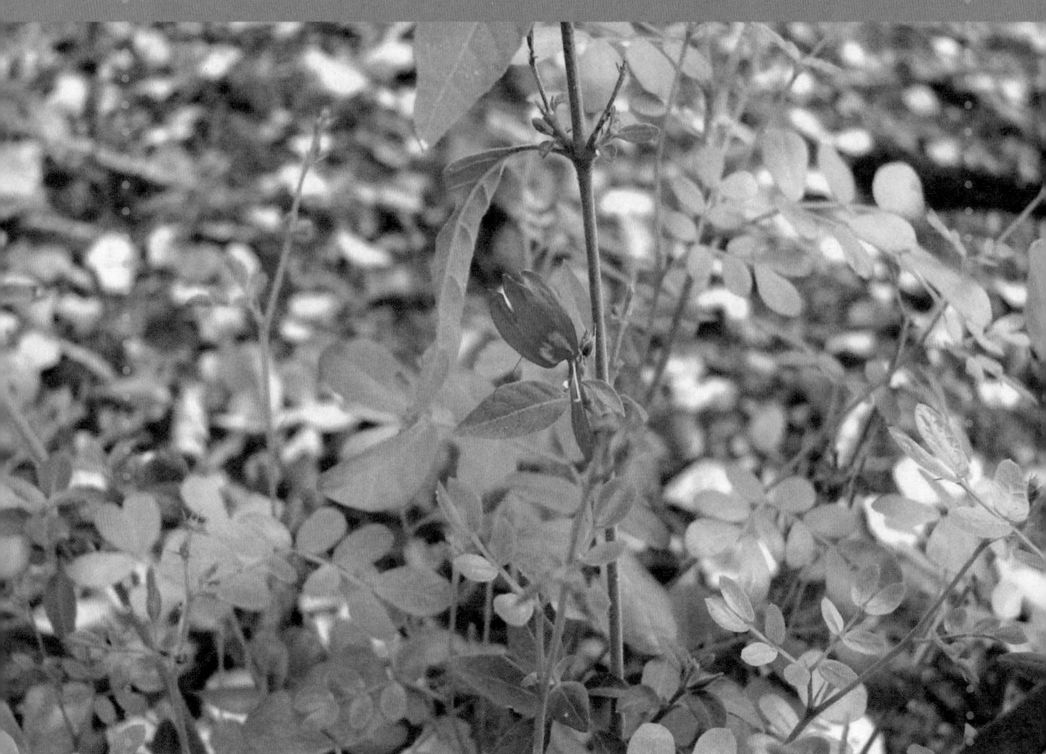

Scientific Name *Hypoestes floribunda* R.Br.

Common Names Bunu, Native Holly.

Aboriginal Name Bunu ninya (Kwini) (Cheinmora et al., 2017; Crawford, 1982).

Field Notes Bunu is a perennial herb or shrub that grows to around 1.5 m in height. Its leaves are ovate to lanceolate, up to 90 mm by 25 mm, with both surfaces of the leaves being hairy. Its pink-purple or cream-white flowers can be up to 25 mm long and are borne terminally. They appear from April to September. Bunu occurs in sand, clay, skeletal or loamy soils, in seasonally wet areas, gullies, on screes and plateaus, on coastal dunes and on creek banks across the top end of Australia from the Pilbara and Kimberley regions of Western Australia to the Northern Territory and Queensland as far south as the Gold Coast (ALA, 2022; ATRP, 2020; WAH, 2022).

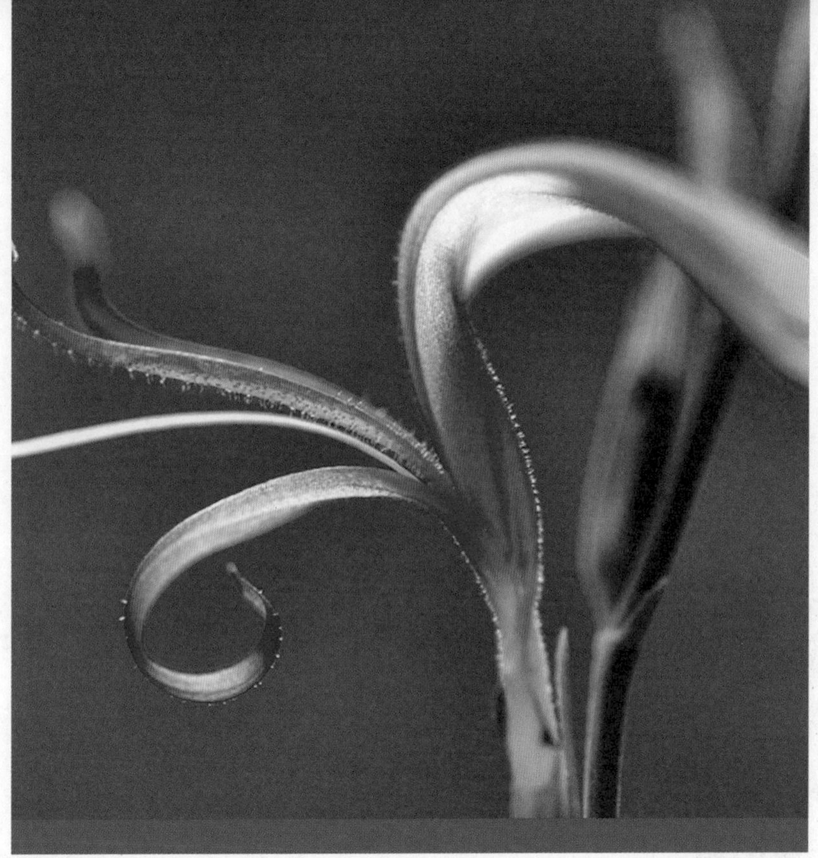

Medicinal Uses The whole plant was mashed and applied as a poultice to wounds, cuts and sores to aid healing (Low, 1990). The plant was sometimes dried and ground to a powder for the same purpose. The name 'Bunu' in Kwini literally translated means 'native powder' (Crawford, 1982). The powder was also used as a talcum powder substitute (Cheinmora et al., 2017).

Bunu Bunu

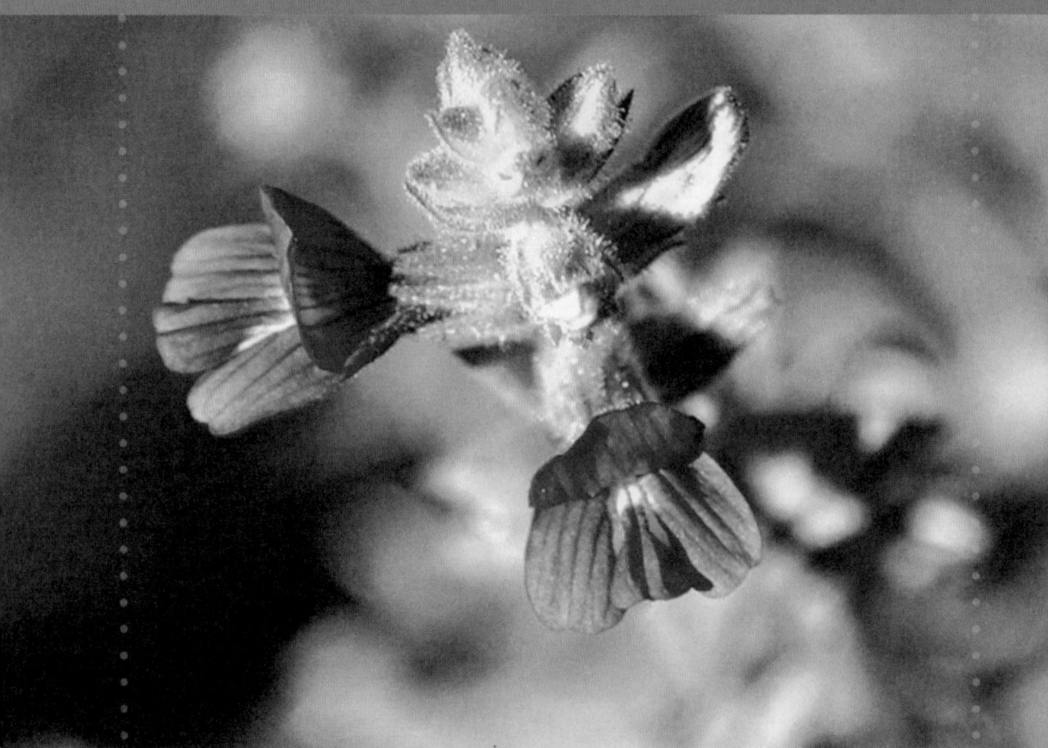

Scientific Name *Stemodia lythrifolia* Benth.

Common Name Bunu Bunu.

Aboriginal Names Jilindi, Wunyarnji (Wunambal, Gaambera) (Karadada et al., 2011), Gilala (Bardi) (Smith & Kalotas, 1985), Ngalil (Bardi) (Kenneally et al., 1996), Bunu Bunu ninya (Kwini) (Cheinmora et al., 2017; Crawford, 1982), Gooroongoony or Kurunguny (Gija) (Purdie et al., 2018), Birlbabirlbany, Birlbany, Birlbabirlinyi (Jaru) (Wightman, 2003).

Field Notes Bunu Bunu is an aromatic, robust, perennial herb that only grows to around 1 m in height. It has hairy, ovate leaves with obvious mid veins and purple, blue-purple or white tubular flowers that have four petals. Flowering can occur any time from February to November. Bunu Bunu occurs in sandy shallow soils over sandstone and laterite in rock crevices, near creeks and around springs across the top end of Australia from Broome in the

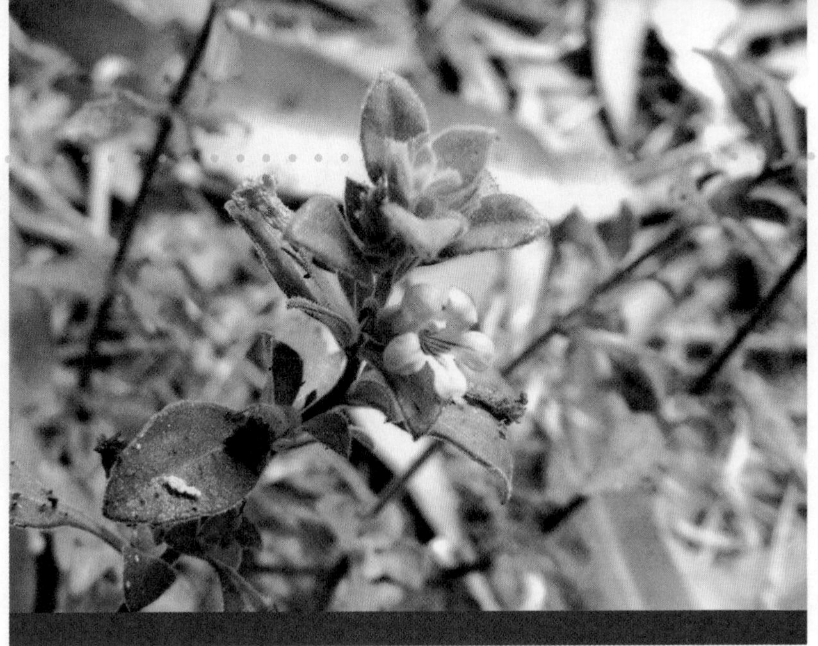

Kimberley region of Western Australia to Far North Queensland (ALA, 2022; ATRP, 2020; WAH, 2022).

Medicinal Uses Infusions of the whole Bunu Bunu plant were used to bathe the head to treat headaches and the symptoms of colds and influenza (Cock, 2011; Crawford, 1982; Lassak & McCarthy, 2001; Low, 1990; Purdie et al., 2018; Reid, 1986; Wightman, 2003). Alternatively, the leaves can be crushed, held under the nose and the vapours inhaled for the same purpose (Karadada et al., 2011). The Gija put the smelly leaves inside the pillow of babies and adults at night to make them feel stronger (Wightman, 2003).

Other Uses The leaves of Bunu Bunu were dried and used as chewing tobacco when regular tobacco was scarce (Clarke, 2007; Wightman, 2003).

Burny Bean

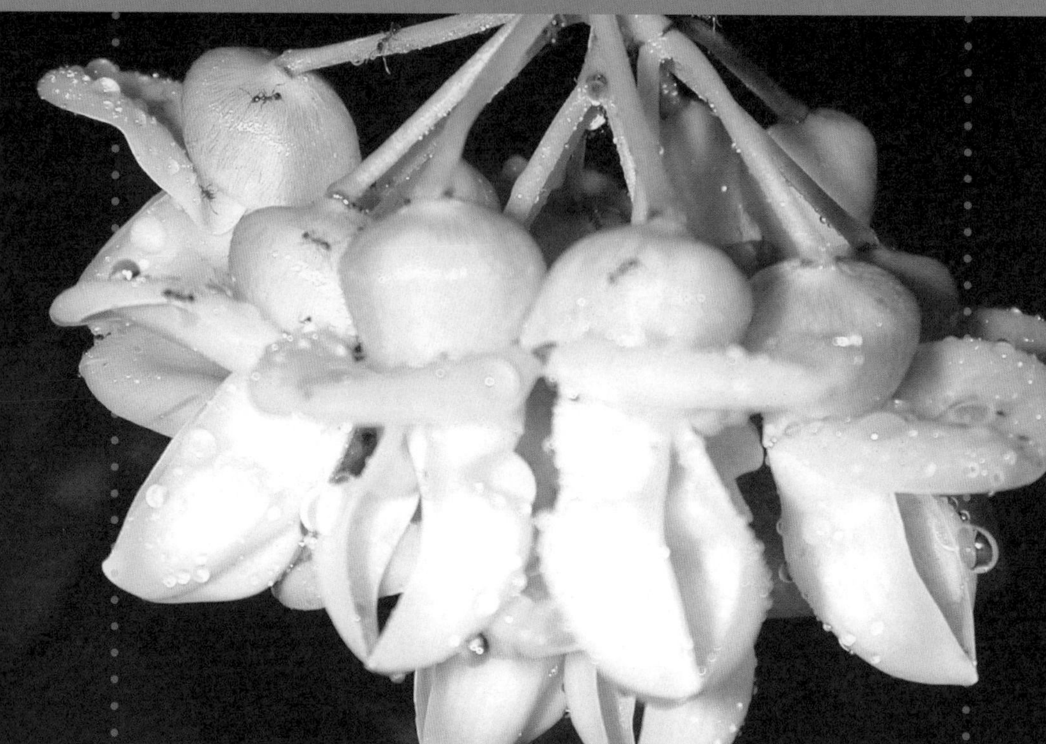

Scientific Name *Mucuna gigantea* (Willd.) DC.

Common Names Burny Bean, Burney Bean, Burny Vine, Velvet Bean, Black Sea Bean.

Field Notes Burny Bean is a woody, climbing vine that has compound leaves with three leaflets, the central leaflet being up to 150 mm long by 75 mm wide. Its inflorescence is an umbel on a peduncle that is up to 120 mm long with pale green, pea-shaped flowers. In Australia, flowering occurs from June to July. Its fruit are brown, flattened, winged pods that are up to 150 mm long and 50 mm wide. The pods are covered with irritant hairs that contain the enzyme mucunain, which can cause itchy blisters when they come in contact with the skin. The pods usually contain three seeds. The seeds are saltwater tolerant and can drift for months (or even years) in the sea, eventually washing ashore on a distant coast and germinating. Burny Bean is very coastal, occurring in freshwater

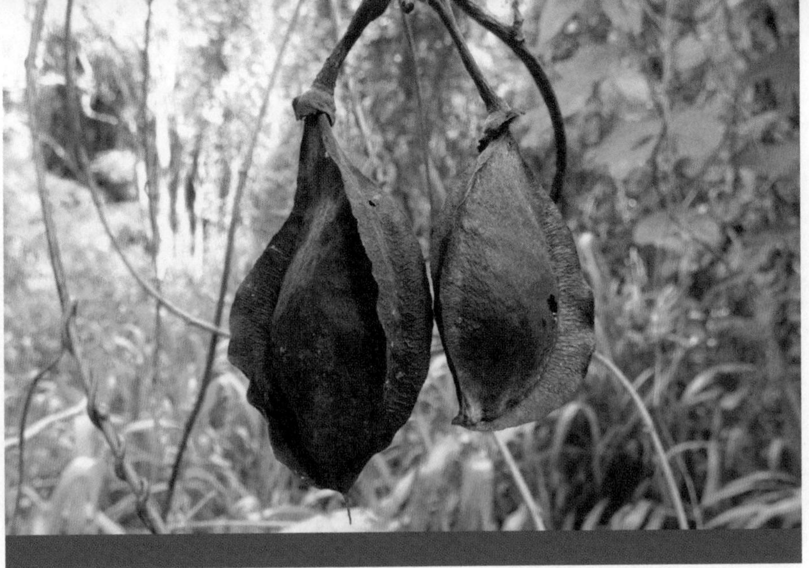

swamps and seepage areas in the top end of the Kimberley region of Western Australia, the Northern Territory, Queensland and as far south as the top coast of New South Wales. It also occurs in sub-Saharan Africa, India, tropical southern Asia, the Philippines, New Guinea and some Pacific islands including Hawaii (ALA, 2022; James Cook University, 2022; SMIP, 2022; WAH, 2022).

Medicinal Uses Burny Bean is used in folk medicine in Africa and some Asian countries. In Africa, decoctions of the roots were taken internally to treat gonorrhoea and schistosomiasis (bilharzia, a disease caused by parasitic flatworms called schistosomes). The bark is pulverised and mixed with ginger powder and rubbed over affected parts to ease rheumatic pain. The bark is crushed and applied externally as a poultice for the same purpose (BRAIN, 2022; Fern, 2021).

Other Uses Traditionally, Aboriginal groups in Australia heated the seeds of Burny Bean on hot stones or in hot sand next to a fire, removed the peel and then ground them to a flour, which they then mixed with water to make a cake that was then wrapped in leaves and baked. The seeds are boiled and eaten as a pulse in some Asian countries (BRAIN, 2022; Fern, 2021). Fern (2021) advises that: 'Because of the presence of toxic compounds in the plant, it seems advisable to eat the seed only after prolonged soaking and boiling.'

Bush Potato

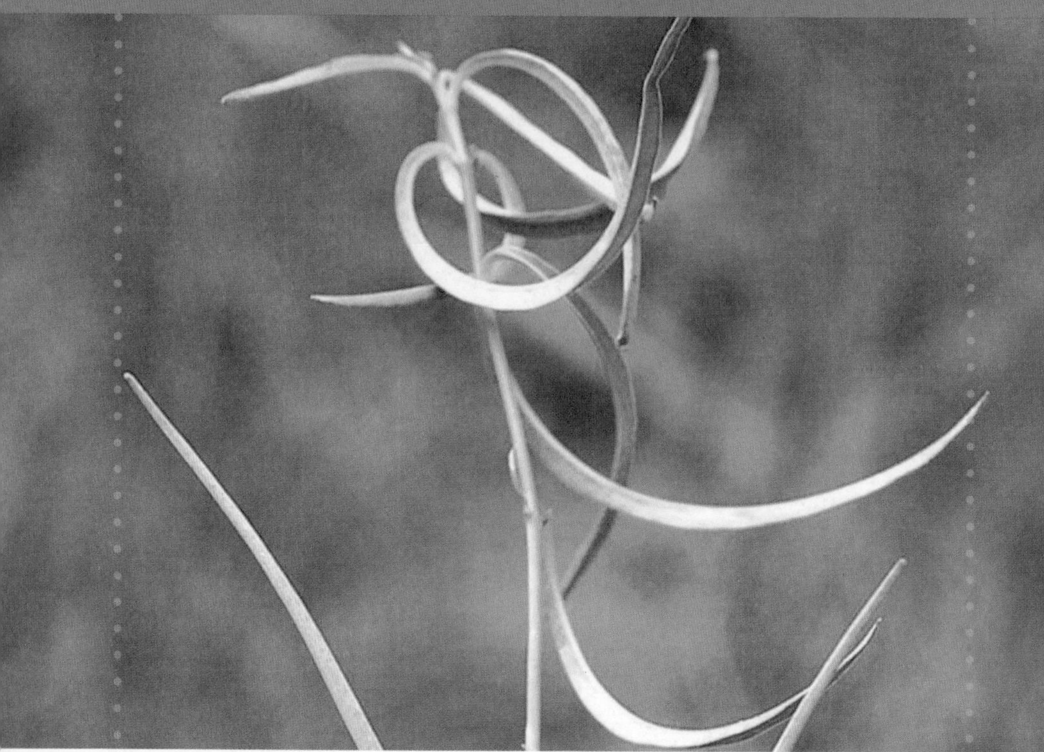

Scientific Name *Brachystelma glabriflorum* (F.Muell.) Schltr., previously known as *Microstemma tuberosum* R. Br.

Common Names Bush Potato, Sweet Round Yam, Bawujin.

Aboriginal Names Barding, Gelinymeng (Mirawoong) (Mirima Dawang Woorlab-gerring, 2013), Karnti (Ngardi) (Cataldi, 2004), Karnti, Pungka (Walmajarri) (Richards & Hudson, 2012), Banariny or Panariny (Gija) (Purdie et al., 2018), Banari (Jaru) (Wightman, 2003), Manganda (Wunambal, Gaambera) (Karadada et al., 2011), Manganda manya (smaller type), Walarnda manya, Darlku manya (larger type) (Kwini) (Cheinmora et al., 2017; Crawford, 1982).

Field Notes The Bush Potato is a tuberous, erect, slender, grass-like plant that grows to around 600 mm in height. It has thin lanceolate leaves and small purple-black flowers that are present from November to January. The Bush Potato occurs in red clay over basalt and sandy soils, often in damp situations, on flats and sandstone

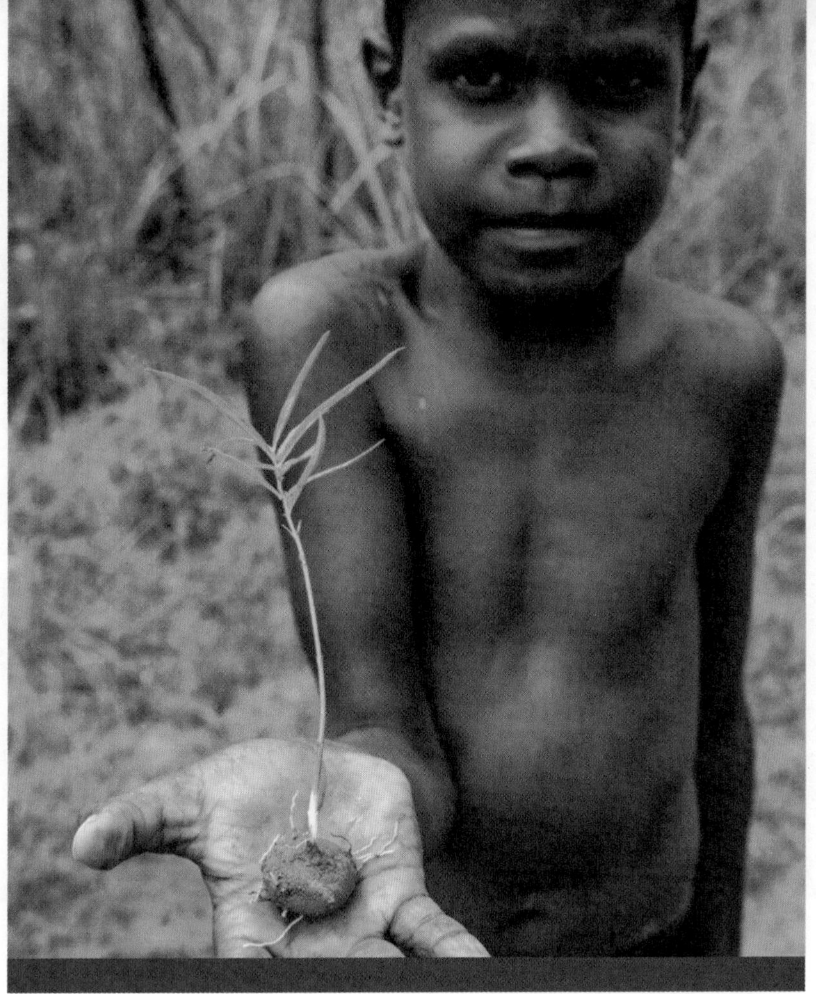

ridges across the far north of Australia from the Kimberley region of Western Australia through the Northern Territory to Far North Queensland (ALA, 2022; eFlora.SA, 2022; WAH, 2022).

Medicinal Uses In Far North Queensland, the thirst-quenching tubers were eaten by Aboriginal groups to treat general malaise (Edwards, 2005).

Other Uses The potato-like tubers can be eaten raw but are occasionally roasted and mixed with green ants to make them more palatable when food is scarce (Cheinmora et al., 2017; Crawford, 1982; Edwards, 2005; Fox & Garde, 2018; Hiddins, 2001; Isaacs, 1987; Kapitany, 2020; Karadada et al., 2011; Wightman, 2003). The bulbs are usually dug up in the late wet and early dry season when they are fat and juicy after the rains (Wightman, 2003).

Cajanus Pea

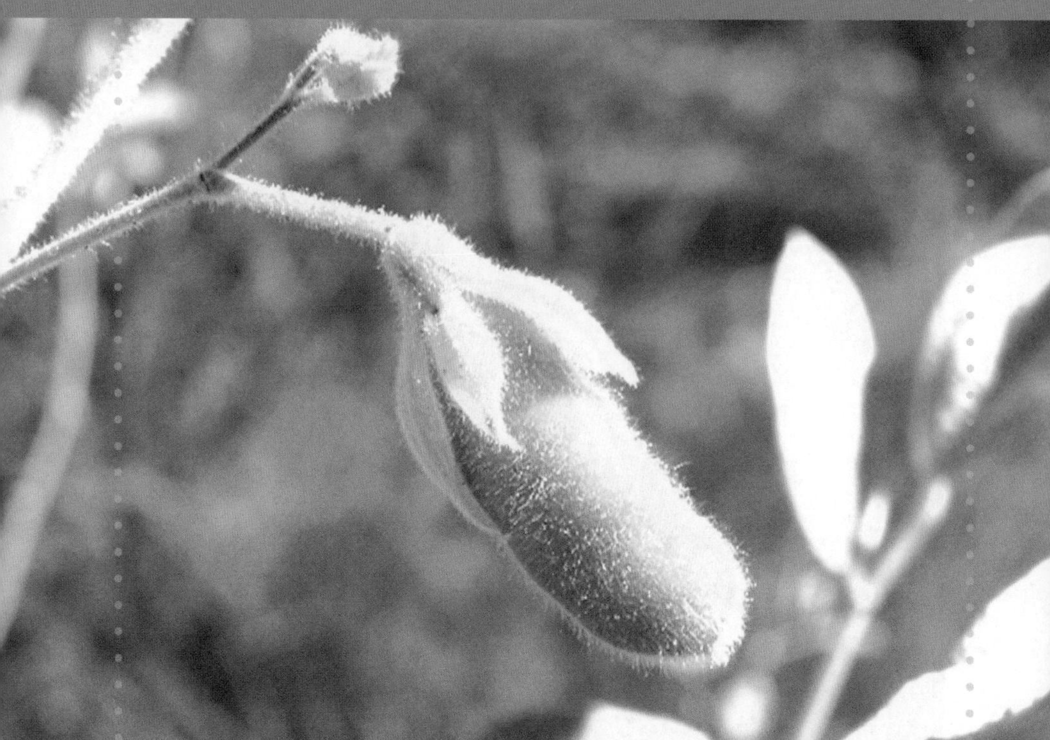

Scientific Name *Cajanus latisepalus* (Reynolds & Pedley) Maesen.

Common Name Cajanus Pea.

Aboriginal Name Warimirri (Kwini) (Cheinmora et al., 2017).

Field Notes Cajanus Pea is an erect or sprawling shrub that grows to 2 m in height. It has hairy rhomboid leaves 35 mm long. Yellow, pea-type flowers are present between March and August. Its fruit are flat, hairy, compressed between the seeds and around 20 mm long and 10 mm wide. Cajanus Pea occurs in sandy or gravelly soils over sandstone, basalt on sandplains, and on rocky slopes in the Kimberley region of Western Australia and the Northern Territory (ALA, 2022; WAH, 2022).

Medicinal Uses Decoctions of the leaves were used externally as an antiseptic wash to treat skin sores, cuts and other wounds (Cheinmora et al., 2017).

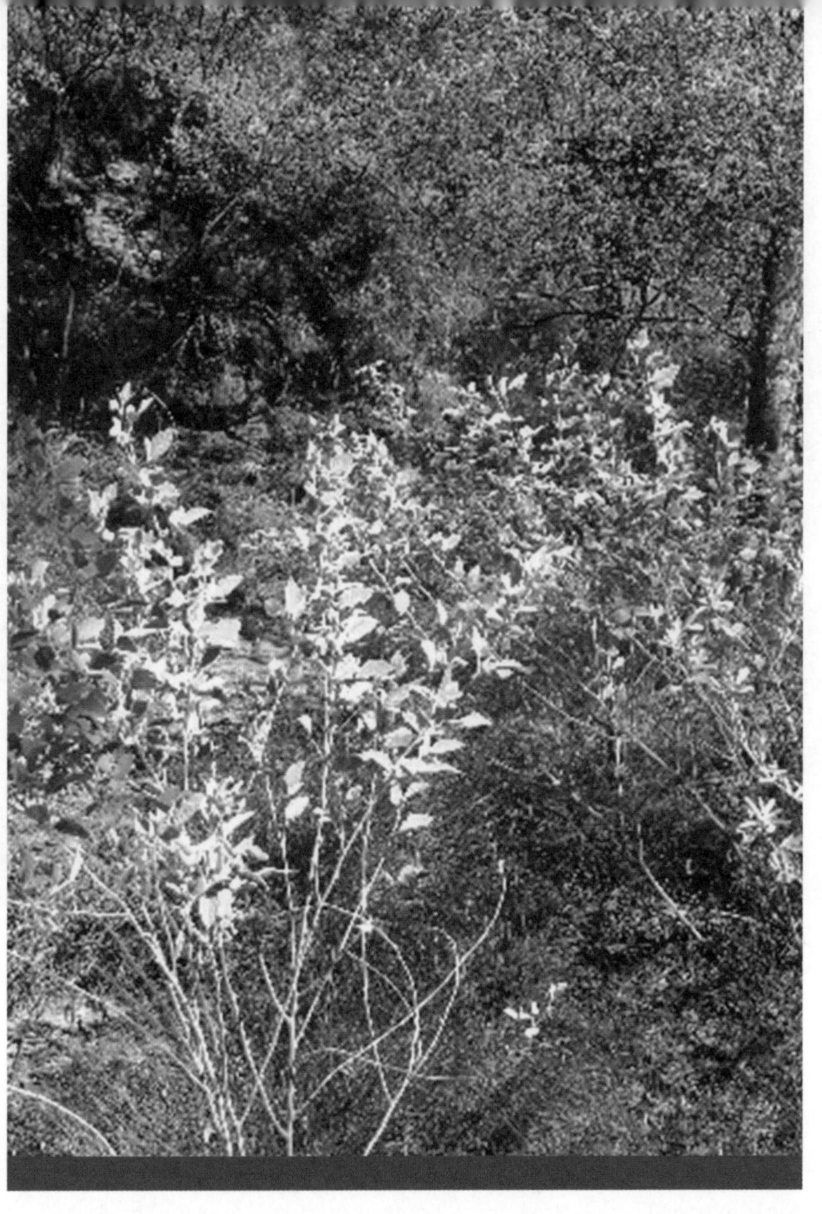

Camel Bush

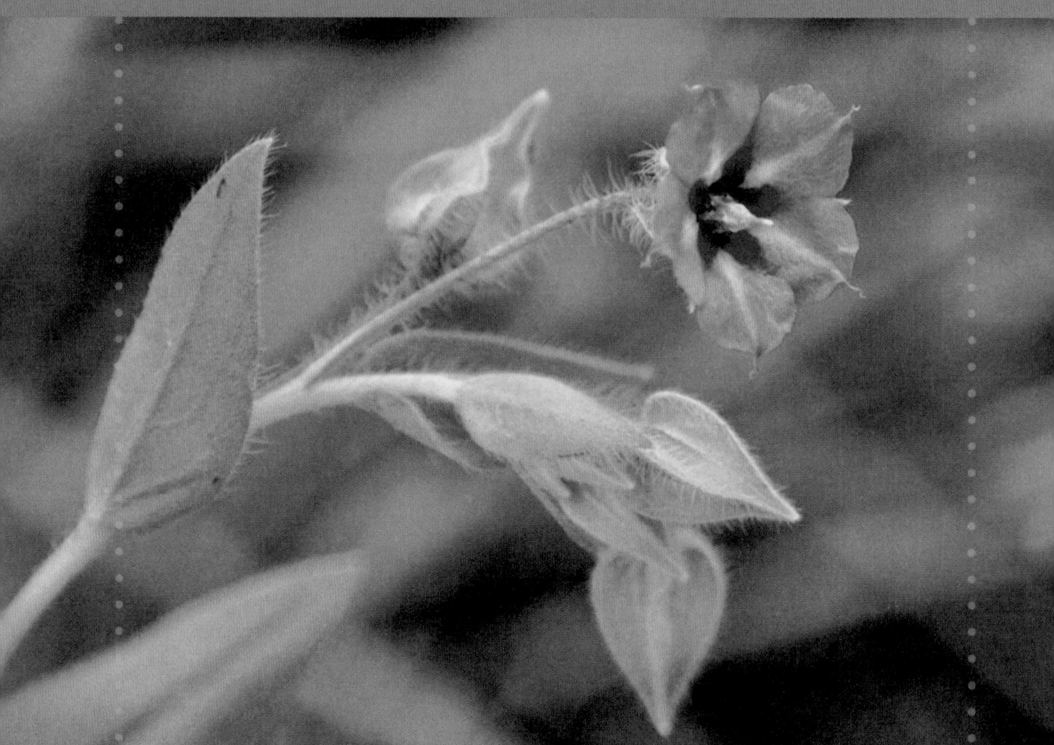

Scientific Name *Trichodesma zeylanicum* (Burm.f.) R.Br.

Common Names Camel Bush, Cattle Bush.

Aboriginal Names Jilarga (Bardi, Nyul Nyul) (Kenneally et al., 2018), Marira, Maritji, Ngumpana-ngumpana, Pakalpa, Winturlka, Yungkumarta (Kukatja) (Valiquette, 1993).

Field Notes Camel Bush is an erect annual or perennial herb or shrub that can reach 2 m in height. It has a well-developed taproot, green lanceolate leaves and round, blue-white flowers that appear between April and December. Its fruit are nutlets about 4 mm long. Camel Bush occurs in sand and skeletal soils over granite or sandstone, on rocky hills and coastal sand dunes on most of mainland Australia, excluding the south-west corner and Victoria (ALA, 2022; ATRP, 2020; WAH, 2022). Other areas where this plant occurs include eastern tropical Africa, India, Sri Lanka, the Malay Peninsula and New Guinea (SMIP, 2022).

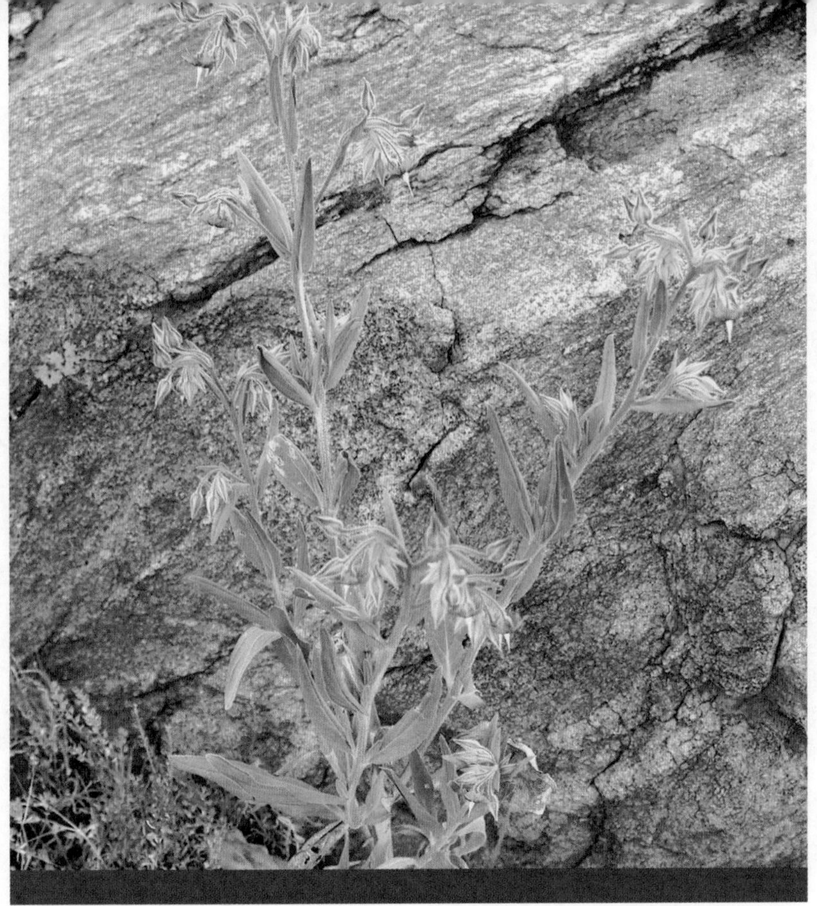

Medicinal Uses Decoctions of the whole plant were rubbed on wounds and sores to aid healing (ATRP, 2020; Cock, 2011; Lassak & McCarthy, 2001; Reid, 1986; Native Tastes of Australia, 2022; Webb, 1959). Infusions of the roots were taken internally as a remedy for tuberculosis, stomach ache, diarrhoea, poisoning and snakebite. A powder made from the dried roots is applied externally to wounds to relieve the pain. The green leaves and roots were chewed and used as a poultice for both fresh and infected wounds, boils and snakebite. Decoctions of the whole plant were taken internally as a treatment for fevers and dysentery (Cock, 2011; Fern, 2021).

Other Uses In other countries the young leaves and shoots are cooked with coconut and eaten as a vegetable (Fern, 2021). The dried leaves have been used by some Aboriginal groups as bush tobacco (Wiynjorrotj et al., 2005).

Candelabra Wattle

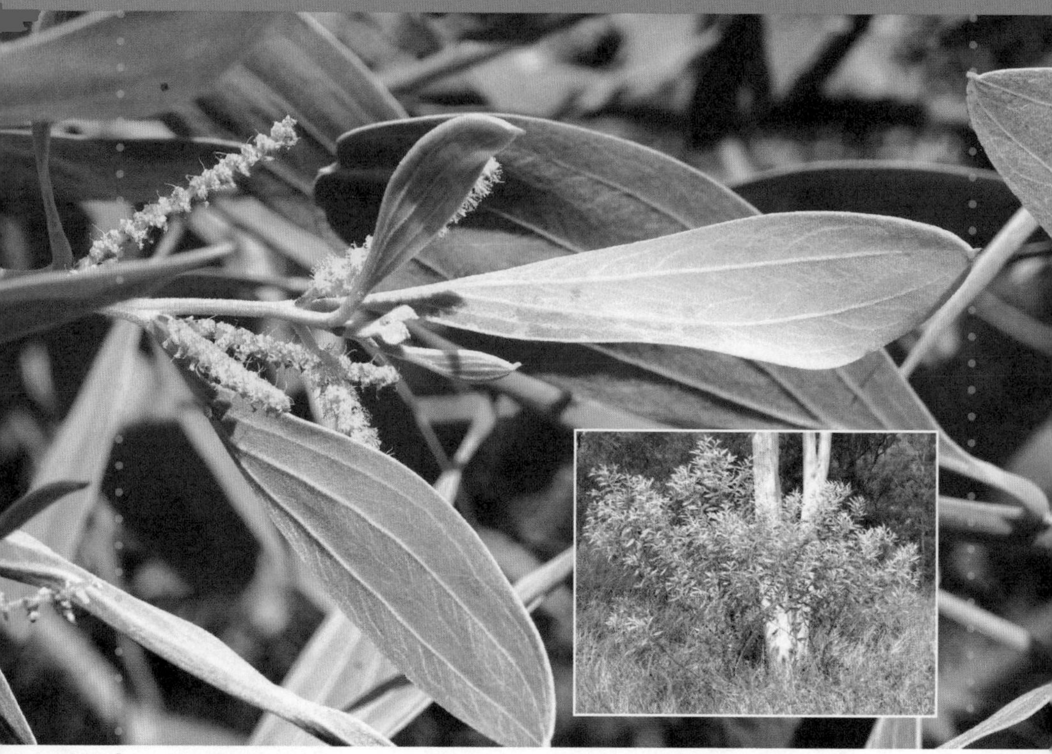

Scientific Name *Acacia holosericea* A.Cunn. ex G.Don.

Common Names Candelabra Wattle, Fish Poison Tree, Soapbush Wattle, Soapbush, Strap Wattle, Silver Wattle, Silky Wattle.

Aboriginal Names Garnkoorlng (Miriwoong) (Mirima Dawang Woorlab-gerring, 2013), Warrgali (Bunuba) (Oscar et al., 2019), Lulurr (Wunambal, Gaambera) (Karadada et al., 2011), Liringgin (Nyigina) (Lassak & McCarthy, 2001; Reid, 1986), Lirrirngirn (Yawuru), Lomoorrkood or Numorgudgud (Bardi) (Smith & Kalotas, 1985), Nimarrkoodkood (Nyul Nuyl), Lirrirnkirn (Nyangumarta), Lirrirnkirn (Karajarri) (Kane, 2022), Parta (Walmajarri) (Richards & Hudson, 2012), Barrawi or Barrabi (Gija, Jaru) (Wightman, 2003), Kilikiti (Kukatja), Bawaju (Kwini) (Cheinmora et al., 2017).

Field Notes Candelabra Wattle is a slender shrub or tree that grows up to 4 m in height. Its leaves, or more correctly phyllodes, are large and up to 200 mm long by 30 mm wide. Its rod-like flower spikes are bright yellow and up to 50 mm long. Flowering is from May to August. Candelabra Wattle is found in a variety of soils, often alongside creeks and rivers, across the top of Australia from the Pilbara and Kimberley regions of Western Australia, through the Northern Territory to the eastern Queensland seaboard (ALA, 2022; Maslin et al., 2010; WAH, 2022).

Medicinal Uses Infusions of mashed roots were sipped to relieve sore throats and laryngitis (Isaacs, 1987; Lassak & McCarthy 2008; Reid, 1986; Williams, 2011). Infusions of the bark or roots were taken to ease the symptoms of coughs and colds (Williams, 2011). Infusions of the phyllodes, bark and pods were used as a wash to treat skin disorders, wounds, sores and headache (Williams, 2011). Infusions of the bark, being high in tannins, were taken internally to relieve diarrhoea and dysentery, and were probably helpful in cases of internal bleeding (Fern, 2021).

Other Uses The seeds of Candelabra Wattle are edible and were eaten boiled or roasted (Native Tastes of Australia, 2022). The seeds can also be ground to a flour and mixed with water to make damper, which is baked in hot ashes (Darwin City Council. n.d.; RFCA, 1993). The Bardi people around Broome do not eat the seeds (Kane, 2022). Some Aboriginal groups ate the young roots of Candelabra Wattle after roasting them (Lindsay, 1997). Bush soap was made from Candelabra Wattle by crushing the phyllodes or pods, which are rich in saponin (Cheinmora et al., 2017; Low, 1990; Maslin et al., 2010; Oscar et al., 2019). The leaves, stems and pods were crushed and used as 'fish poison' so the fish floated to the top of the water and were easy to catch (Cheinmora et al., 2017; Darwin City Council, n.d.; Kimberley Specialists, 2020).

Candlestick Cassia

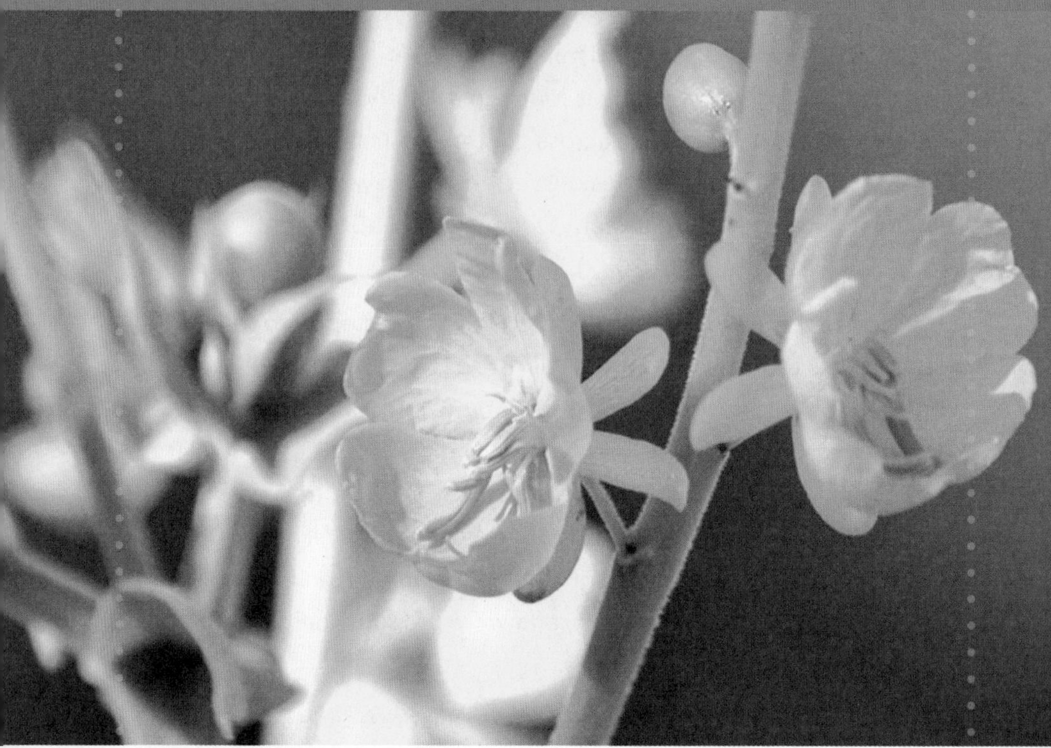

Scientific Name *Senna venusta* (F.Muell.) Randell.

Common Names Candlestick Cassia, Cockroach Bush, Lambi-lambi.

Aboriginal Names Lambi-lambi (Gooniyandi) (Dilkes-Hall et al., 2019), Ganbirr-ganbirr, Yijarda (Jaru) (Deegan et al., 2010; Wightman, 2003).

Field Notes Candlestick Cassia grows as a spindly or spreading shrub to around 2 m in height. Its light green, ovate leaves with a sharp point on their apex are opposite on the stems. Its bright yellow, buttercup-type flowers appear between March and October. Its seed pods are green, flat and contain around eight seeds. Candlestick Cassia occurs in sand, stony soils and laterite over sandstone in rocky areas and on river flats in the Pilbara and Kimberley regions of Western Australia, the Northern Territory and north-west Queensland (ALA, 2022; WAH, 2022).

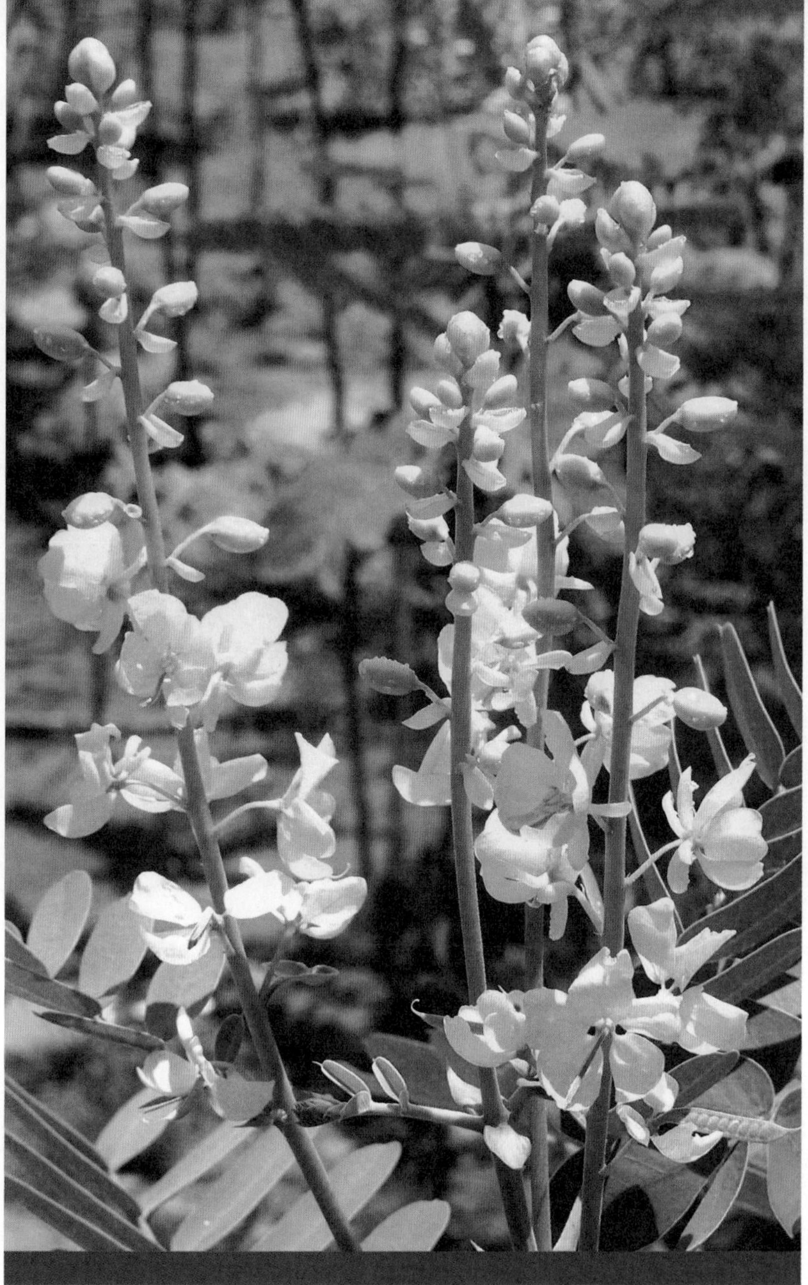

Medicinal Uses The young stems and leaves of Candlestick Cassia were crushed and the resulting liquid was rubbed directly onto the skin to relieve itchy skin and as a treatment for fungal infections of the skin, such as dermatophytosis (ringworm and tinea) (Smith, 1991) and skin sores (Wightman, 2003). Alternatively, decoctions of the leaves were used for the same purpose (Deegan et al., 2010).

Caustic Bush

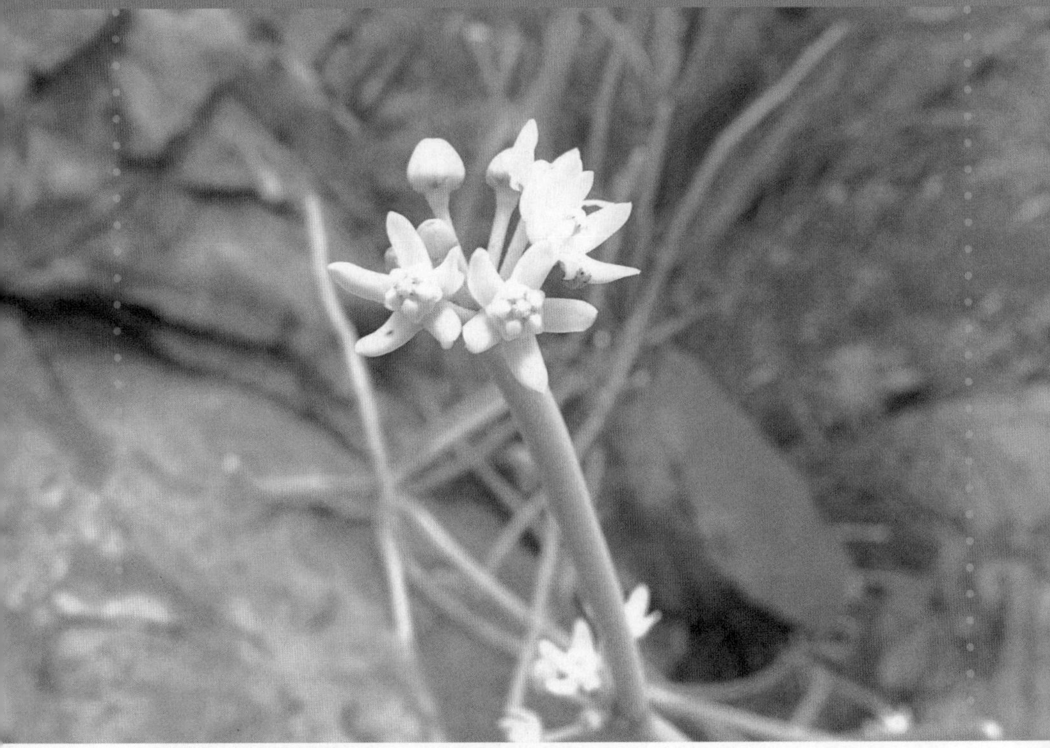

Scientific Names *Cynanchum viminale* subsp. *australe* (R.Br.) Meve & Liede, previously known as *Sarcostemma australe* R.Br.

Common Names Caustic Bush, Caustic Plant, Pencil Caustic, Milk Bush, Milk Vine.

Aboriginal Names Gurrngarl (Wunambal, Gaambera) (Karadada et al., 2011), Ngamalu, Wiliny, Pipirtipirti (Walmajarri) (Richards & Hudson, 2012), and Kanyjewuny or Karnjiwuny (Gija), Ngabulungabulu, Ngabuluyaru (Jaru) (Wightman, 2003), Ngamalu (Kukatja) (Valiquette, 1993), Ngaamungaamu manya, Ngamulngamul manya (Kwini) (Cheinmora et al., 2017; Crawford, 192).

Field Notes Caustic Bush is a trailing or climbing plant with stems up to 6 m long. It is sometimes found as a compact, much-branched shrub up to 2 m in height. Its small leaves are opposite and scale-like. Its small, star-shaped flowers have five petals and form in clusters. Caustic Bush occurs over most parts of mainland

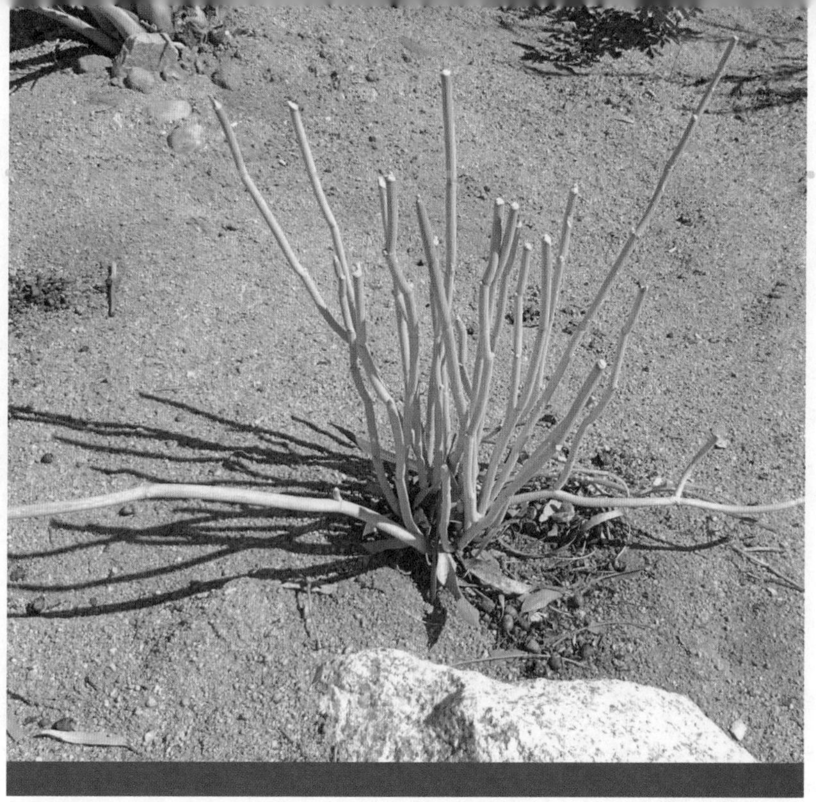

Australia except for the far south-west and Victoria (ALA,2022; Lassak & McCarthy, 2001; PlantNET, 2022).

Medicinal Uses The sap or latex of Caustic Bush was used as an astringent to stop bleeding, and was applied to sores, dermatophytosis (tinea and ringworm) and skin rashes to aid healing. The Jaru also used the sap to treat skin cancer (Cheinmora et al., 2017; Karadada et al., 2011; Richards & Hudson, 2012; Webb, 1959; Wightman, 2003). It was also used as a liniment for sprains. The whole plant was warmed and used as a poultice on the breasts of new mothers to induce lactation (Cheinmora et al., 2017; Clarke, 2008; Crawford, 1982; Isaacs, 1987; Lassak & McCarthy, 2001; Low, 1991; Richards & Hudson, 2012). Infusions of the stems were used as a medicinal wash to treat itchy skin, conjunctivitis, rashes and scabies infestations (Cock, 2011; Devanesen, 2000; Smith, 1991).

Other Uses The leaves of Caustic Bush were crushed and used as 'fish poison', which made the fish float to the surface of the water where they could be easily collected (Wightman, 2003).

Caustic Weed

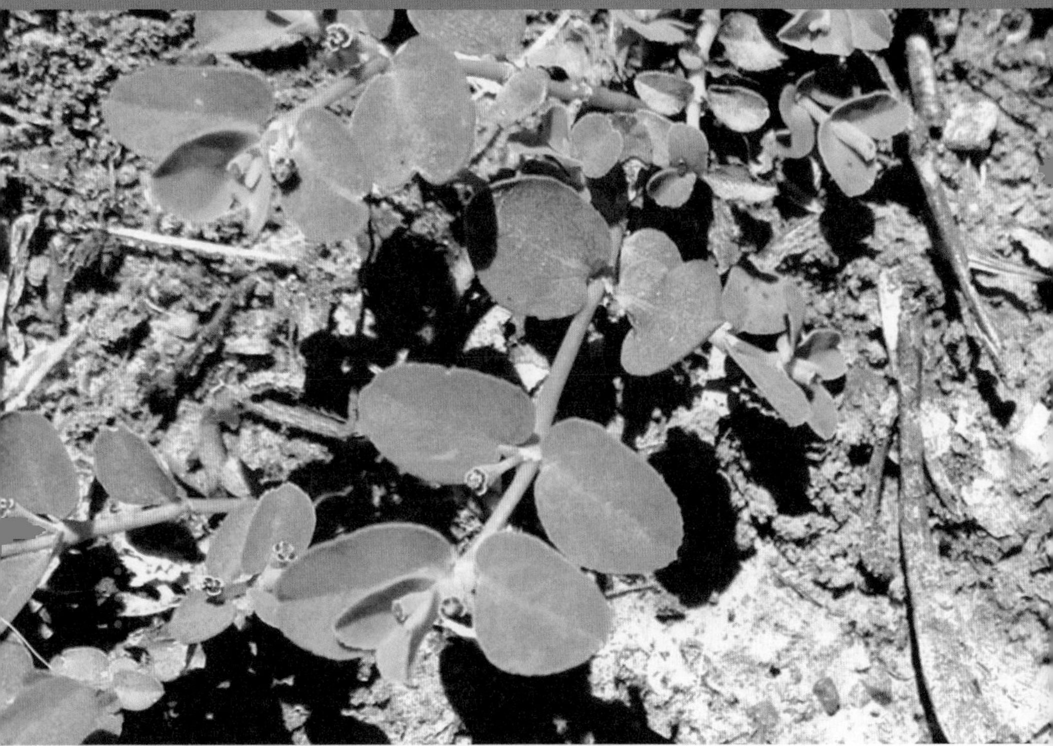

Scientific Name *Euphorbia drummondii* Boiss.

Common Names Caustic Weed, Caustic Creeper, Milk Plant, Pox Plant, Creeping Caustic, Mat Spurge.

Field Notes Caustic Weed is a small, low-lying, short-lived herb that spreads to around 300 mm in diameter. It has a corrosive, milky sap when its red stems are broken. Its small, ovate leaves are blue-green in colour. Small flowers appear from March to September and can range from green-white to red-pink in colour. Caustic Weed occurs on disturbed ground in a range of soils, including clay and sand, throughout the Australian mainland from the tropics to the more temperate regions (Lassak & McCarthy, 2001; WAH, 2022).

Medicinal Uses The milky sap was used as a treatment for non-melanoma skin cancer, sores, cuts and scabies infestations. Infusions of the stems and leaves were used by Aboriginal people

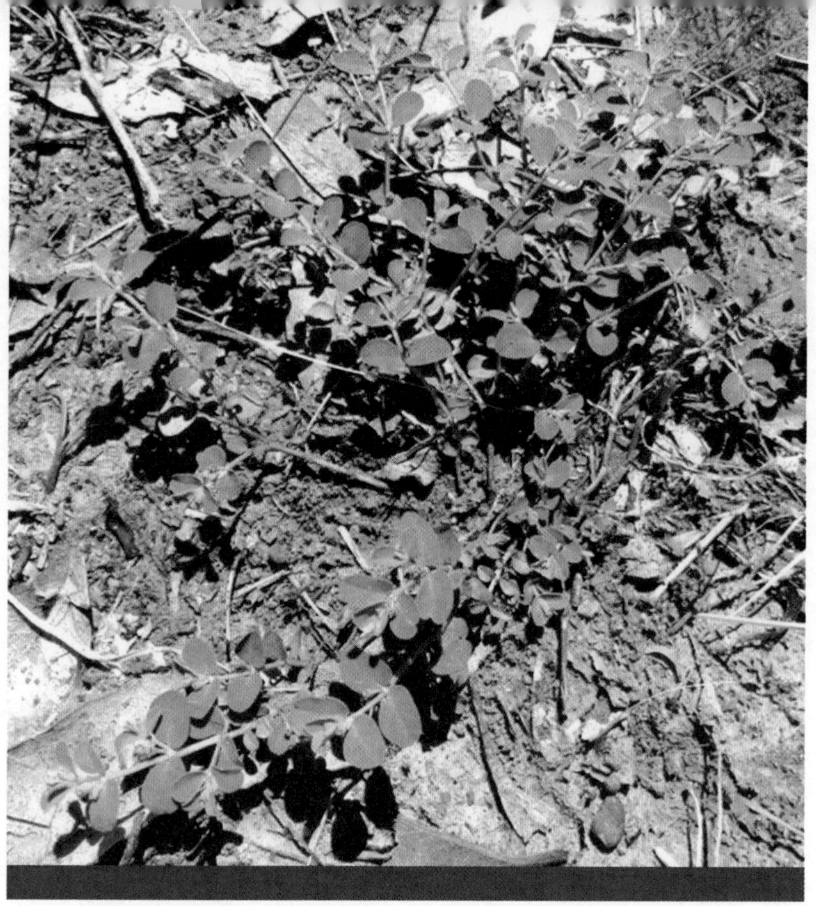

as a treatment for diarrhoea, dysentery and low fever. Decoctions of the stems and leaves were used as a wash for itchy skin, sores and scabies infestations (Cock, 2011; Lassak & McCarthy, 2001). The milky latex was also used topically by women to enlarge their breasts and to promote the flow of milk for breastfeeding (Peile, 1997).

Cedar Mangrove

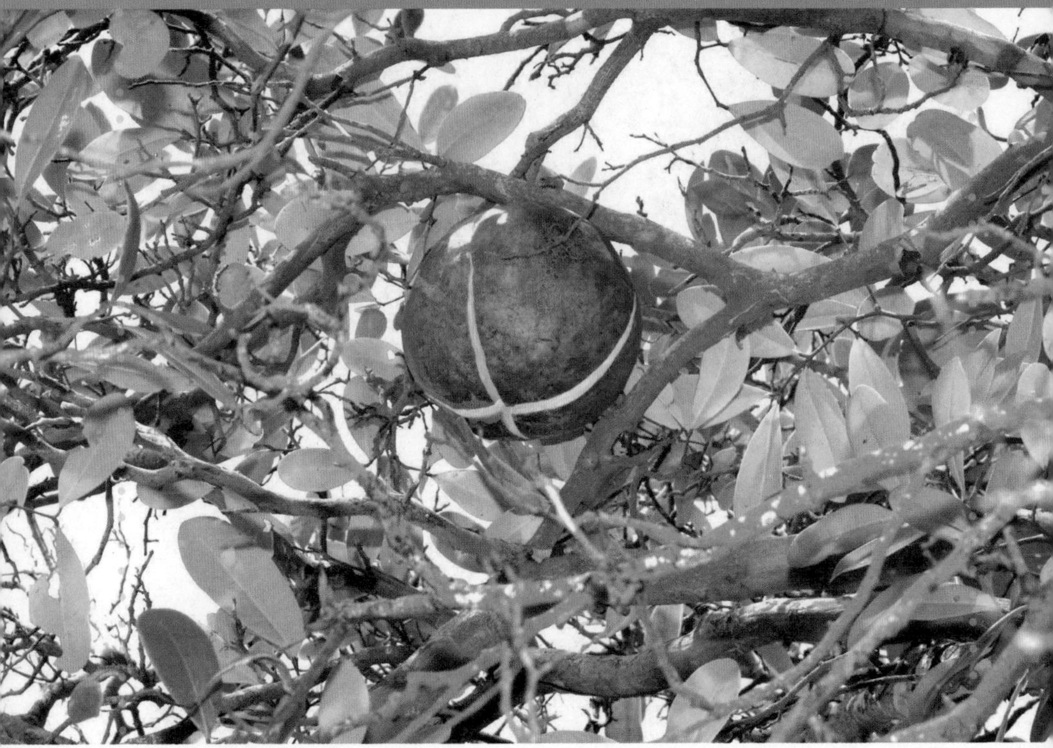

Scientific Name *Xylocarpus granatum* J.Koenig, and *Xylocarpus moluccensis* (Lam.) M.Roem.

Common Names Cedar Mangrove, Cannonball Mangrove, Puzzle Fruit Tree, Monkey-Puzzle Nut, Puzzlenut Tree.

Aboriginal Name Kulii (*Xylocarpus moluccensis*) (Kwini) (Cheinmora et al., 2017).

Field Notes There are two Cedar Mangroves related to each other with the same distribution and same medicinal properties. *Xylocarpus granatum* grows up to 5 m in height, whereas *Xylocarpus moluccensis* has been found growing up to 22 m high. Both have well-developed buttresses and an elaborate above-ground root system. The branches of *X. granatum* are grey, smooth and glabrous. Both have elliptic to obovate-oblong, sub-leathery, glabrous leaflet blades up to 90 mm long by 50 mm wide. Their flowers are creamy-white with five petals and red-

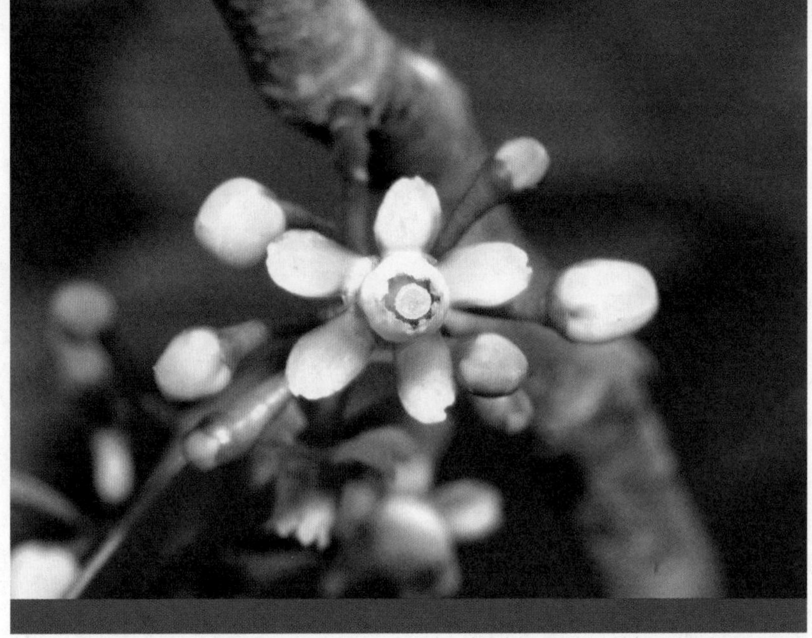

tipped stamens. In Australia, flowering is from June to August. The fruit of *X. granatum* are globose, pendulous, woody capsules up to 250 mm in diameter and weighing up to 3 kg. The fruit of *X. moluccensis* are smaller in size and weight. In Australia, Cedar Mangroves occur naturally along the coast in the northern Kimberley, the Northern Territory and Queensland. They also occur in coastal regions of the Old World tropics, from East Africa and Madagascar through tropical Asia to Polynesia (ALA, 2022; WAH, 2022).

Medicinal Uses Decoctions or infusions of the astringent bark of both varieties of Cedar Mangrove are used in traditional medicine in Australia, tropical Africa and South-east Asia to treat dysentery, diarrhoea, other abdominal troubles and fever. Powders or decoctions of the fruit or seeds are used for the same purpose. Decoctions of the crushed fruit of *X. granatum* are drunk as an aphrodisiac in tropical Africa (Bailey, 1881; Fern, 2021). In Tonga, decoctions of the bark were used to treat candidiasis, scabies infestations, baby rash, stomach pains and constipation. In Fiji, decoctions of the bark, or bark and leaves, were used to treat headaches, fatigue, candidiasis, joint pain, chest pain and buccal (cheek) pain (Philippine Medicinal Plants, 2020).

Centipede Fern

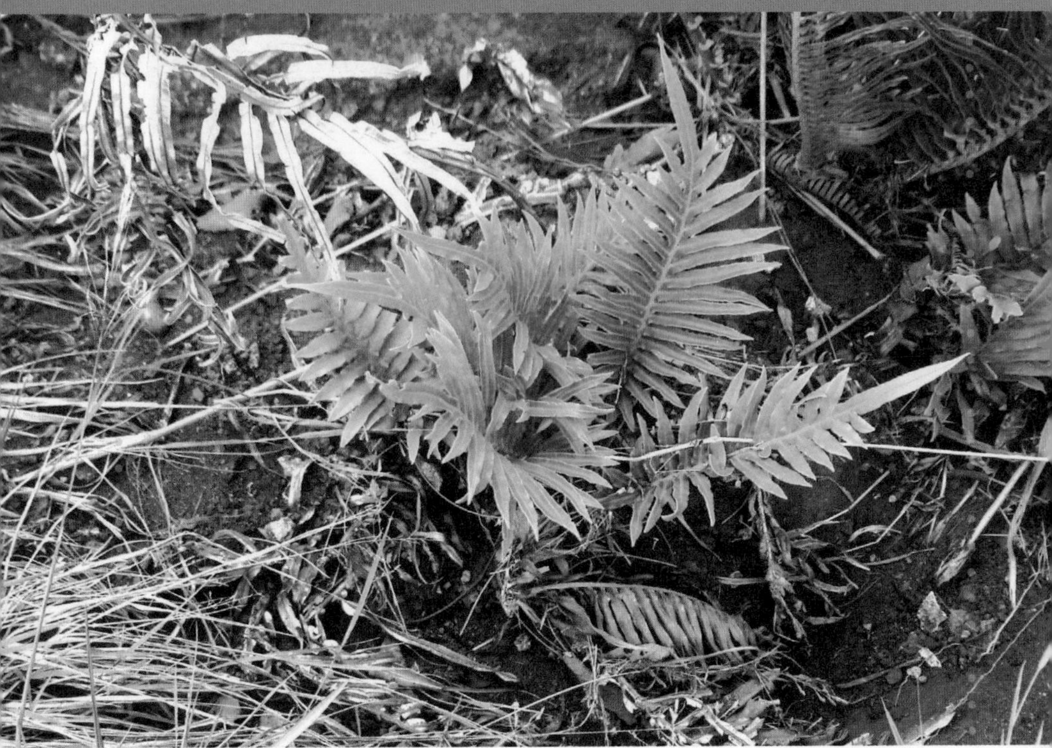

Scientific Name *Blechnopsis orientalis* (L.) C.Presl., previously known as *Blechnum orientale* L.

Common Names Centipede Fern, Eastern Water Fern.

Field Notes Centipede Fern is a rhizomatous, perennial fern forming a clump of arching fronds, originating from a thick rhizome, that rises to an erect trunk up to 2 m in height. The fronds are pinnate and rarely simple. The pinnae are linear, entire or dentate (having a toothlike or serrated edge). Centipede Fern occurs in black loam near creeks, in moist vine thickets and on rock ledges of cliffs or waterfalls across the far north of Australia. It also occurs in parts of South-east Asia (ALA, 2022; Kumar et al., 2015; WAH, 2022).

Medicinal Uses Centipede Fern is used in folk medicine in South-east Asia. According to Kumar et al., (2015), 'The plant has been found to possess promising antioxidant, anticancer, antidiabetic, antimicrobial and wound healing activities'. In Malaysia and the

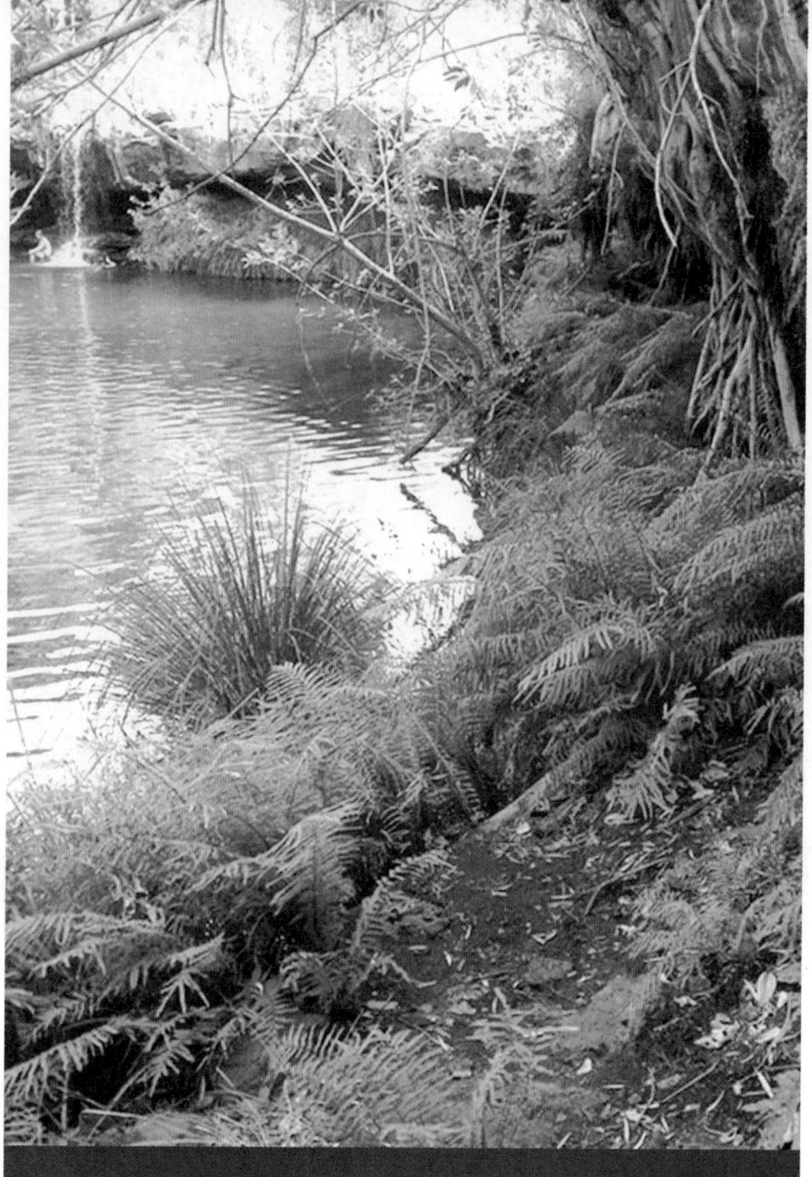

Philippines, a paste of the young fronds is applied externally to treat abscesses and fungal skin infections, to staunch bleeding and to treat blisters, boils, carbuncles and sores (Fern, 2021). The leaves are also reported to be used in treating stomach pain and urinary tract infections. The rhizomes are reported to be anthelmintic and have been used to expel intestinal parasites (Kumar et al., 2015).

Other Uses The young shoots or fiddles of the Centipede Fern are edible and are eaten cooked as a vegetable (Barker, 1991; Fern, 2021; Kumar et al., 2015).

Chaff Flower

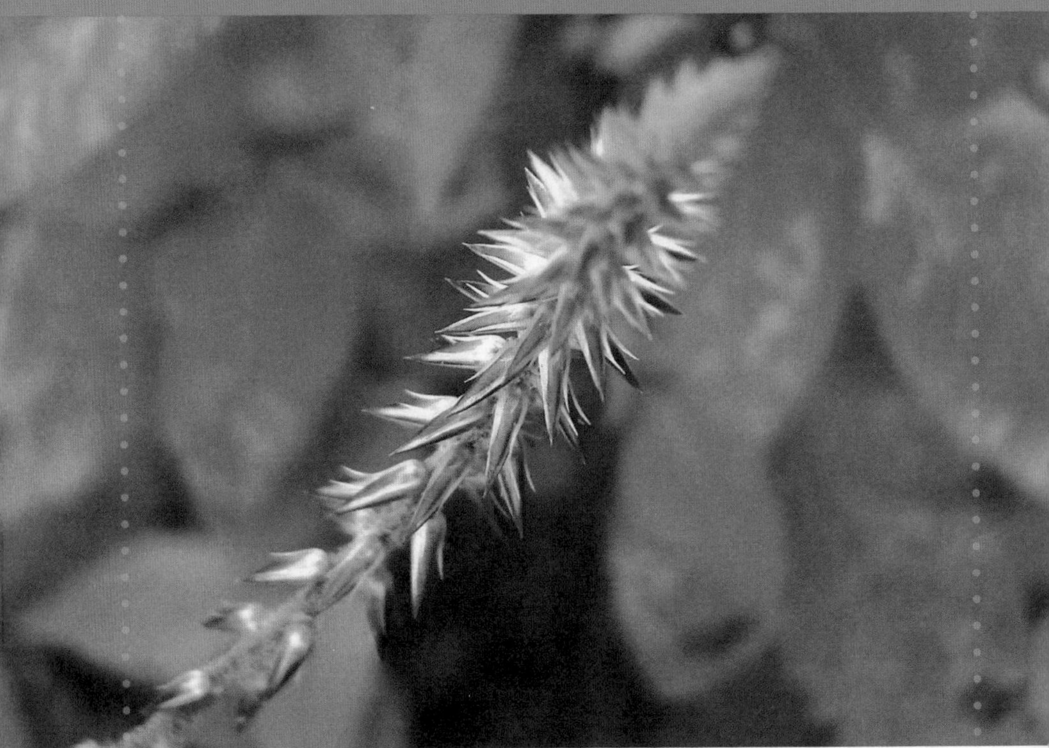

Scientific Name *Achyranthes aspera* L.

Common Names Chaff Flower, Prickly Chaff Flower, Devil's Horsewhip.

Field Notes Chaff Flower is an erect perennial herb that grows to a height of 1 m or more. Its short-stalked, ovate leaves have a broad end at the base and are up to 100 mm long by 80 mm wide. Its small, cream-green-pink flowers form on spikes up to 600 mm long from March to August. Its sharp-pointed fruit are orange to reddish-purple or straw-brown capsules. Chaff Flower occurs in sandy soils and alluvium alongside rivers and creeks over most of the top half of Australia. It is also found either growing naturally or as an introduced species throughout the tropical world (ALA, 2022; WAH, 2022).

Medicinal Uses Although there is no record of it being used medicinally in Australia, the whole plant has medicinal properties and is used in Ayurvedic medicine as an astringent, diuretic

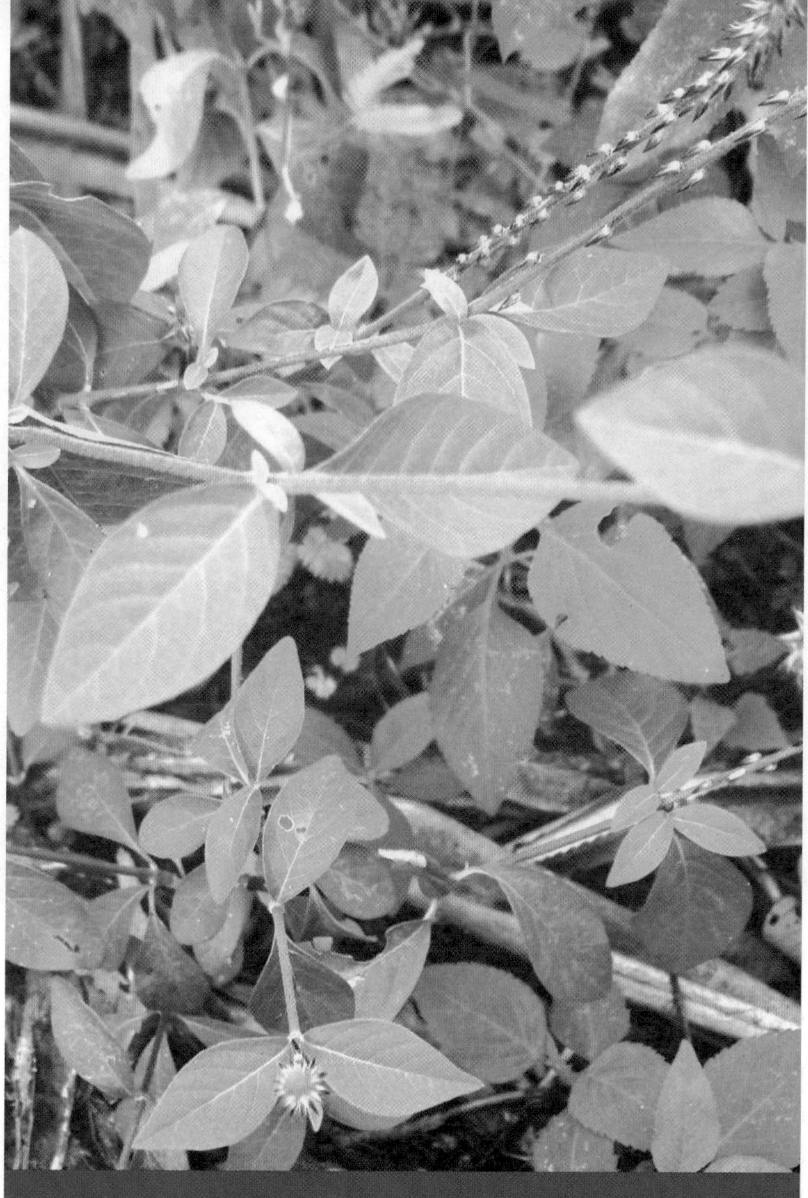

and antispasmodic digestive, diuretic, laxative, purgative and stomachic. The root is used to treat oedema, rheumatism, stomach problems, cholera, skin diseases and rabies. The juice of the plant is used in the treatment of boils, diarrhoea, dysentery, haemorrhoids, rheumatic pain, itches and skin eruptions (Fern, 2021).

Other Uses The young leaves are edible and are cooked and eaten similar to spinach. The seeds are also edible (Barker, 1991; Cribb & Cribb, 1981; Fern, 2021; Glasby, 2018; Hiddins, 2001).

Chain Fruit

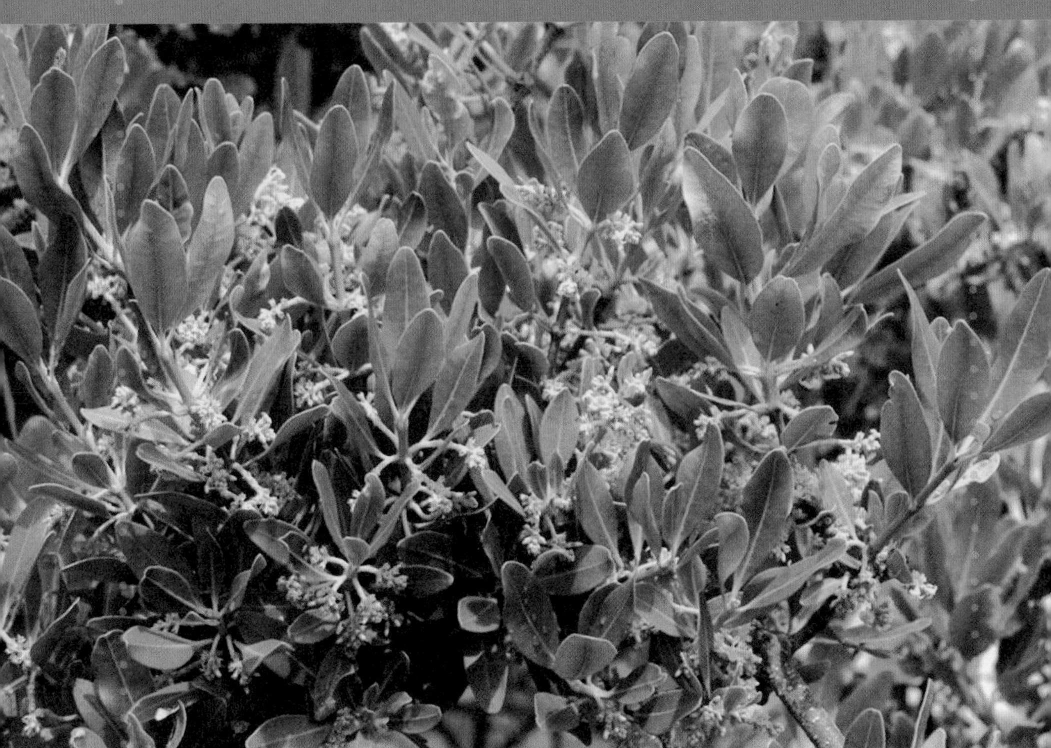

Scientific Name *Alyxia spicata* R.Br.

Common Name Chain Fruit.

Field Notes Chain Fruit grows as a shrub or climber up to 4 m in height. Its leaves are large, ovate and up to 80 mm long. Its small, cream-white flowers are tubular with cream lobes and are only 4 mm in diameter. Flowering is between May and September. Its fruit are ovoid drupes, about the size of olives, that form in chains, hence the common name, Chain Fruit. They are initially green and turn black when ripe. Chain Fruit occurs in basalt and loam over laterite, on cliffs and in vine thickets in the northernmost parts of the Kimberley region of Western Australia, the Northern Territory and north-east Queensland. It also occurs in Papua New Guinea (ALA, 2022; ATRP, 2020; WAH, 2022).

Medicinal Uses Decoctions of the roots of Chain Fruit were taken internally for breathlessness due to asthma or bronchitis.

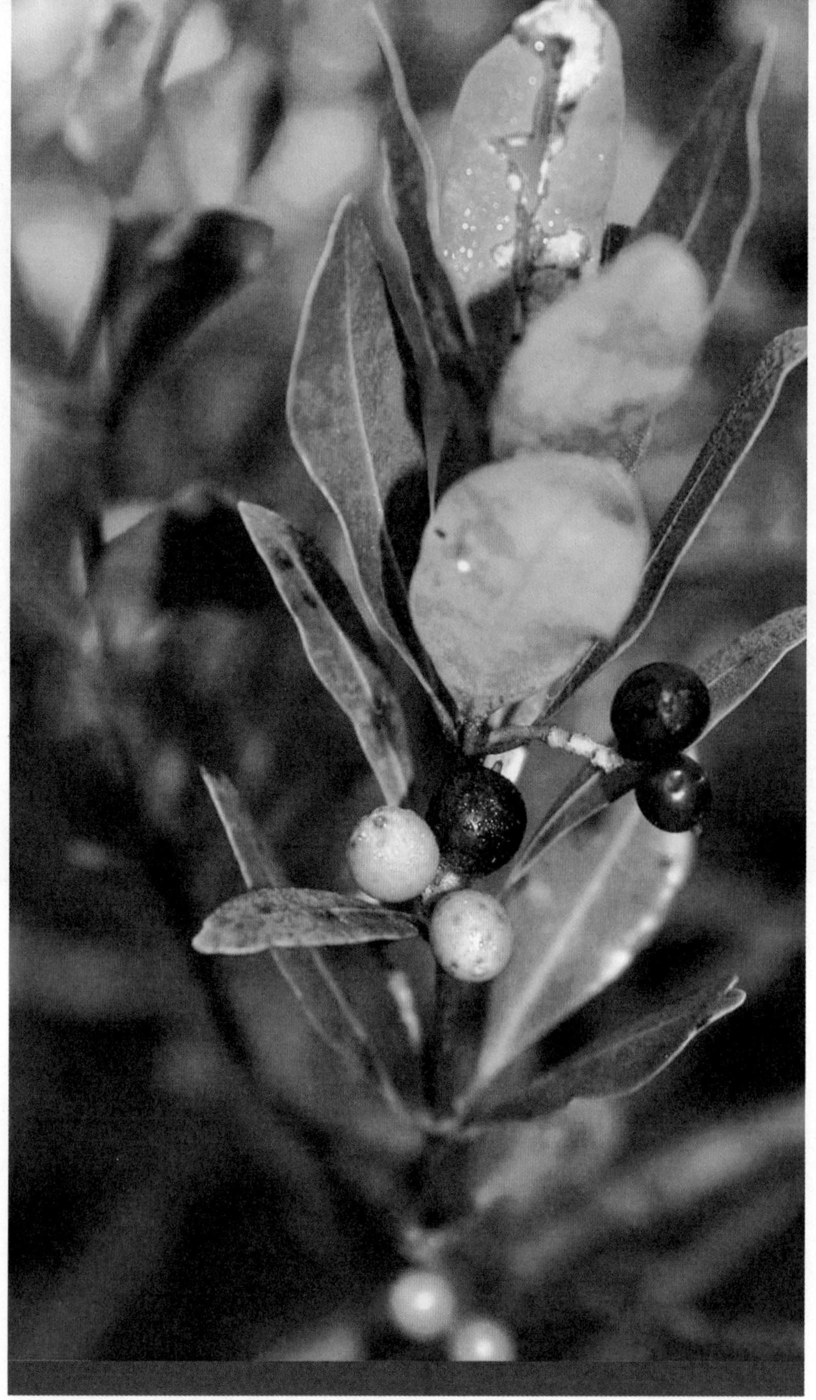

Drunk daily, it was reported to relieve symptoms after two days (Lassak & McCarthy, 2001; Fern, 2021; Webb, 1959). Decoctions of the roots were also used to expel intestinal worms (Fern, 2021).

Chinese Salacia

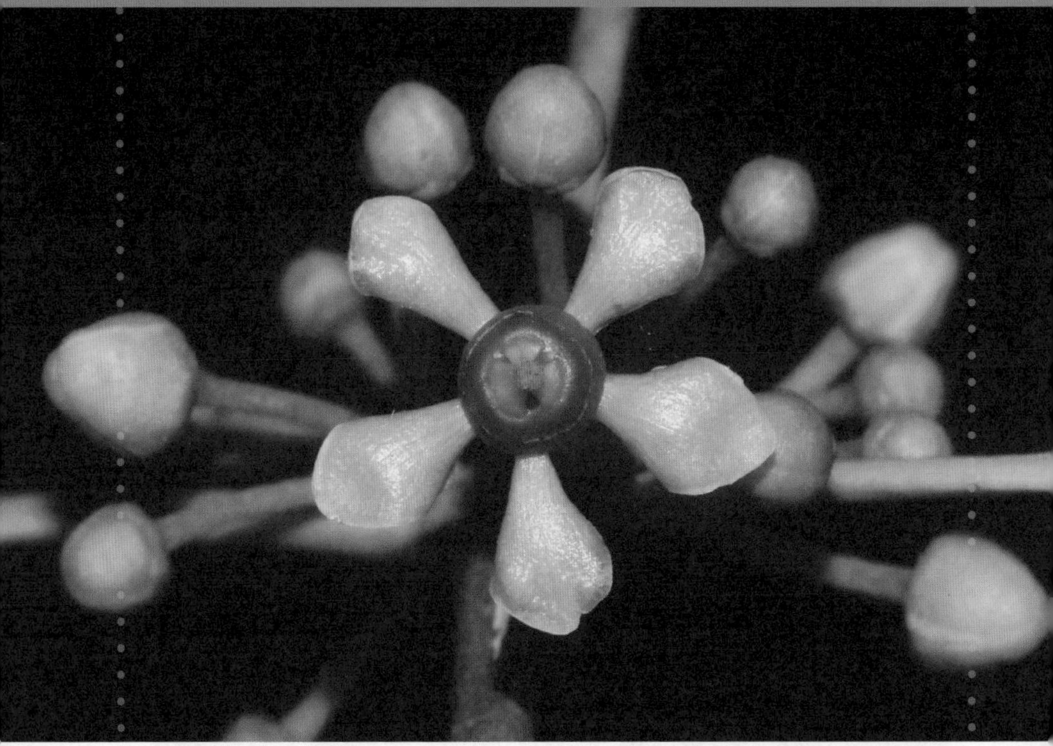

Scientific Name *Salacia chinensis* L.

Common Names Chinese Salacia, Lolly Vine, Lolly Berry.

Field Notes Chinese Salacia is a climber, or more rarely a tree, that can reach up to 5 m in height. It has glossy, ovate, mostly opposite leaf blades that are up to 200 mm long and 120 mm wide. Its small, yellow or yellow-green, propellor-like flowers are around 6 mm in diameter and emit a rather unpleasant odour. Its subglobose to ellipsoid fruit are up to 23 mm in diameter and are red when ripe. Chinese Salacia occurs close to the sea, often found where mangroves are near to rainforests around Wyndham in the Kimberley region of Western Australia, the Northern Territory and the Cape York Peninsula in Queensland. It also occurs in tropical Africa, Cambodia, China, India, Indonesia, Laos, Malaysia, Myanmar, Papua New Guinea, the Philippines, Sri Lanka, Vietnam and some islands in the south-west Pacific (ALA, 2022; ATRP, 2020; WAH, 2022).

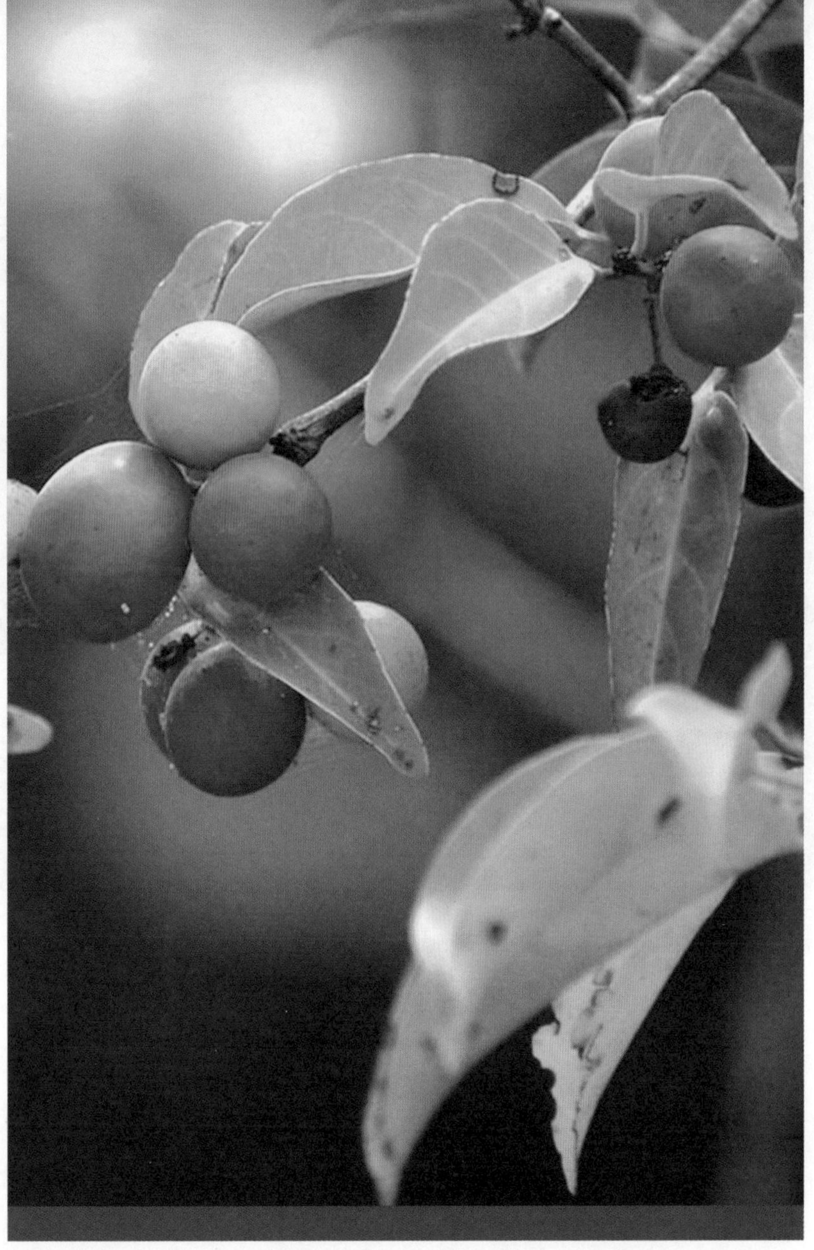

Medicinal Uses Chinese Salacia is used in folk medicine in some Asian countries. Decoctions are used as a treatment for amenorrhoea to normalise menstruation and are also given to revitalise the circulation (Fern, 2021).

Other Uses The ripe fruit of Chinese Salacia, once peeled, are edible raw (Bindon, 2014; Fern, 2021).

Climbing Deeringia

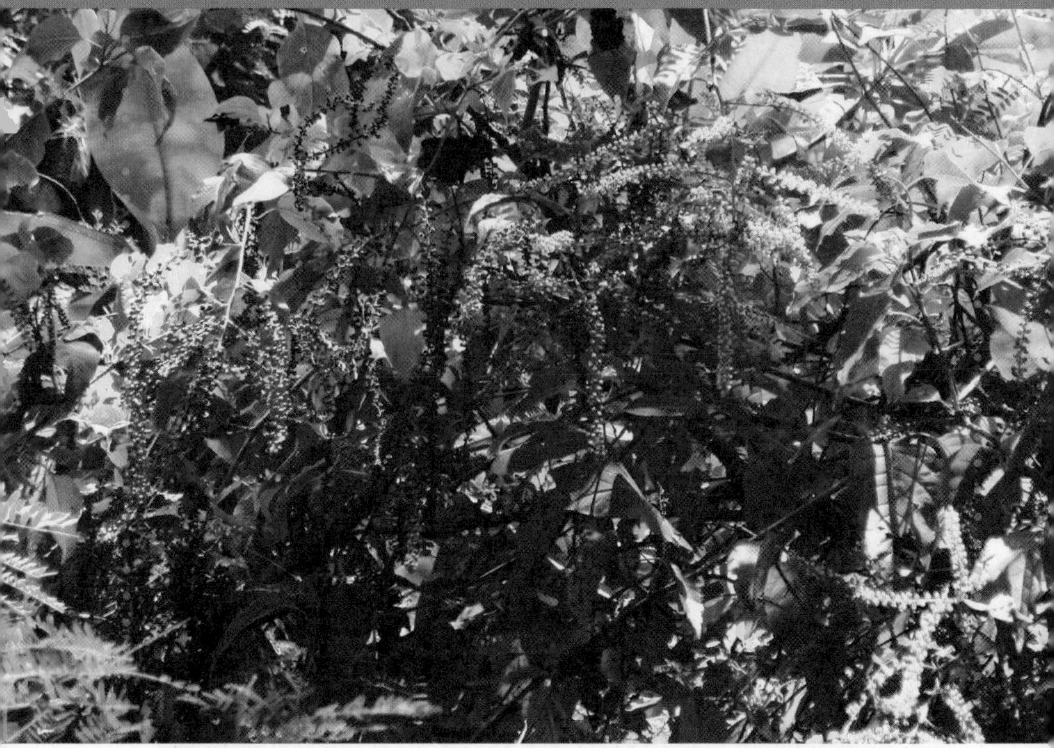

Scientific Name *Deeringia amaranthoides* (Lam.) Merr.

Common Names Climbing Deeringia, Shrubby Deeringia. There are many other local vernacular names for this plant in other countries.

Field Notes Climbing Deeringia is a slightly hairy climbing vine with drooping branches and stems reaching a length of up to 6 m. Its leaves are dark green, heart-shaped and up to 140 mm long. Its small numerous greenish-white flowers are about 1.5 mm long and are borne on racemes. Its fruit are ovoid, fleshy red berries about 4 mm in diameter which grow on long spikes. Climbing Deeringia occurs in rainforests, on rainforest margins and in coastal scrub in the Kimberley region of Western Australia and right down the east coast. It also occurs in Bhutan, China, India, Indonesia, Laos, Malaysia, Myanmar, Nepal, Thailand, the Philippines and Vietnam (ALA, 2022; WAH, 2022).

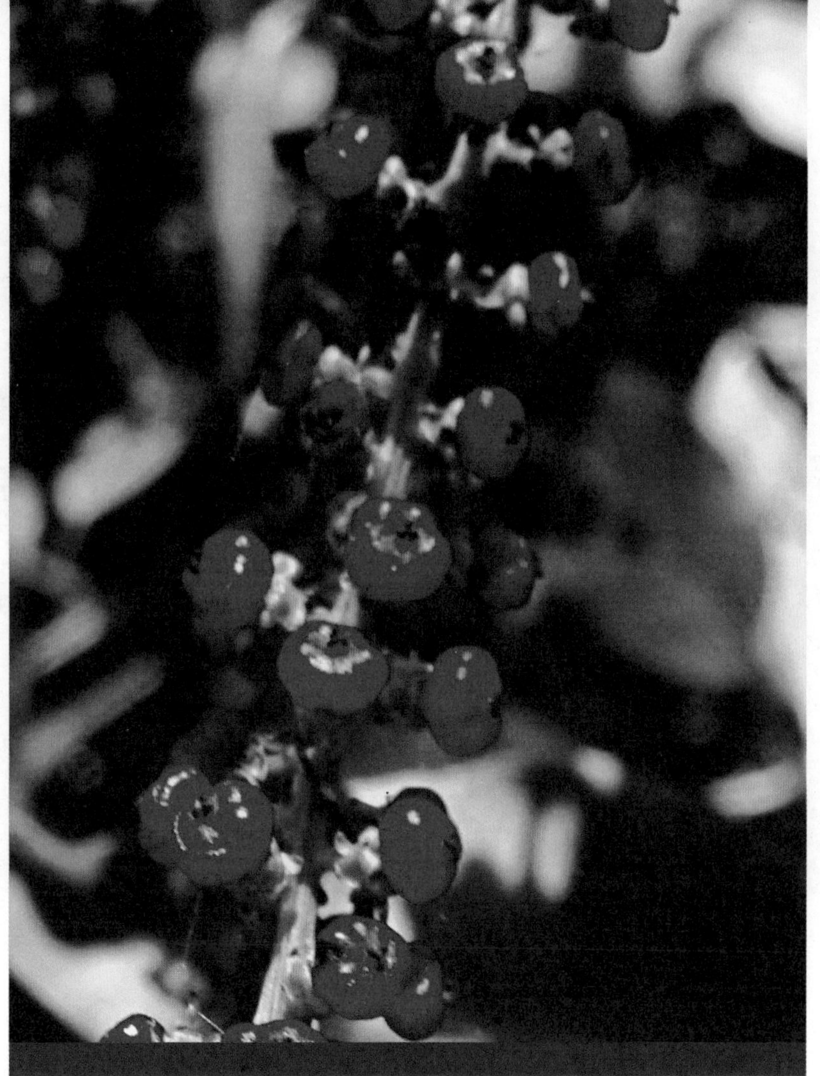

Medicinal Uses Climbing Deeringia is used in folk medicine throughout South-east Asia. Decoctions of the leaves were taken internally to treat diarrhoea and dysentery. Infusions of the leaves were given to children to treat chickenpox. Poultices of the leaves were applied to boils, sores, placed on the stomach to treat stomach ache, and on the forehead to treat fever and headache. A powder made from dried roots is inhaled in some countries to cause sneezing, which clears the nose (Fern, 2021). Infusions of the root mixed with vinegar and alum are inhaled through the nose for the same purpose (Philippine Medicinal Plants, 2022).

Climbing Fern

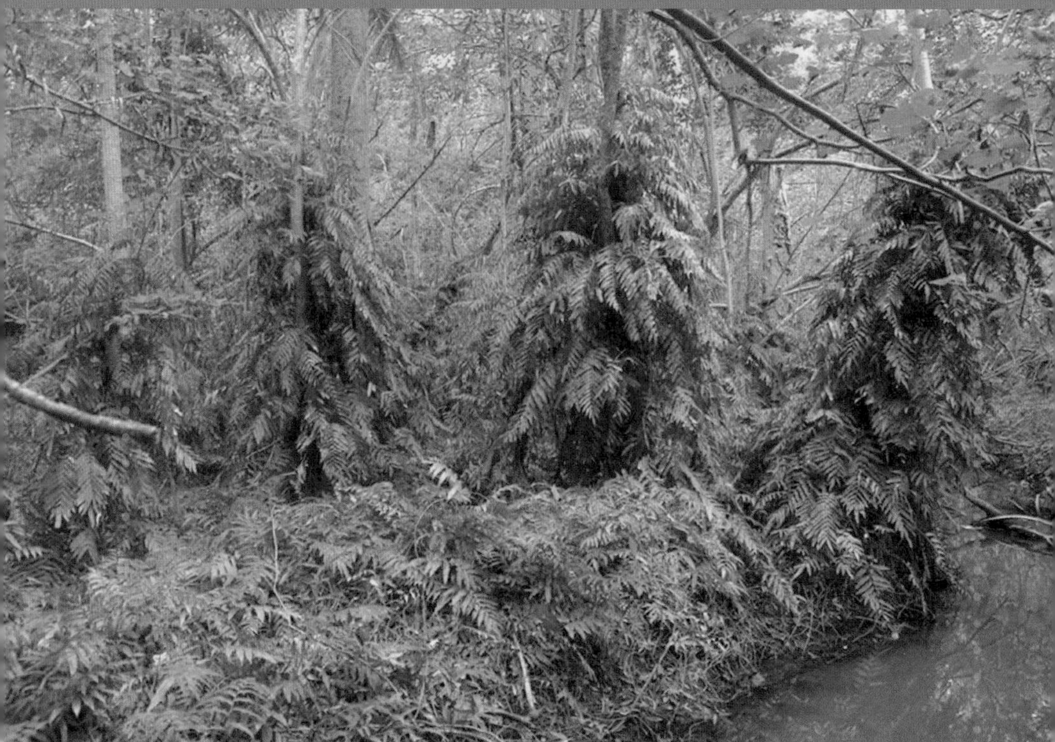

Scientific Name *Stenochlaena palustris* (Burm.f.) Bedd.

Common Names Climbing Fern, Climbing Swamp Fern.

Field Notes Climbing Fern is a rhizomatous, perennial fern that can climb up to 20 m in height. Its fronds are up to 1 m long and comprise numerous shiny alternate leaflets tapering to a fine point. In Australia it occurs in vine thickets, on sandstone rock faces, in swamps and beside creeks across the very top end from the Kimberley region of Western Australia through the Northern Territory to Far North Queensland (ALA, 2022; Calvert, 2016; WAH, 2022). It also occurs in India, Laos, Malaysia, southern China, Thailand, the Philippines, Vietnam and on some Pacific islands (Fern, 2021).

Medicinal Uses Climbing Fern is used in Ayurvedic medicine in India and Sri Lanka and in folk medicine in Malaysia. Decoctions of the leaves were used externally to treat fever, skin diseases,

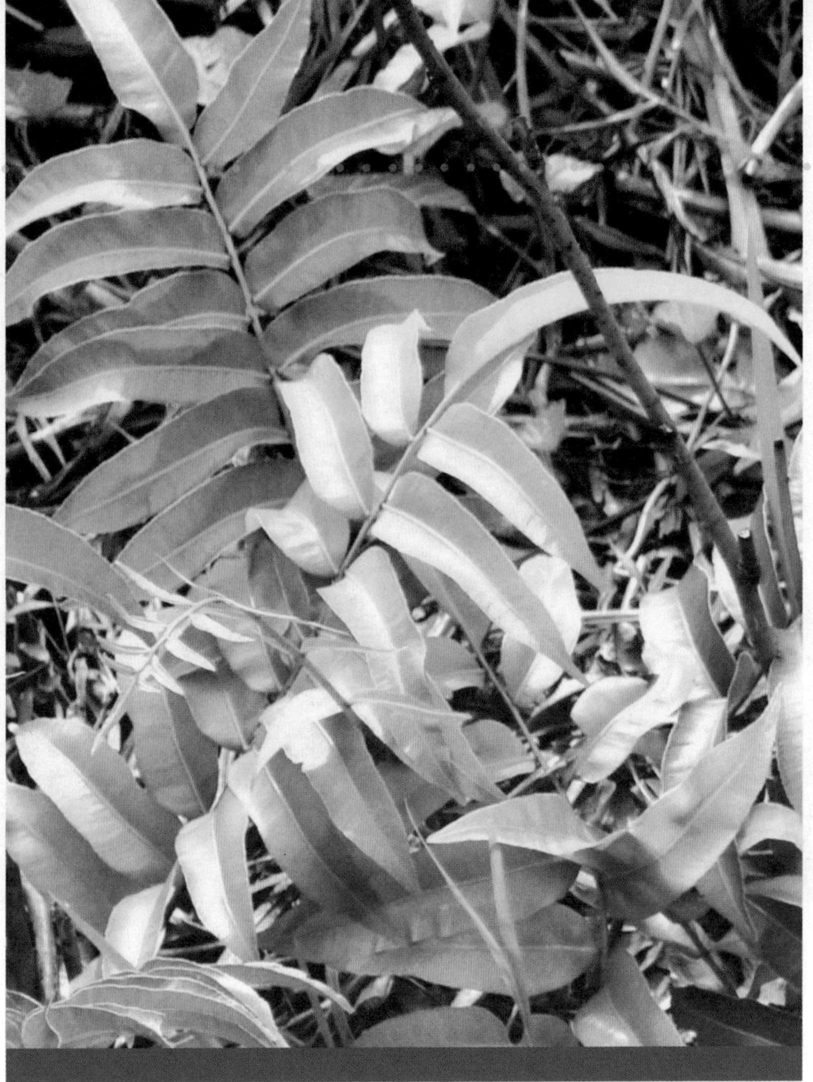

leg ulcers and stomach ache (Benjamin & Manickam, 2007; Herbal Medicine Research Centre, 2002). Indonesian people eat the vegetable as a gentle laxative. Malaysian people use the young shoots to treat diarrhoea. Decoctions or the juice of the young shoots are taken internally for fever (Pl@ntUse, 2022).

Other Uses The young shoots and leaves of the Climbing Fern are edible raw or cooked in a soup but should not be eaten in large amounts because of the laxative properties of the leaves (Calvert, 2016; Fern, 2021). The tuberous underground rhizomes are edible and are roasted in hot ashes before they are eaten (Calvert, 2016).

Climbing Maidenhair Fern

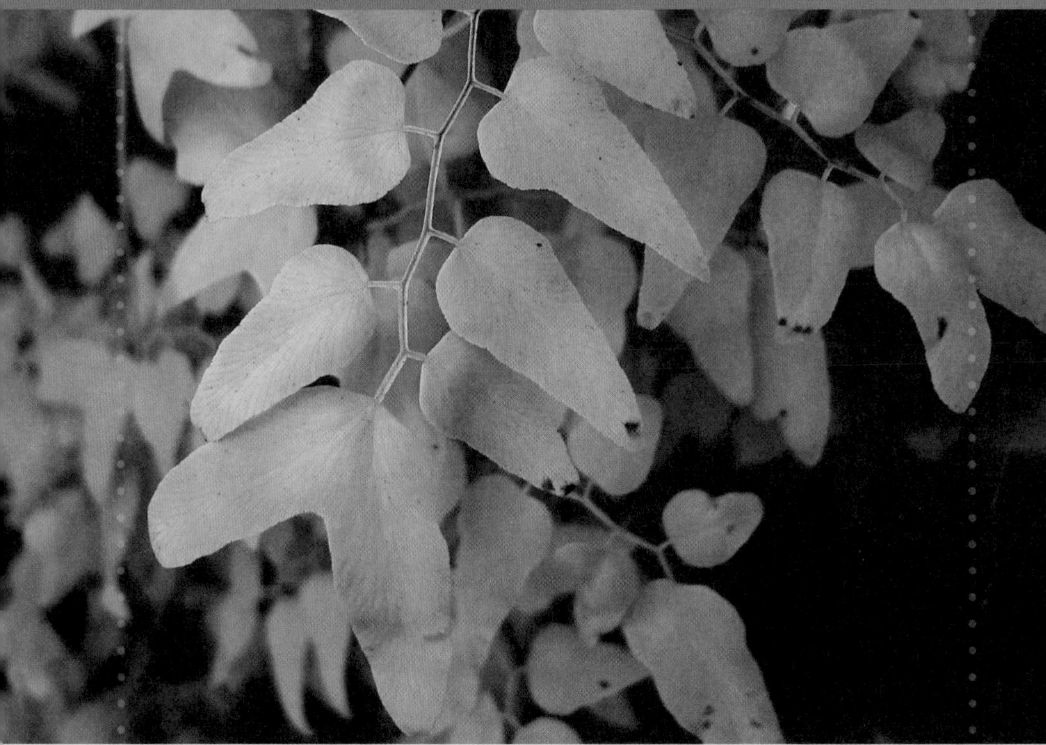

Scientific Name *Lygodium microphyllum* (Cav.) R.Br.

Common Name Climbing Maidenhair Fern, Climbing Maidenhair, Old World Climbing Fern, Small-leaf Climbing Fern, Snake Fern.

Aboriginal Name Gurrngarl (Wunambal, Gaambera) (Karadada et al., 2011).

Field Notes Climbing Maidenhair Fern is a rhizomatous, perennial fern with stems that can reach up to 15 m in length using surrounding trees for support. Its leafy branches off main rachis are up to 120 mm long. Ferns do not have flowers or fruit but produce spores on the backs of their leaves. Climbing Maidenhair Fern occurs in black or brown loam in wet areas such as swamps and near creeks, waterfalls and wet rock crevices in the Kimberley region of Western Australia, the Northern Territory and the east coast of Queensland and New South Wales (ALA, 2022; WAH, 2022). It also occurs in Africa and South-east Asia, including Indonesia, Malaysia and the Philippines (Fern, 2021).

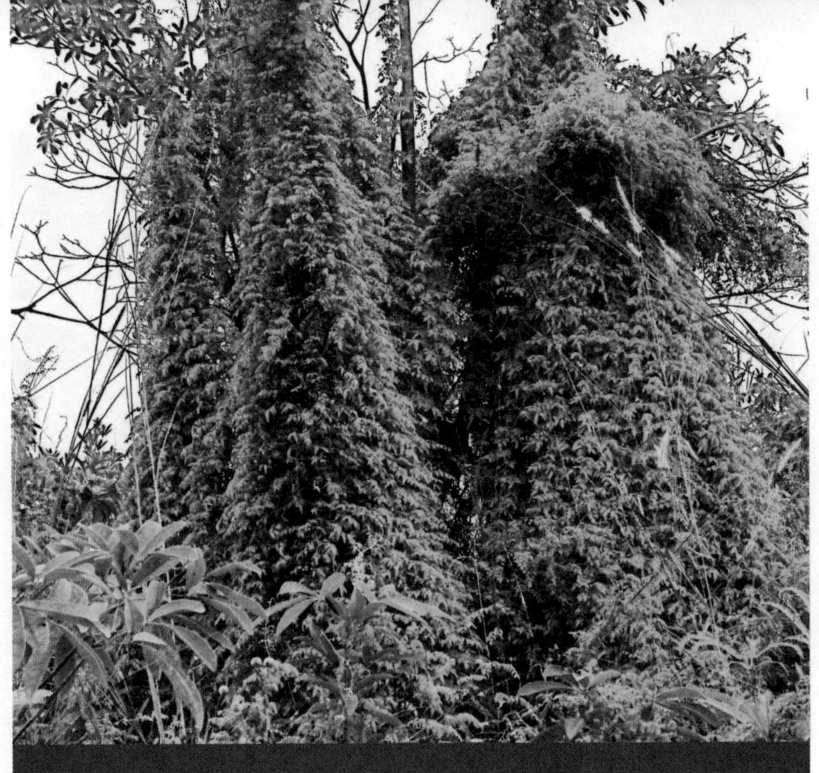

Medicinal Uses Climbing Maidenhair Fern is used in folk medicine in some countries. Decoctions of the leaves are taken internally to treat dysentery. Crushed leaves are applied externally as a poultice to treat skin diseases and swellings (Fern, 2021).

Other Uses The leaves and underground rhizomes are edible but are reported to taste like 'boiled newspaper' and are only eaten when other foods are scarce (Glasby, 2018; Noosa's Native Plants, 2022). The underground rhizomes have only a meagre amount of white starch (Noosa's Native Plants, 2022).

Clubleaf Wattle

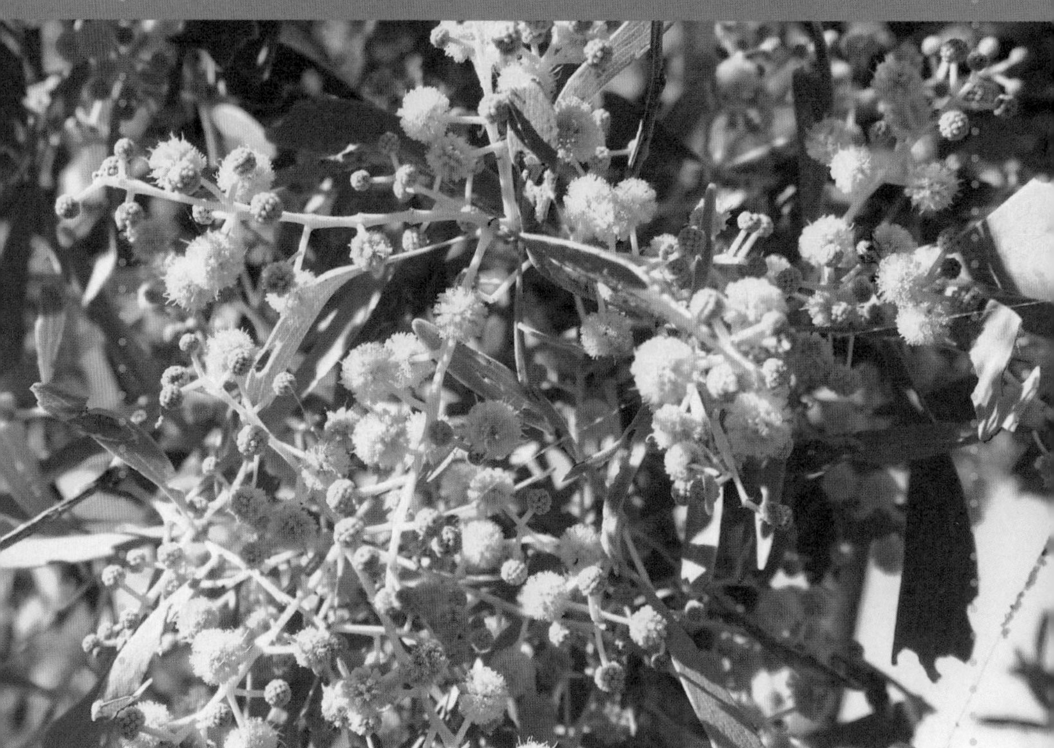

Scientific Name *Acacia hemignosta* F.Muell.

Common Name Clubleaf Wattle.

Aboriginal Names Warrayayi (Gija and Jaru) (Wightman, 2013), Ngalkarnpa, Nyurilpa (Kukatja) (Valiquette, 1993).

Field Notes Clubleaf Wattle is a shrub or tree that grows up to 7 m in height. Its bark is rough, corky and fissured. Its green to yellowish-green to grey-green phyllodes are oblanceolate to narrowly oblanceolate in shape, and are straight to shallowly recurved. The phyllodes are up to 150 mm long and 30 mm wide. Its bright yellow, globular flower heads appear between June and October. Seed pods are flat, straight, narrowly oblong up to 80 mm long and 12 mm wide and appear after flowering. Clubleaf Wattle occurs in flat or undulating country in sandy and lateritic soils, and in heavier soils around watercourses in the Kimberley region of

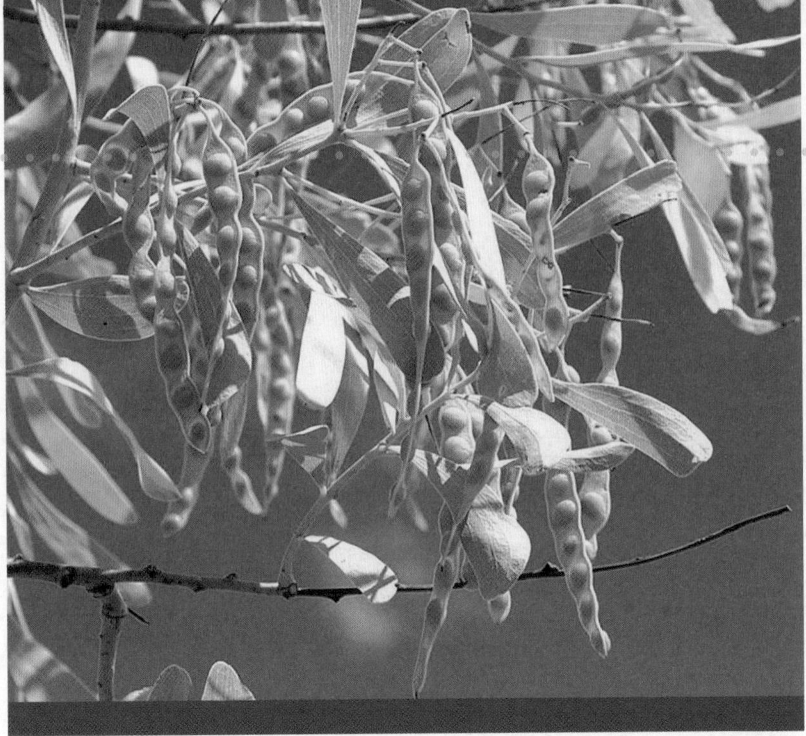

Western Australia, the Northern Territory and northern Queensland (ALA, 2022; WAH, 2022; World Wide Wattle, 2022).

Medicinal Uses Bark from the Clubleaf Wattle was burnt on a fire and the black ash was rubbed onto the sore lips and tongues of babies. If the baby had a sore throat, the ash was rubbed onto the mother's nipples before the baby was breastfed. Ash was also rubbed on the shoulders, neck and chest of adults as an analgesic to ease pain in those areas. Alternatively, the ash was mixed with animal fat and used as an analgesic ointment for the same purpose (Williams, 2011).

Other Uses The gum that oozes from wounds in the branches of Clubleaf Wattle is edible (Deegan et al., 2010; Wightman, 2003). The seeds are also edible and are usually ground to a flour for making Johnny cakes or damper or used as a tasty additive to wheat flour (Fern, 2021; Queensland Bushfoods Association, 2022).

Clump Yellow Pea Bush

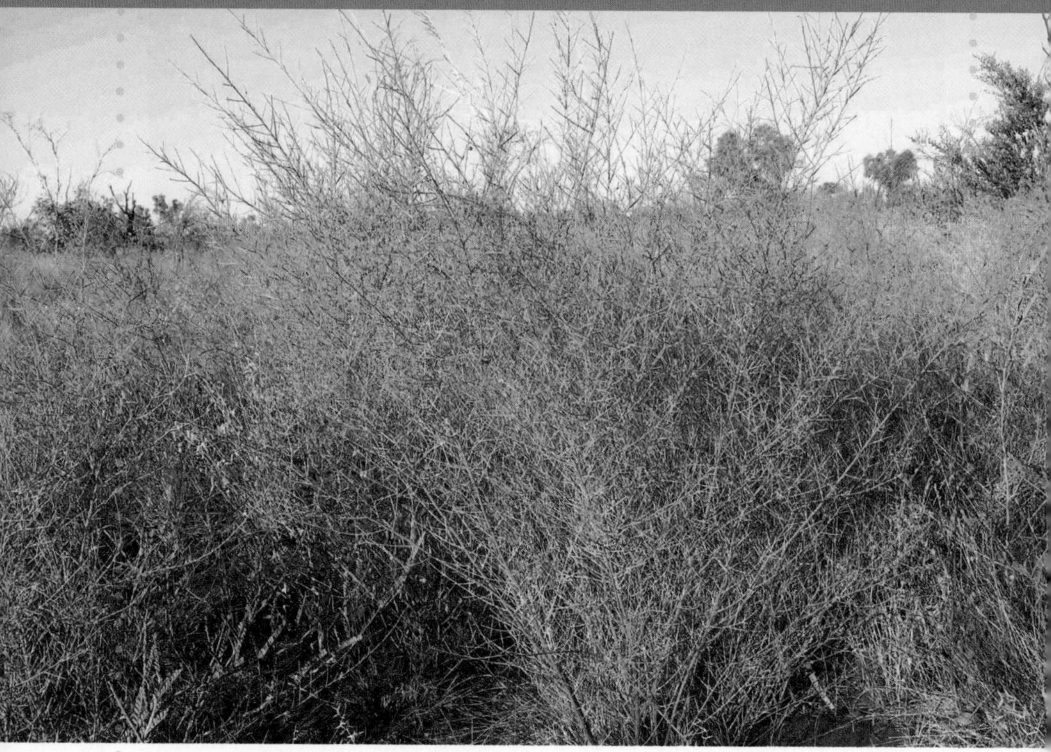

Scientific Name *Mirbelia viminalis* (Benth.) C.A.Gardner

Common Name Clump Yellow Pea Bush.

Aboriginal Names Rangkarrpa, Yilli-yilli, Yungu-yungu (Kukatja) (Valiquette, 1993).

Field Notes Clump Yellow Pea Bush is an erect to spreading, much-branched, spiny shrub that grows to around 2 m in height. Its leaves or phylloclades are glabrous, alternate and up to 45 mm long and 1.5 mm wide. Its pea-type, yellow flowers are present between March and October. Its fruit or seed pods are round in cross-section and break open when mature to disperse the seeds. Clump Yellow Pea Bush occurs in sand, sandstone and stony loam, on rocky outcrops, screes, plateaus and hills in the Pilbara and Kimberley regions of Western Australia, the Northern Territory and Queensland (ALA, 2022; WAH, 2022).

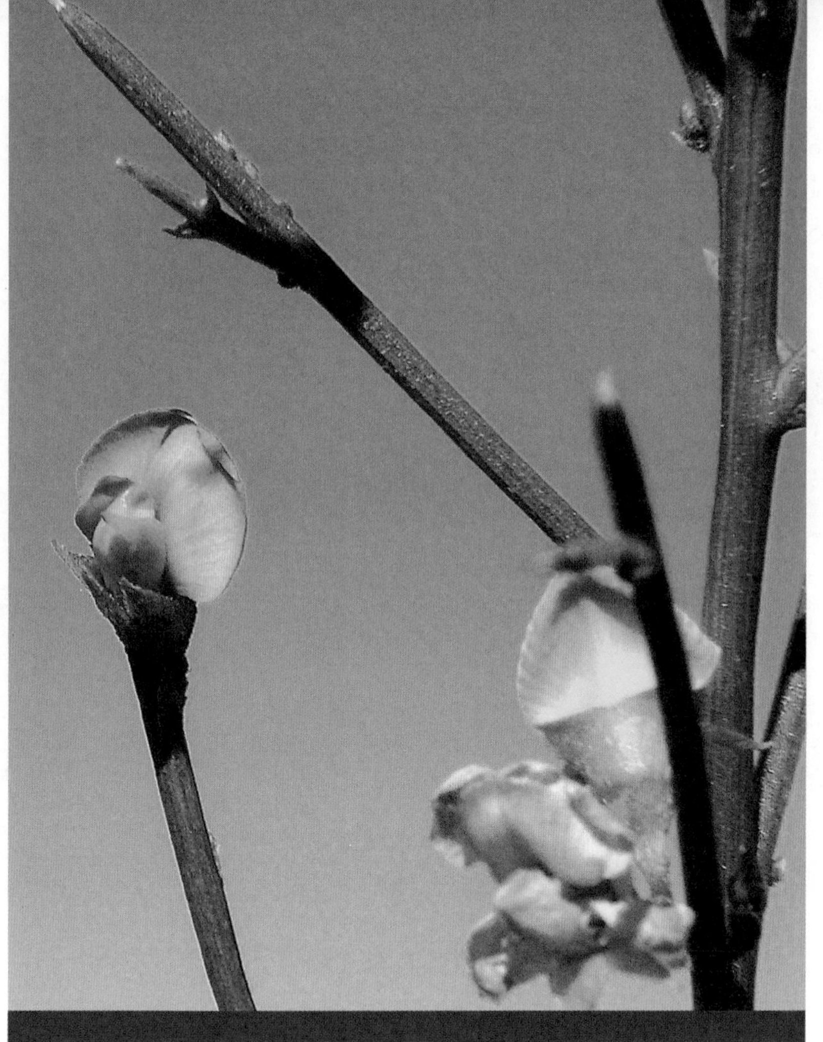

Medicinal Uses The leaves of Clump Yellow Pea Bush were mixed with those of Shrubby Samphire (*Tecticornia halocnemoides*) then ground to a paste and applied to wounds and sores to aid healing (Valiquette, 1993).

Coast Roly-poly

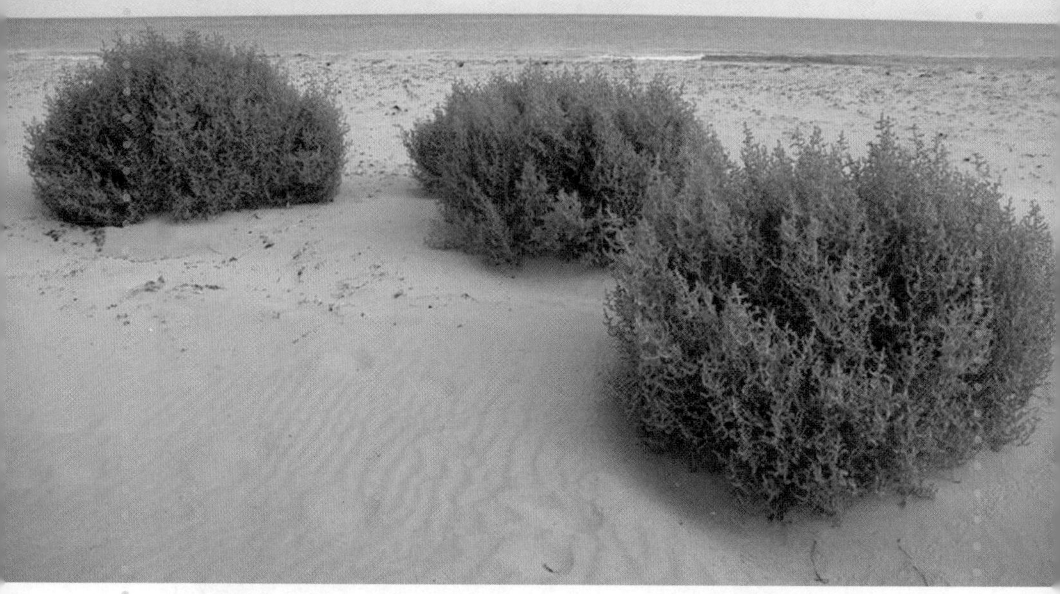

Scientific Name *Salsola australis* R.Br., previously known as *Salsola tragus* L. (misapplied).

Common Names Coast Roly-poly, Prickly Saltwort, Buckbush, Prickly Roly-poly, Roly-poly, Russian Thistle, Saltwort, Soft Roly-poly, Tumbleweed.

Aboriginal Names Jijil (Jaru) (Deegan et al., 2010), Jantara (Karajarri) (Willing, 2014), Djilar (Bardi) (Smith & Kalotas, 1985) or Jilarr (Bardi), Putunarri (Ngardi) (Cataldi, 2004), Tjilka-tjilka, Yili-yili (Kukatja) (Valiquette, 1993), Yandara (Yawuru) (Kenneally et al., 1996).

Field Notes Coast Roly-poly is an erect, compact, somewhat fleshy shrub, branching from the base, that grows to 1 m in height or more. Its leaves are fleshy, flattish, short and tipped with sharp spines. Its flowers are solitary and unstalked with five narrow whitish petals. Its older branches are snake-like and purplish in colour.

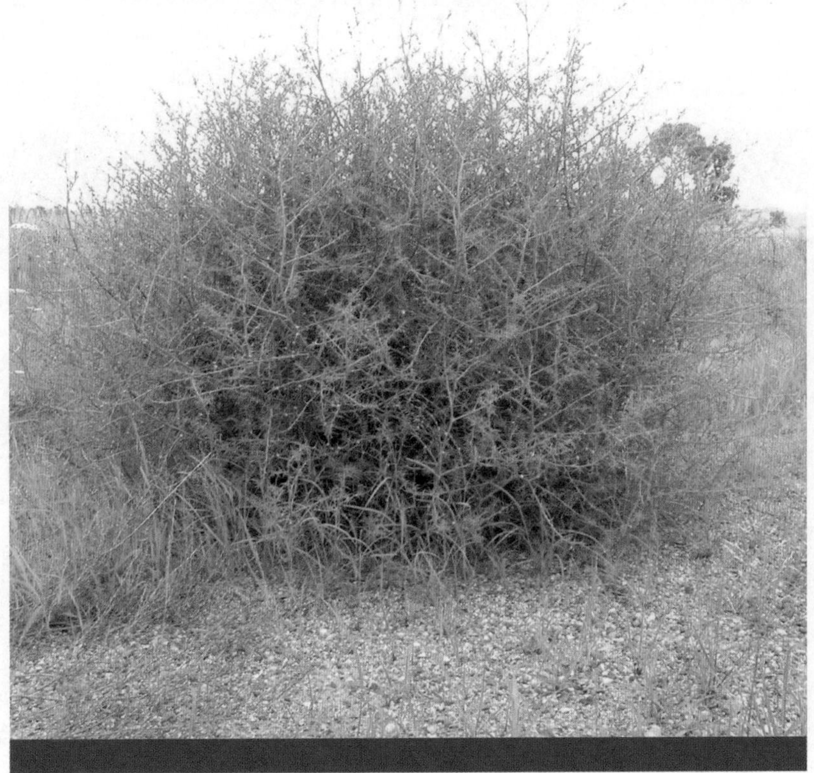

In Western Australia, flowering is between March and September. Its fruit, present from spring to autumn, are dry, flattened capsules up to 7 mm wide with papery wings. The plant breaks off at the base in dry conditions and is blown about in the wind like tumbleweed. Coast Roly-poly occurs in rocky red sandy loam, red-brown or grey sandy clay, and sandstone on seasonal wetlands, creek beds, rocky rivers, bases of sand ridges and hills all over mainland Australia. It is also found in Europe and North America (ALA, 2022; Herbiguide, 2022; NACC, 2022; WAH, 2022).

Medicinal Uses Decoctions of the leaves of Coast Roly-poly were taken internally as a diuretic and anthelmintic to treat intestinal parasites (NACC, 2022). The leaves and stems were chewed or crushed and were used as a poultice to treat ant, bee and wasp stings. Infusions of the plant ashes have been used both internally to treat colds and influenza and as a wash in the treatment of rashes and other skin conditions (PFAF, 2022).

Other Uses The leaves and shoots of the Coast Roly-poly can be eaten raw or cooked as a vegetable (NACC, 2022).

Coastal Caper

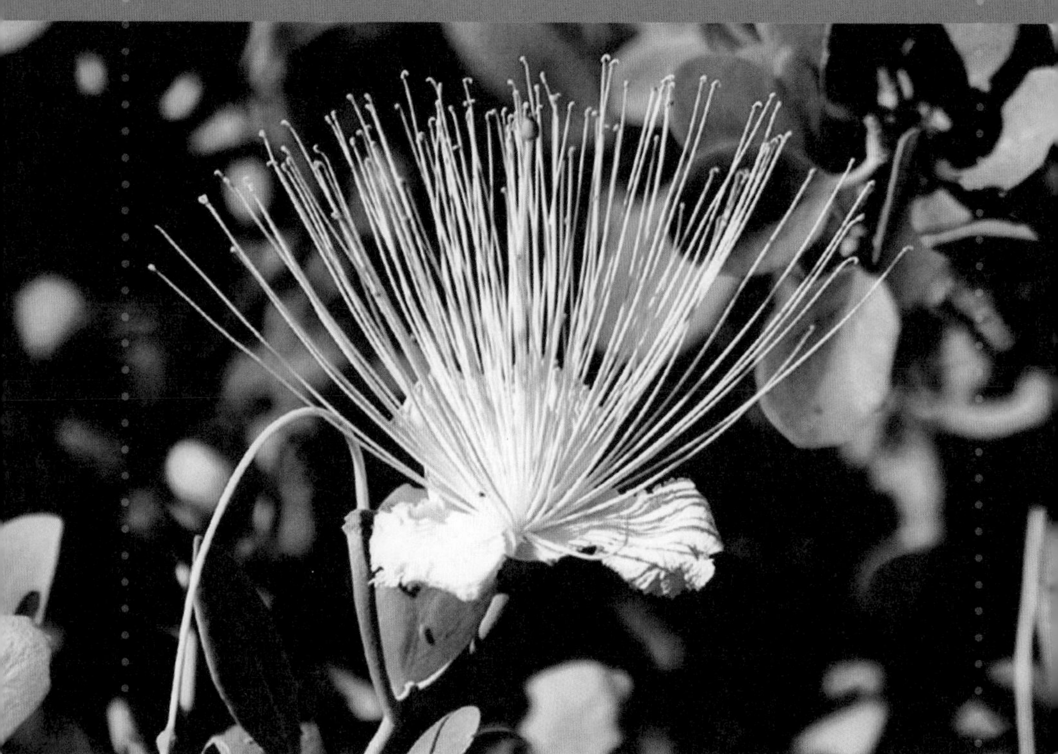

Scientific Names *Capparis spinosa* L., *Capparis spinosa* subsp. *nummularia* (DC.) Fici.

Common Names Coastal Caper, Caper Bush, Split Arse, Splitjack, Flinders Rose, Wild Passionfruit.

Field Notes Coastal Caper is the plant grown in most sub-tropical and temperate parts of the world for the flower buds, the capers, which are usually pickled and used in the cuisine of many countries. *Capparis spinosa* subsp. *nummularia* is a sub-species that has adapted to desert conditions. It is a prostrate or scrambling shrub that grows up to 3 m in height, with a spread of around 2 m. The species is hermaphroditic (that is, it has both male and female organs on the same tree). It has ovate leaves and white flowers with large petals and long white stamens. The flowers can be present all year round. Coastal Caper prefers a good annual rainfall but is also drought tolerant. In Australia it occurs in sandy

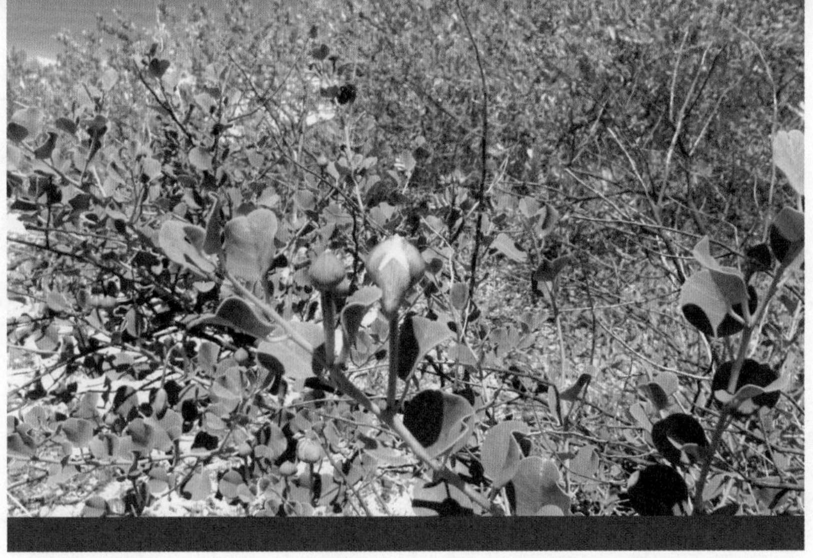

soils on and around the coast and inland in the Gascoyne, Pilbara and Kimberley regions of Western Australia, in the Northern Territory and most of Queensland (ALA, 2022, Preedy et al., 2011, WAH, 2022).

Medicinal Uses Traditionally, Coastal Caper was used for coughs, asthma and toothache. Thomson (2018) reports that 'there is ongoing research into its antioxidant, anticancer and antibacterial effects'. Parts of the plant have been used in folk medicine, including Ayurvedic medicine, in many parts of the world for centuries. Decoctions of the plant were used externally to treat vaginal thrush. The leaves were crushed and applied externally as a poultice to treat gout. The root-bark is known for its analgesic, anthelmintic, antihaemorrhoidal, aperient, deobstruent, depurative, diuretic, emmenagogue, expectorant, tonic and vasoconstrictor properties. Decoctions of it were taken internally to treat gastrointestinal infections, diarrhoea, gout and rheumatism. The decoctions are used externally to treat skin conditions and capillary weakness (Fern, 2021). The flower buds have laxative properties (Fern, 2021; Preedy et al., 2011).

Other Uses The attractive flowers and flower buds (capers) of Coastal Caper are edible (Thomson, 2018). Fern (2021) reports that 'the young fruit and tender branch tips can also be pickled and used as a condiment and steamed and eaten as a vegetable'.

Coastal Jack Bean

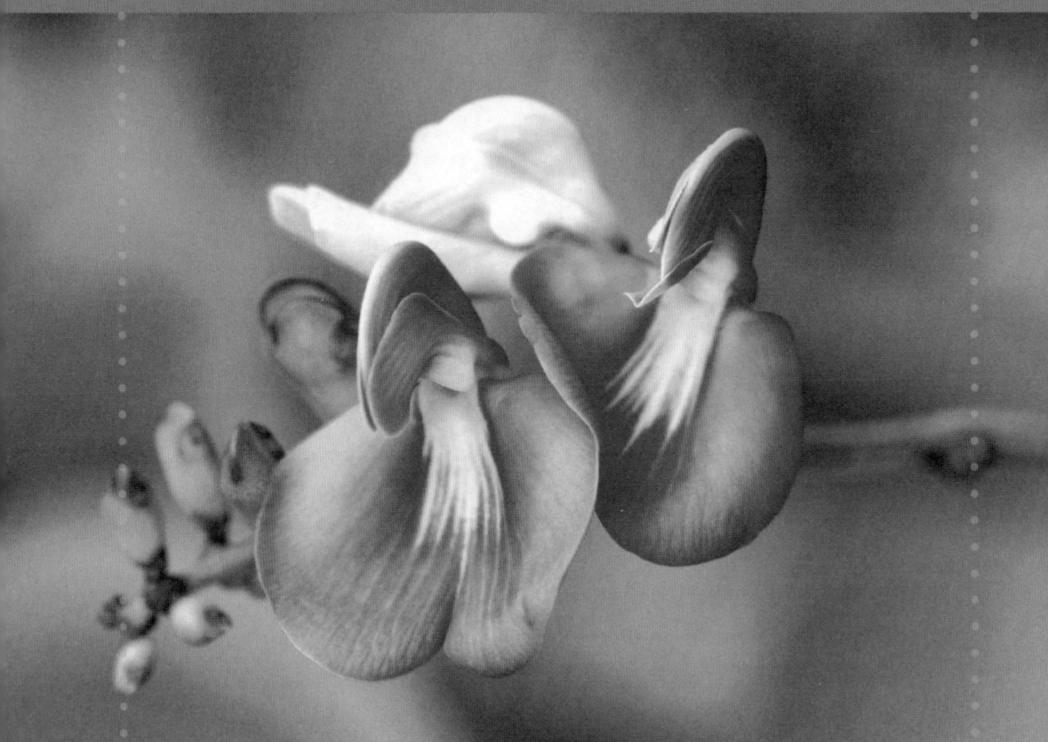

Scientific Name *Canavalia rosea* (Sw.) DC.

Common Names Coastal Jack Bean, Wild Jack Bean, Beach Bean, Bay Bean, Seaside Jack-bean, MacKenzie Bean.

Aboriginal Names Windi (Yawuru), Gudayun (Bardi) (Smith & Kalotas, 1985), Goordayun (Bardi) (Kenneally et al., 1996).

Field Notes Coastal Jack Bean grows as a prostrate, trailing perennial herb or climber with stems up to 10 m long. Its compound leaves are made up of three leaflets and are up to 76 mm in diameter. Its purple to pink flowers appear in clusters on stalks between February and October. Its flat seed pods are up to 150 mm long. Coastal Jack Bean occurs in sand on coastal beaches and sand dunes, and among limestone rocks around the northern coastline of Australia from Carnarvon in Western Australia to the border between New South Wales and Victoria. It also occurs in tropical parts of other countries including Africa, the Americas,

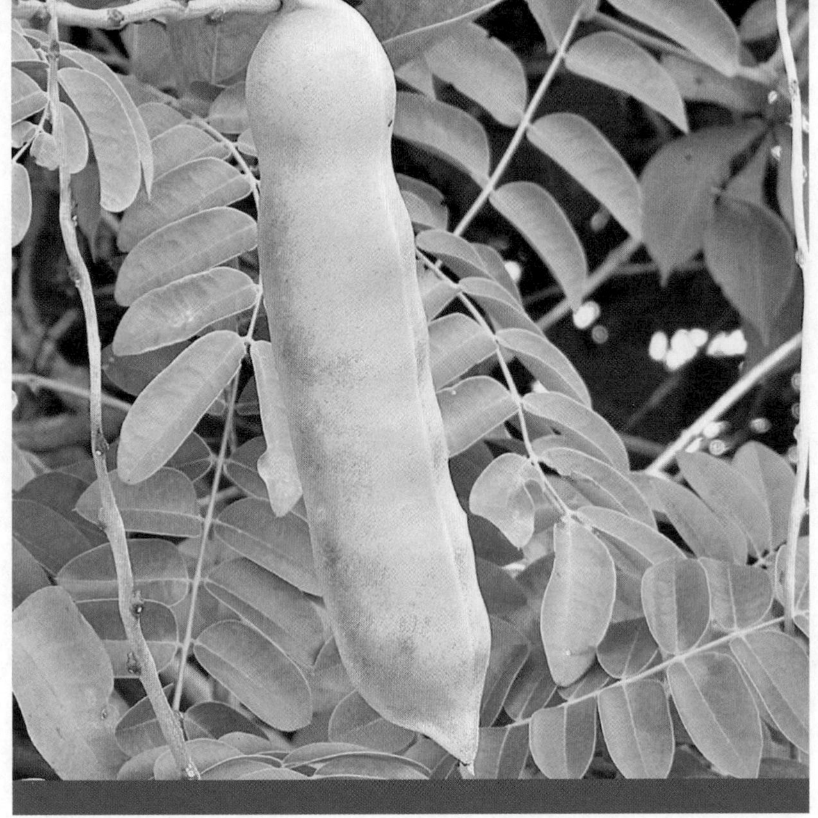

Indonesia, Malaysia and the Pacific islands (ALA, 2022; Fern, 2021; Lassak & McCarthy, 2001; WAH, 2022).

Medicinal Uses Infusions or decoctions of the mashed roots were used externally as a liniment for rheumatic pain, broken bones, colds and as an antiseptic wash to treat leprosy (CMKB, 2019; Cock, 2011; Fern, 2021; Kenneally et al., 1996; Lassak & McCarthy, 2001; Low, 1990; Native Tastes of Australia, 2022; Reid, 1986; Steptoe & Passananti, 2012; Webb, 1959; Williams, 2012).

Other Uses The young bean pods of Coastal Jack Bean are edible and make a pleasant vegetable but must be cooked before eating to avoid the emetic effects of the raw bean. Low (1991) and Cribb & Cribb (1981) report that the seeds inside the beans are very tasty after roasting. Malaysians make a porridge from the beans. There are scant records of Aboriginal groups from the top end eating this bean (Australian Plants Society SA Region, 2022; Fern, 2021; Low, 1991; Williams, 2010).

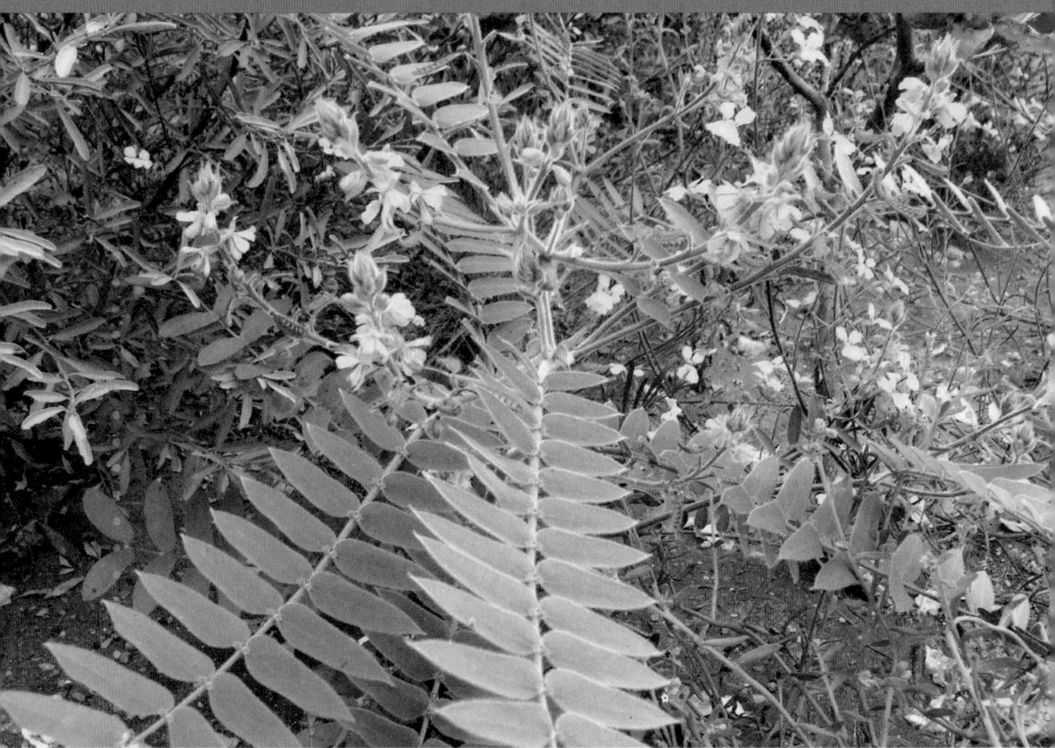

Scientific Names *Senna notabilis* (F.Muell.) Randell, also known as *Cassia notabilis* F.Muell.

Common Names Cockroach Bush, Tinki Tink.

Aboriginal Names Kalpirr-kalpirr, Marnapulyka, Pakarlpa, Pitarl-pitarlpa (Kukatja) (Valiquette, 1993), Lumbilumbi (Bunuba) (Oscar et al., 2019), Lampilampi (Walmajarri) (Richards & Hudson, 2012), Wangalji (Gija) (Purdie et al., 2018), Birralbirral (Nyikina) (Milgin, 2009), Girriliny (Jaru) (Wightman, 2003).

Field Notes Cockroach Bush is an annual or perennial spreading shrub that rarely grows above 1.5 m in height. It has light green, lanceolate leaves with a pointed tip that are up to 20 mm long. Yellow flowers appear in dense terminal racemes between April and October. Its brown, flat seed pods are up to 40 mm long and 15 mm wide and faintly resemble cockroaches, hence the common name. Cockroach Bush occurs in red sand, clay or stony soils in the

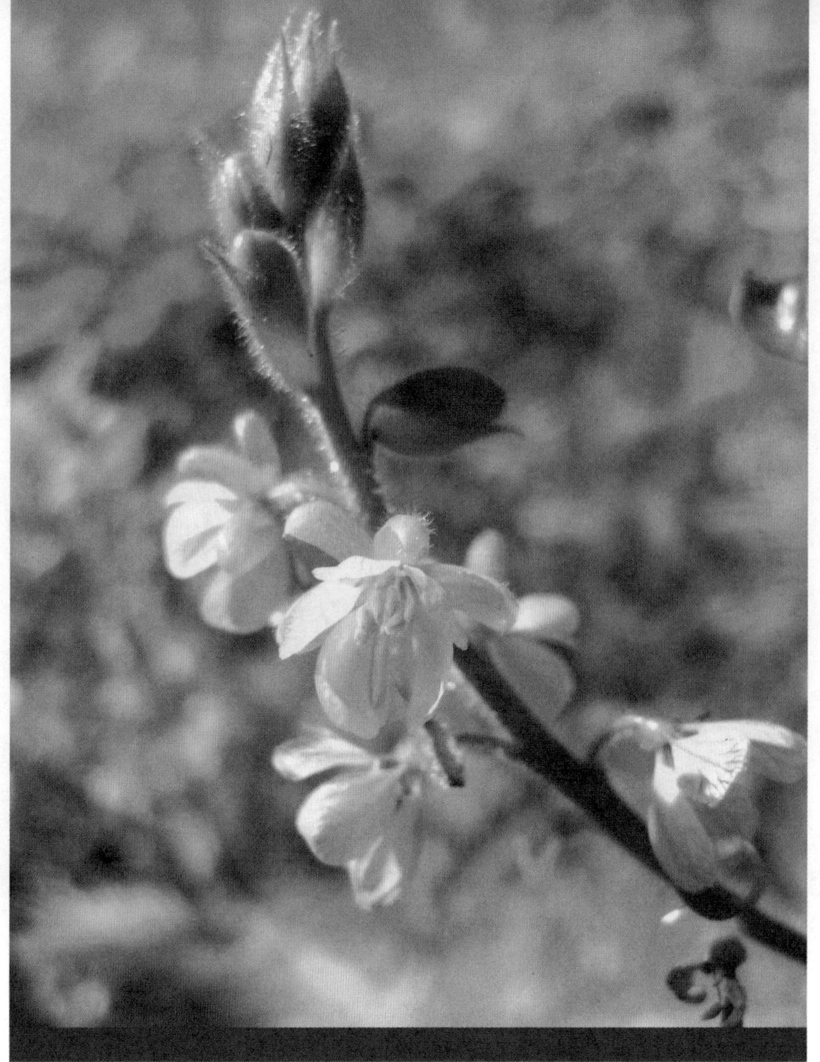

Pilbara and Kimberley regions of Western Australia, the Northern Territory and Queensland (ALA, 2022; Flora of Australia Online, 2022; WAH, 2022).

Medicinal Uses Decoctions of the branches and leaves of Cockroach Bush were used externally as a medicinal wash to help reduce high fever, and as a treatment for skin sores and fungal infections of the skin, such as dermatophytosis (tinea and ringworm) (Oscar et al., 2019; Smith, 1991; YMAC, 2016).

Other Uses The sap of the Cockroach Bush is edible. Witchetty Grubs are dug up from under this plant and eaten raw or slightly roasted (YMAC, 2016).

Coffee Bush

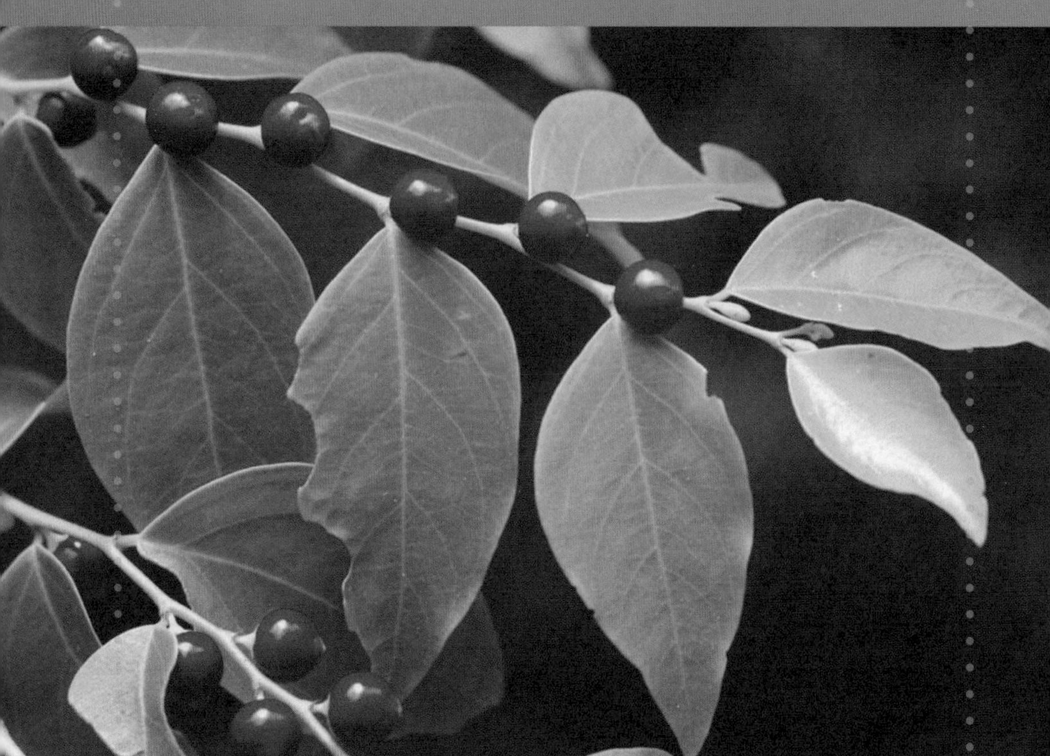

Scientific Name *Breynia cernua* (Poir.) Müll.Arg.

Common Names Coffee Bush, Fart Bush, Bird Apple.

Field Notes Coffee Bush grows as a shrub or small tree up to 3 m in height. Its leaves are ovate coming to a slight point at the tip. Its small green-yellow or white flowers are tubular with spreading petals. They can be present in Australia any time between December and June. Its fruit are small red berries. Coffee Bush is found in sandy soils, often on sandstone or limestone, in a variety of habitats across the north from the Kimberley region of Western Australia, through the Northern Territory and Queensland and down the east coast as far as the Victorian border with New South Wales. It also occurs in Malaysia, New Guinea, the Philippines and the Solomon Islands (ALA, 2022; Fern, 2021; WAH, 2022).

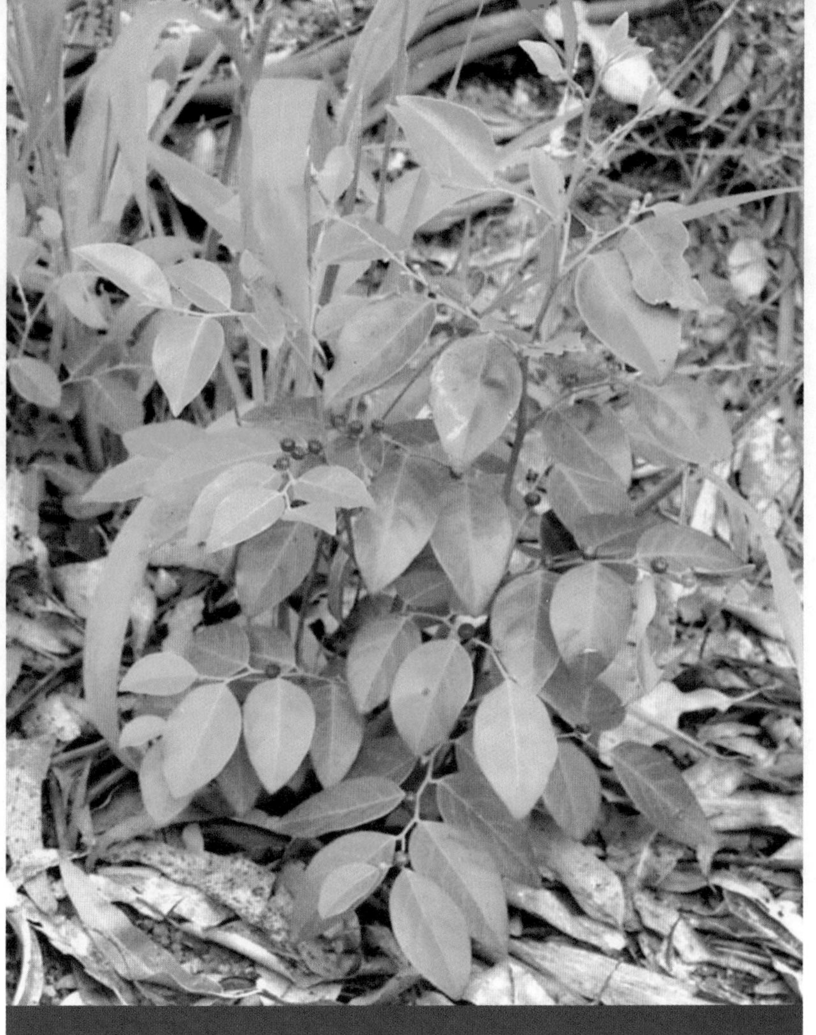

Medicinal Uses Decoctions of the leaves of Coffee Bush have been used by some Aboriginal groups to bathe sore eyes due to conjunctivitis (Cock, 2011; Lassak & McCarthy, 2001). The leaves were crushed and the juice drunk as a cough suppressant. Pounded leaves were applied as a poultice to swollen legs and other painful areas. Decoctions of the leaves made with salt water were mixed with lime and applied externally to wounds, sores and ulcers to aid healing. Infusions of the bark were taken internally to stem diarrhoea (Cock, 2011; Fern, 2021).

Other Uses The berries of the Coffee Bush are edible and were a common bushfood for many Aboriginal groups across the top end of Australia (BushcraftOz, 2022; Fox & Garde, 2018).

Comet Grass

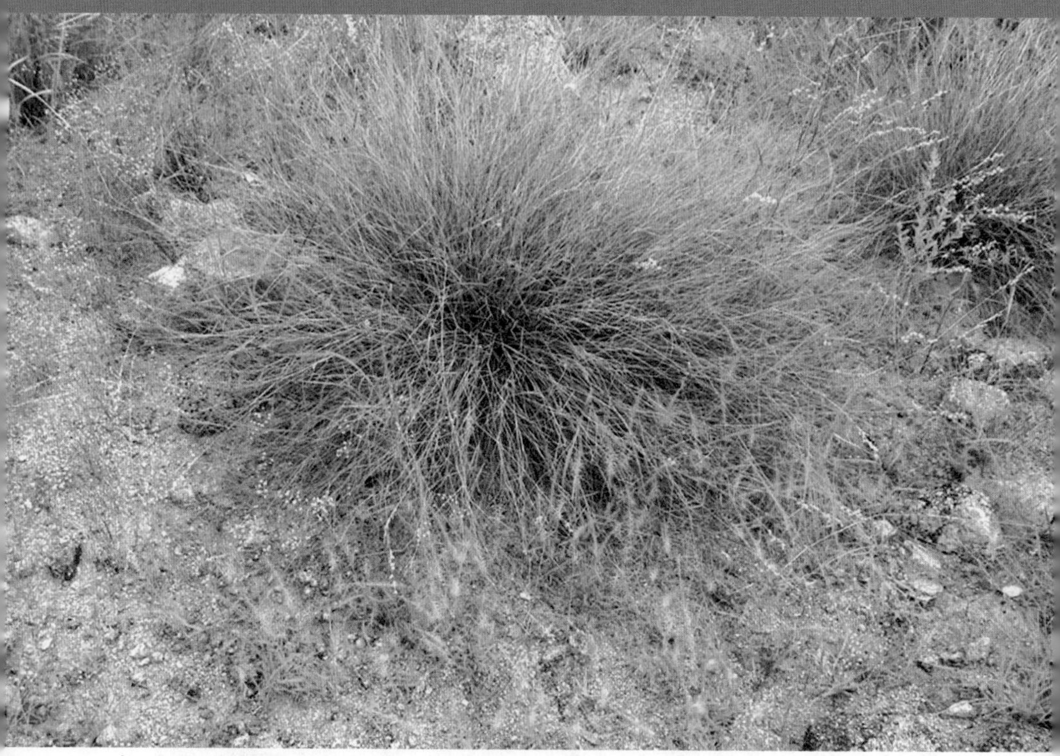

Scientific Name *Perotis rara* R.Br.

Common Name Comet Grass.

Aboriginal Name Garawal (Bardi) (Kenneally et al., 1996).

Field Notes Comet Grass is a tufted annual or perennial (short-lived) grass that grows to around 300 mm in height. Its leaf blades are lanceolate and approximately 30 mm long by 4 mm wide. Its green flower heads appear as a single terminal raceme up to 100 mm long between February and June. Comet Grass occurs in red, yellow or white sand and alluvium all over the top half of Australia. It also occurs in parts of China, New Guinea, the Philippines, Thailand and Vietnam (ALA, 2022; AusGrass2, 2022; WAH, 2022).

Medicinal Uses Aboriginal groups chewed the plant, but did not swallow it, as a treatment for upset stomachs. Decoctions of the whole plant were used as eyedrops to treat conjunctivitis and as an antiseptic wash to bathe sores and wounds (Edwards, 2005).

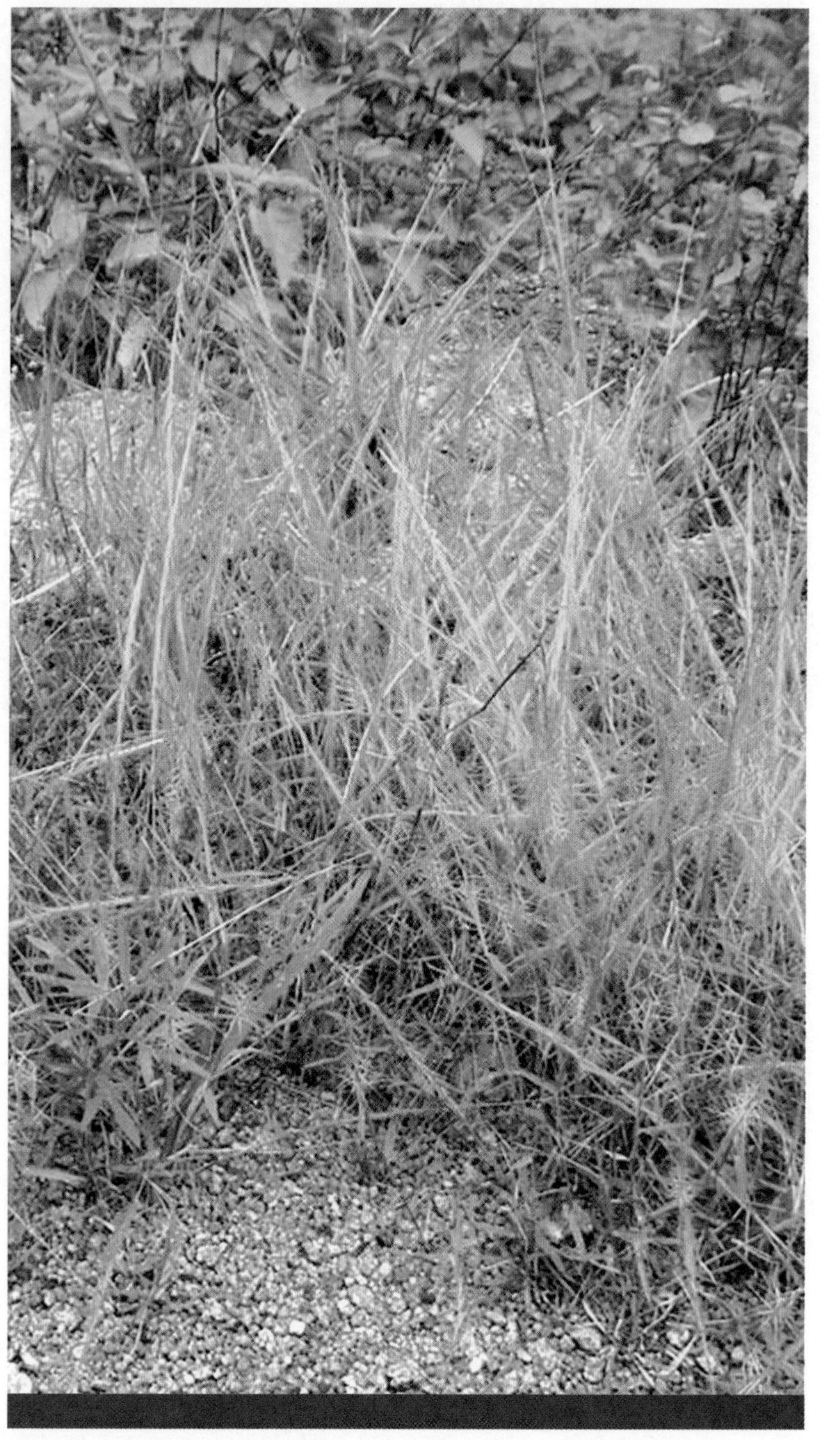

Common Hakea

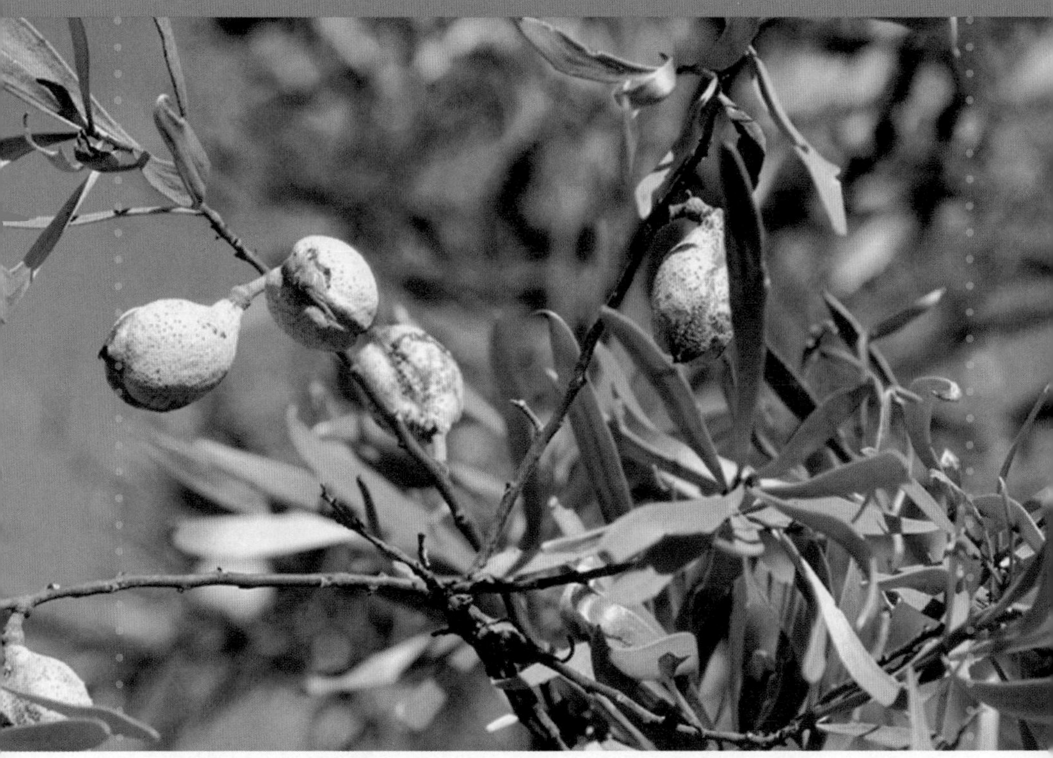

Scientific Name *Hakea arborescens* R.Br.

Common Names Common Hakea, Yellow Hakea, Boomerang Tree.

Aboriginal Names Jirrindi (Bunuba) (Oscar et al., 2019), Irrgil (Bardi) (Smith & Kalotas, 1985; Paddy et al., 1993), Jaarni, Jarangkarr, Yirrkili (Walmajarri) (Richards & Hudson, 2012), Yirrkili (Nyikina) (Smith & Smith, 2009), Jirrindiny (Gija) (Purdie et al., 2018), Booroowa (Gooniyandi) (Dilkes-Hall et al., 2019), Jirrirndi, Wadaruru, Jawilyi (Jaru) (Wightman, 2003), Bambura (Kwini) (Cheinmora et al., 2017).

Field Notes Common Hakea grows as a tall shrub or tree to 7 m in height. Its bark is black or grey and deeply fissured. Its leaves are flat, linear, narrowly elliptic or narrowly obovate and up to 170 mm long. The flowers are white or yellow pedicels and claws up to 4.5 mm long. Flowering occurs between January and June. The fruit are obliquely ovate and up to 55 mm long. Common Hakea

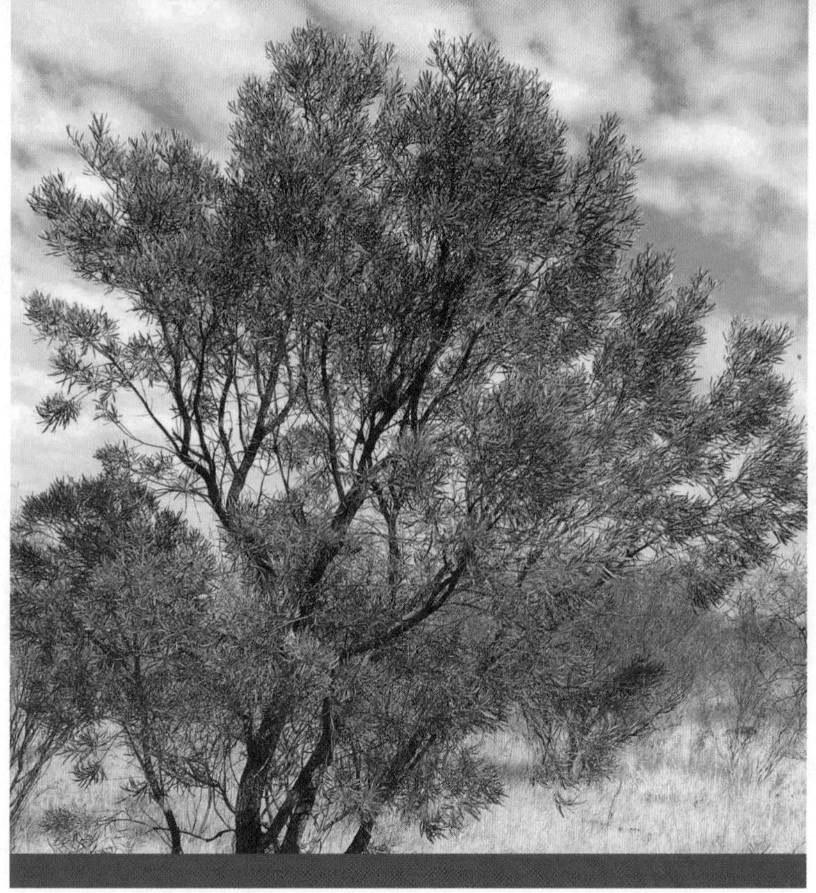

occurs in basalt or laterite over basalt and sandstone in the Kimberley region of Western Australia, the Northern Territory and northern part of Queensland (ALA, 2022, eFlora.SA, 2022; Flora of Australia Online, 2022; WAH, 2022).

Medicinal Uses Decoctions of the inner bark were used as a wash to treat itchy skin and scabies infestations (Smith, 1991). The Jaru rubbed the ash from burnt bark and wood on small babies 'to make them strong and healthy in later life' (Wightman, 2003).

Other Uses The seeds of the Common Hakea are edible (RFCA, 1993). The Gija, Jaru and Kwini used the wood from the Common Hakea to make boomerangs (Cheinmora et al., 2017; Purdie et al., 2018; Wightman, 2003).

Conkerberry

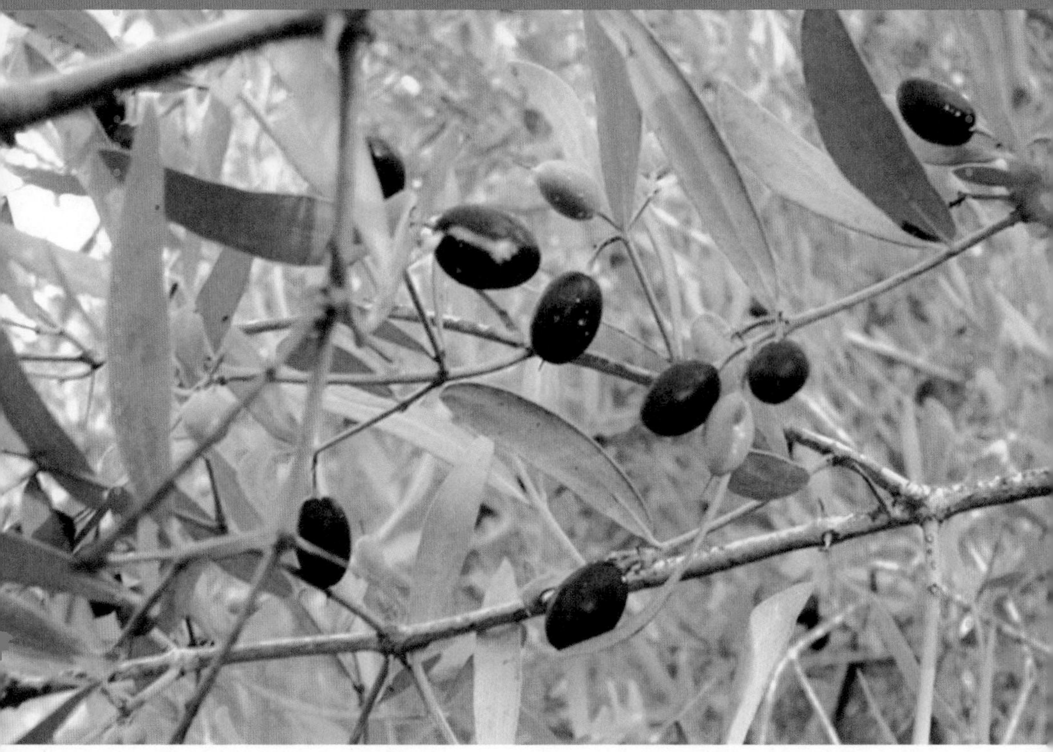

Scientific Names *Carissa lanceolata* R.Br., also known as *Carissa spinarum* L.

Common Names Conkerberry, Konkerberry, Concle Berry, Bush Plum, Kungsberry Bush.

Aboriginal Names Boodbarung (Mirriwoong) (Leonard et al., 2013), Gungkara (Yawuru), Goonggar or Goonggara (Bardi), Jima (Nyangumarta) (Lands, 1997), Koongkoora (Nyul Nyul), Jima (Nyangumarta), Kungkura (Karajarri) (Kane, 2022), Marnuwiji (Walmajarri) (Richards & Hudson, 2012), Biriyaldji, Maboorany (Gija) (Purdie et al., 2018), Mapura (Miwa) (Kimberley Specialists, 2020), Biriyali (Gooniyandi, Bunuba) (Dilkes-Hall et al., 2019), Burnungarna, Mabura (Jaru) (Wightman, 2003), Briyal (Kwini) (Cheinmora et al., 2017), Marnakiji (Walpiri) (Northern Tanami IPA, 2015), Kitjiparnta, Marnukitji, Purnuwana, Walalpa (Kukatja) (Valiquette, 1993), Koongkara (Nyikina) (DAWE, n.d.).

Field Notes Conkerberry grows as a small spreading and prickly shrub or small tree up to 3 m in height. Its leaves are bright green, lanceolate blades that are thick and leathery, measuring up to 30 mm long and 15 mm wide. Its small, scented, star-shaped flowers (appearing around October) are white and up to 7 mm in diameter. The fruit are green, changing to a bluish-black when ripe, and look similar to black olives. Conkerberry trees occur near creeks, on open floodplains, on cliff faces and in rocky patches in the Pilbara and Kimberley regions of Western Australia as well as the Northern Territory, north-east Queensland, and southwards to Grafton in New South Wales (ALA, 2022; Laasak & McCarthy, 2008; SKIPA, 2022; WAH, 2022).

Medicinal Uses The whole plant was crushed and the sap applied externally as a liniment for rheumatic pain. Decoctions of the wood pulp were taken internally to relieve the symptoms of colds and influenza. The leaves were used to smoke adults to give them strength for long walks (Fern, 2021; Lassak & McCarthy, 2001; Low, 1990; SKIPA, 2022), babies to make them strong and able to walk, or to treat diarrhoea (Kenneally et al., 2016; Wightman, 2003). Infusions of the orange inner bark were used as a wash for skin problems and to treat conjunctivitis (Olive Pink Botanic Garden, 2010). Decoctions of crushed wood were used as a mouthwash to relieve the pain of toothache. A hot compress soaked in the liquid was held against the face to relieve the pain of toothache (Smith, 1991). A small piece of the root was inserted into a cavity in a tooth to ease the pain of toothache (Cheinmora et al., 2017). Oily sap from the roots can be rubbed on skin to ease rheumatic pain (Kane, 2022). In Western Australia, the leaves and branches were used as smoke medicine to treat children with stomach ache, coughs and colds (Purdie et al., 2018; Wightman, 2003). Decoctions of the crushed roots were used as a wash to treat scabies infestations (Northern Territory Department of Health, 1981).

Other Uses The fruit of the Conkerberry are edible when ripe (soft and black) and were eaten by most Aboriginal groups across the top end of Australia between December and mid-March. The dried berries under the bush were also collected and were soaked in water before eating (Cheinmora et al., 2017; Fox & Garde, 2018; Kane, 2022; Low, 1991; Oscar et al., 2019; Purdie et al., 2018; RFCA, 1993; Wheaton, 1994; Wightman, 2003). Aboriginal people in the Kimberley burnt the wood of this plant in campfires to repel mosquitoes and other insects (Cheinmora et al., 2017; Kane, 2022; Low, 1990; Oscar et al., 2019; Purdie et al., 2018; SKIPA, 2022). The Gija used the hook part of branches to make the hook part of woomeras (throwing sticks) (Purdie et al., 2018).

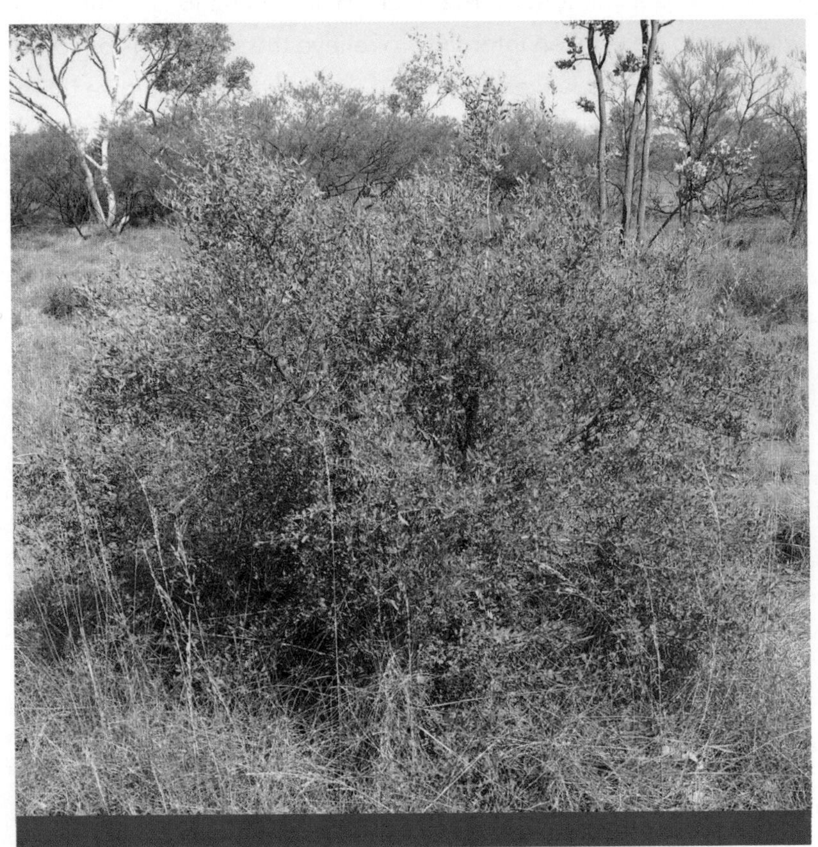

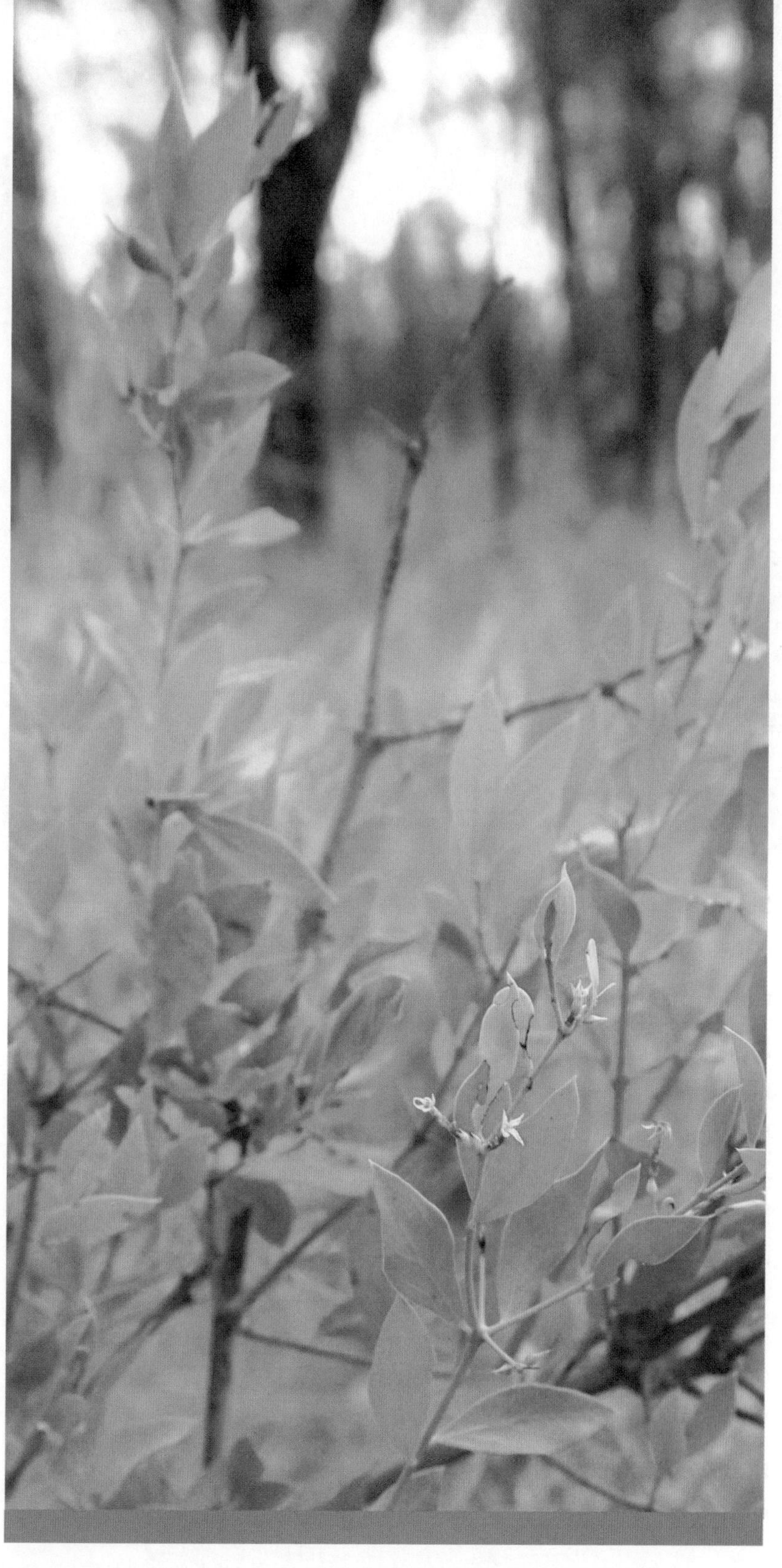

Coolibah Mistletoe

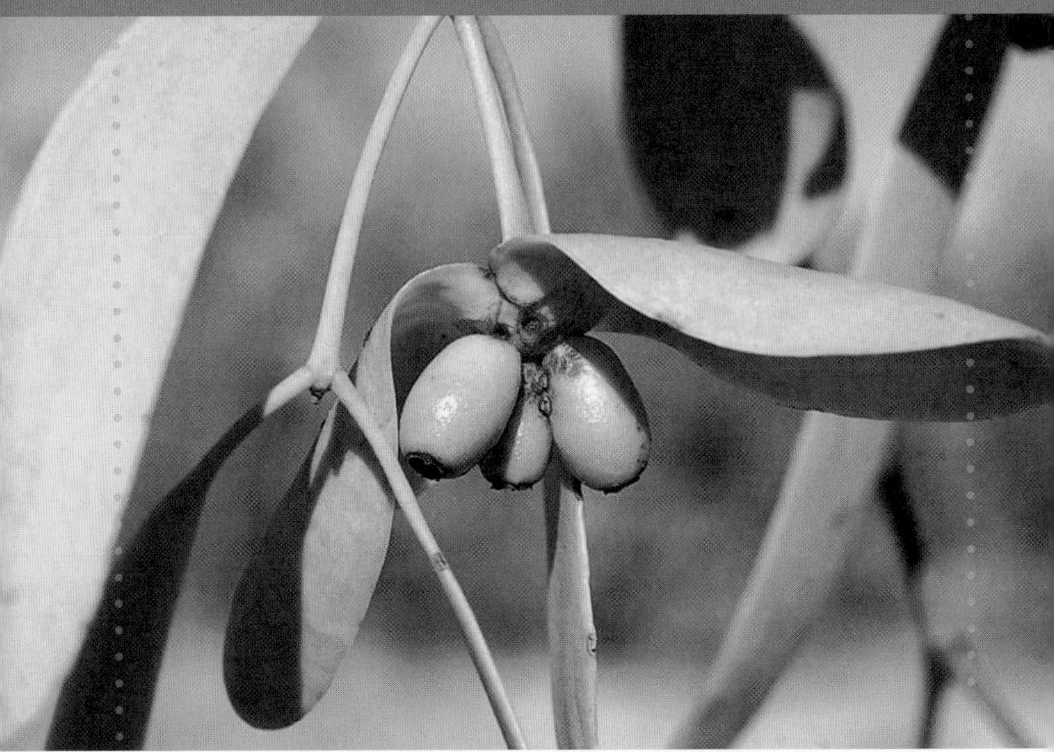

Scientific Names *Diplatia grandibractea* (F.Muell.) Tiegh., also known as *Loranthus grandibracteus* F. Muell.

Common Name Coolibah Mistletoe.

Field Notes Coolibah Mistletoe is an aerial shrub that is hemiparasitic on the stems on host trees. Its leaves are lanceolate to oblong and up to 120 mm long. Its flowers are typical green and red, pendulous, mistletoe-type and can be present any time between February and December. Its fruit are yellow-green, ovoid drupes around 10 mm long. Coolibah Mistletoe occurs on eucalypts and melaleucas in the Pilbara and Kimberley regions of Western Australia, the Northern Territory, South Australia, Queensland and New South Wales (ALA, 2022; eFlora.SA, 2022; WAH, 2022).

Medicinal Uses Decoctions of the leaves of Coolibah Mistletoe were taken internally or used as an antiseptic wash to treat sores

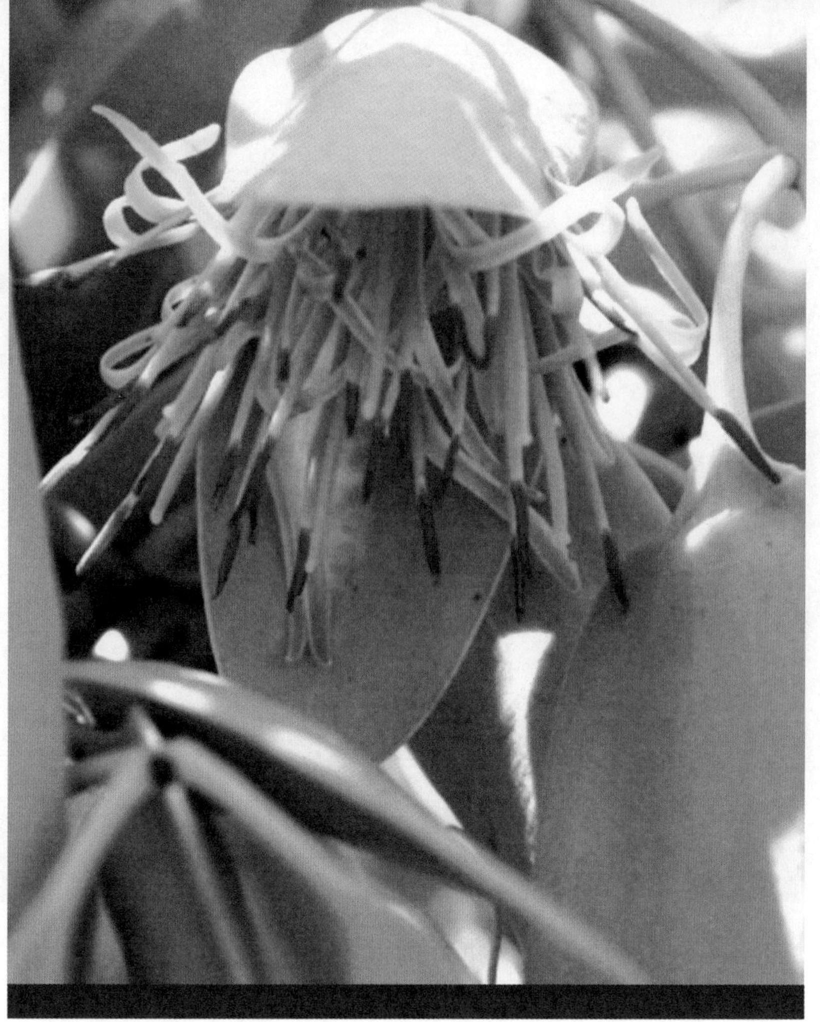

and infected wounds (Austin & Nathan, 1998).

Other Uses The fruit of the Coolabah Mistletoe are edible. The flesh was eaten and the seeds were discarded (Nyinkka Nyunyu Art and Culture Centre, n.d.).

Cordia Tree

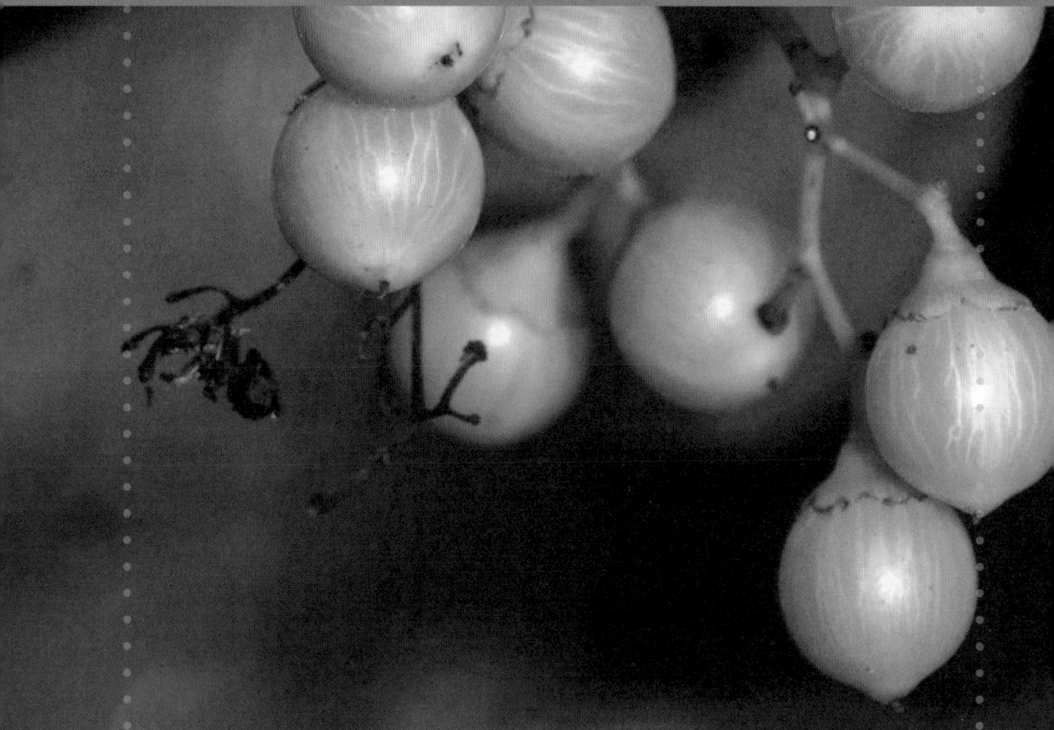

Scientific Name *Cordia dichotoma* G.Forst.

Common Names Cordia Tree, Glue Berry Tree, Clammy Cherry, Fragrant Manjack, Snotty Gobbles.

Field Notes The Cordia Tree is a deciduous shrub or tree growing up to 10 m in height. Its large, dark green, lanceolate leaves are up to 210 mm long. In Western Australia, its small, white flowers are present from November to December or from January to March. Its globose fruit are yellow or pinkish-yellow and shiny, turning black as they ripen. The pulp is sticky when the fruit are ripe. In Australia, the Cordia Tree occurs on moist sites, often along watercourses, along the coast in the Kimberley region of Western Australia, the Northern Territory and along the Queensland coast as far south as Townsville. It also occurs in India, New Caledonia and South-east Asia (ALA, 2022; ATRP, 2020; WAH, 2022).

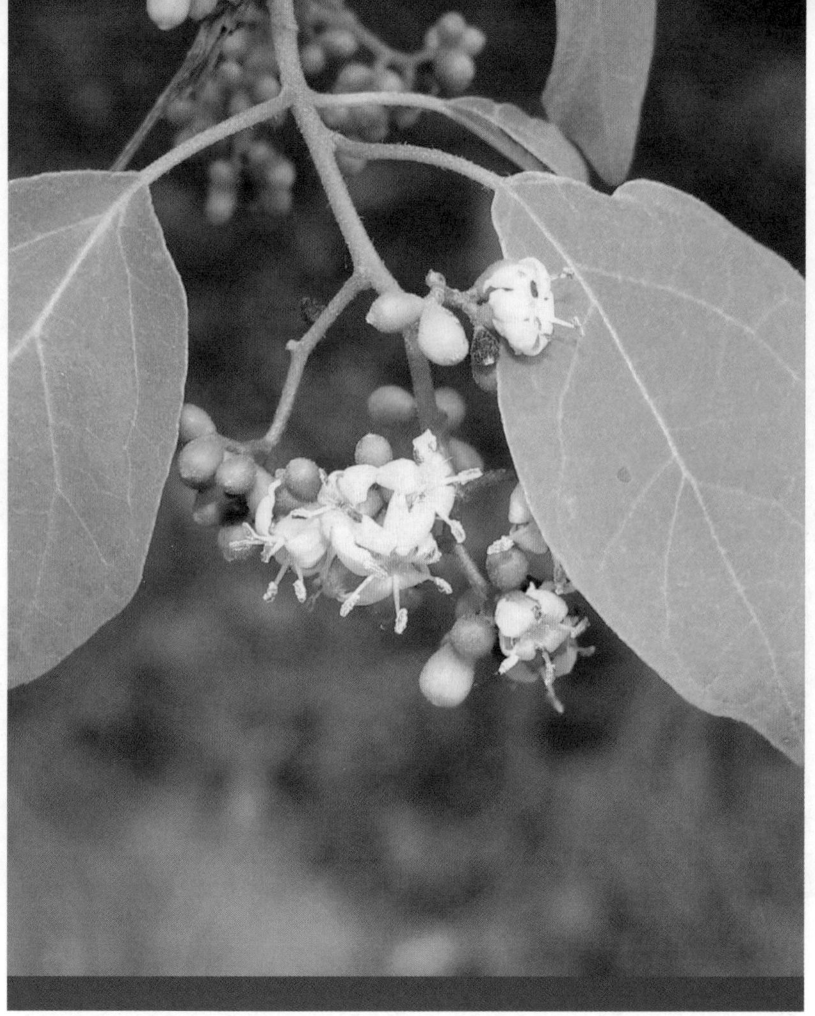

Medicinal Uses Parts of the plant are used in folk medicine in some Asian countries. The powdered seeds are mixed with oil and applied to skin eruptions and dermatophytosis (ringworm and tinea corporis). Decoctions of the stem bark are taken internally to treat dyspepsia, diarrhoea, dysentery, headache, stomach ache and as a tonic. Moistened bark is applied as a poultice to boils and swellings. The leaves are crushed and applied externally as a poultice to treat migraine, inflammation and swellings. The fruit is used to treat coughs and pulmonary diseases (Fern, 2021).

Other Uses The fruit of the Cordia Tree are edible raw or cooked. The green fruit are pickled in some countries (Fern, 2021; Jackes, 2010; Maiden, 1889). The kernel is also edible (Maiden, 1889).

Crab's Eyes

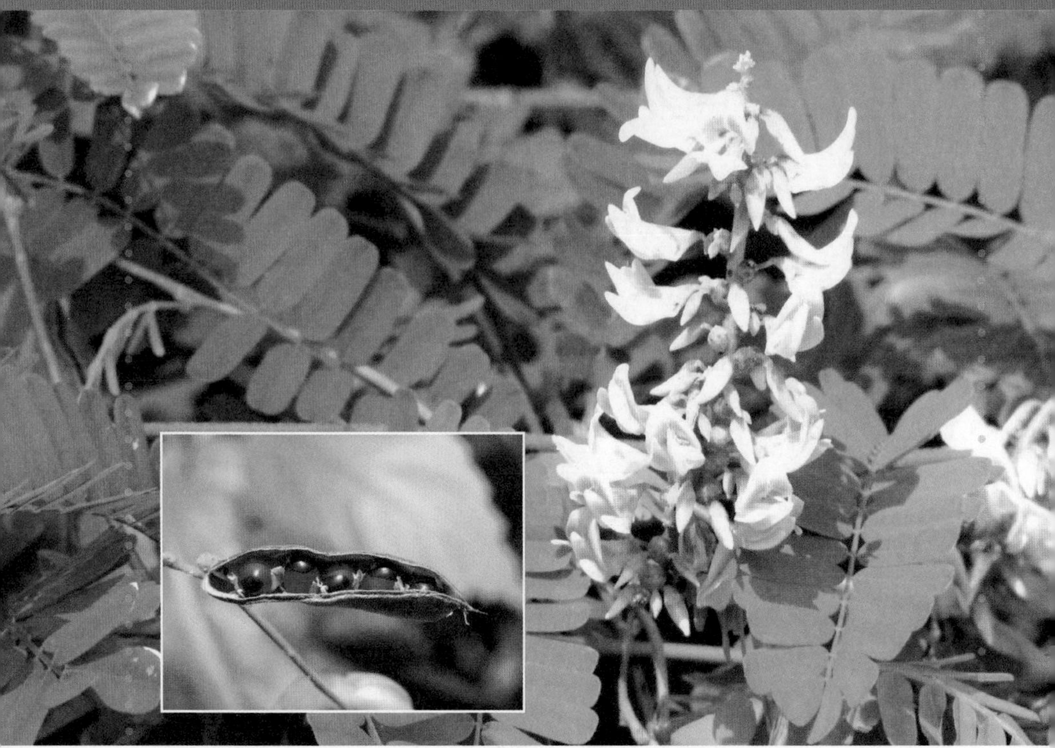

Scientific Name *Abrus precatorius* L.

Common Names Crab's Eyes, Crab's Eye Bean, Crab's-eye Creeper, Giddee-Giddee, Indian Liquorice, Jequirity Bean, Rosary and many other colloquial names.

Aboriginal Names Ngaminy-ngaminy (Bardi) (Smith & Kalotas, 1985), Ngaming-ngaming (Bardi) (Kenneally, 2018), Jinjalgurany (Yawuru) (Kenneally et al., 1996), Jirrindi (Gija, Jaru) (Wightman, 2003), Ngarwaluwali (Bunuba) (Moss et al., 2021).

Field Notes Crab's Eyes is a herbaceous, slender, perennial climbing plant that twines around trees and shrubs. It has up to 36 leaflets per compound leaf, each leaflet blade measuring up to 25 mm by 8 mm, with the underside of each sparsely covered in prostrate hairs. Its pale pink, pea-type flowers are borne in dense racemes up to 50 mm long and can be present for most of the year in Australia. Its fruit are pods up to 50 mm long by 15 mm wide, containing up to seven very poisonous seeds that look like a crab's eyes, as the common name suggests. In Australia, Crab's Eyes occurs in sand, sandstone, limestone and basalt in coastal areas and inland, sometimes along creek lines, in the Kimberley region of Western Australia, the Northern Territory and along the Queensland coast as far as the border with New South Wales. It also occurs in Africa, China, India, Indonesia, Malaysia, New Guinea, the Philippines and the Western Pacific (ALA, 2022; ATRP, 2020; WAH, 2022).

Medicinal Uses Crab's Eyes is used in folk medicine in some countries. The seeds are dried and ground to a paste, which is applied externally to treat sciatica, hair loss, skin diseases, leprosy, nervous debility and paralysis. Decoctions of the leaves are taken internally to treat sore throats and a range of chest conditions, including asthma, bronchitis and dry coughs. A paste made from the roots is applied to boils and carbuncles to draw them out. Decoctions of the bark are taken internally to treat stomach ache, thrush, colds, coughs, sore throats and asthma (ATRP, 2020; Fern, 2021).

Other Uses The thoroughly cooked seeds of Crab's Eyes are sometimes eaten in times when food is scarce, though they are reported to remain hard and are not very digestible. Apparently, heat over 65 degrees Celsius 'breaks down the toxic principles' in the seeds (Fern, 2021). The seeds are used to make beads and in percussion instruments (Fern, 2021).

CAUTION: Ingestion of a single well-chewed seed that has not been heated and prepared for consumption can be fatal to both children and adults (Fern, 2021).

Crocodile Tree

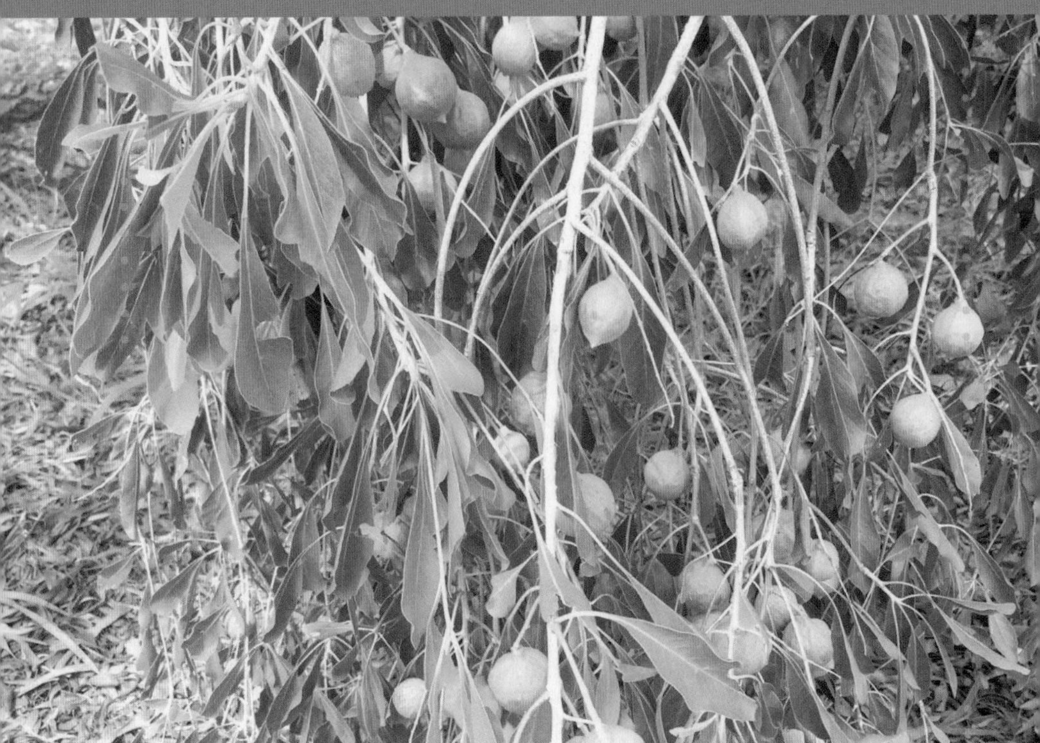

Scientific Name *Terminalia arostrata* Ewart & O.B.Davies.

Common Names Crocodile Tree, Bush Peanut, Nutwood.

Aboriginal Names Bardiging (Miriwoong) (Mirima Dawang Woorlab-gerring, 2021), Baregel, Bardigil, Bardiginy (Gija) (Purdie et al., 2018), Bardigi, Miyany, (Jaru) (Wightman, 2003), Bardigi (Miwa) (Kimberley Specialists, 2020).

Field Notes The Crocodile Tree is a deciduous or semi-deciduous tree that grows to around 12 m in height. It has ovate leaves that are up to 130 mm long and beaked fruit that are present the whole year round. Its white, orange or red flowers are present between July and November. Crocodile Trees are found in heavy soils and alluvium in seasonal swampy areas and basaltic plains in the central Kimberley region around Halls Creek, the north-west corner of the Northern Territory and the north-east corner of Queensland (ALA, 2022; WAH, 2022).

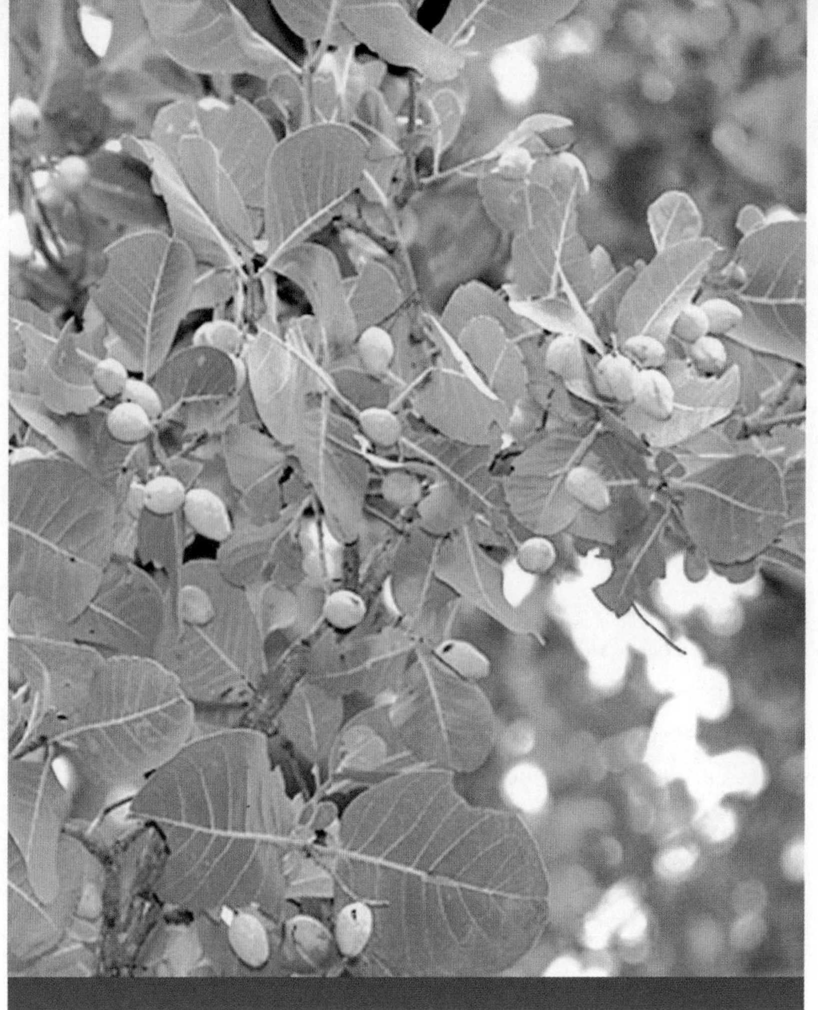

Medicinal Uses Decoctions of the fresh leaves and twigs were used as a medicinal wash to help draw out boils and carbuncles, and to reduce a high fever (Smith, 1991). The leaves were used by the Gija for the 'steaming treatment of colds and influenza' (Purdie et al., 2018).

Other Uses The kernels of the seeds of the Crocodile Tree are edible and were eaten raw (ALA, 2022; Purdie et al., 2018; Smith, 1991; Wightman, 2003). The fruit are usually collected from the ground early in the dry season and are cracked between stones to remove the kernels (Kimberley Specialists, 2020; RFCA, 1993).

Croton

Scientific Name *Croton tomentellus* F.Muell.

Common Name Croton.

Aboriginal Name Ankoolmarr (Bardi) (Paddy et al., 1993).

Field Notes Croton is a monoecious (having male and female flowers on the same plant) shrub, growing up to 4 m in height. Its ovate leaf blades are up to 100 mm long. Its Inflorescences are up to 130 mm long with yellow male and female flowers that are approximately 3 mm in diameter. Flowering is between November and March. The fruit are capsules about 6–8 mm in diameter, clothed in star-shaped scales. Croton occurs on granite, sandstone and basalt, in vine thickets and monsoon forest in the Kimberley region of Western Australia. It also occurs in Brunei, Indonesia, Malaysia, New Guinea and the Philippines (ATRP, 2020; WAH, 2022).

Medicinal Uses Crushed leaves of Croton were applied as a poultice to areas of arthritic and rheumatic pain (Paddy et al., 1993).

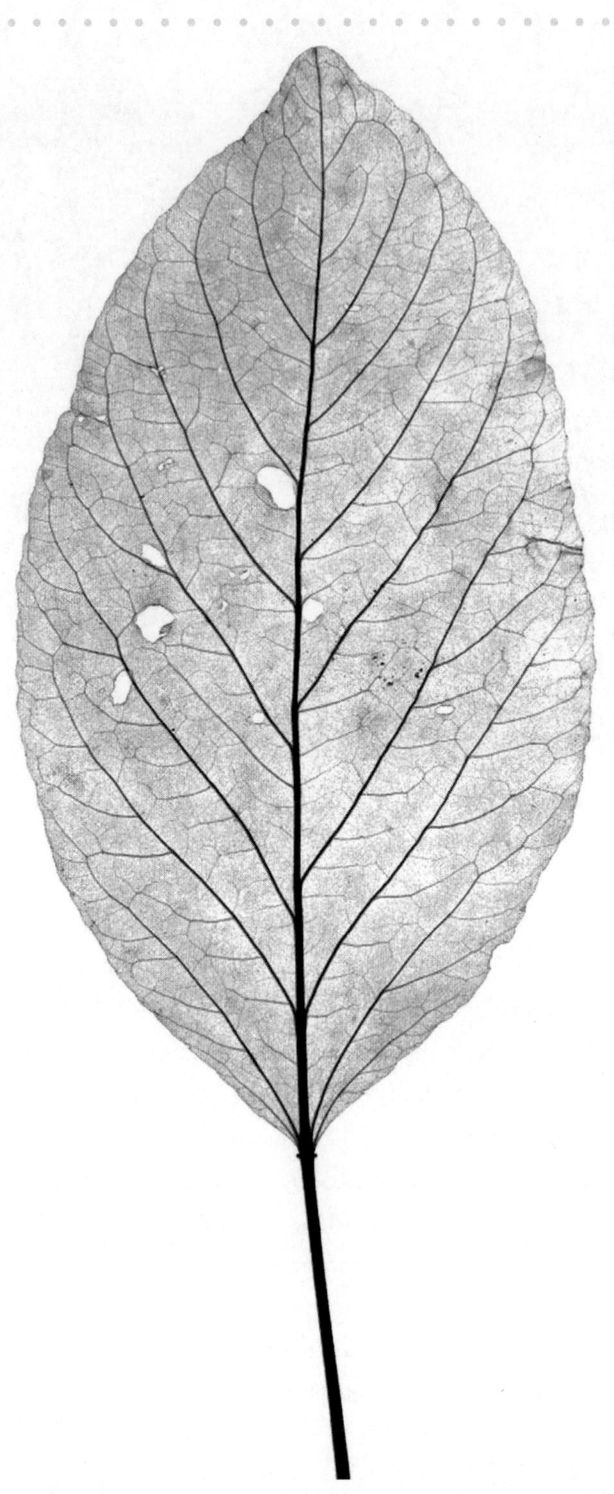

Cucumis

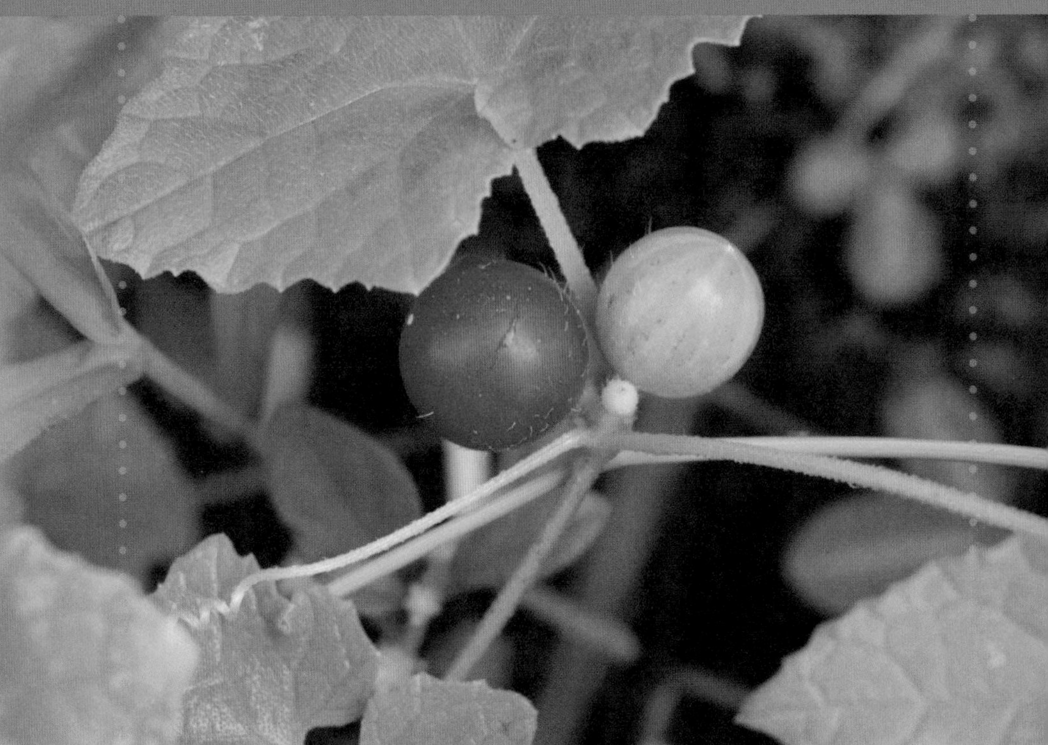

Scientific Name *Cucumis althaeoides* (Ser.) P.Sebastian & I.Telford.

Common Name Cucumis.

Field Notes Cucumis is a trailing or climbing perennial vine that is monoecious (having both the male and female reproductive organs on the same plant) with stems up to 3 m long. Most of its vegetative parts are covered with hairs or bristles. Its leaves are arrowhead-shaped and are up to 75 mm long. It has small, yellow, star-shaped flowers. Its male flowers occur in crowded bundles of up to 15. Its female flowers occur in groups of up to four. Its fruit are spherical, pale green with darker green linear markings, and up to 18 mm in diameter, turning red as they mature. Cucumis occurs in the Pilbara and Kimberley regions of Western Australia, the Northern Territory, Queensland and northern New South Wales. It is pantropical and occurs in Africa, India, South-east Asia and the Pacific (ALA, 2022; eFlora.SA, 2022).

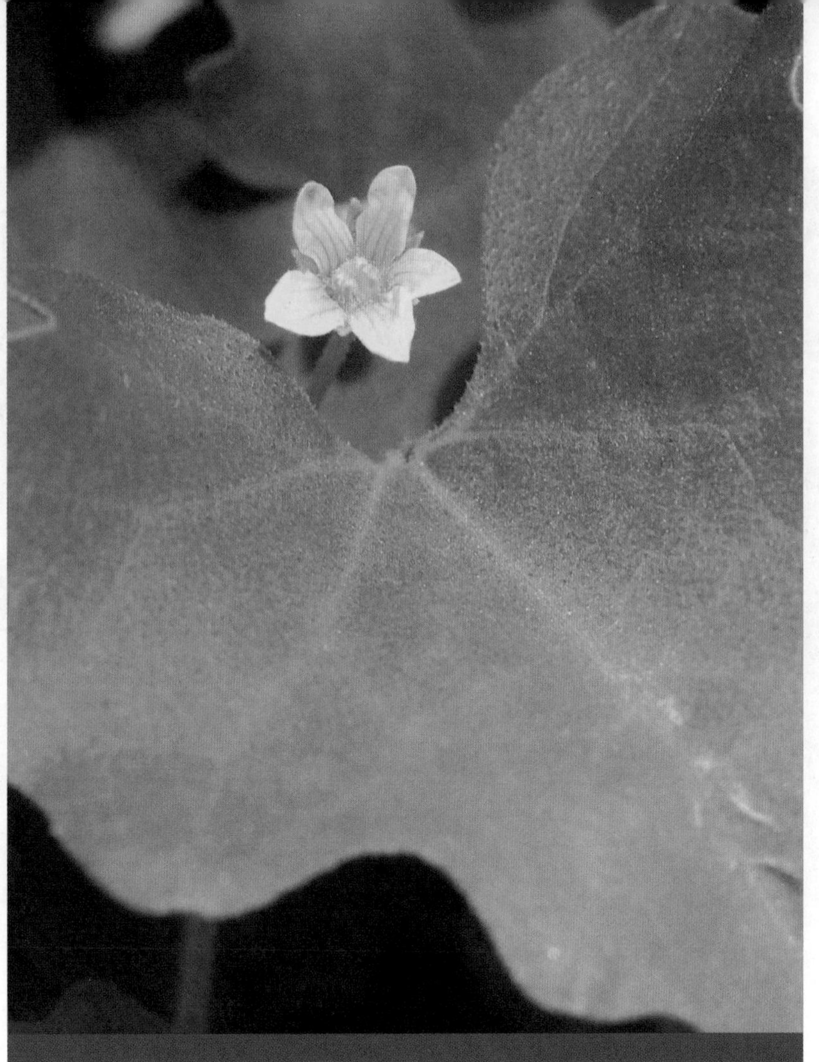

Medicinal Uses The leaves of Cucumis were pulped, wetted and applied as a compress to the head to treat headaches and insomnia (Morse, 2005).

Other Uses The fruit, leaves and tender shoots of Cucumis are edible and eaten in some Asian countries (Nutrition Security, 2020).

Currant Bush

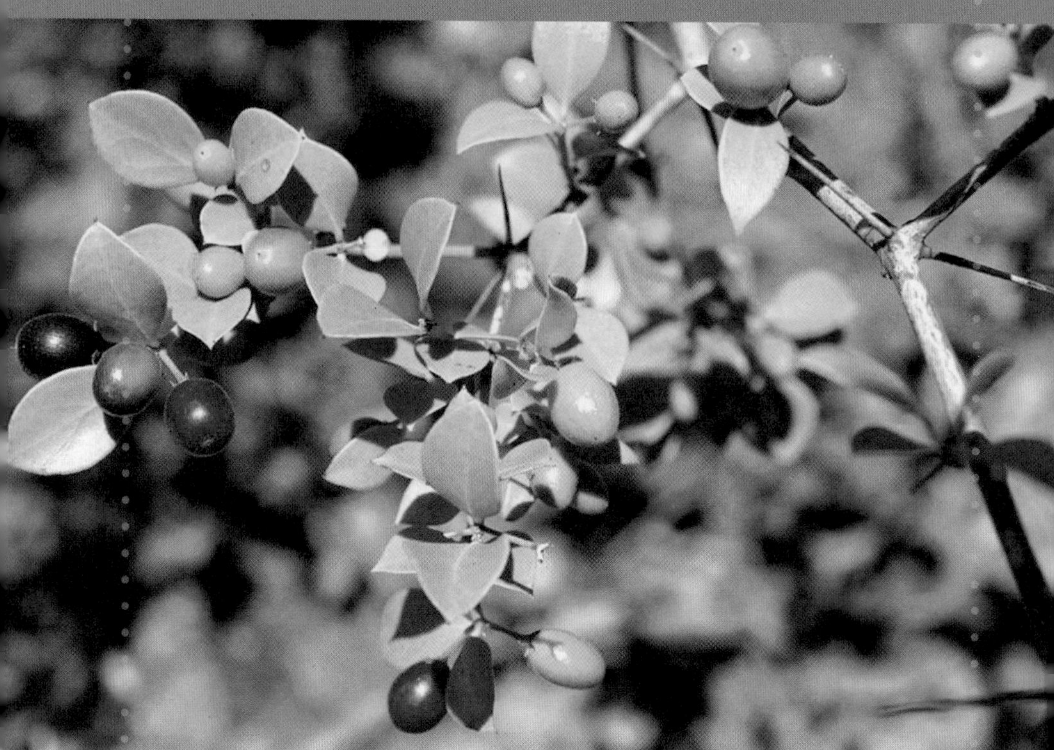

Scientific Name *Carissa spinarum* L., previously known as *Carissa ovata* R.Br.

Common Names Currant Bush, Bush Plum, Conkerberry, Kunkerberry.

Field Notes Currant Bush is an open, spiny shrub with thorny stems that grows to around 3 m in height in good conditions. Its leaves are glossy, ovate, opposite and up to 40 mm long. Its white, perfumed, star-shaped flowers are approximately 10 mm across. Its ovoid fruit are black when ripe and are approximately 10 mm long. Currant Bush occurs in sandy soil among sandstone rocks and dolerite boulders on rocky sites and at the foot of scree slopes in the Pilbara and Kimberley regions of Western Australia and on nearby islands. It also occurs in the Northern Territory, Queensland and eastern New South Wales (ALA, 2022; Noosa's Native Plants, 2022; Save Our Waterways Now, n.d.; WAH, 2022).

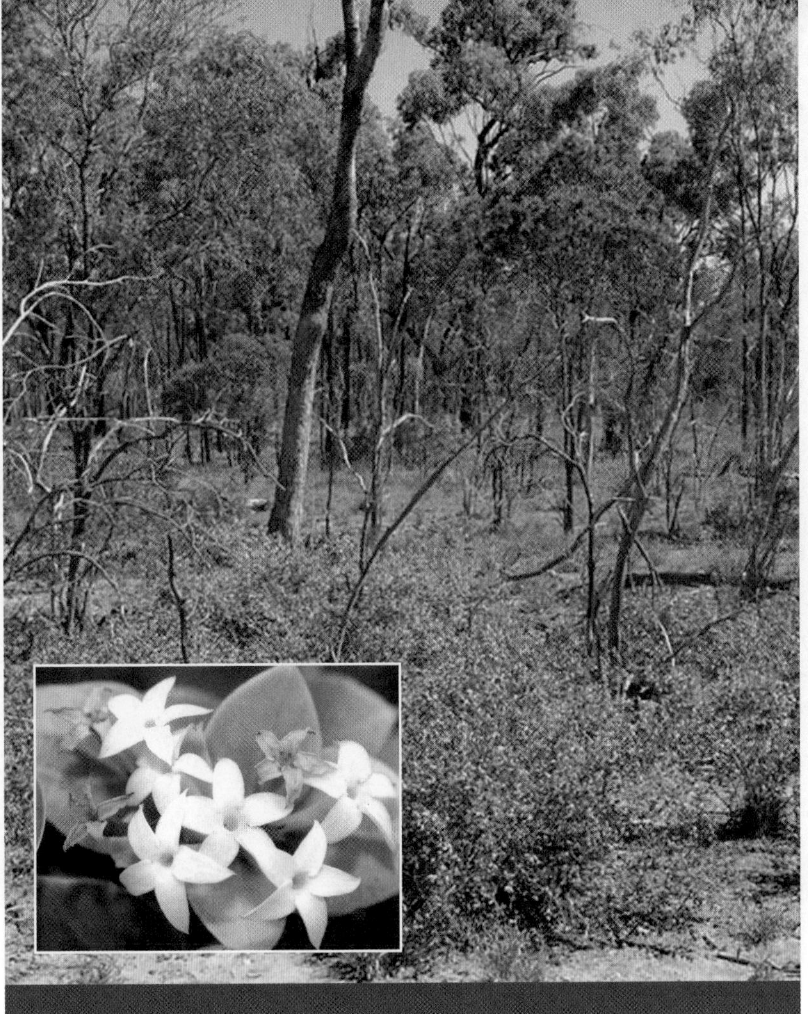

Medicinal Uses Webb (1959) relates that 'the whole plant, including roots, is chipped into small pieces to get an oily sap which is rubbed on for rheumatism', presumably to ease rheumatic pain. Infusions of the inner bark of the roots were used as a wash to treat skin conditions and conjunctivitis (Morse, 2005).

Other Uses The fruit of the Currant Bush are edible when black and ripe.

CAUTION: The fruit should not be eaten before they are ripe or when there is discernible milky sap oozing from them, as they are poisonous at this stage (Fern, 2021; Jackes, 2010; Maiden, 1889; Vigilante et al., 2013).

Cuthbertson's Wattle

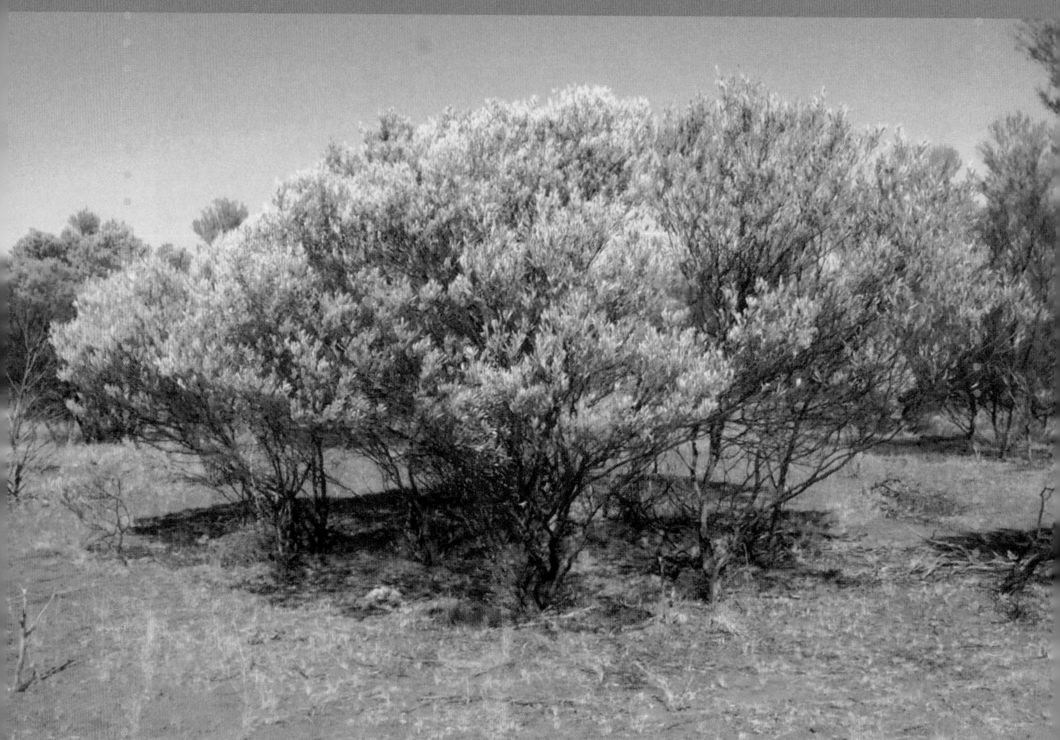

Scientific Name *Acacia cuthbertsonii* Luehm.

Common Name Cuthbertson's Wattle.

Aboriginal Names Kalirrma, Wilpiya, Yarlpirri (Kukatja) (Valiquette, 1993), Matu (Ngardi), Wilpiya (Ngardi, Kukatja) (Cataldi, 2004).

Field Notes Cuthbertson's Wattle is a bushy, often gnarled shrub or tree that grows up to 5 m in height. It has fissured bark that flakes off in brittle pieces. Its phyllodes are elliptic to narrowly elliptic or linear and up to 110 mm long. Its yellow, globular flower heads are present in January or from April to December. The fruit or seed pods are narrowly oblong to linear, shallowly constricted between seeds, sometimes curved and up to 140 mm long. Cuthbertson's Wattle occurs in rocky sand or clay, on gibber plains, stony rises and along creeks and drainage lines in the Pilbara and southern Kimberley regions of Western Australia, and in the Northern Territory (ALA, 2022; WAH, 2022; World Wide Wattle, 2022).

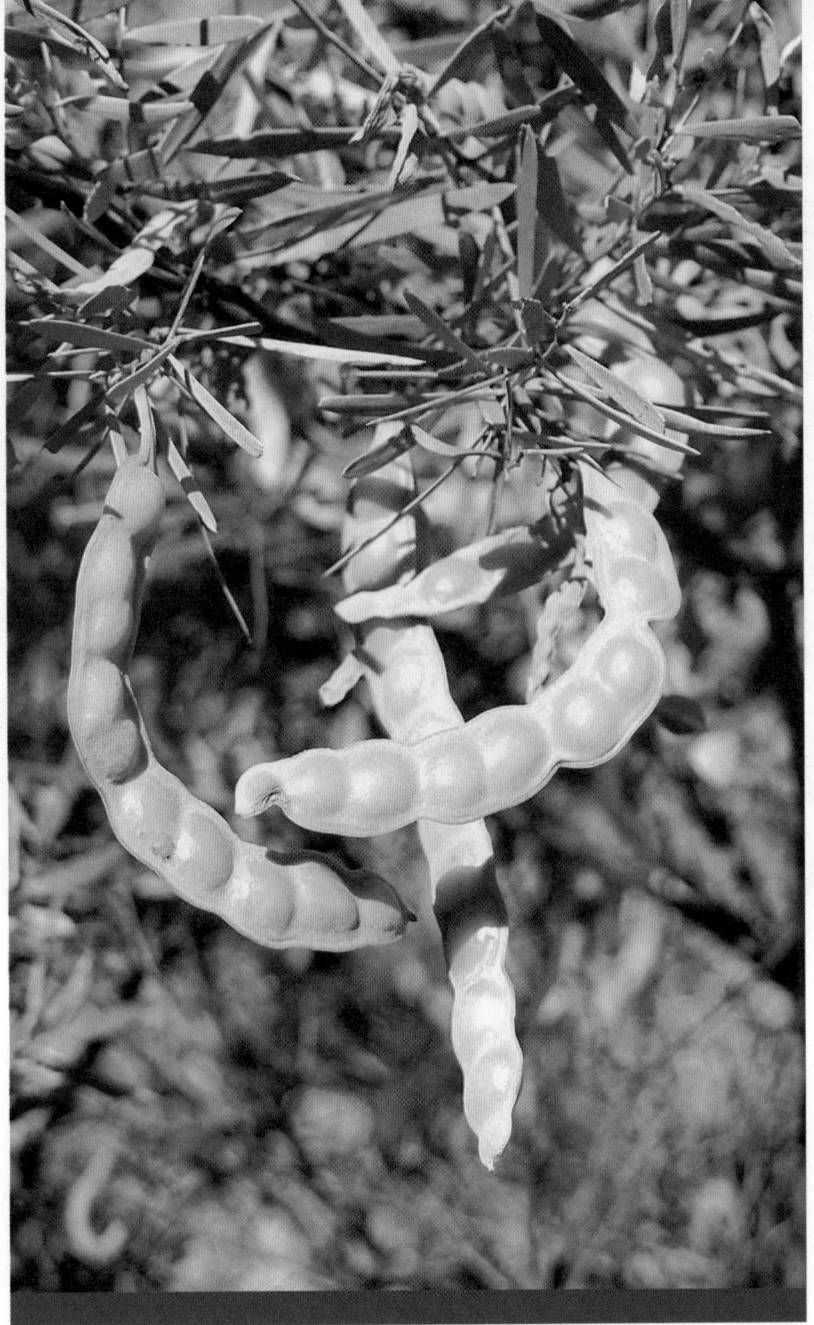

Medicinal Uses The bark of Cuthbertson's Wattle is used by some Aboriginal groups to treat toothache (Australian Native Edible & Medicinal Seed Service, n.d.).

Daly River Satinash

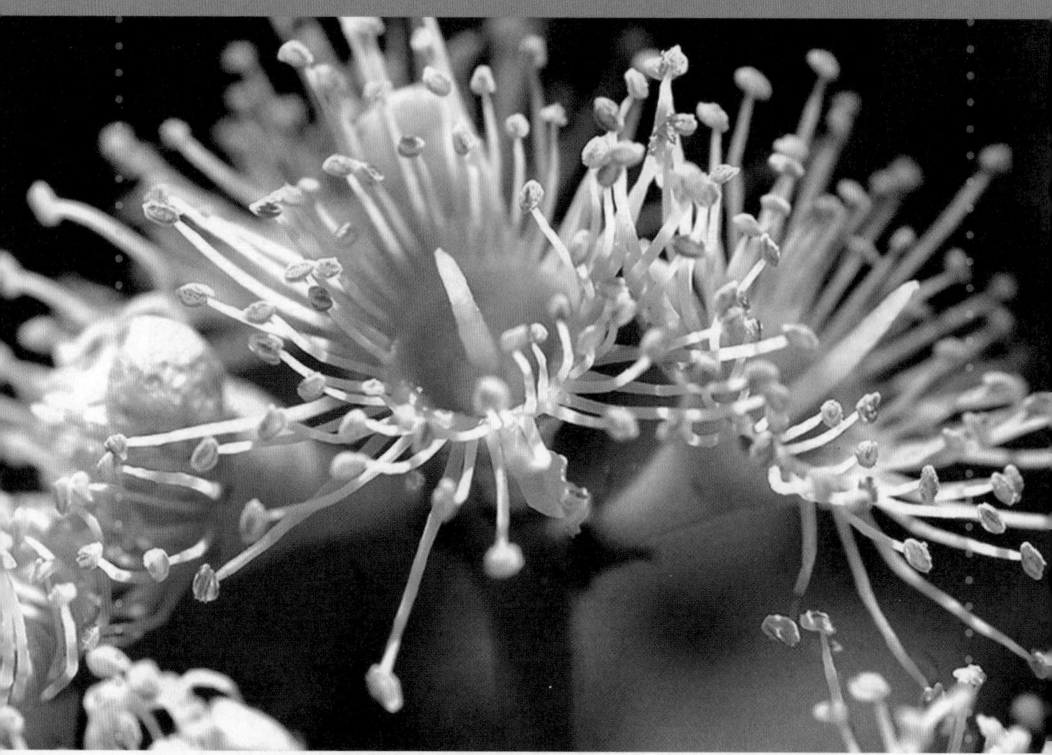

Scientific Name *Syzygium nervosum* DC.

Common Name Daly River Satinash.

Field Notes Daly River Satinash is a many-branched, evergreen tree that grows up to 15 m in height. The bark is brown or reddish brown and coarsely flaky. The leaves are obovate with a pointed apex and base and are up to 180 mm long. Its white, spiky flowers have long stamens but no petals. Its fruit are purple ellipsoid berries with white flesh, and are roughly 18 mm long and 12 mm in diameter. In Australia, Daly River Satinash is found in forests, on the sides of streams, in rainforests, around the margins of swamps or near perennial creeks in the top end of the Kimberley region of Western Australia and the Northern Territory (ALA, 2022; ATRP, 2020; WAH, 2022). It also occurs in southern China, on the Indian subcontinent, in Indonesia, Malaysia, Myanmar, Thailand, Vietnam and the Philippines (Fern, 2021).

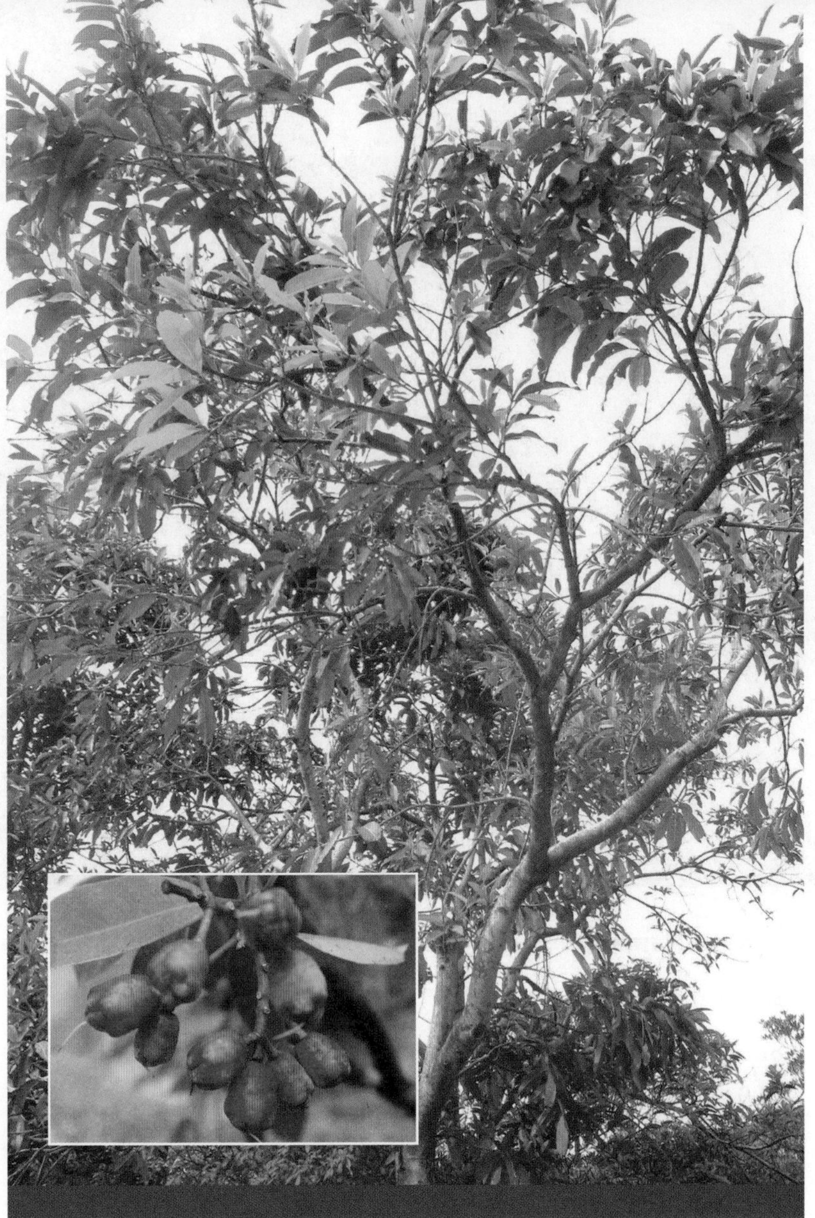

Medicinal Uses In Vietnam, the leaves and buds of Daly River Satinash are brewed as a herbal tea known as *nước vối* that is reported to stimulate the appetite and assist digestion (Nguyen, 1993).

Other Uses The fruit of the Daly River Satinash are eaten raw when they are purple and ripe after the wet season or made into drinks and preserves (Australian Bushfoods, 2022; Territory Native Plants, 2022).

Damson Plum

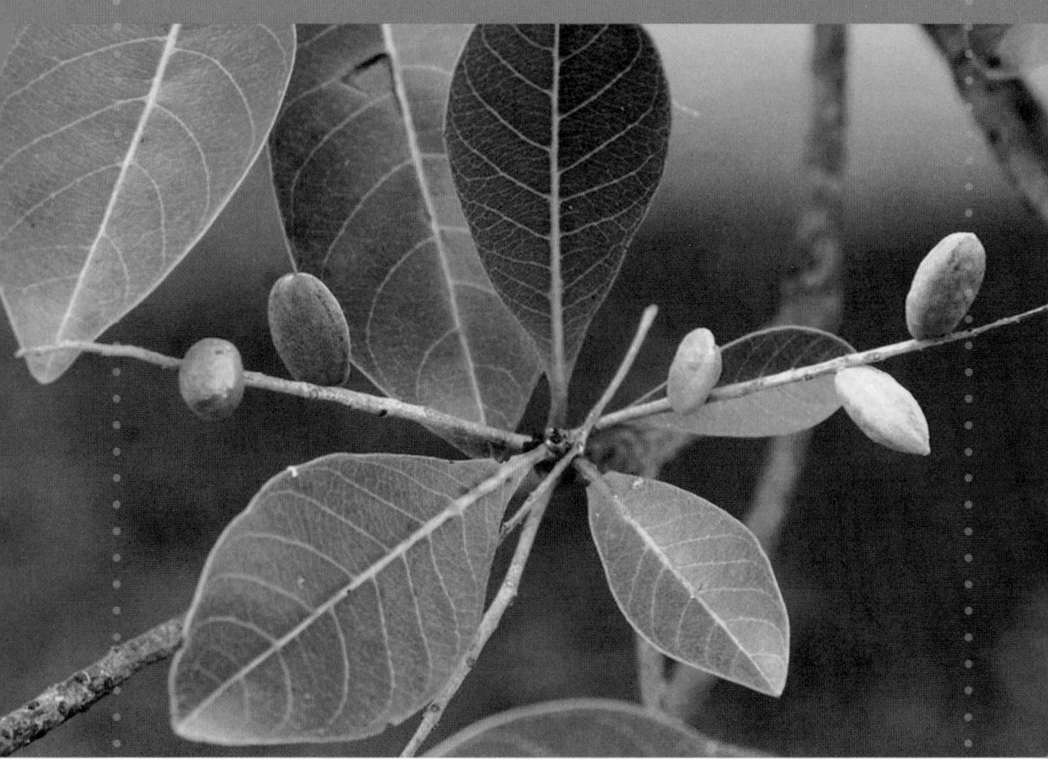

Scientific Name *Terminalia microcarpa* Decne.

Common Names Damson Plum, Bandicoot, Sovereign Wood.

Aboriginal Names Gundulu (Wunambal, Gaambera) (Karadada et al., 2011), Kundulu (Kwini) (Cheinmora et al., 2017).

Field Notes Damson Plum is a deciduous tree that grows up to 30 m in height. Its large, obovate, alternate leaves are up to 135 mm long with a shiny upper surface, but with some small, silky hairs present on the lower surface. Its small, cream flowers that form on racemes are present from September to October. The plum-like, ovoid fruit are approximately 50 mm long, and are dark purple when ripe. Damson Plum occurs around springs and swamps or on rocky creek beds in the Kimberley region of Western Australia, the top end of the Northern Territory and in Queensland from the Cape York Peninsula down the coast to Cairns (ALA, 2022; James Cook University, 2022; WAH, 2022). It also occurs in Indonesia, Malaysia,

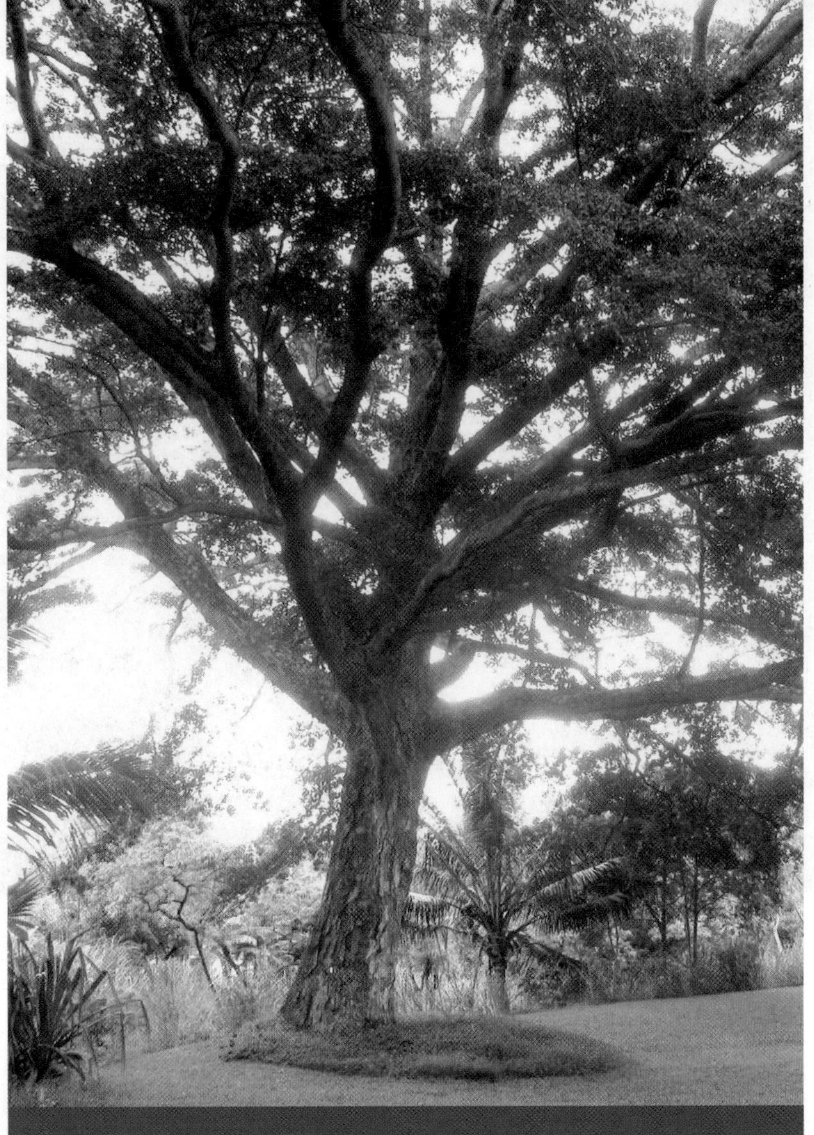

New Guinea and the Philippines (Fern, 2021).

Medicinal Uses The fruit of Damson Plum have been used in folk medicine in some Asian countries. Infusions of the fruit are used as an eyewash to treat conjunctivitis. The fruit are also used in lotions to treat humid herpetic lesions and eczema (Fern, 2021).

Other Uses The fruit of the Damson Plum are edible when purple and ripe. They are available after flowering finishes in November (Bindon, 2014; Cheinmora et al., 2017; City of Darwin, 2013; Fox & Garde, 2018; Karadada et al., 2011; RFCA, 1993; Territory Native Plants, 2022; Top End Native Plants Society, 2020).

Desert Cassia

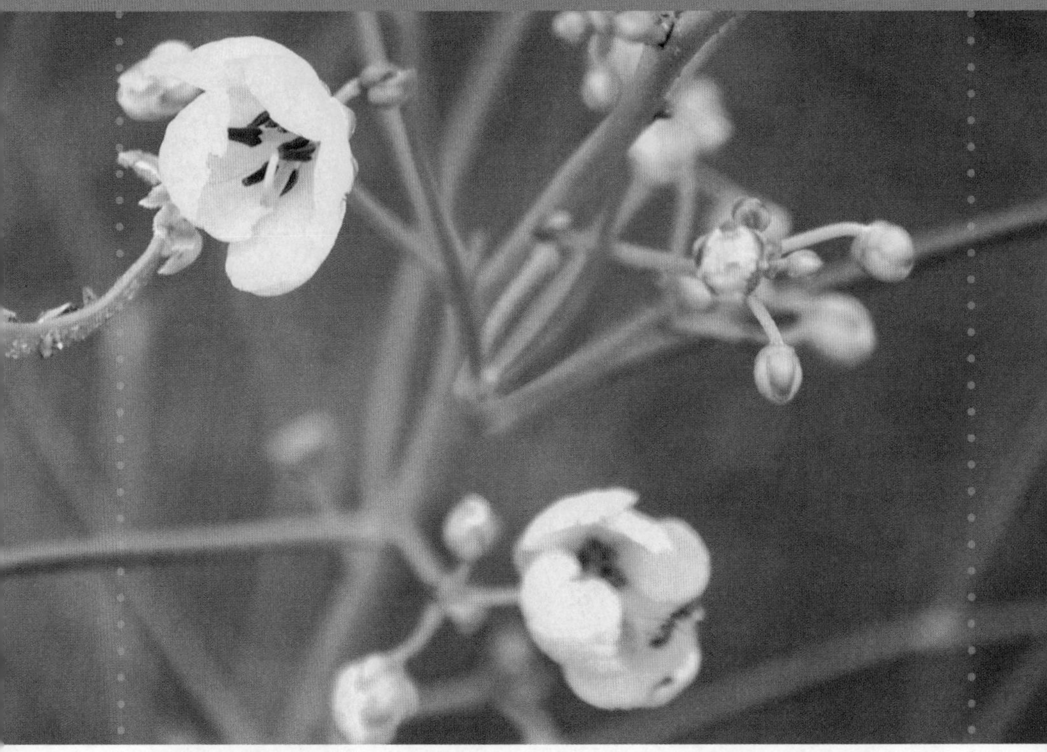

Scientific Name *Senna artemisioides* (DC.) Randell, previously known as *Cassia artemisioides* DC.

Common Names Desert Cassia, Silver Senna, Silver Cassia, Feathery Cassia, Wormwood Senna.

Field Notes Desert Cassia is a shrub that grows up to 3 m in height. It has grey-green, pinnate leaves approximately 50 mm long and yellow flowers up to 15 mm in diameter that are present most of the year. Flowering is followed by the appearance of flat, green pods that are up to 70 mm long, and which age to dark brown. Desert Cassia occurs in sand, loam or in stony or gravelly soils in a variety of habitats over most of Australia, including Tasmania (ALA, 2022; WAH, 2022).

Medicinal Uses Decoctions of the leaves of the Desert Cassia were used as a wash to aid the healing of sores and wounds (McDonald, 1988; Olive Pink Botanic Garden, 2013; Wild, 2020).

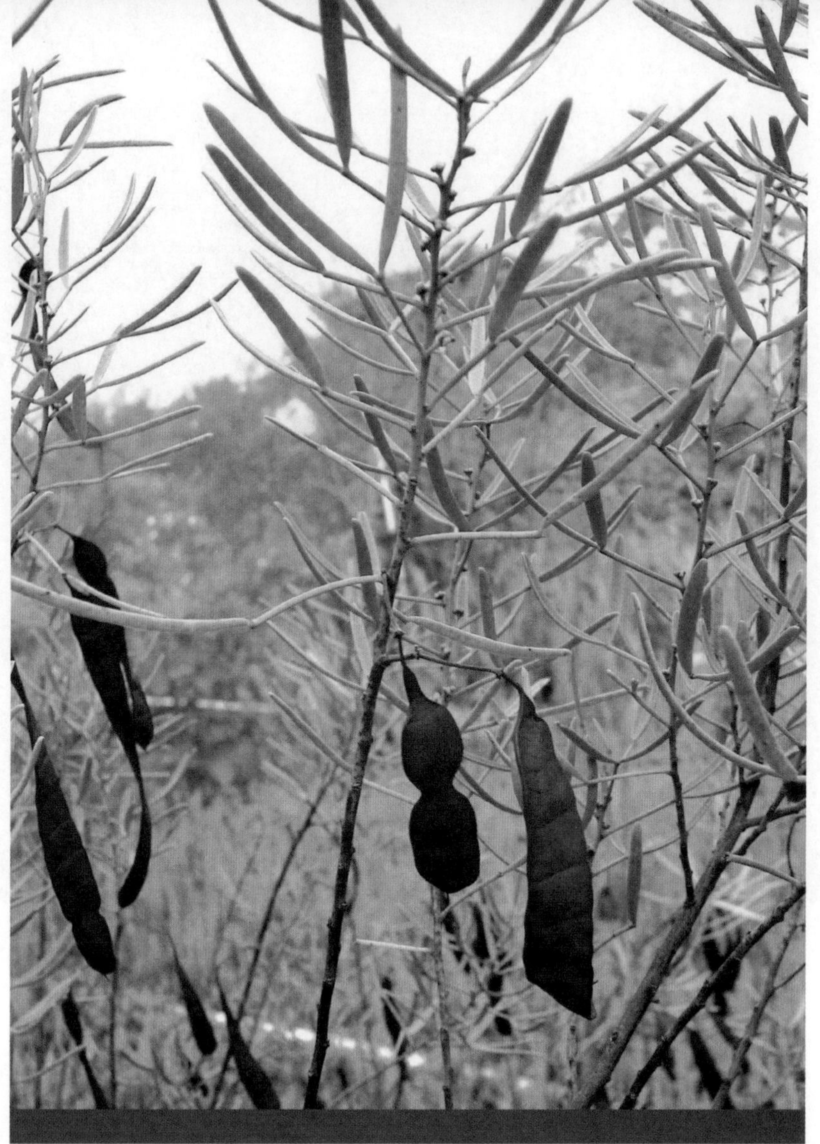

Other Uses The seeds of the Desert Cassia are edible (Wild, 2020). Edible grubs can be found in the roots of the tree in some areas (Olive Pink Botanic Garden, 2013).

Desert Oak

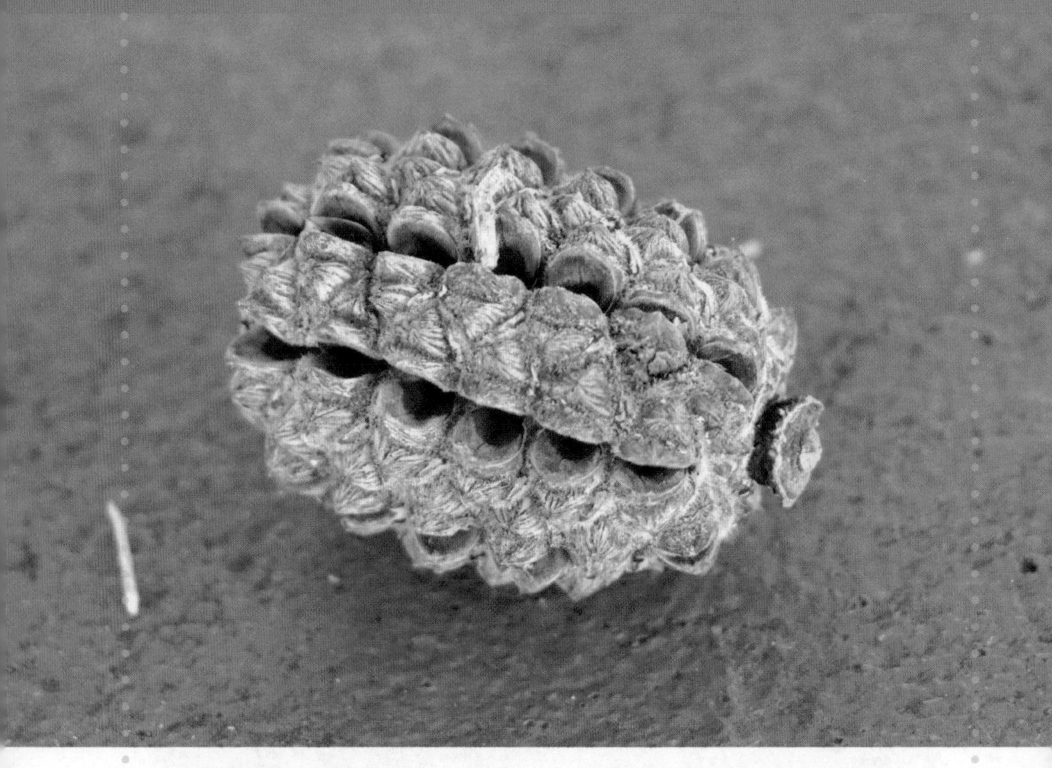

Scientific Name *Allocasuarina decaisneana* (F.Muell.) L.A.S.Johnson.

Common Names Desert Oak, Desert She-oak.

Aboriginal Names Yarnandi (Gija, Jaru) (Wightman, 1993), Kyurrkapi, Kurrkara, Ngurrarangka, Nyinyirrpalangu, Nyirrpi, Parka-parrka, Tjangkapi, Tjangkatimara, Witulawu-lawu (Kukatja) (Valiquette, 1993), Kurrkara, Kurrkapi, Kurrkayi, Jangkardi (Ngardi) (Cataldi, 2004).

Field Notes Desert Oak is a dioecious tree that grows up to 16 m or more in height. Instead of leaves the tree has long, olive green, segmented branchlets, known as cladodes, that resemble pine needles. Small, fluffy red or brown flowers form between March and June. Its large cylindrical cones are the largest of all the species, measuring up to 100 mm long. Desert Oak occurs in red sand in swales between sand dunes in the dry desert regions of Western

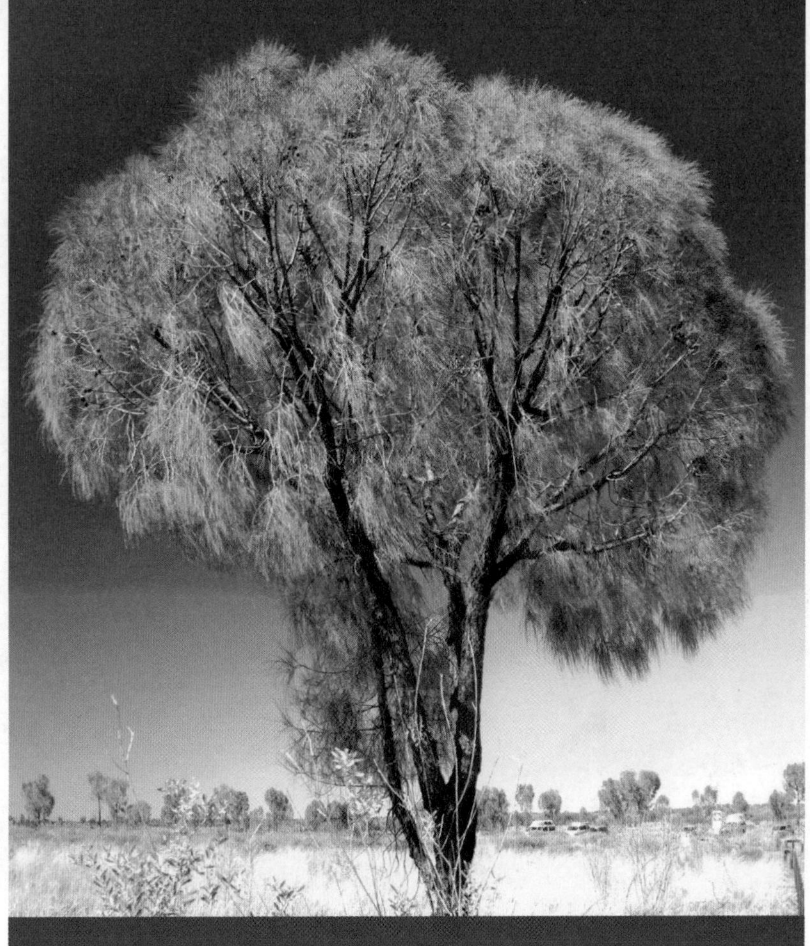

Australia, the Northern Territory and South Australia. In Western Australia it occurs in the east Pilbara, Halls Creek, Ngaanyatjarraku and Wiluna Local Government Areas (ALA, 2022; WAH, 2022).

Medicinal Uses The leaves of the Desert Oak are burnt and the white ash is applied to wounds and sores as an antiseptic powder. The moist inner surface of the bark is used for the same purpose (Valiquette, 1993).

Other Uses The seeds and gum of the Desert Oak are edible. The seeds are extracted from the woody cones and are roasted before they are eaten (Barker, 1991; Uluru-Kata Tjuta National Park, n.d.; Valiquette, 1993). The cones reportedly exude a sweet, white fluid in the warmer months that is good for drinking (Uluru-Kata Tjuta National Park, n.d.; Valiquette, 1993). The roots of the Desert Oak are a good source of water (Williams, 2020).

Desert Spurge

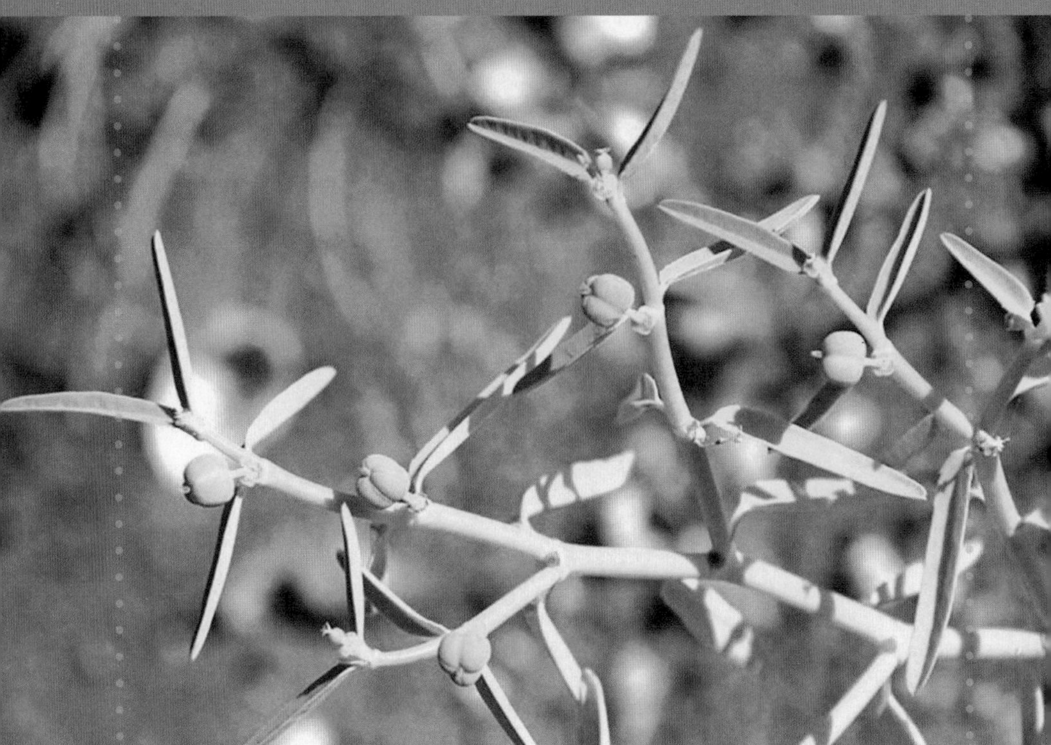

Scientific Name *Euphorbia tannensis* Spreng.

Common Name Desert Spurge.

Field Notes Desert Spurge is an erect annual or perennial herb or shrub that grows to 1 m in height. Its leaf blades are linear, up to 70 mm long and 7 mm wide, with toothed margins. Its small, green-yellow flowers appear between January and September. Its fruit are oblong to ovoid, three-lobed and up to 5 mm long. Desert Spurge occurs in stony or sandy soils all over most of mainland Australia except for south-east Victoria and the south-west of Western Australia (ALA, 2022; SMIP, 2022; WAH, 2022).

Medicinal Uses The whole plant was heated on a fire until soft then, when cool, rubbed over the body to treat scabies infestations. Alternatively, the latex was squeezed out and boiled in water and the decoction used for the same purpose (Smith, 1991).

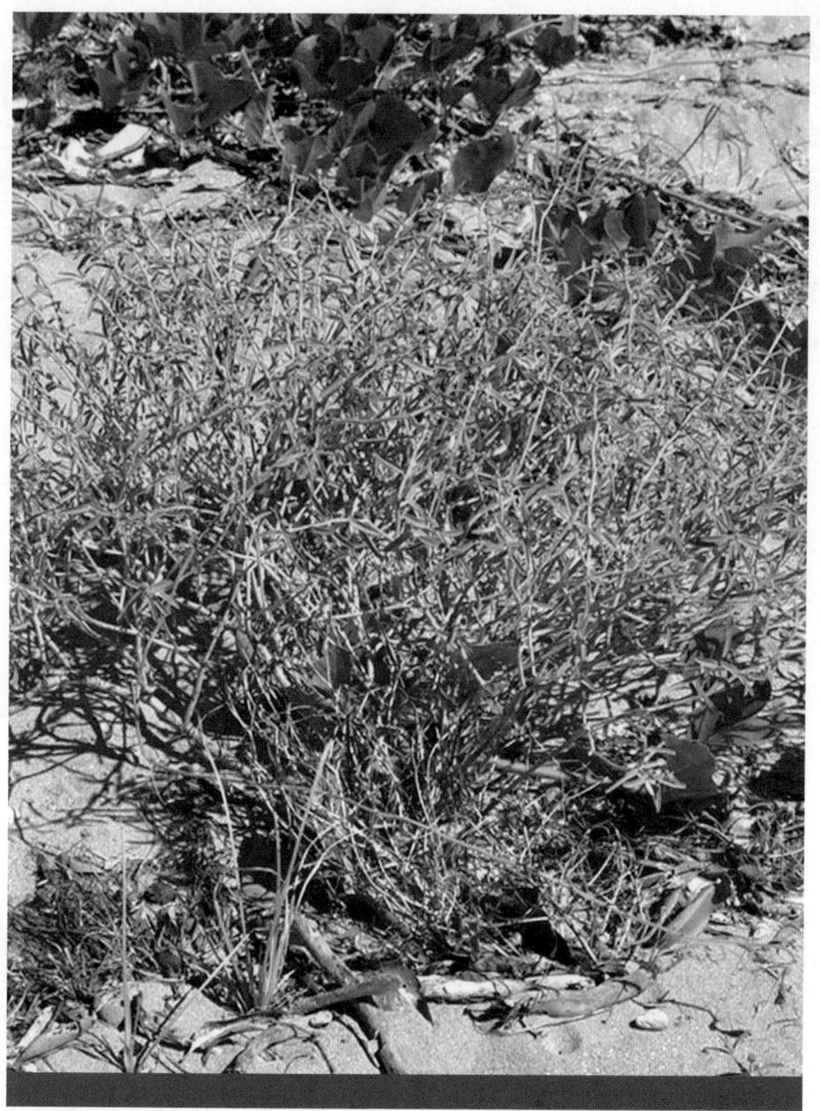

Djabaru

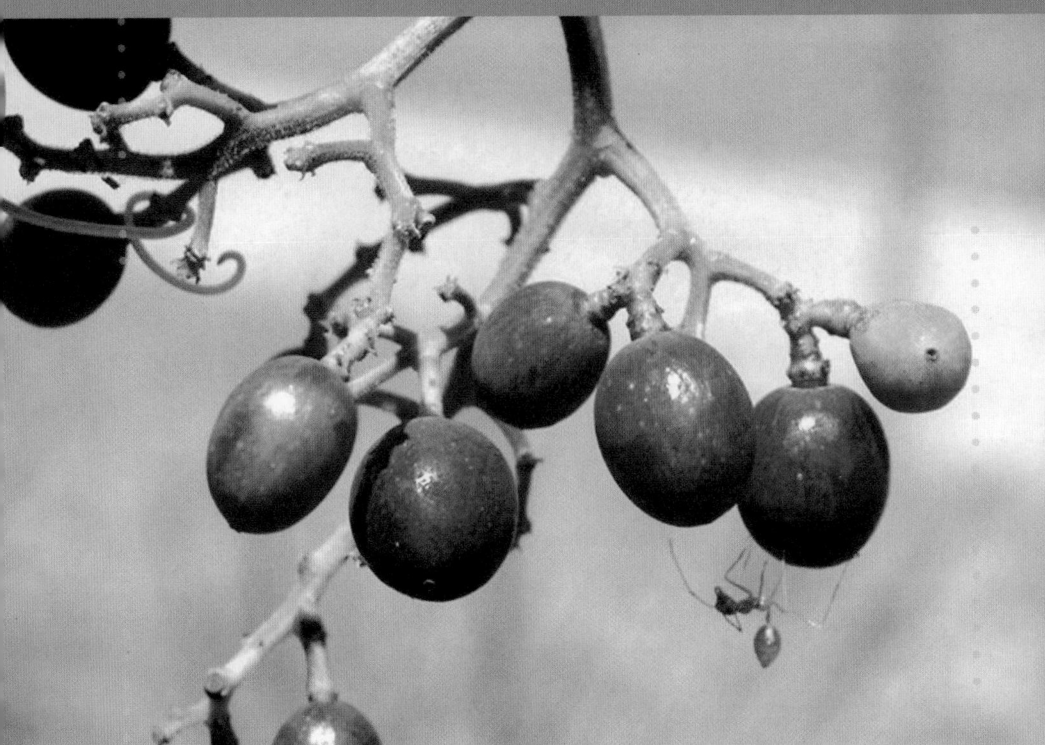

Scientific Name *Ampelocissus acetosa* (F.Muell.) Planch.

Common Names Djabaru, Bush Grape, Wild Grape, Native Grape.

Aboriginal Names Marawalay (Bunuba) (Oscar et al., 2019), Goolmerrng (Miriwoong) (Leonard et al., 2013), Mawalaga (Wunambal, Gaambera) (Karadada et al., 2011), Mbau-nu (Batavia River), Giwalwal (Mangarrayi), Midyurun (Miwa) (Kimberley Specialists, 2020), Kaarnurra wunu (Worrorra) (Clendon et al., 2000), Jaburru winya (Kwini) (Cheinmora et al., 2017; Crawford, 1982).

Field Notes Djabaru (more commonly known outside Western Australia as Wild or Native Grape) is a dense and tangled climbing vine. Each leaf is made up of five to seven ovate leaflets that are up to 120 mm long. Its red-brown flowers, which are made up of five petal-like segments, are present between September and February. The fruit are sour-tasting, globular berries that are up to 12 mm in diameter and available from February to April. Djabaru is found

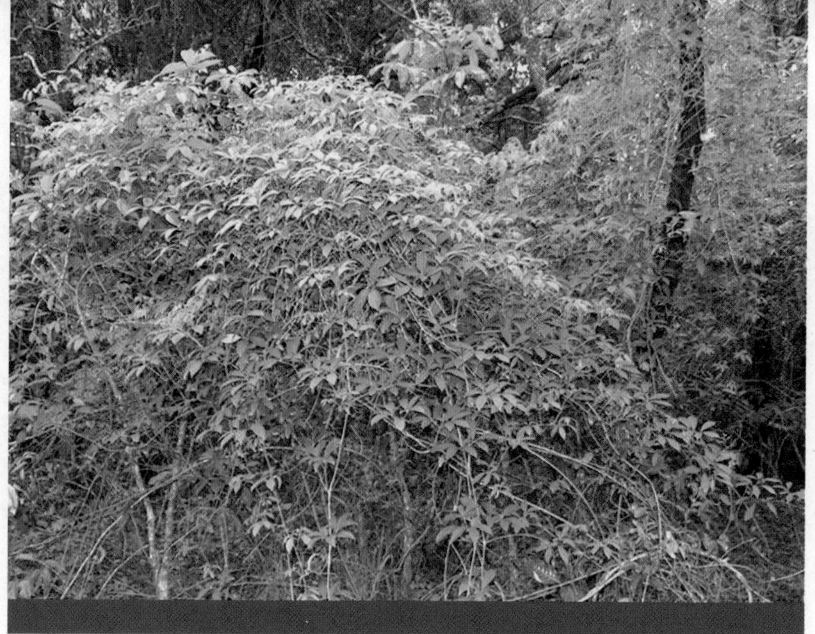

growing in a variety of soils across the far tropical north of Australia from the Kimberley region in Western Australia to Cape York Peninsula (ALA, 2022; Lassak & McCarthy, 2001; WAH, 2022).

Medicinal Uses The juice of the fruit has reportedly been used as an antidote for snakebite, including the bite of the death adder, by some Aboriginal groups in Queensland (Cock, 2011; Hiddins, 2001; Lassak & McCarthy, 2001; Williams, 2012). Its efficacy has not been recorded.

Other Uses The fruit and new growth roots of Djabaru are edible and were eaten by Aboriginal groups across the top end of Australia. After eating, the consumer suffers a slight burning sensation in the throat that soon passes. The fruit are available from late February to April. The roots are cooked over a fire or roasted in hot ashes before they are eaten. The tubers can cause an itchy throat, even after they are roasted. The roots were harvested during the dry season from the end of April to November. The leaves were used as a wrap for cooking meat in ground ovens (Barker, 1991; Cheinmora et al., 2017; Crawford, 1982; Fox & Garde, 2018; Hiddins, 2001; Karadada et al., 2011; Low, 1991; Isaacs, 1987; McMahon, 2006; Oscar et al., 2019; Vigilante et al., 2013; Wightman, 2017; Williams, 2012).

Dog's Balls

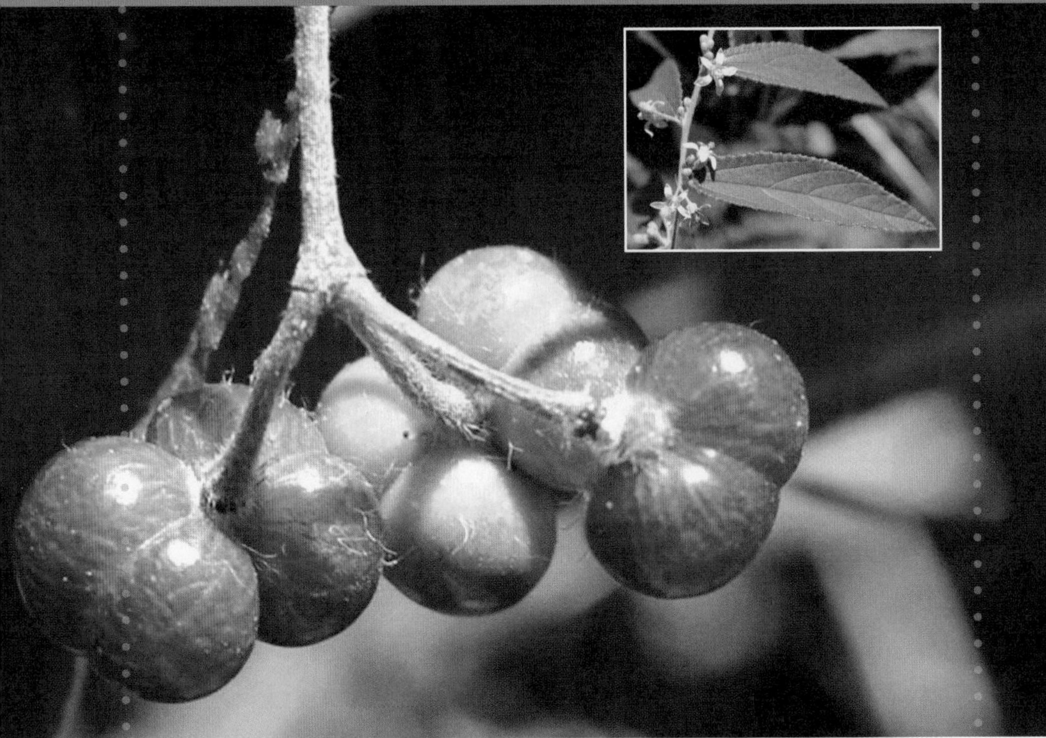

Scientific Names *Grewia savannicola* R.L.Barrett, previously known as *Grewia retusifolia* Kurz (misapplied).

Common Names Dog's Balls, Dysentery Plant, Plain Currant, Dog Nuts, Jack's Joy, Emu Berry.

Aboriginal Names Worlula (Wunambal, Gaambera) (Karadada et al., 2011), Wombanyilinyli (Nyul Nyul) (Kenneally et al., 1996), Garrawoony, Ngoowardiny, Ngoojal, Ngoojany (Gija) (Purdie et al., 2018; Wightman, 2003), Kara ninya or Kaara ninya (Kwini) (Cheinmora et al., 2017; Crawford, 1982).

Field Notes Dog's Balls is a small straggling shrub with hairy, alternate, oblong to broadly spoon-shaped leaves that are up to 50 mm long, usually with toothed margins and three prominent veins. Its small, white, star-shaped flowers with five petals appear any time from September to May. Its fruit are two-lobed, rather hard, with a brownish skin and are approximately 10 mm in diameter. Dog's Balls occur in a variety of soils in the Kimberley region of Western Australia, the Northern Territory and Queensland. It also occurs in Papua New Guinea (ALA, 2022; Fern, 2021; WAH, 2022).

Medicinal Uses The fruit of Dog's Balls can be eaten to relieve diarrhoea and dysentery. Infusions made from the mashed roots were drunk to treat diarrhoea and dysentery. The leaves were chewed for the same purpose (Williams, 2010). The infusions were also used as an eyewash to treat conjunctivitis. Decoctions of the roots were used externally on swollen limbs, on boils to help draw them out and to treat scabies infestations. Sometimes the crushed root was put onto a boil to draw it out. The leaves were chewed without swallowing the juice to relieve toothache (Cock, 2011; Edwards, 2005; Isaacs, 1987; Lassak & McCarthy, 2001; Low, 1990; Smith, 1991; Webb, 1959). Alternatively, a 'root was debarked and the inner silky part rolled into a small ball' then inserted into the tooth cavity for the same purpose (Edwards, 2005). Decoctions of the roots were also used as an eyewash for conjunctivitis and tired eyes. Decoctions of the root bark were drunk to treat bad headaches or as a 'pick me up' for extreme fatigue. Decoctions of the roots and stems were drunk to treat diarrhoea and high fever. Decoctions of the leaves were drunk to relieve stomach upsets and diarrhoea (Cock, 2011; Edwards, 2005; Isaacs, 1987; Smith, 1991; Wightman, 2003).

Other Uses The fruit of Dog's Balls, together with the seeds, are edible and were eaten raw when ripe by Aboriginal groups across the top end of Australia. They are rich in vitamin B1 (thiamine) and they also contain vitamin C (ascorbic acid). The fruit are available between May and August (Cheinmora et al., 2017; Karadada et al., 2011; Kenneally et al., 1996; Low, 1991; Smith, 1991; Vigilante et al., 2013; Wightman, 2003).

Dogwood

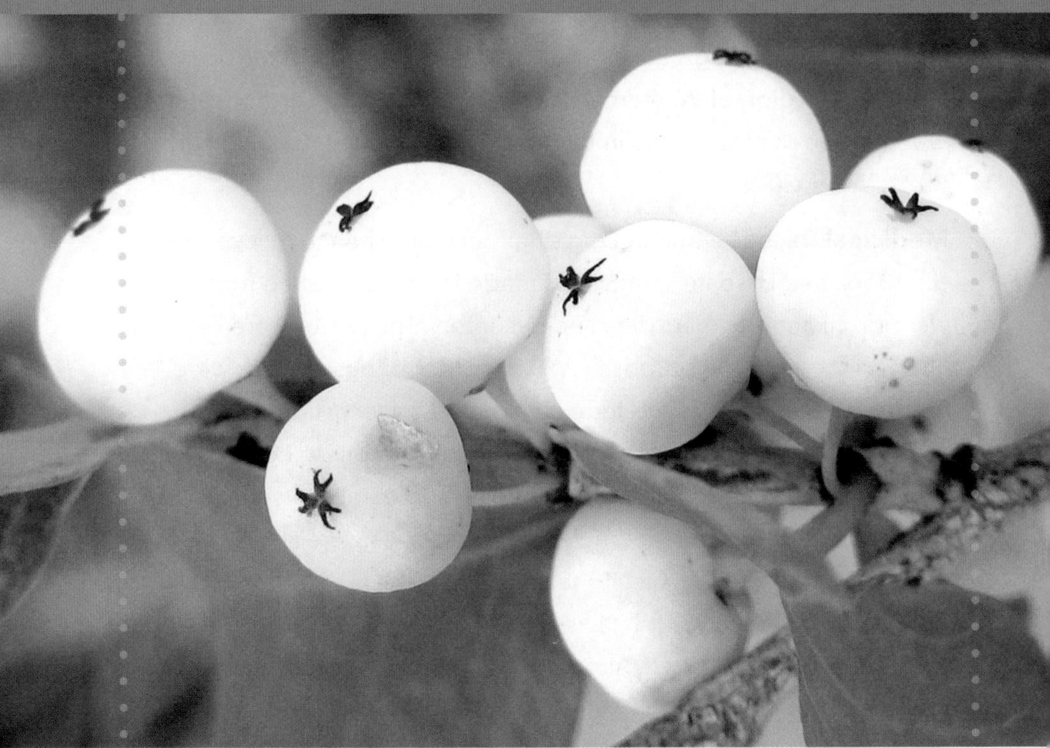

Scientific Name *Flueggea virosa* subsp. *melanthesoides* (F.Muell.) G.L.Webster, previously known as *Securinega melanthesoides* (F.Muell.) Airy Shaw.

Common Names Dogwood, White Raisin, White Berry Bush, White Currant, Snowberry.

Aboriginal Names Wooloo-wooleng (Miriwoong) (Leonard et al., 2013), Guwal (Yawuru and Nyigina), Anbamar (Kwini) (Crawford, 1982), Koowal Ngooji, Guralga (Bardi) (Smith & Kalotas, 1985), or Goorralgar (Bardi) (Paddy et al., 1993), Witulurru, Karnku (Walmajarri) (Richards & Hudson, 2012), Woolawoolun (Miwa) (Kimberley Specialists, 2020), Guwarl (Djugan), Koowal Ngooji (Nyikina) (Young et al., 2012), Kuwal (Nyangumarta, Karajarri) (Lands, 1997), Berenggarrji, Goowarroolji (Gija) (Barney et al., 2013).

Field Notes Dogwood grows as a shrub or tree to 5 m in height. The leaves are green, papery, oblong, obovate or orbicular, and up

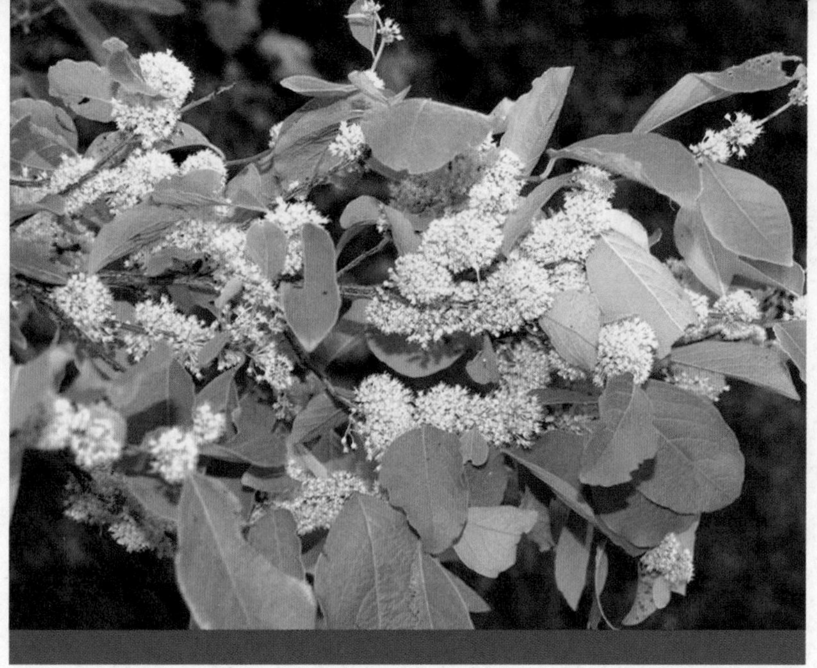

to 50 mm long. Its white-yellow flowers are very small and appear in clusters any time from August to April. The fruit are small, white, spherical berries that are 3 mm or more in diameter. Dogwood occurs in a variety of soils, on floodplains, hillsides and sand dunes across the top half of Australia from the Pilbara and Kimberley regions of Western Australia through the Northern Territory and down into Queensland as far as Rockhampton (ALA, 2022; Lassak & McCarthy, 2001; SMIP, 2022; WAH, 2022).

Medicinal Uses Infusions of the young leaves were taken internally for internal pain and for severe sickness. They were also applied externally for itchy skin, heat rash, chickenpox rash, open sores and leprosy (Cock, 2011; Lassak & McCarthy, 2001; Reid, 1986; Webb, 1959). Poultices of crushed bark and roots were applied to areas of rheumatic pain (Paddy et al., 1993). In Far North Queensland, decoctions of the root were used as a mouthwash to treat toothache. Alternatively, small pieces of root were packed into the tooth cavity for the same purpose (Edwards, 2005).

Other Uses The small fruit of the Dogwood are edible and quite sweet when ripe. The fruit are available from mid-November to February (Crawford, 1982; Jackes, 2010; Lands, 1997; Low, 1991; RFCA, 1993; SMIP, 2022; Young et al., 2012).

Dogwood Hakea

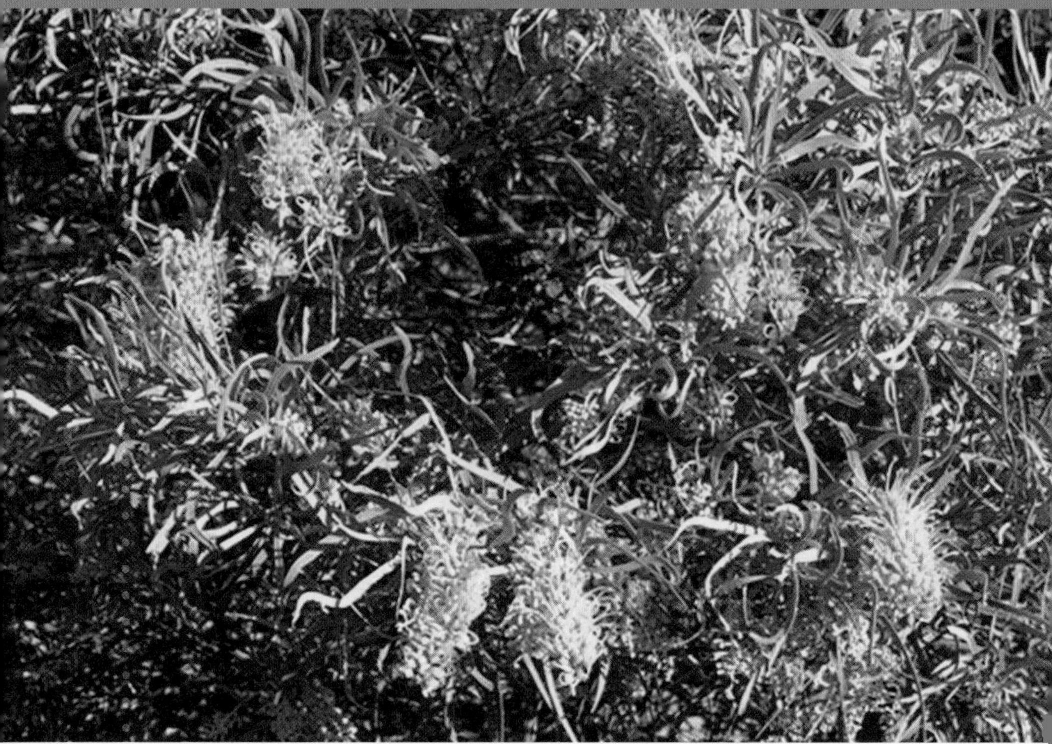

Scientific Name *Hakea macrocarpa* R.Br.

Common Names Dogwood Hakea, Boomerang Tree (Broome area), Gnarled Hakea.

Aboriginal Names Goonanderoony, Jawoolyi, Jawoolyiny (Gija) (Purdie et al., 2018), Jarridany (Nyikina) (Smith & Smith, 2009), (Bardi) (Smith & Kalotas, 1985), Jarradiny (Bardi) (Paddy et al., 1993), Jarangkarr, Jirrmi (Walmajarri) (Richards & Hudson, 2012), Koolooloo (Nyikina) (Young et al., 2012), Piruwa, Tjituwangalpa (Kukatja) (Valiquette, 1993), Kurlulu (Karajarri) (Willing, 2014).

Field Notes Dogwood Hakea grows as a tall shrub or tree up to 6 m in height. Its leaves are a curved or sickle shape and up to 30 mm long by 10 mm wide. The flower heads are cream or greenish yellow, pendulous racemes up to 150 mm long. Flowering is followed by the appearance of woody seed pods about 40 mm long. Flowering is between May and August. Dogwood Hakea

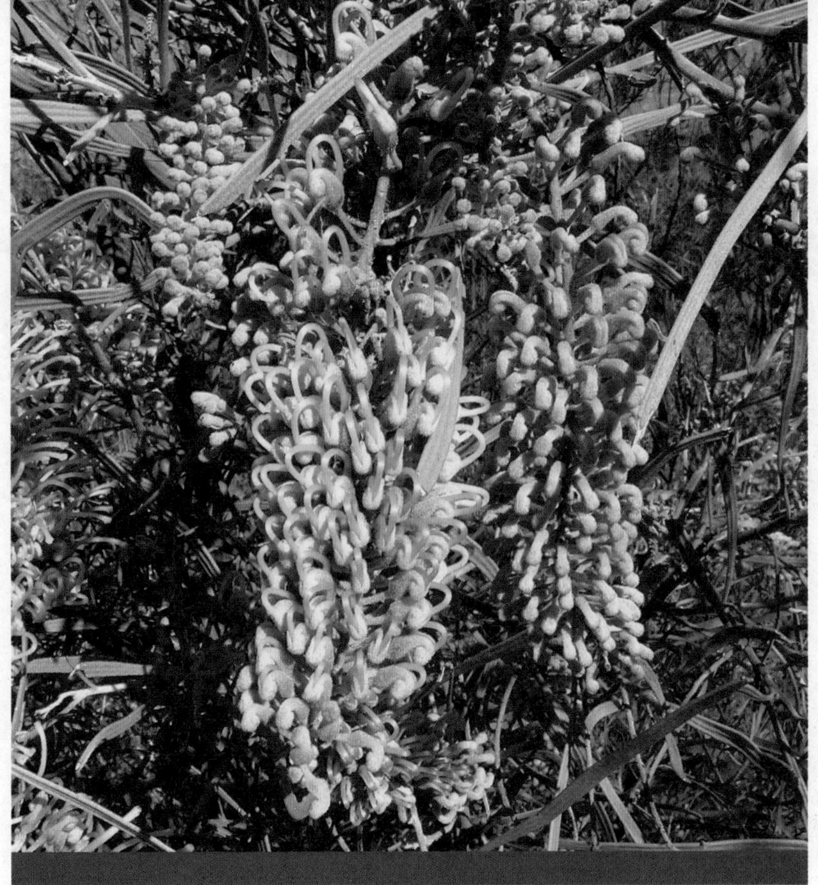

occurs in red, sandy soils on coastal sand dunes, rocky ridges and sandplains in the more arid area of northern Western Australia, the Northern Territory and Western Queensland (ALA, 2022; ANPSA, 2022; WAH, 2022).

Medicinal Uses Aboriginal groups across the Kimberley, the Northern Territory and western Queensland burnt the wood from Dogwood Hakea and the resulting charcoal was powdered and rubbed into cuts, sores and cracked lips to promote healing (Devanesen, 2000; Kane, 2022; Lassak & McCarthy, 2001; Reid, 1986; Smith, 1991; Webb, 1959).

Other Uses Aboriginal people of the Kimberley sucked nectar directly from the flowers of Dogwood Hakea or soaked the flowers in water to make a sweet drink (Kane, 2022). The Gija used the wood of the Dogwood Hakea to make boomerangs and fighting clubs they call 'wirigi' (Purdie et al., 2018).

Droopy Leaf

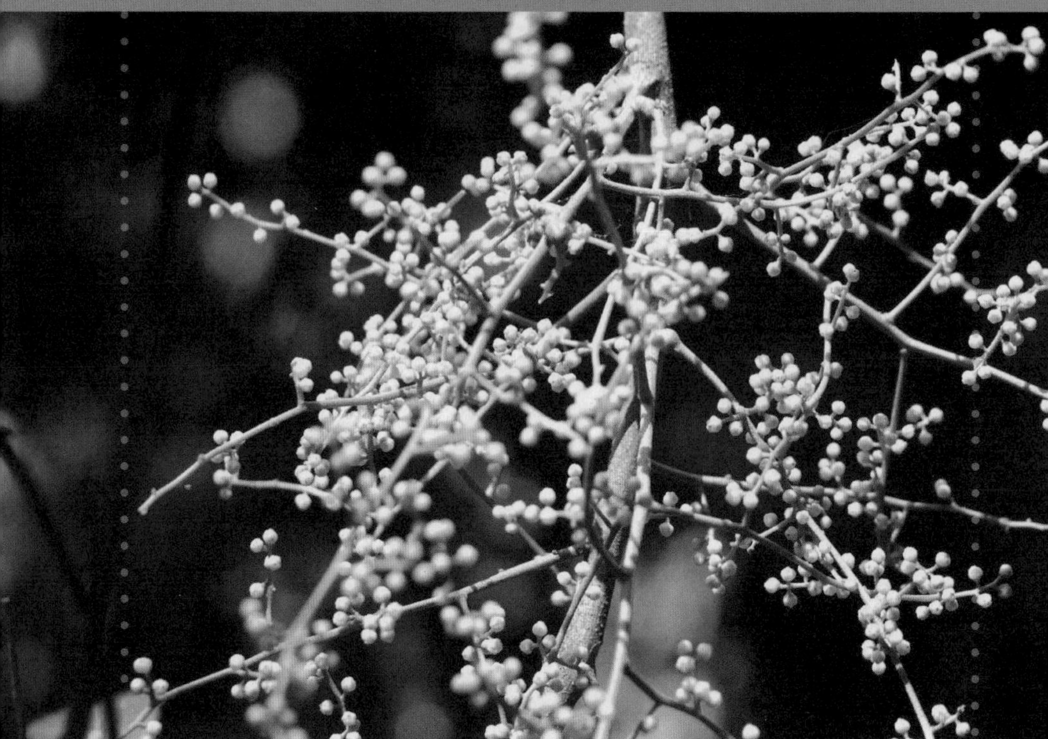

Scientific Name *Aglaia elaeagnoidea* (Juss.) Benth., with synonyms too numerous to list here.

Common Names Droopy Leaf, Coastal Boodyarra.

Field Notes Droopy Leaf is a tree that grows up to 15 m in height. Its ovate leaflet blades are 130 mm long and 50 mm wide. Its small, cream-yellow-white male flowers are only 2 mm in diameter. The female flowers are slightly larger. Flowering in Australia occurs between April and September. Its fruit are scaly berries that are nearly globose, up to 15 mm in diameter and contain two seeds. Droopy Leaf occurs in clay, basalt and sandstone on cliffs, scree slopes, along rivers and in gullies. It is endemic to coastal areas of the Kimberley region of Western Australia, Arnhem Land in the Northern Territory and Far North Queensland. It also occurs in Cambodia, India, Indonesia, Malaysia, Myanmar, New Guinea,

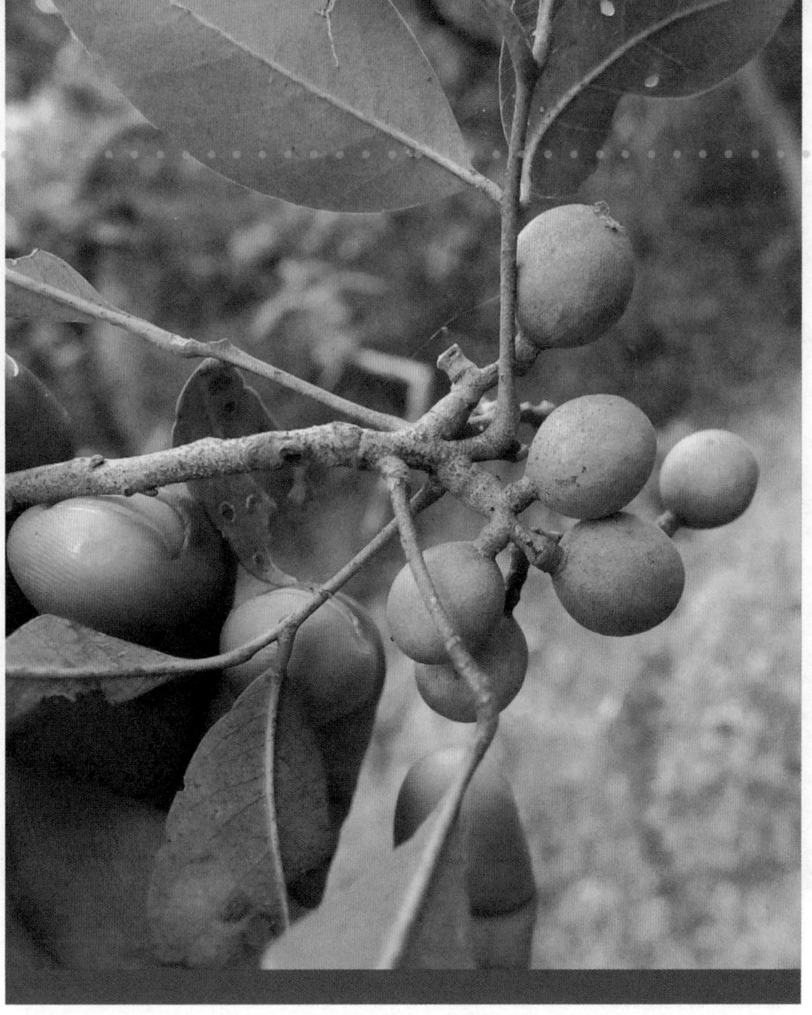

Sri Lanka, Thailand, the Philippines, Vietnam and the western Pacific (ALA, 2022; ATRP, 2020; Biodiversity India, 2022; WAH, 2022).

Medicinal Uses Droopy Leaf is used in Ayurvedic medicine for its antipyretic, astringent, antidiarrhoeal, antidysenteric and anti-inflammatory properties. The fruit are considered to be astringent and cooling and are used in the treatment of inflammation and fever. The seeds are used to treat painful micturition due to urinary tract infection (Fern, 2021; Manjari et al., 2017).

Other Uses The fruit of Droopy Leaf are edible, usually eaten raw and reported to have a slight tart flavour. The gelatinous flesh (aril) around the seed is sweeter and tastier (Fern, 2021).

Dumara Bush

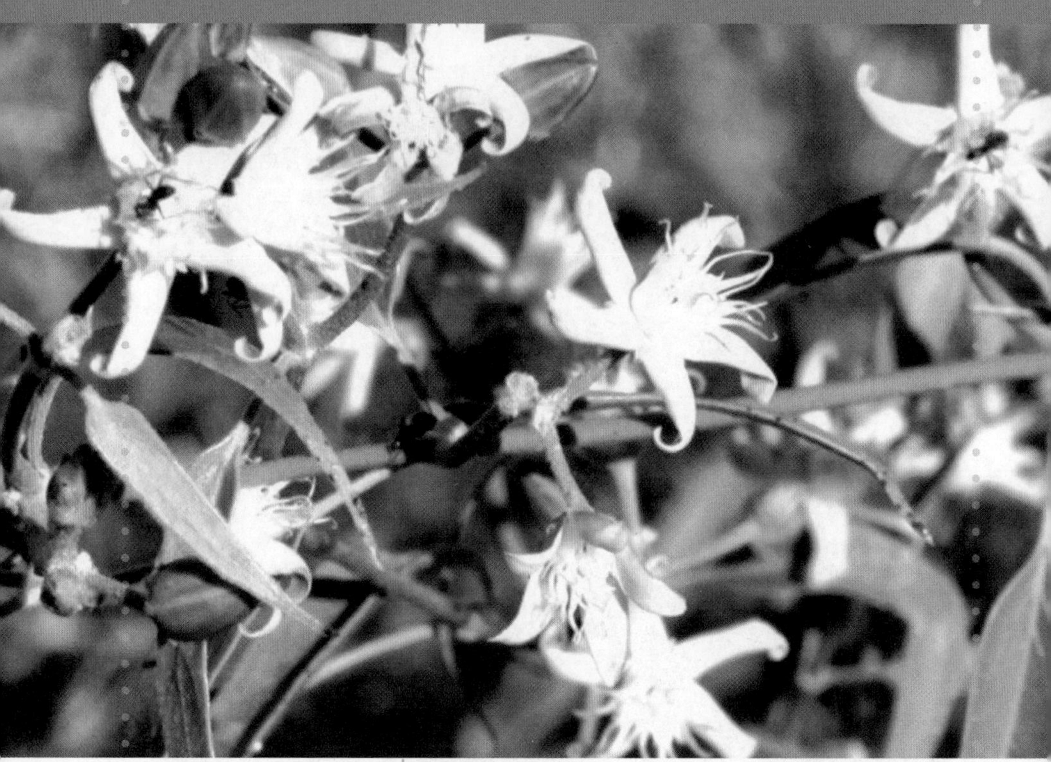

Scientific Name *Cynanchum floribundum* R.Br.

Common Names Dumara Bush, Desert Cynanchum, Ngiltha, Native Pear.

Field Notes Dumara Bush is a perennial herb that reaches around 1 m in height. Its leaves are broad and tapered at the ends. Its flowers are white and spiny with five petals that are curled at the ends, and with long stamens. Flowering is between March and October. Its small fruit are tubular and quite un-pear-like although they are slightly pear-shaped. Dumara Bush occurs in sandy soils along drainage lines, on coastal dunes and amongst granite rocks in the Murchison, Gascoyne, Pilbara and Kimberley regions of Western Australia, the Northern Territory, Queensland, and the western part of New South Wales (ALA, 2022; Lassak & McCarthy, 2001; Native Tastes of Australia, 2022; WAH, 2022).

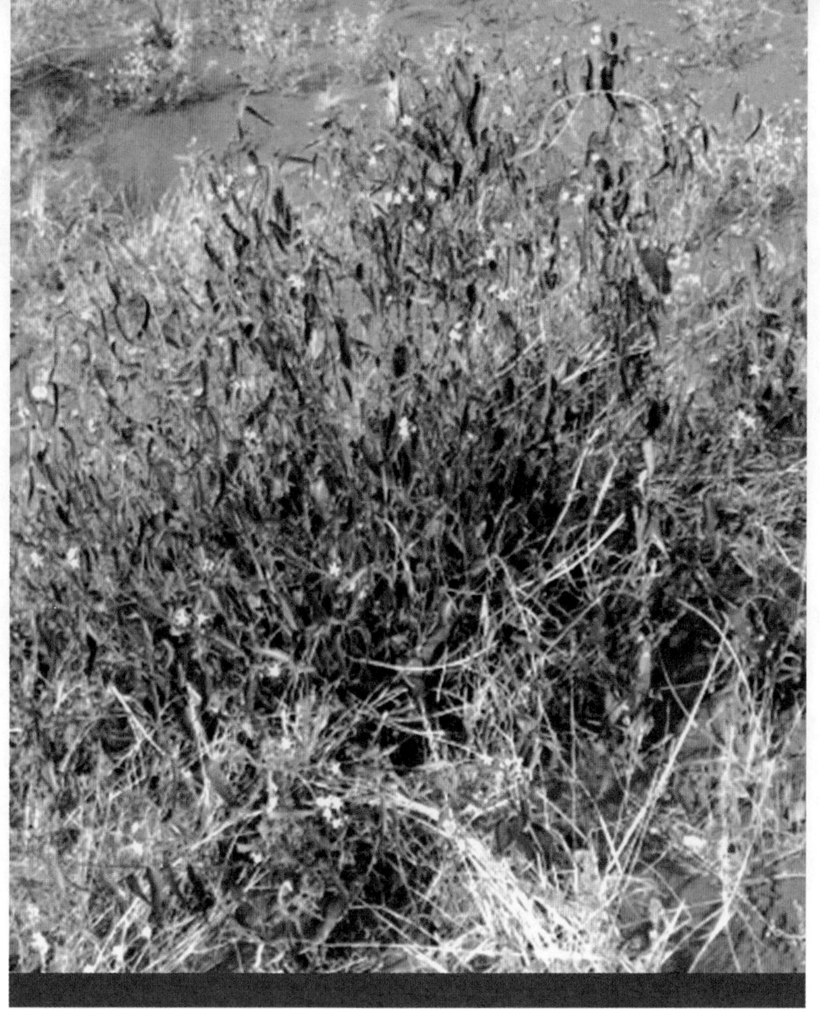

Medicinal Uses Some Aboriginal groups rubbed the latex (milky sap) of Dumara Bush on their bodies to raise their temperature in cold weather (Lassak & McCarthy, 2001; Native Tastes of Australia, 2022).

Other Uses: The young green fruit or seed pods of Dumara Bush were eaten whole and are reported to taste slightly sweet (Cribb & Cribb, 1981; Glasby, 2018; Reid, 1986). Older pods were eaten after steaming (Low, 1991). The fibrous inner stem bark was spun into string that was reportedly quite strong (Low, 1991).

Emu Apple

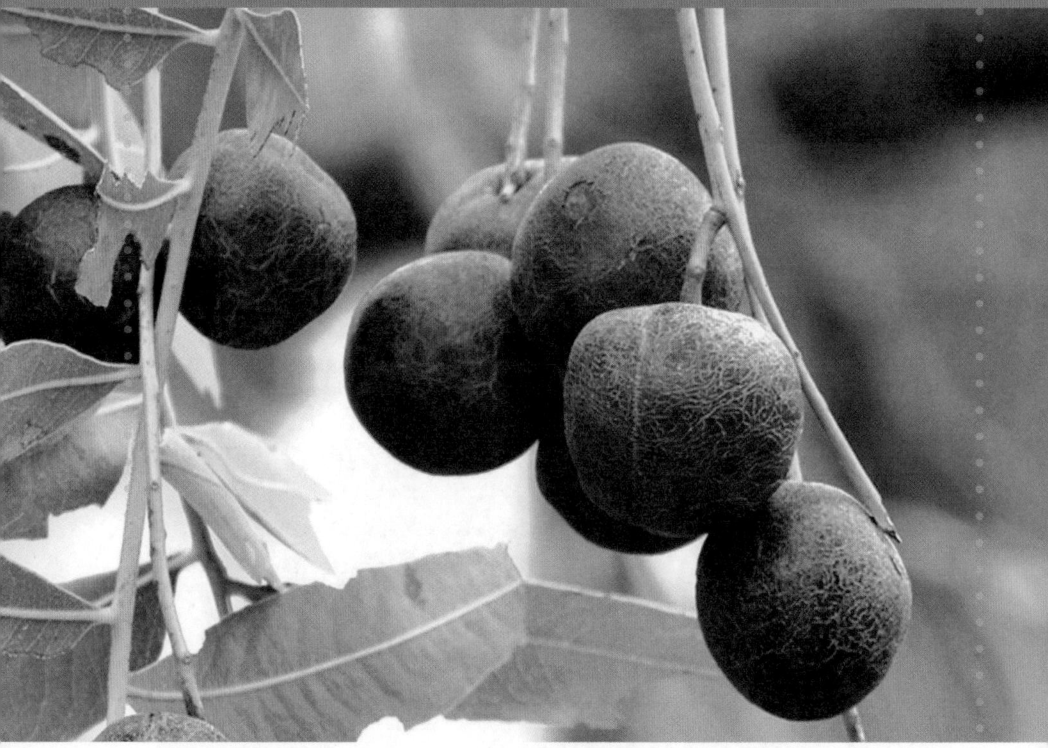

Scientific Name *Owenia vernicosa* F.Muell.

Common Names Emu Apple, Black Cocky Apple.

Aboriginal Names Bandanyi (Bunuba) (Oscar et al., 2019), Yermuna (Wunambal, Gaambera) (Karadada et al., 2011), Ngooyoo, Nguyu, Nyarerrji (Gija) (Purdie et al., 2018; Wightman, 2003), Bardigi (Miwa) (Kimberley Specialists, 2020) Yirrmana (Kwini), Debildebil taka (the fruit of the devils) (Kriol) (Cheinmora et al., 2017).

Field Notes Emu Apple is a tree that grows up to 10 m in height. It has grey-orange, flaky bark and pinnate leaves usually 200–300 mm long. Its red-maroon, globose fruit grow up to 40 mm in diameter. Its small, white-cream-green flowers appear from October to November. Emu Apple occurs in black clay loam over sandstone or alluvial sand on rocky ridges, scree slopes and along creek lines in the northern half of the Kimberley region of Western Australia, the

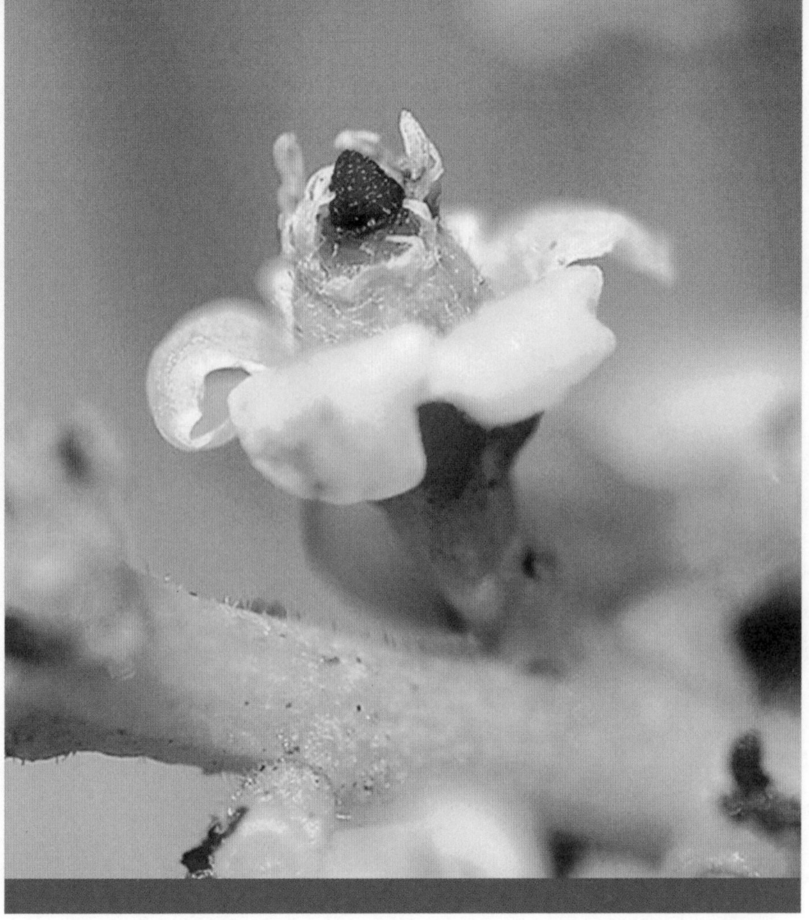

top portion of the Northern Territory and the Cape York Peninsula in Far North Queensland (ALA, 2022; FloraNT, 2022; WAH, 2022).

Medicinal Uses Decoctions of the red inner bark of Emu Apple were used as an antiseptic wash for open cuts and sores to aid the healing process (Hiddins, 2001; Smith, 1991). Infusions of shavings of the inner bark were taken internally to treat coughs and colds (Hiddins, 2001). Leaves were heated and placed over the eyes to treat conjunctivitis and placed on the forehead to treat headaches (El Questro, n.d.).

Other Uses The seeds inside the hard green to red fruit of Emu Apple are edible. The fruit are cracked open to allow access to seeds that are cooked and ground then made into damper. The fruit are available in the middle of the dry season (Kimberley Specialists, 2020). The bark was used by some Aboriginal groups as a 'fish poison' (El Questro, n.d.; Hiddins, 2001; Smith, 1991).

Entire-leaf Wild Grape

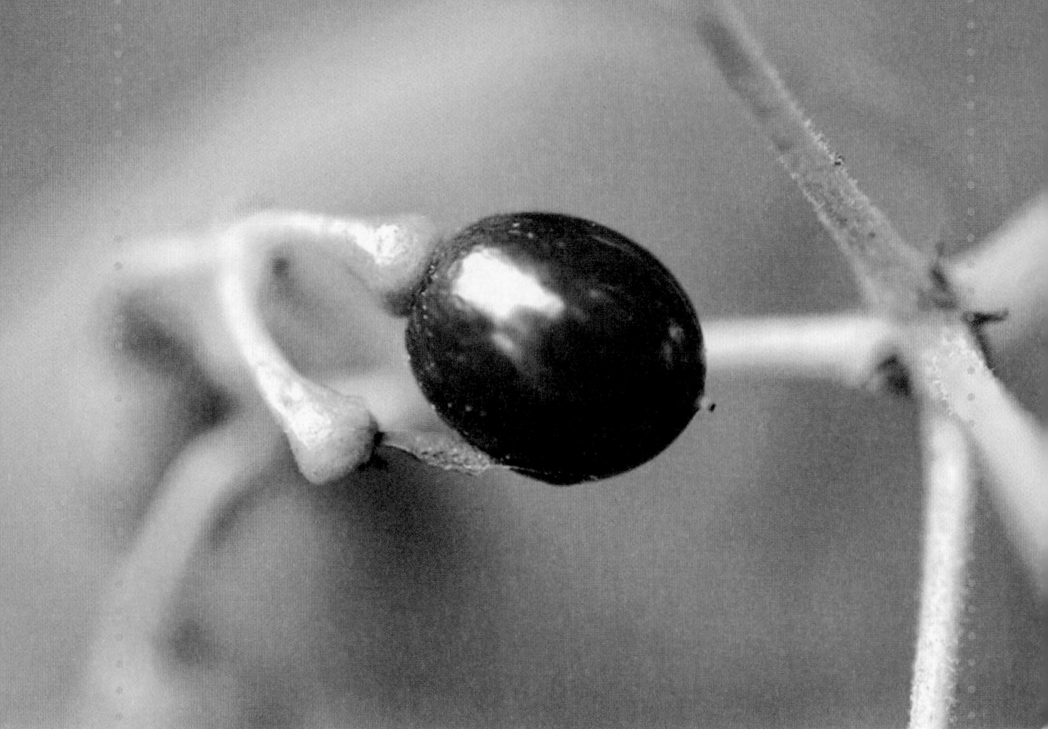

Scientific Name *Cissus adnata* Roxb.

Common Name Entire-leaf Wild Grape.

Field Notes Entire-leaf Wild Grape is a scrambling or climbing perennial, herb or shrub or climber that grows up to 8 m in height in good conditions. Its heart-shaped leaves are up to 180 mm long by 190 mm wide. Its small, pale-green flowers are only 2 mm in diameter, forming in inflorescences up to 70 mm long. Flowering is between January and March. Its globular, grape-like fruit are approximately 7 mm in diameter with one round seed. In Australia, Entire-leaf Wild Grape occurs in loam, sandstone, limestone and sand along rocky creek lines, on rocky hills and in gullies in the Kimberley region of Western Australia, the Northern Territory and northern Queensland (ALA, 2022; Fox & Garde, 2018; WAH, 2022). It also occurs in southern China, India, Sri Lanka, through South-east Asia to Indonesia, and New Guinea (Fern, 2021).

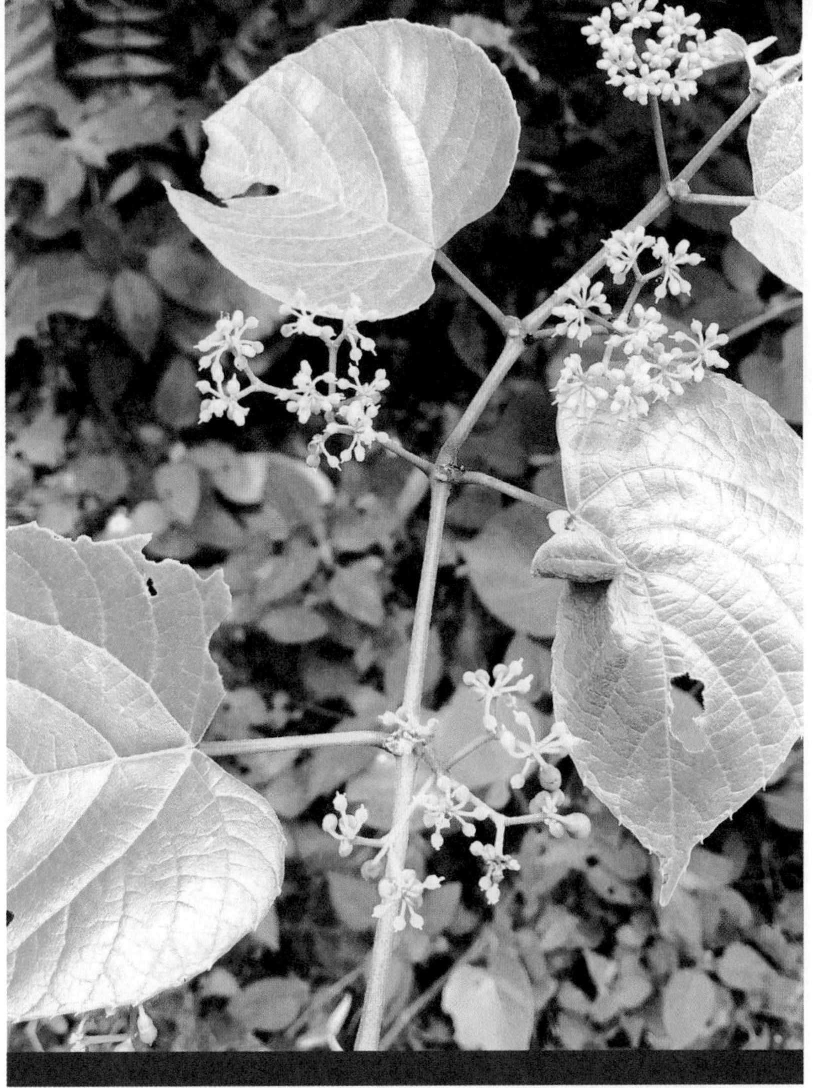

Medicinal Uses Entire-leaf Wild Grape is used in folk medicine in some Asian countries. The roots are alterative and diuretic, and are used as a detoxifying agent. Infusions of the pounded root are taken internally as a treatment for coughs. Poultices made from crushed roots are heated and applied externally on cuts and fractures to aid healing. The juice from the stem is taken internally as a treatment for coughs and diarrhoea. Poultices of the leaves are applied to boils and carbuncles to help draw them out (Fern, 2021).

Other Uses The fruit of Entire-leaf Wild Grape are edible when they are black and ripe (Fox & Garde, 2018; Williams, 2012).

Eucalypts

Family Myrtaceae Juss.

There are over 900 species of eucalypts, or gum trees, of the Myrtaceae family in Australia, a large proportion of which are only found in Western Australia. The term eucalypt - meaning well (eu) covered (calyptos) – was coined by French botanist Charles Louis L'Héritiert de Brutelle in 1788. Eucalypts come in all shapes and sizes from small bushes to giant trees. Eucalypts are divided into three different groups: Eucalyptus, which make up the bulk of the species; Corymbia, the bloodwood eucalypts mainly found in the north; and Angophora. Their leaves, bark, seed capsules (gumnuts) and flowers are also varied. One thing they have in common is that their flowers do not have petals but rather large, colourful stamens which are full of nectar (Euclid, 2020). Some of the more useful eucalypts that are native to the Kimberley region of Western Australia are listed on the following pages.

Common Name	Scientific Name	Aboriginal Names
Apple Gum	*Corymbia clavigera*	Boonbang (Miriwoong), Garnbala (Wunambal, Gaambera), Warra manya, Karlarl manya, Kornbo manya (Kwini)
Broome Bloodwood	*Corymbia zygophylla*	Kurtany (Walmajarri), Jugudany (Yawuru), Jukurtany (Nyangumarta), Jukutany (Karajarri)
Cabbage Ghost Gum	*Corymbia flavescens*	Warlarri, Wiliwirrel, Wiliwoorrool, Wiliwirrirrel (Gija), Kunurru, Yanagurru (Karajarri), Gunurru (Yawuru), Koorrbiji (Nyikina)
Cable Beach Ghost Gum	*Corymbia paractia*	Gunurru (Yawuru)
Coolibah	*Eucalyptus microtheca*	Kampalana, Malanpa, Walytji (Kukatja), Goonjalng (Miriwoong), Waran, Warrpul (Walmajarri), Jaroowenyji (Gija), Dinyjil (Jaru), Arnkurru minya (Kwini), Tinyjil (Ngardi)
Darwin Box	*Eucalyptus tectifica*	Gunjali (Bunuba), Gawuja, Jon (Wunambal, Gaambera), Noorda (Bardi), Kardoo-kardoo (Bardi), Jon, Yuulan (Kwini), Ngarrban (Yawuru), Ngarraban (Nyikina)
Dampier's Bloodwood	*Corymbia greeniana*	Jugudany (Yawuru) and Bilawal (Nyul Nyul), Biilarl (Bardi, Nyikina), Pilawal, Langkarn (Karajarri)
Darwin Stringybark	*Eucalyptus tetrodonta*	Yakmin (Wunambal, Gaambera), Barurru winya, Balangurr winya (Kwini)
Desert Bloodwood	*Corymbia opaca*	Kurntupungu (Walmajarri), Muraga (Bunuba)

Common Name	Scientific Name	Aboriginal Names
Ghost Gum	*Corymbia dendromerinx*	Warlarri (Walmajarri, Bunuba), Jalabari (Bardi)
Glossy-leaved Bloodwood	*Corymbia bleeseri*	Burunkurr, Maranguda (Kwini)
Kimberley White Gum	*Eucalyptus houseana*	Warlarring (Miriwoong), Walarriy (Nyikina)
Long-fruited Bloodwood	*Corymbia polycarpa*	Muraga (Bunuba), Bunja, Binda (Wunambal, Gaambera), Ngalngoorr (Jawi) Gaardga or Ngalngoorroo (Bardi), Kardgu (Yawuru), Mawoorroony (Gija), Bûnda winya, Bûrndal winya, Burrku winya, Burku manya (Kwini), Kardkoo (Nyikina)
Paper-fruited Bloodwood	*Corymbia bella*	Walarri (Bunuba), Gwiyili (Wunambal, Gaambera), Warlarr (Jaru), Kwiyili manya, Karlal manya, Kornbo manya (Kwini), Jukulu, Marroolal (Bardi), Warlarriny, Lawoorany (Gija), Goonoorr (Nyul Nyul) Gunurru (Yawuru), Kunurru (Karajarri)
River Gum	*Eucalyptus camaldulensis*	Dimalan (Miriwoong), Garringga (Bunuba), Garlarl (Wunambal, Gaambera), Malarn (Walmajarri), Wurangara (Nyangumarda), Bilirnji, Bilirn, Bilirnbe, Garranggany (Gija), Malarn, Dimalarn (Jaru), Yaawarl (Kwini), Ngapiri (Walpiri), Jalipari Malarn, Walarri (Ngardi), Ngapiri, Yapalinypa (Kukatja), Libirrar (Nyikina)

Common Name	Scientific Name	Aboriginal Names
Rough Leaf Cabbage Gum	*Corymbia confertiflora*	Punpany, Boonbany (Gija), Warlarri (Jaru), Warra manya, Karlarl manya, Kornbo manya (Kwini)
Rough-leaved Ghost Gum	*Corymbia aspera*	Kily-Kily (Kukatja), Mawurru, Garndirri (Jaru)
Round-leaved Bloodwood	*Corymbia latifolia*	Guulunggurr, Burunggu (Wunambal, Gaambera), Manjirra (Kwini)
Scraggy Bloodwood	*Corymbia abbreviata*	Marlambeny, Marlampeny (Gija)
Snappy Gum	*Eucalyptus brevifolia*	Thalngarrng (Miriwoong), Thalngarri (Bunuba),Thalngarrji, Thalngarr (Gija) Lunja, Wumbard (Jaru), Nurlku (Walpiri), Mangkapuru, Wumpart (Ngardi), Pantapi, Wumparlpa (Kukatja)
Sturt Creek Mallee	*Eucalyptus odontocarpa*	Wartaruru (Ngardi), Parlpinpa, Tjipari (Kukatja)
Swamp Bloodwood	*Corymbia ptychocarpa*	Wawulu (Wunambal, Gaambera), Booniny (Gija)
Variable-barked Bloodwood	*Corymbia dichromophloia*	Gardgu (Nyigina), Palgarri (Njiijapli), Walgalu (Ngarluma), Mardaudhu (Jindjiparndi), Punaangu (Roebourne area), Mawoorrool (Gija), Bunba (Jaru)

Common Name	Scientific Name	Aboriginal Names
Western Bloodwood	*Corymbia terminalis*	Kunturrpungu, Munmurrpa, Murr-murrpa, Tjarra, Walytji, Wakalpuka (Kukatja), Bilal (Bardi), Garndirri (Jaru), Gunjirrd (Nyul Nyul), Wirrkali (Walpiri), Thelinyjeng (Mirawoong), Mawoorroony (Gija)
Woollybutt	*Eucalyptus miniata*	Woolewoorrng (Miriwoong), Arngurru (Wunambal, Gaambera), Manawan or Manuan (Bardi), Booniny, Marlarriny (Gija), Wiliwarra, Manawan manya, Wuluwurr, Unkurru (Kwini), Manoowan (Kyikina)

Medicinal Uses of Eucalypts

The crushed inner bark of the **Coolibah (*Eucalyptus microtheca*)** was used by some Aboriginal groups across the top end as a poultice for snakebite and headaches (Lassak & McCarthy, 2001: 172; Native Tastes of Australia, 2022; Williams, 2020). Decoctions of the leaves mixed with native honey were a cure-all in Queensland for influenza, internal pain, aching joints and sores (Williams, 2020).

Infusions of the inner bark and sapwood of **Darwin Stringybark (*Eucalyptus tetrodonta*)** and **Woollybutt (*Eucalyptus miniata*)** were ingested for diarrhoea. Infusions of the young leaves were drunk for fevers and headaches. Decoctions of the leaves were drunk for influenza (Lassak & McCarthy, 2001; Low, 1990; Webb, 1959). Decoctions of **Darwin Stringybark (*Eucalyptus tetrodonta*)** leaves were used to treat sores, and scabies infestations (Smith, 1991; Williams, 2010).

The kino (gum) of **Paper-fruited Bloodwood (*Corymbia bella*)** and **Glossy-leaved Bloodwood (*Corymbia bleeseri*)** was

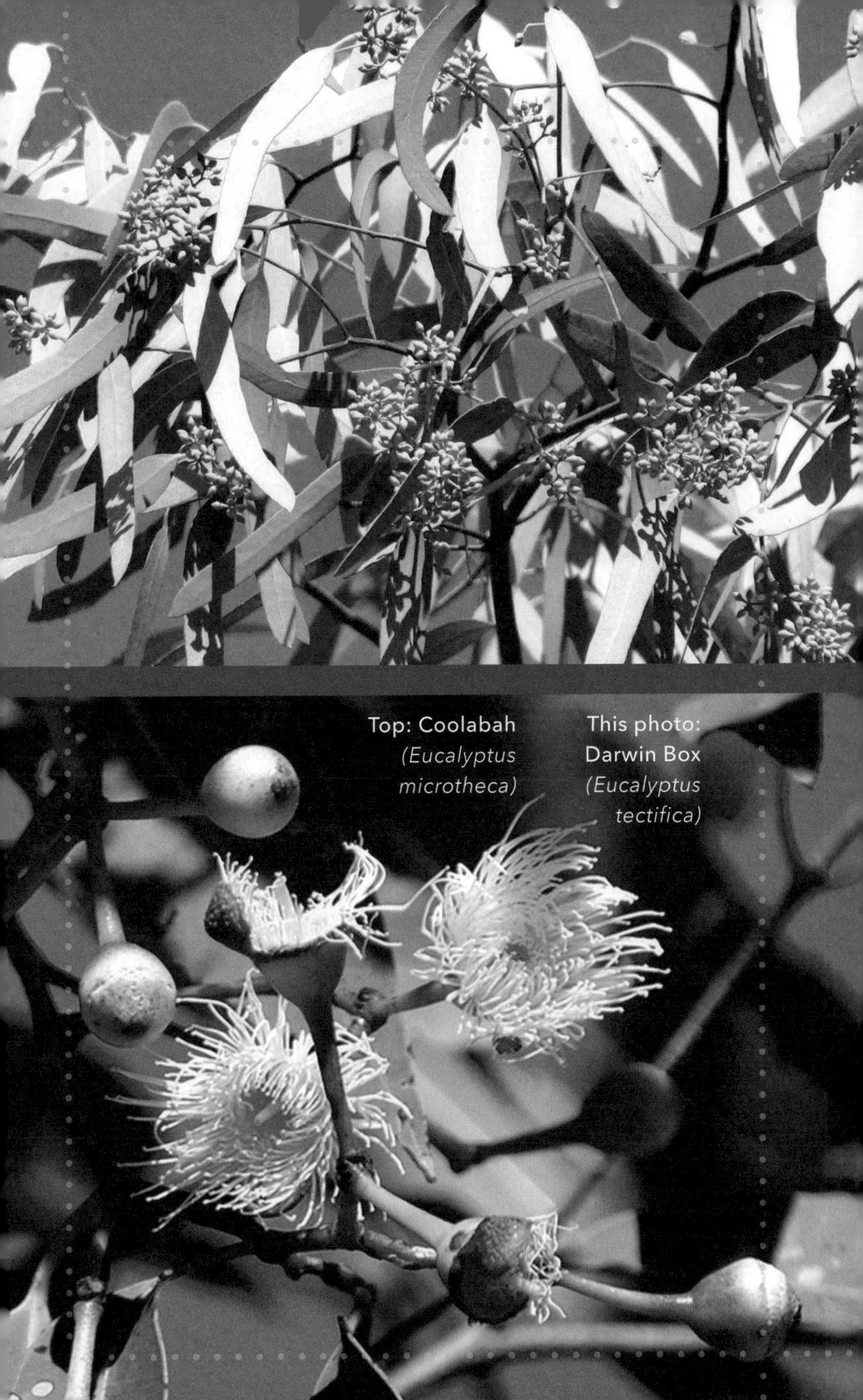

Top: Coolabah *(Eucalyptus microtheca)*

This photo: Darwin Box *(Eucalyptus tectifica)*

applied directly to sores and wounds to aid healing. If the kino had dried it would be powdered and applied as an antibiotic powder (Kenneally et al., 1996; Williams, 2020). The kino (gingba) of **Desert Bloodwood (*Corymbia opaca*)**, **Long-fruited Bloodwood (*Corymbia polycarpa*), Cabbage Ghost Gum (*Corymbia flavescens*)** and **Western Bloodwood (*Corymbia terminalis*)** was eaten to stop diarrhoea in dysentery (Lassak & McCarthy, 2001; Richards & Hudson, 2012). The gum was applied directly to sore teeth to treat toothache. The kino from **Long-fruited Bloodwood (*Corymbia polycarpa*)**, **Dampier's Bloodwood (*Corymbia greeniana*)** and **Urn-fruited Bloodwood (*Corymbia pachycarpa*)** was also rubbed directly on the area of the pain, or the gum was placed in the cavity, to ease the pain of toothache (Paddy et al., 1993).

A small amount of **River Gum (*Eucalyptus camaldulensis*)** kino (resin) ground to powder and dissolved in water was drunk to treat diarrhoea. Infusions of leaves and twigs were used to bathe the heads of people with colds (Lassak & McCarthy, 2001). Arrernte people around Alice Springs pounded the bark of River Gum to make an antiseptic paste that was used to treat wounds (Olive Pink Botanic Garden, 2010).

The Jaru boiled the kino or gum from the **Rough-leaved Ghost Gum (*Corymbia aspera*)** and **Paper-fruited Bloodwood (*Corymbia bella*)** and drank the decoction to treat the symptoms of colds and influenza.

Decoctions of the bark of **Snappy Gum (*Eucalyptus brevifolia*)** were a good antiseptic healing agent when applied to burns (Gija Bush Food and Medicine, n.d.).

The Ngardi used decoctions of the leaves of **Sturt Creek Mallee (*Eucalyptus odontocarpa*)** as an antiseptic wash to bathe sores. They also used the leaves to make 'smoke medicine' to relieve the symptoms of colds and influenza (Cataldi, 2004).

The flowers of many eucalypts, including **Variable-barked Bloodwood (*Corymbia dichromophloia*)** and **Dampier's Bloodwood (*Corymbia greeniana*)**, contain various amounts of nectar and were dipped in water to extract the nectar, with the resulting sweet liquid drunk for coughs and colds, or just to quench one's thirst. A small grain of the sap or kino was sucked or a weak solution was ingested as a tonic, and for coughs, colds and bronchitis. Small pieces of the kino were used to plug cavities in the teeth to stop toothache (Lassak & McCarthy, 2001; Reid, 1986; Webb, 1959).

The leaves of all eucalypts were crushed and used as antibacterial poultices for healing wounds. They were also used in steam pits to relieve rheumatism. Crushed leaves were held under the nose to relieve congestion due to colds and influenza. The kino (gum) of most eucalypts was ground and used as an antiseptic powder on sores. It was also eaten to relieve diarrhoea and dysentery (Clarke, 2007; Hansen & Horsfall, 2016; Lassak & McCarthy, 2001; Reid, 1986).

Other Uses of Eucalypts

Manna or Sugarleaf, which comes from the activity of Lerps, is sometimes present on **Desert Bloodwood (*Corymbia opaca*)**, **Dampier's Bloodwood (*Corymbia greeniana*)** and **Western Bloodwood (*Corymbia terminalis*)**.

The seeds of **Bloodwood (*Corymbia terminalis*), Rough Leaf Cabbage Gum (*Corymbia confertiflora*)**, **Rusty Bloodwood (*Corymbia confertiflora*), Woollybutt (*Eucalyptus miniata*)**, **Swamp Bloodwood (*Corymbia ptychocarpa*)** and **Coolabah (*Eucalyptus microtheca*)** are edible and are eaten raw (ANBG, 2020; El Questro, n.d.; Fox & Garde, 2018; Kane, 2021;RFCA, 1993; Smith & Kalotas, 1985; Territory Native Plants, 2022; Vigilante et al., 2013; Williams, 2010; Willing, 2014).

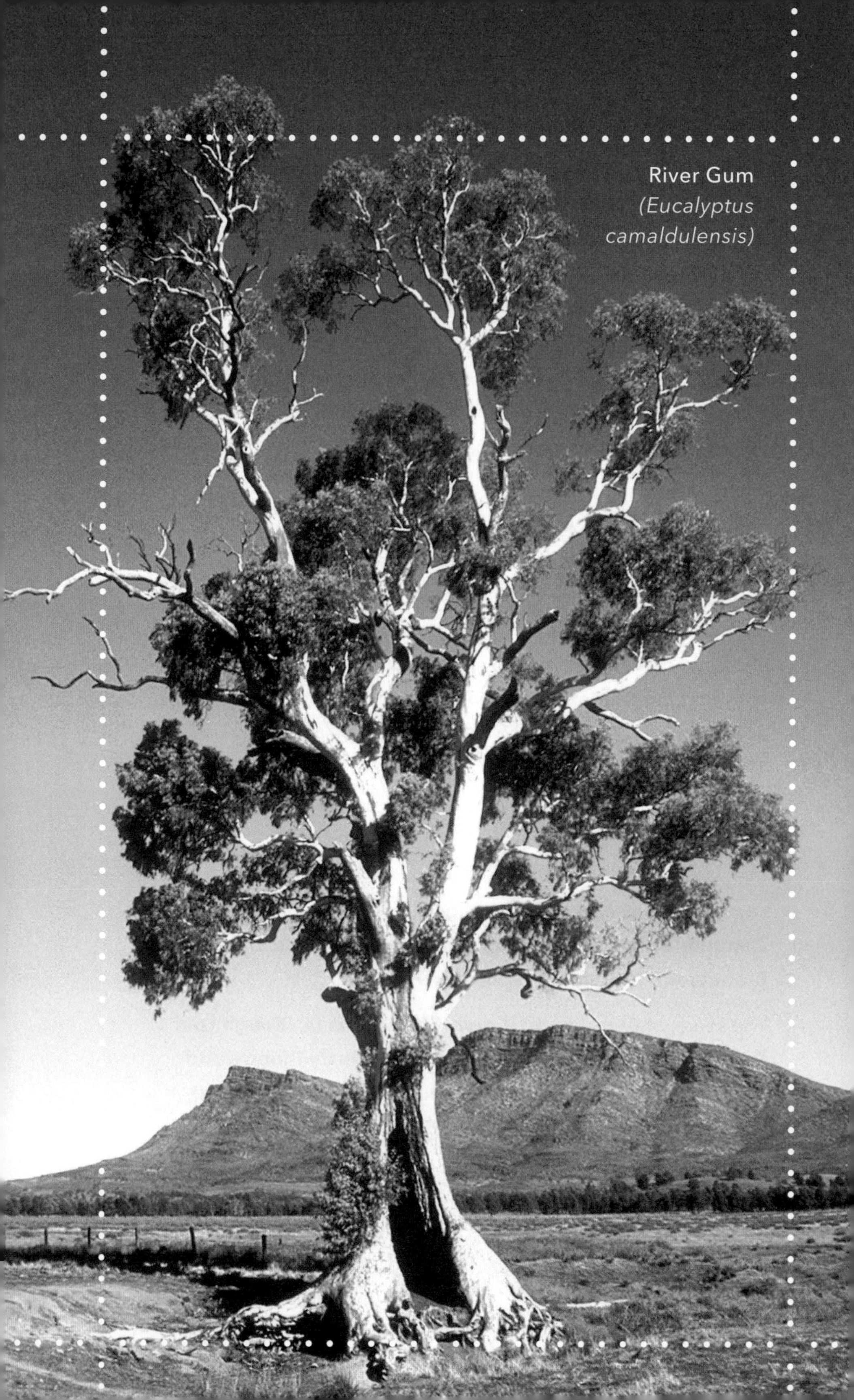

River Gum
(Eucalyptus camaldulensis)

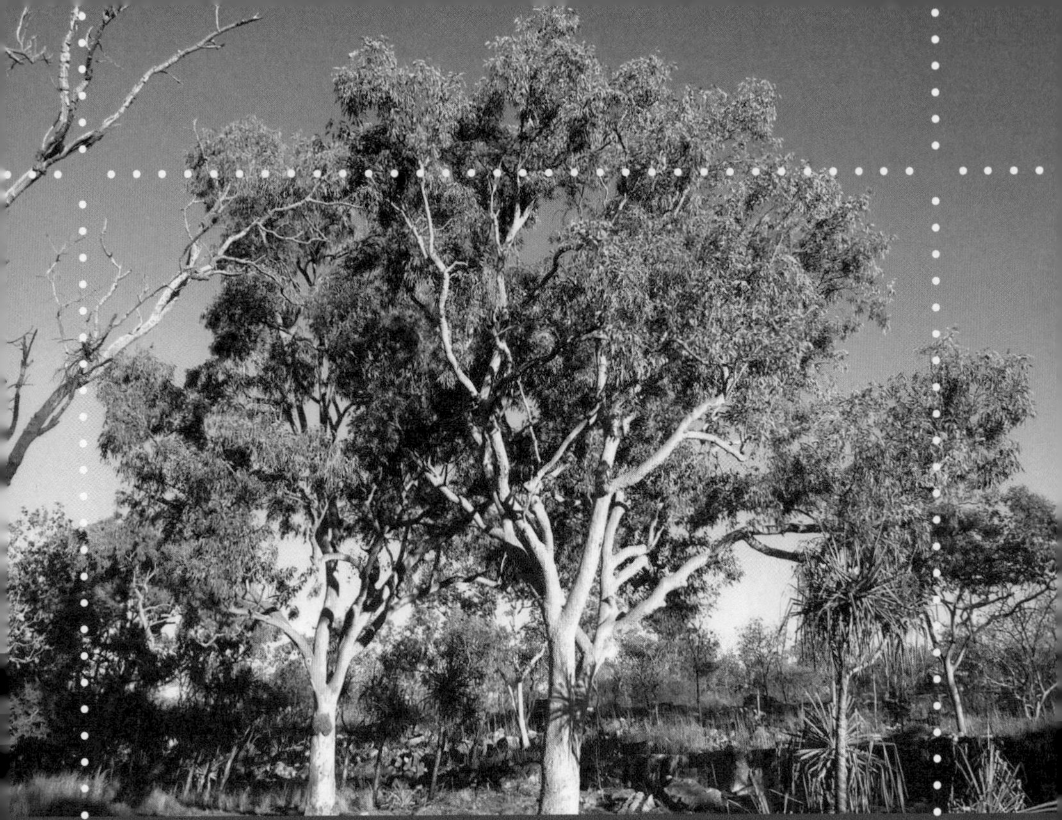

Top: Kimberley White Gum *(Eucalyptus houseana)*

This photo: Snappy Gum *(Eucalyptus brevifolia)*

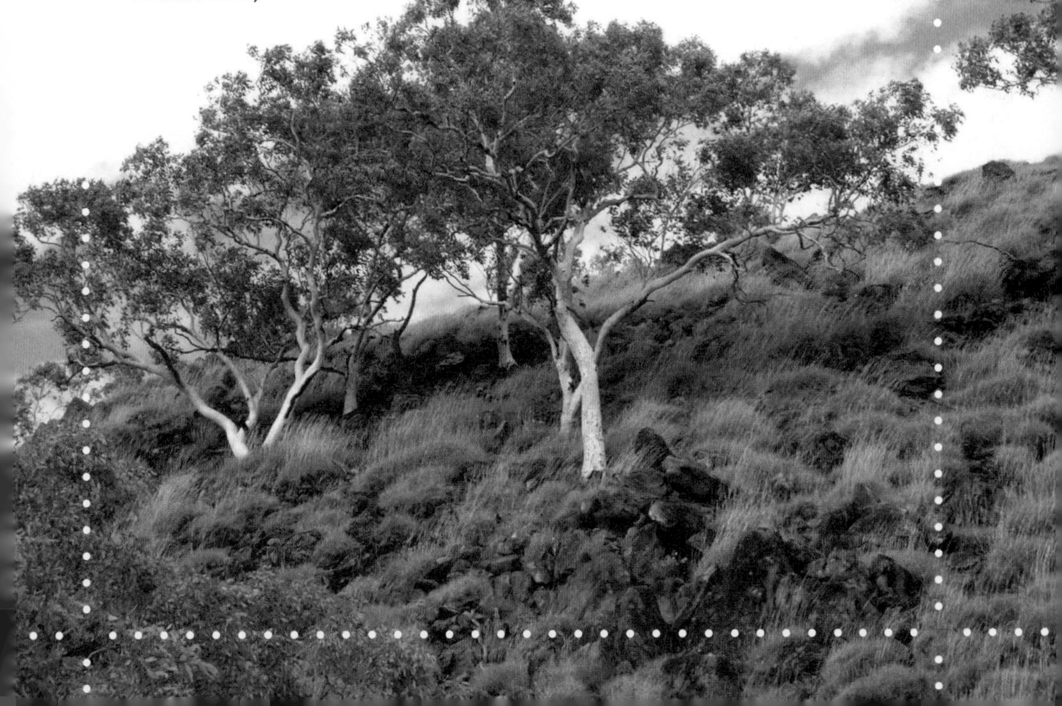

False Cedar

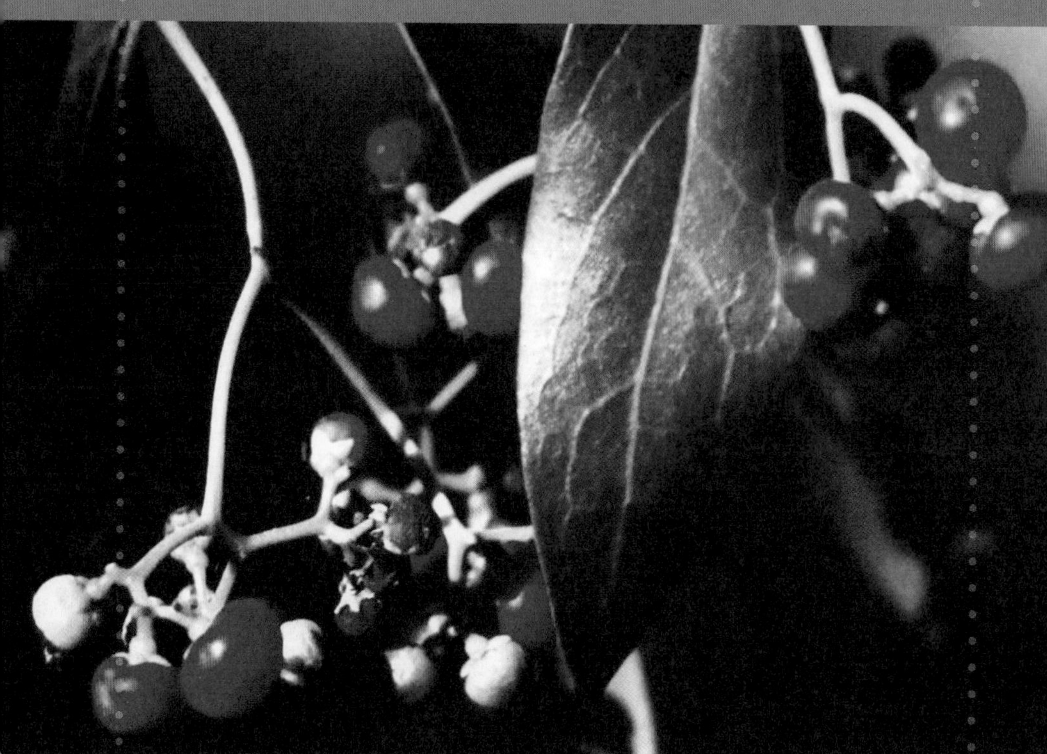

Scientific Name *Ehretia saligna* R.Br.

Common Names False Cedar, Peach Bush, Native Willow, Peachwood.

Aboriginal Names Bundawurra (Bunuba) (Oscar et al., 2019), Jiimany (Bardi), Miganiny (Yawuru) (Kenneally et al., 1996), Malkarniny or Mikarniny (Nyikina) (Smith & Smith, 2009).

Field Notes False Cedar grows as a shrub or weeping tree up to 6 m in height. Its leaves are lanceolate and up to 250 mm long. Its small, white-cream to green flowers appear in clusters at the end of branchlets from March to May or August to November. The fruit are globular berries up to 6 mm in diameter. False Cedar occurs in alluvial soil, or sandy and clayey soils on coastal dunes, along drainage lines, on rocky outcrops and claypans along the north-west coast from Exmouth in the Pilbara, through the Kimberley, the Northern Territory and Queensland and down into northern

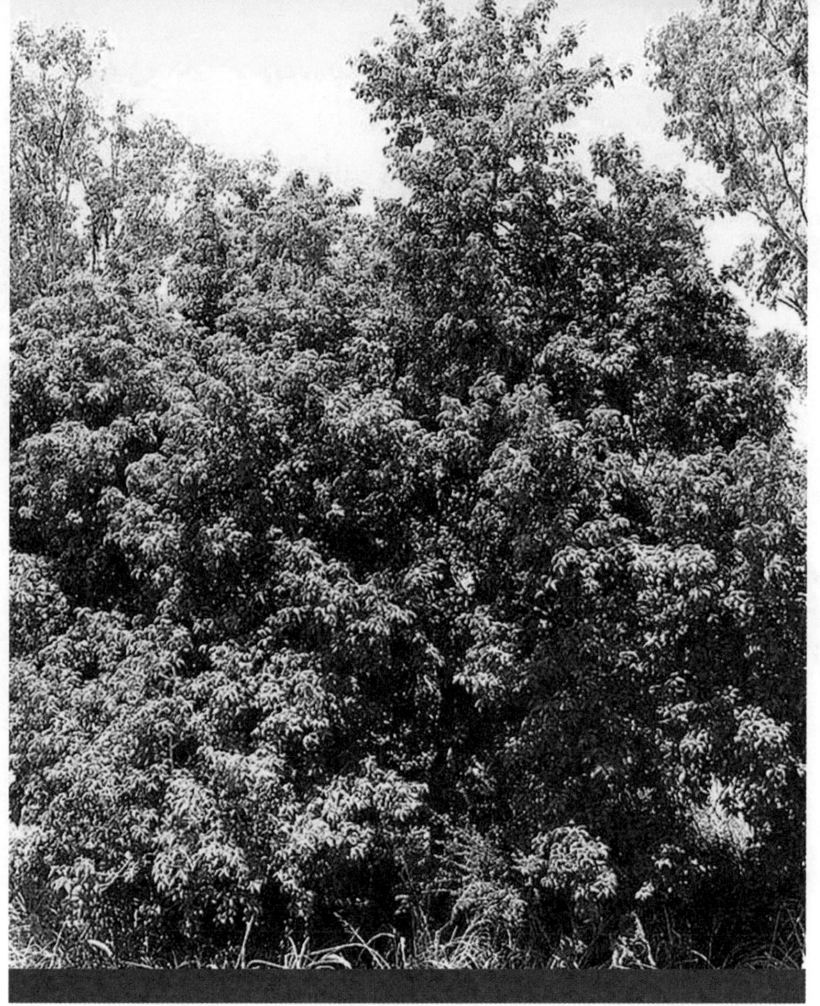

New South Wales (ALA, 2022; ATRP, 2020; Lassak & McCarthy, 2001; WAH, 2022).

Medicinal Uses Decoctions of the wood of False Cedar were taken internally by Aboriginal groups as an analgesic for aches and pains (Lassak & McCarthy, 2001; Webb, 1959).

Other Uses The fruit of False Cedar are edible and were an important food source for Aboriginal Australians, especially in more arid regions where food was scarcer. The fruit are available from November to February (Kane, 2022; Kenneally et al., 1996; Revoly, 2020; Vigilante et al., 2013).

Fibrebark

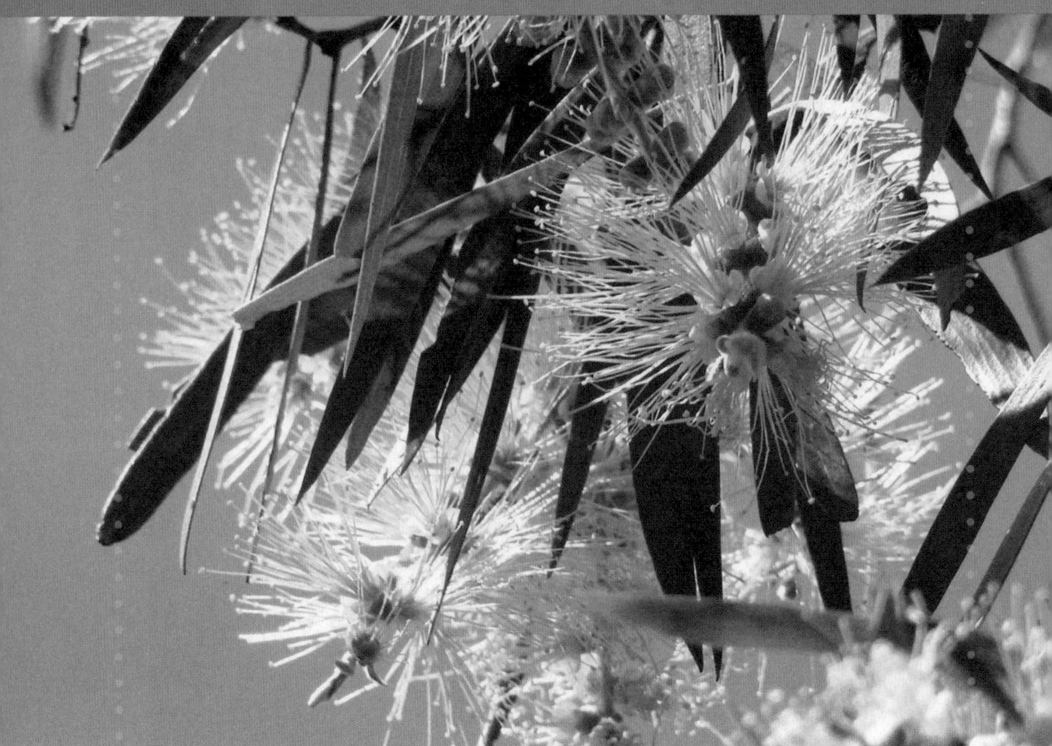

Scientific Name *Melaleuca nervosa* (Lindl.) Cheel.

Common Names Fibrebark, Stunted Paperbark.

Aboriginal Names Nimalgoon (Nyul Nyul) (Dobbs et al., 2015), Dangai (Wanambal, Gaambera) (Karadada et al., 2011), Biido (Bardi) (Kenneally et al., 1996), Bidor (Bardi) (Smith & Kalotas, 1985), Banderanil, Panteranil (Gija) (Purdie et al., 2018), Lambu (Jaru) (Wightman, 2003), Nimarlkarn (Nyikina) (Smith & Smith, 2009).

Field Notes Fibrebark grows as a shrub or tree up to 15 m in height. Its ovate leaves are dull grey-green, stiff, leathery and up to 105 mm long. Its creamy-green, cream, yellow-green or occasionally red flowers are borne on dense cylindrical spikes approximately 100 mm long and carried in groups of one to four. Flowering occurs between March and September. The fruit are cup-shaped, woody capsules approximately 3 mm in diameter. Fibrebark occurs in alluvium and sandy soils, along watercourses, in

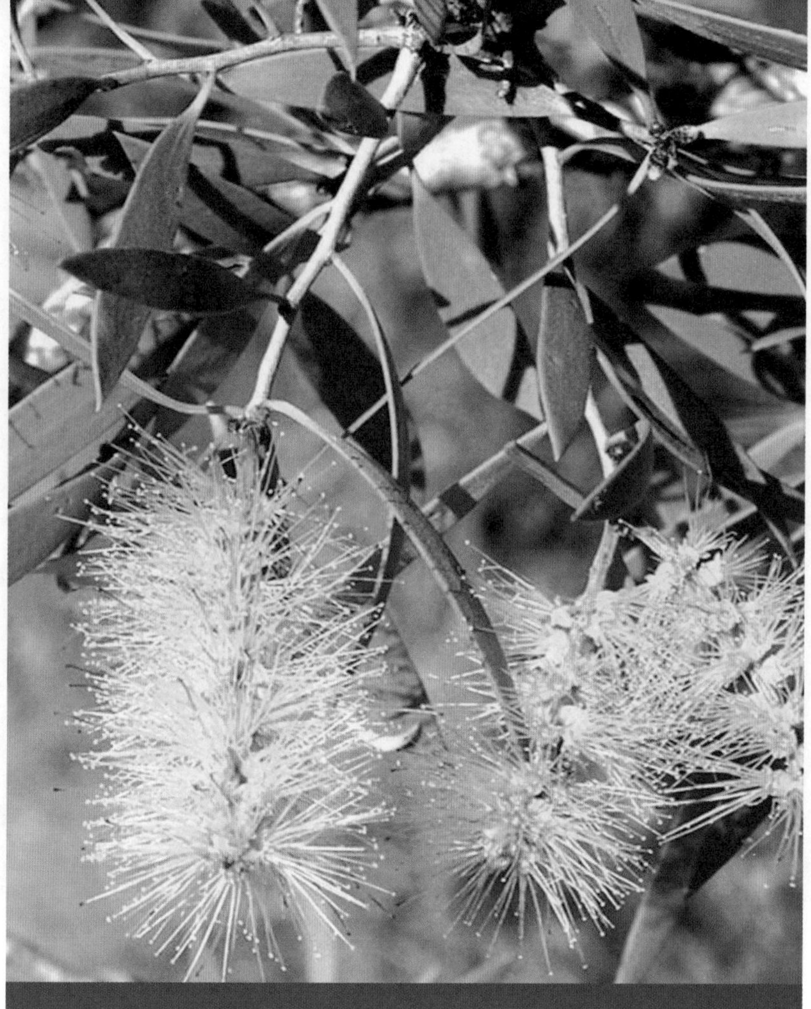

damp depressions and on red sand dunes across the northern part of Australia from the Kimberley region of Western Australia and the Northern Territory extending south in Queensland to the Wide Bay area (ALA, 2022; Native Plants Queensland - Townsville Branch, 2022; WAH, 2022).

Medicinal Uses Infusions of crushed leaves of Fibrebark were drunk for 'cold sick', presumably to ease the symptoms of colds and influenza (Smith & Kalotas, 1985; Williams, 2011). Alternatively, fresh leaves were crushed and the vapours inhaled, and crushed leaves were rubbed on the forehead or used as 'steaming' medicine for the same purpose (Webb, 1959; Wightman, 2003; Williams, 2011). Infusions of the inner bark were drunk to treat depression (efficacy unknown) or vomiting (Williams, 2011).

Fitzroy Wattle

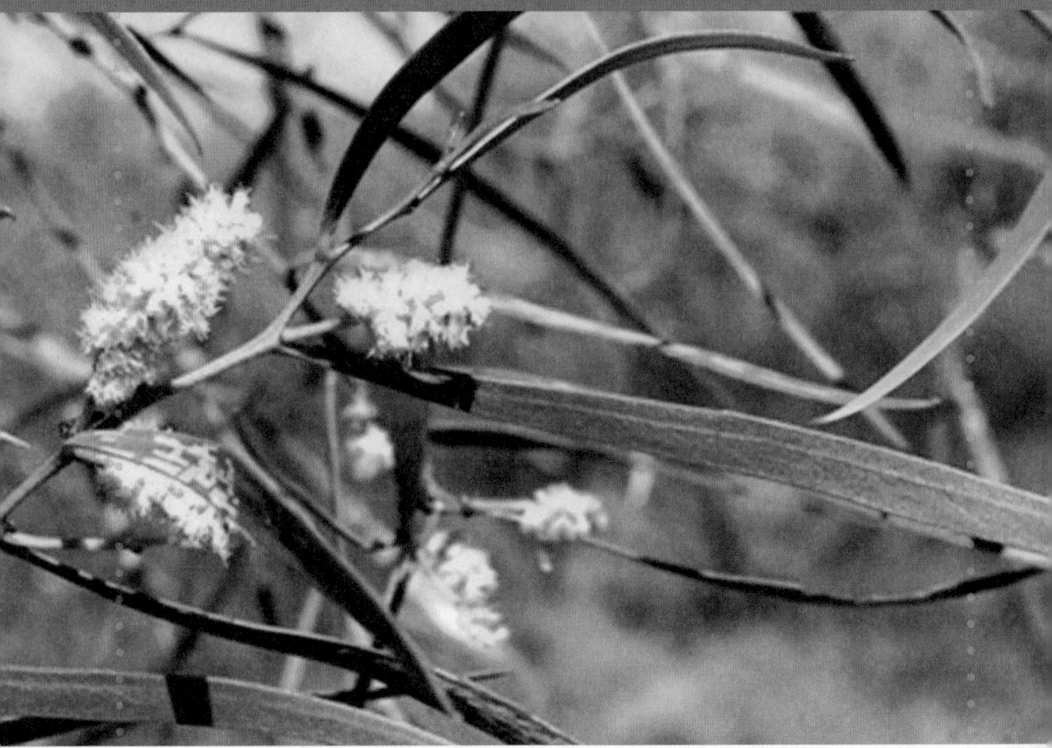

Scientific Name *Acacia ancistrocarpa* Maiden & Blakely.

Common Names Fitzroy Wattle, Fish-hook Wattle, Pindan Wattle, Shiny Leaved Wattle.

Aboriginal Names Kampuka (Ngardi) (Cataldi, 2004), Parlpi (Nyangumarta, Karajarri), Kampuka, Palpiny (Walmajarri) (Richards & Hudson, 2012), Kampuka, Palpirrpa, Parlpinpa, Watarurru (Kukatja) (Valiquette, 1993).

Field Notes Fitzroy Wattle grows as a spreading shrub or small tree, occasionally to 4 m in height. Its phyllodes are linear to very narrowly elliptic and up to 180 mm long. Its long golden flower spikes appear between March and August. Its fruit or seed pods are narrow and oblong, with a slight curve and are up to 110 mm long. Fitzroy Wattle occurs in red sandy soils along creeks, pindan or stony plains across northern Australia from the Pilbara and Kimberley regions of Western Australia through the Northern

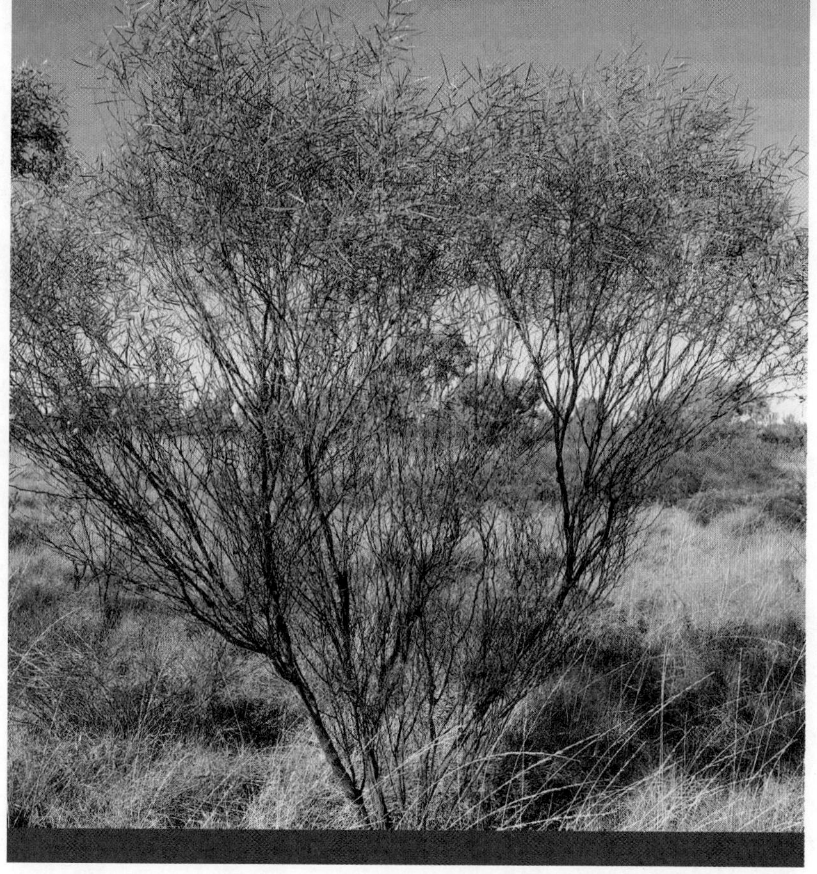

Territory and over the border into Queensland (ALA, 2022; WAH, 2022; World Wide Wattle, 2022).

Medicinal Uses Infusions or decoctions of the mashed phyllodes and twigs of Fitzroy Wattle were used as a wash for skin sores and headaches (Lassak & McCarthy, 2001; Reid, 1986; Williams, 2011). The infusions were also drunk to relieve the symptoms of colds and influenza. Twigs were heated until sweating, then applied to swellings to draw out the fluid and to relieve pain (Maslin et al., 2010; Williams, 2011). The leaves were chewed and the resulting juice was applied to sores and wounds (Richards & Hudson, 2012). The leaves were used as smoke medicine for babies with diarrhoea (Williams, 2011).

Other Uses: The seeds of Fitzroy Wattle are edible and were ground to make flour for damper. The seeds were also eaten raw as a snack. The roots were a good source of edible grubs (Bindon, 2014; Maslin et al., 2010).

Flannel Bush

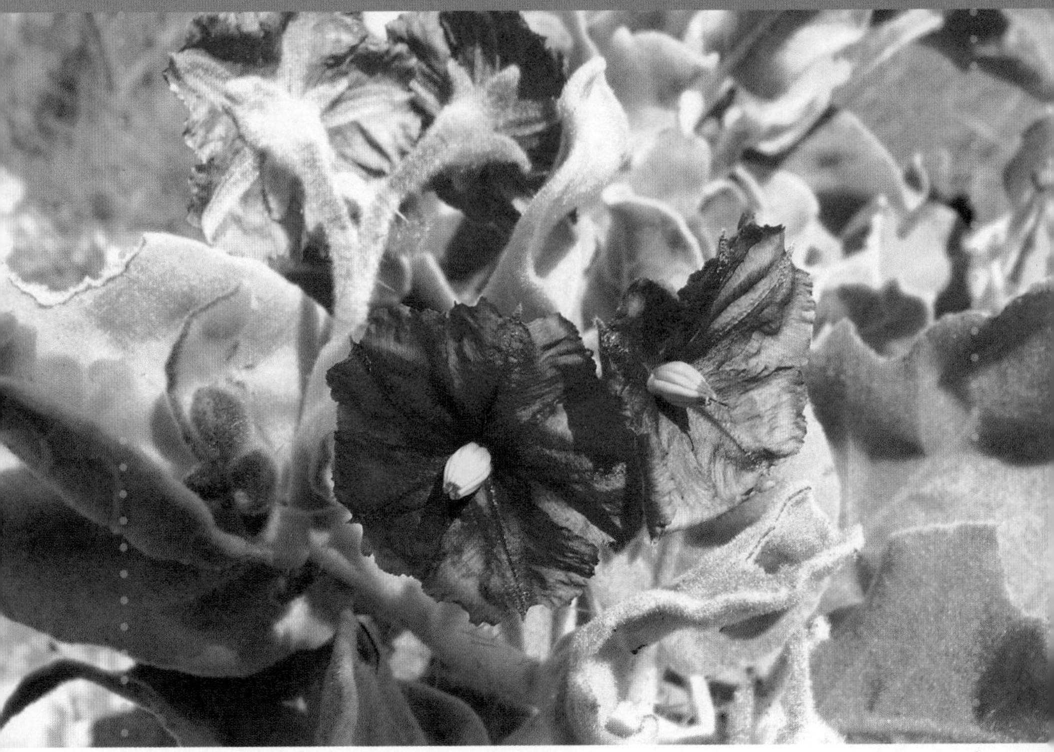

Scientific Name *Solanum lasiophyllum* Poir.

Common Names Flannel Bush, Native Tomato.

Field Notes Flannel Bush is a prickly, bushy shrub of the nightshade family that grows up to 2 m in height. It has round or broadly ovate leaves that are up to 50 mm long and hairy on both sides. Its purple-violet, trumpet-shaped flowers with five pointed petals appear in January or from April to October. Flannel Bush occurs in a variety of soils, including sand and clay, on stony rises all over Western Australia except in the far north and far south. In the Kimberley, it is reported to occur in the Broome and Halls Creek Local Government Areas. It also occurs in parts of the Northern Territory and South Australia (ALA, 2022; eFlora.SA, 2022; Lassak & McCarthy, 2008; WAH, 2022).

Medicinal Uses Decoctions of the crushed roots of Flannel Bush were used as a liniment that was rubbed on swollen legs to reduce

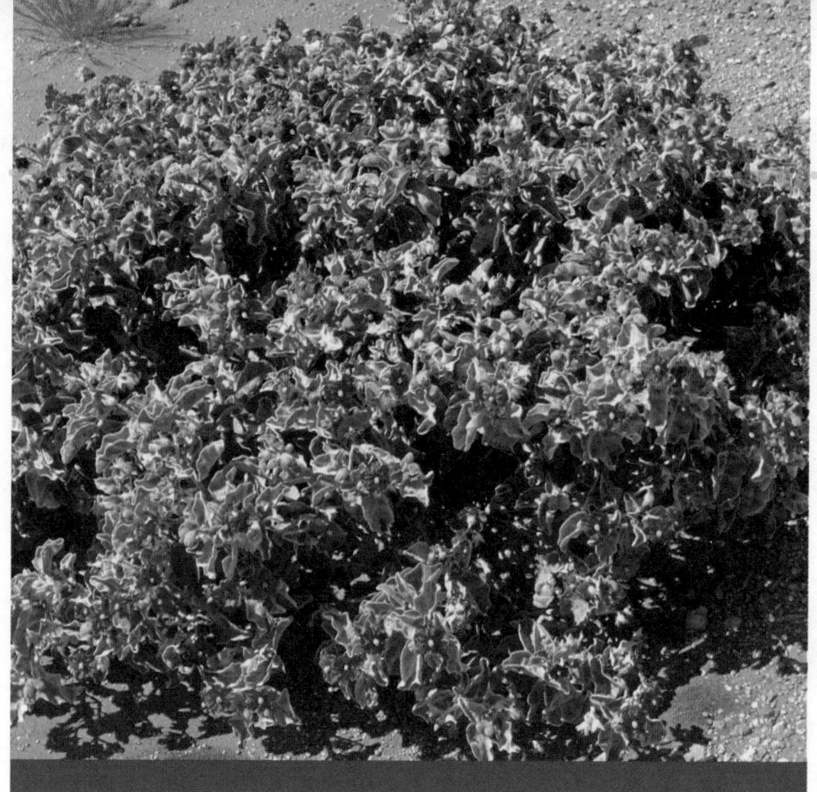

the swelling. Alternatively, crushed roots were applied as a poultice to leg swelling for the same purpose (Lassak & McCarthy, 2008; Webb, 1959; Williams, 2012).

Other Uses The fruit of Flannel Bush are reported to be edible when ripe. Some people remove the bitter skin before eating them (Williams, 2012). Plant Broome (n.d.) describes the fruits as 'hard inedible drupes, fully enclosed by prickly bracts full of small brown-black seeds'.

Flinders River Poison

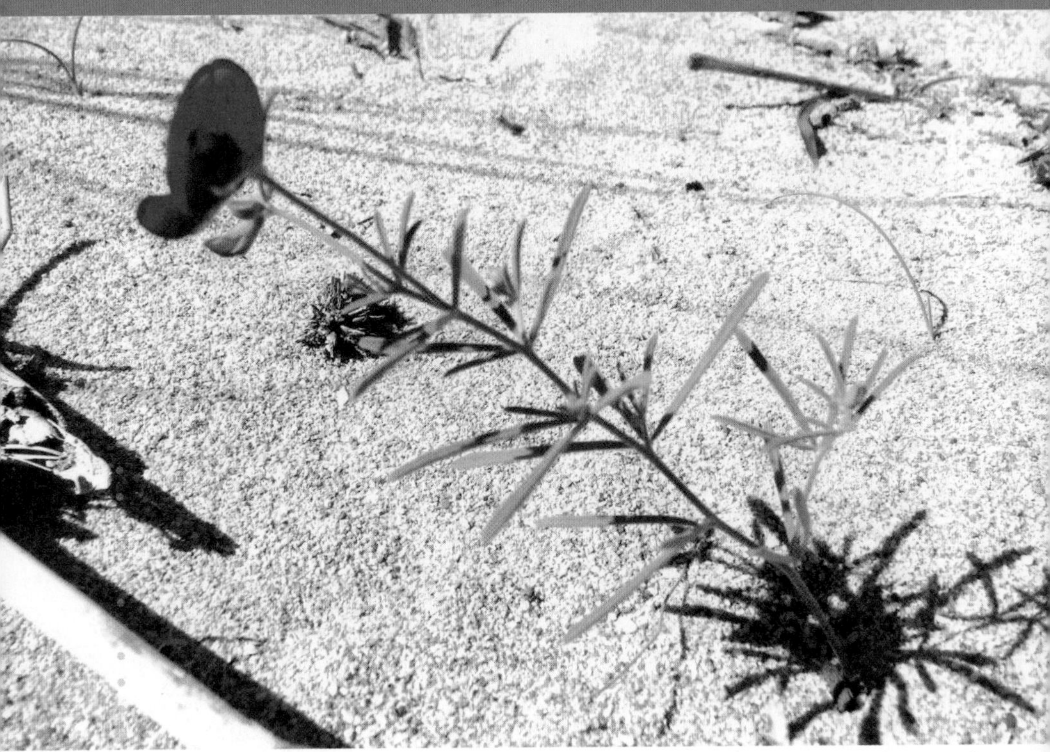

Scientific Names *Tephrosia rosea* Benth., also known as *Tephrosia purpurea* (L.) Pers.

Common Names Flinders River Poison, Fish Poison Pea.

Aboriginal Names Layini (Wunambal, Gaambera) (Karadada et al., 2011), Ilngam (Bardi) (Kenneally et al., 2018), Bidiny (Bardi) (Smith & Kalotas, 1985), Panjurta (Karajarri) (Willing, 2014), Bawulu (Bunuba) (Moss et al., 2021).

Field Notes Flinders River Poison is an erect or sometimes sprawling shrub that grows up to 2 m in height. Its pinnate leaves are up to 52 mm long and 13 mm wide and are covered on both sides by silky hairs. Its pea-type, pink-purple and sometimes red-brown flowers can be present all year round. Its fruit are up to 30 mm long, are densely clothed in silky hairs and contain up to eight seeds per fruit. Flinders River Poison occurs in a variety of habitats in the Pilbara and Kimberley regions of Western Australia, the

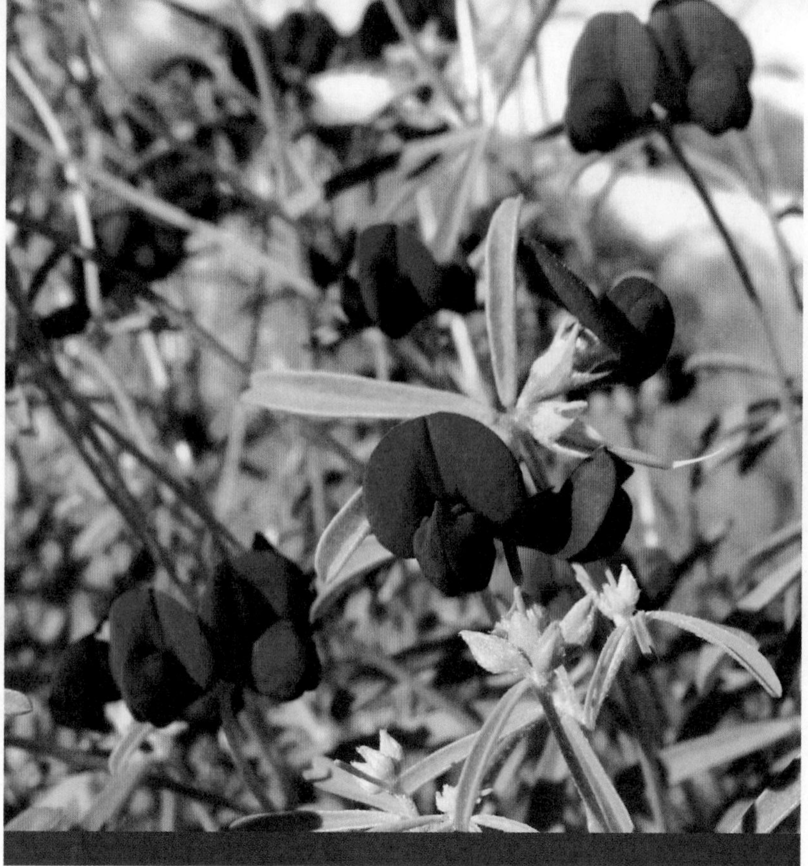

Northern Territory and Queensland. It also occurs in India, Sri Lanka and tropical Africa (ALA, 2022; ATRP, 2020; WAH, 2022).

Medicinal Uses Flinders River Poison is used in Ayurvedic folk medicine as a deobstruent and diuretic, and has proved useful in the treatment of bronchitis, fever and 'obstructions of the liver, spleen and kidneys', as a blood purifier and as a treatment for boils and pimples. Decoctions of the fruit were taken internally to expel intestinal parasites and to relieve bodily pains and inflammation (Sujatha & Renuga, 2014). Decoctions of the bitter roots have been used in India to treat dyspepsia, dysentery and tympanites (abdominal distension due to gas) (Bailey, 1881; Williams, 2012).

Other Uses The Bardi, Karajarri and other groups used preparations of the roots or whole plant as 'fish poison' in reef pools to stun fish that would then float to the top and make them easy to collect (Karadada et al., 2011; Kenneally et al., 2018; Willing, 2014; Williams, 2012).

Forked Mistletoe

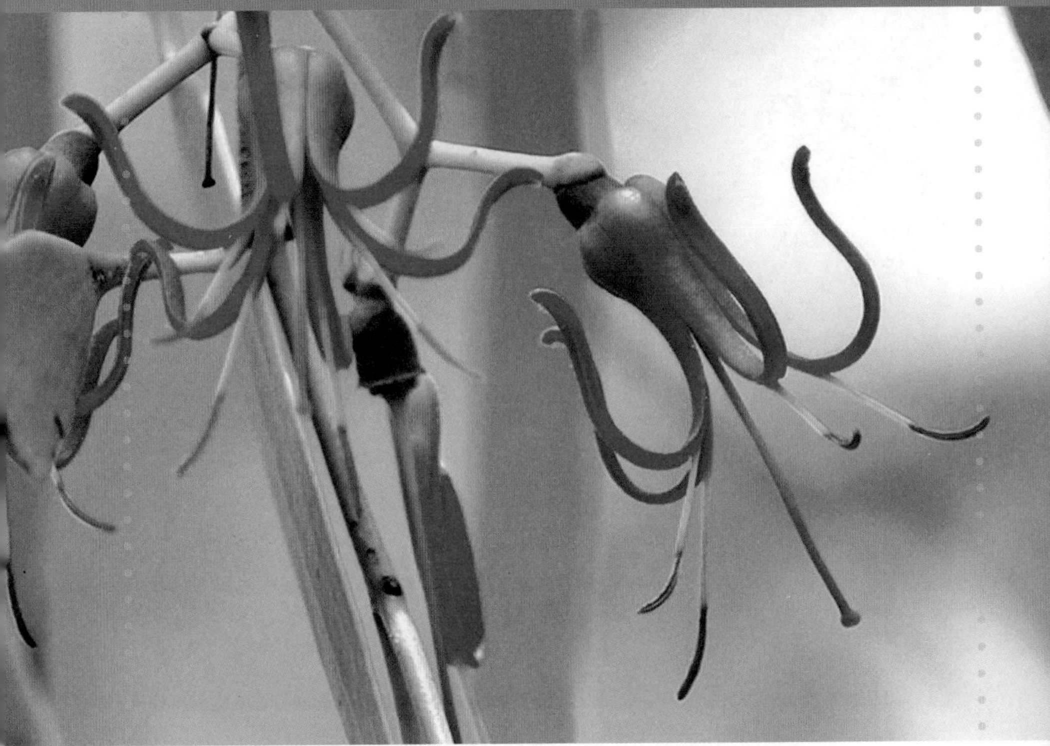

Scientific Name *Amyema bifurcata* (Benth.) Tiegh., previously known as *Amyema bifurcatum* Barlow.

Common Names Forked Mistletoe, Gum Tree Mistletoe.

Aboriginal Names Nyil Nyil (Bardi) (Smith & Kalotas, 1985), Yun-gurrmari (Jaru) (Wightman, 2003).

Field Notes Forked Mistletoe is an aerial shrub that is hemiparasitic on eucalypts. The leaves are linear to lanceolate and can be up to 400 mm long and 25 mm wide. Its orange-red inflorescence is an umbel of paired, tubular flowers that can be up to 40 mm long. Flowers can be present any time between June and January. Its fruit are globose to pear-shaped, cream to orange when ripe and about 9 mm in diameter. Forked Mistletoe is endemic to the Pilbara and Kimberley regions of Western Australia, the Northern Territory, Queensland and north-east New South Wales (ALA, 2022; ATRP, 2020; SMIP, 2022; WAH, 2022).

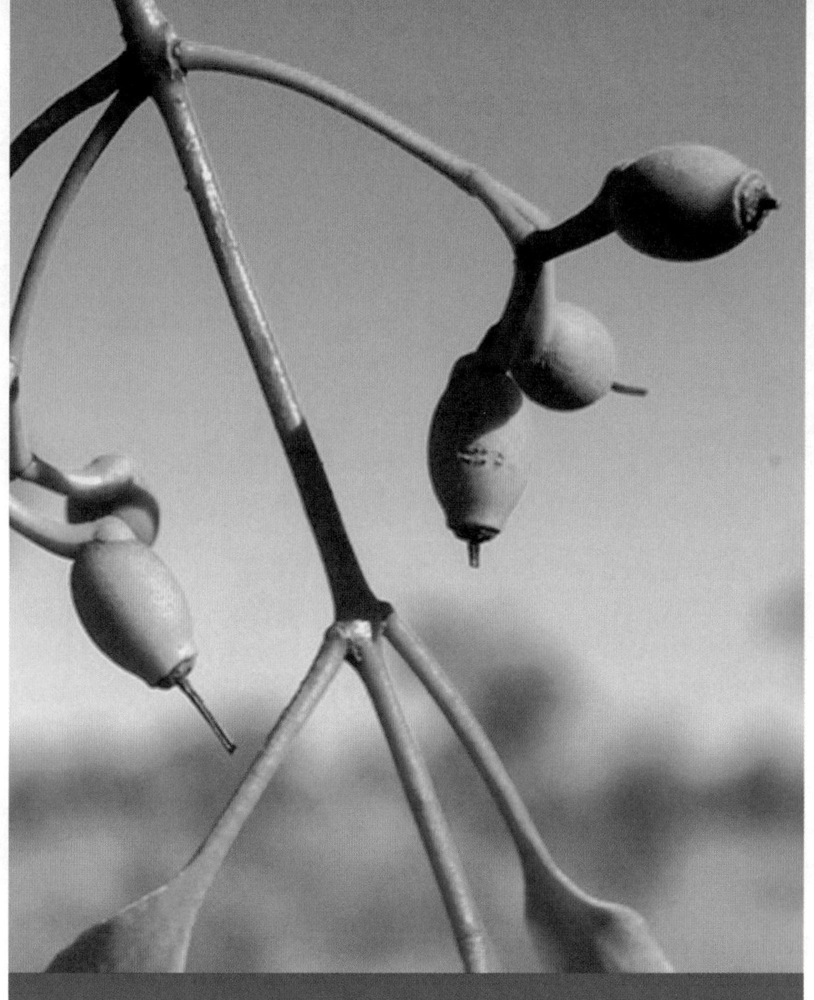

Medicinal Uses Decoctions of the inner wood were sipped to relieve the symptoms of bad colds and influenza. The decoctions were sipped as often as needed (Smith, 1991).

Other Uses The fruit of the Forked Mistletoe can be eaten raw when yellow and ripe. The fruit is reported to be very sticky inside (RFCA, 1993; Wightman, 2003). Children are known to suck the nectar directly from the flowers (Barker, 1991; Smith & Kalotas, 1985).

Fragrant Opilia

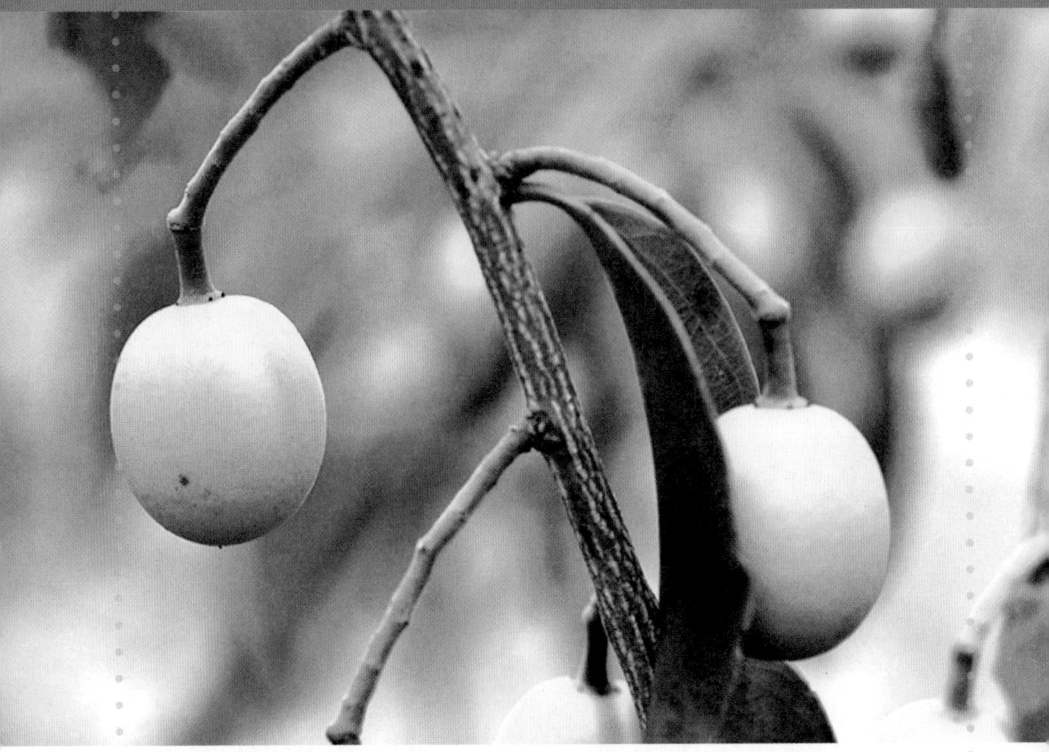

Scientific Name *Opilia amentacea* Roxb.

Common Names Fragrant Opilia, Brown Grape.

Aboriginal Names Wulgujar (Wunambal, Gaambera) (Karadada et al., 2011), Larlamurri (Mangarrayi), Jimirlbil (Gija) (Purdie et al., 2018; Wightman, 2003), Minkal ninya, Mingkurl ninya (Kwini) (Cheinmora et al., 2017).

Field Notes Fragrant Opilia grows as a climber or shrub up to 7 m in height. Its roots are parasitic. The branchlets are warty and brown. Its leaves are leathery, ovate with a pointed tip and up to 90 mm long by 30 mm wide. Its small, green-yellow flowers are borne in racemes of up to five. Its fruit are ovate drupes up to 30 mm long by 18 mm in diameter. In Australia, flowering is from July to October. Fragrant Opilia occurs in sand, on coastal dunes, sandstone screes and riverine habitats across the top of tropical Australia, including the Kimberley region of Western Australia, the north of

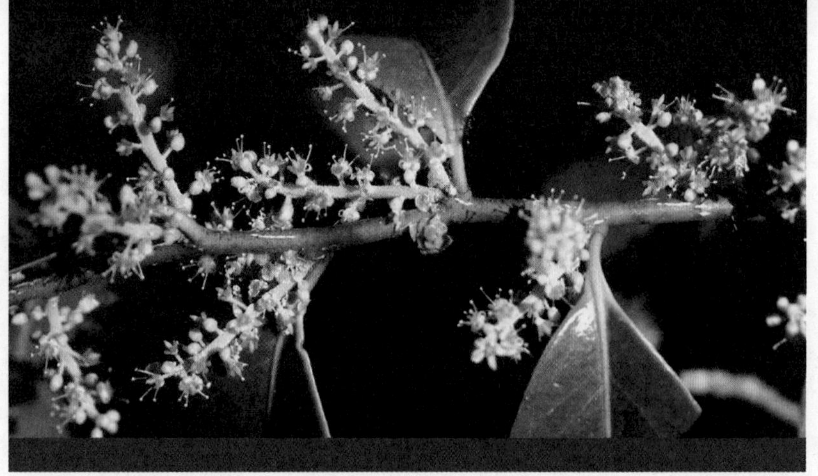

the Northern Territory and the Cape York Peninsula in Queensland. It is also native to tropical Africa, China, the Indian subcontinent, Indochina, Indonesia, Malaysia, Myanmar and Sri Lanka (ALA, 2022; ATRP, 2020; Flowers of India, 2022; WAH, 2022).

Medicinal Uses In Australia, decoctions of the leaves of Fragrant Opilia were used as an external wash to treat fever, colds and general malaise. In other tropical countries, the leaves and roots are used in traditional folk medicine. Decoctions or infusions of the root were drunk for the treatment of fevers, mental illness, headache, influenza and stomach problems. Extracts of the leaves were used to treat intestinal parasites. Infusions of the crushed bark were used to treat malaria (Fern, 2021).

Other Uses The fruit of Fragrant Opilia are edible and are eaten raw when ripe and yellow to red and are reported to be sweet and tasty (Cheinmora et al., 2017; DBCA, 2019; Fern, 2021; Fox & Garde, 2018; Kenneally et al., 1996; Purdie et al., 2018; RFCA, 1993; Vigilante et al., 2013; Wightman, 2003). The fruit are available in December and January (Kenneally et al., 1996). The flexible stems of Fragrant Opilia are used in Asia like rattan for making chairs and storage containers. The wood is soft and easily carved so it is used for making combs, toothbrushes and spoons (Fern, 2021).

CAUTION: eating the pulp and juice of the yellow fruit of Fragrant Opilia can cause stomatitis (inflammation of the mouth) (Wightman, 2017).

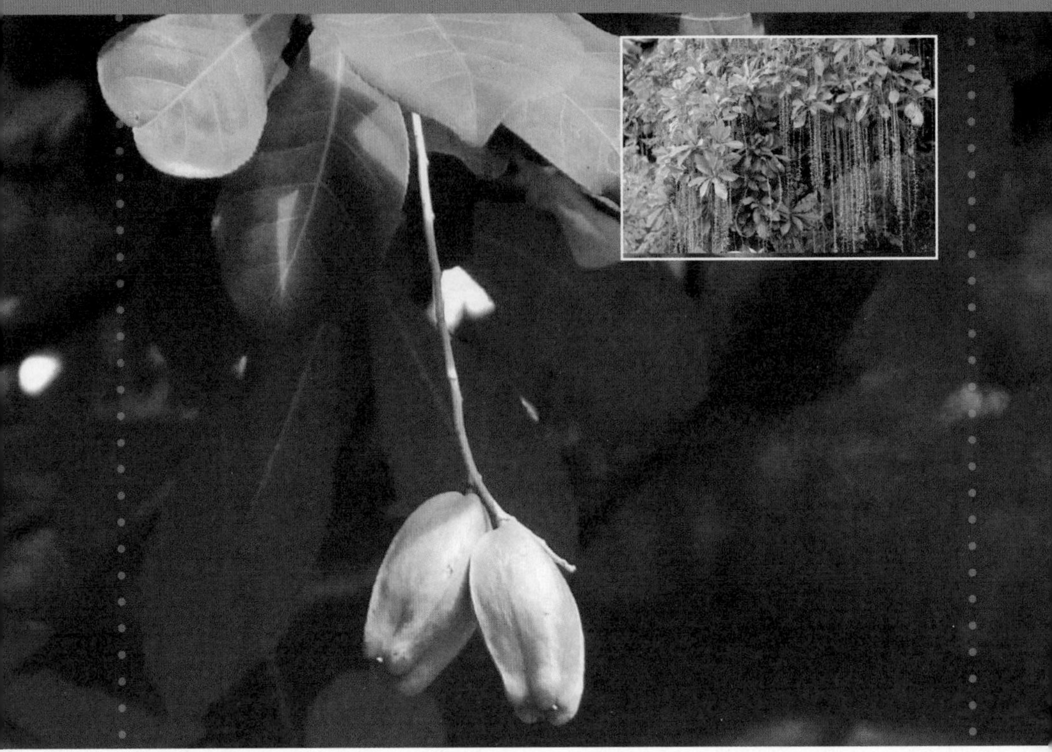

Scientific Name *Barringtonia acutangula* (L.) Gaertn.

Common Names Freshwater Mangrove, Itchytree, Mango-pine.

Aboriginal Names Jinggoolng (Miriwoong) (Leonard et al., 2013), Danbu (Wunambal, Gaambera) (Karadada et al., 2011), Majala, Punyju (Walmajarri) (Richards & Hudson, 2012), Malawanji, Malawani, Mangoonyji (Gija) (Purdie et al., 2018), Gooroo (Gooniyandi) (Dilkes et al., 2019), Mangunyji, Werlarlampalji (Gija) (Wightman, 2003), Danba manya (Kwini) (Cheinmora et al., 2017; Crawford, 1982), Majala (Nyikina) (DAWE, n.d.), Malaa (Bunuba) (Oscar et al., 2019), Mirlbarridi (Yawuru) (Moss et al., 2021).

Field Notes Freshwater Mangrove grows as a shrub or tree to 25 m in height. It has rough, fissured, dark grey bark and thick, smooth, obovate leaves that are up to 120 mm long. Red flowers appear on drooping racemes about 200 mm long, usually from April to May in Australia. Its fruit are four-sided capsules. In Australia, Freshwater

Mangrove occurs in alluvium or sandy clay on the banks of rivers and creeks and on floodplains across the tropical north from the Kimberley region of Western Australia to the Cape York Peninsula in Far North Queensland. It is also native to Afghanistan, Cambodia, the Indian subcontinent, Indonesia, Laos, Malaysia, Myanmar, New Guinea, the Philippines, Thailand and Vietnam (ALA, 2022; Fern, 2021; Flowers of India, 2022; WAH, 2022).

Medicinal Uses In the Kimberley, the bark of Freshwater Mangrove was chewed and applied as a poultice to relieve the pain of a catfish sting, barramundi sting or toothache. The chewed bark applied as a poultice was also used to stop bleeding and to help heal wounds. The only side effect noted was drowsiness (Bush Heritage Australia, 2019; Oscar et al., 2019). Freshwater Mangrove is also used in traditional folk medicine in Asian countries, particularly in India and Sri Lanka where it is used in Ayurvedic medicine. The scraped bark was squeezed with coconut meat and the juice drunk daily for treating pneumonia, diarrhoea and asthma. The scraped bark and coconut meat combination was also used as a poultice to treat wounds, ulcers, sores and itchy skin. Infusions or decoctions of the leaves were taken internally to treat diarrhoea. Decoctions of the bark were given in small doses for anorexia to increase the appetite. Crushed seeds were mixed with water to form a paste that was rubbed on the chest of children suffering from chest colds (Fern, 2021; Flowers of India, 2022; Maiden, 1889).

Other Uses The roots, bark and leaves were used for 'fish poison' by some Aboriginal groups in the Kimberley. The stunned fish would float to the surface where they were easily caught (Cheinmora et al., 2017; Hiddins, 2001; Karadada et al., 2011; Oscar et al., 2019; SKIPA, 2022; Wightman, 2003).

Frogsmouth

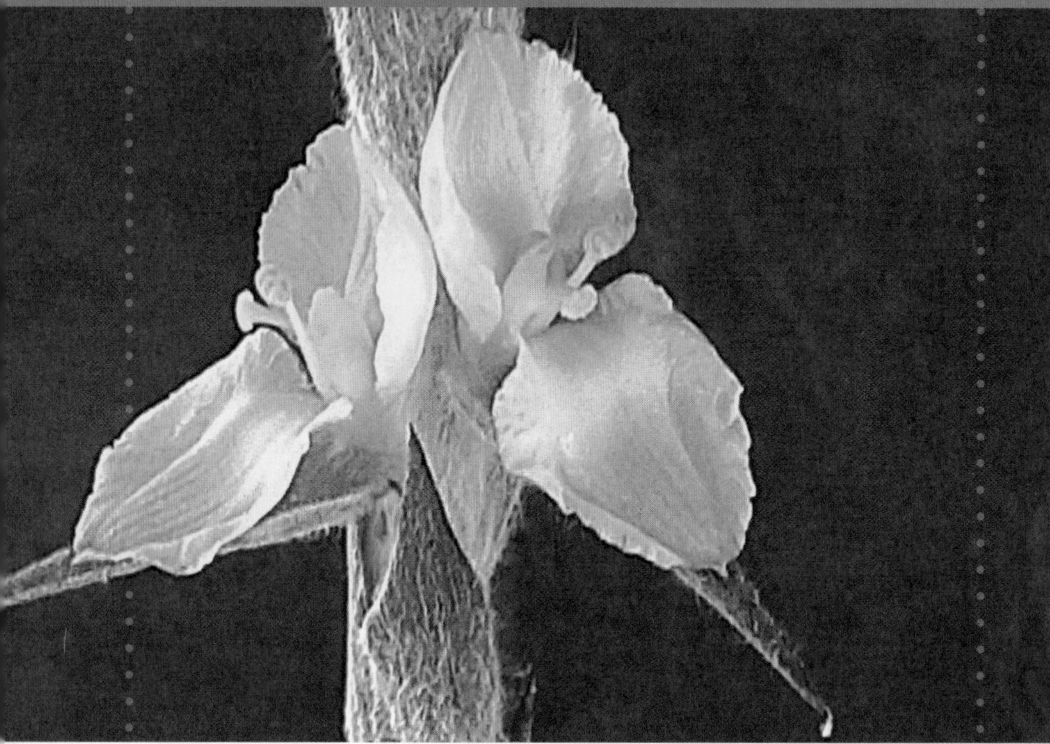

Scientific Name *Philydrum lanuginosum* Gaertn.

Common Names Frogsmouth, Woolly Frogmouth.

Field Notes Frogsmouth is a tuberous, tufted, perennial herb that grows to around 1.25 m in height. Its green leaves arise from the base of the plant and are up to 800 mm long. Its yellow flowers have two large petals, which make the flower look like an open frog's mouth, hence the common name. The flowers are present from March to September. Its fruit are a hairy, triangular to oblong capsule approximately 10 mm long and 5 mm in diameter. Frogsmouth occurs in lateritic wet loam around freshwater swamps and watercourses in the Kimberley region of Western Australia and in all other mainland states and territories, except South Australia. It is also native to the Andaman Islands, India, Japan, Malaysia, Myanmar, Papua New Guinea, Taiwan, Thailand and Vietnam (ALA, 2022; WAH, 2022).

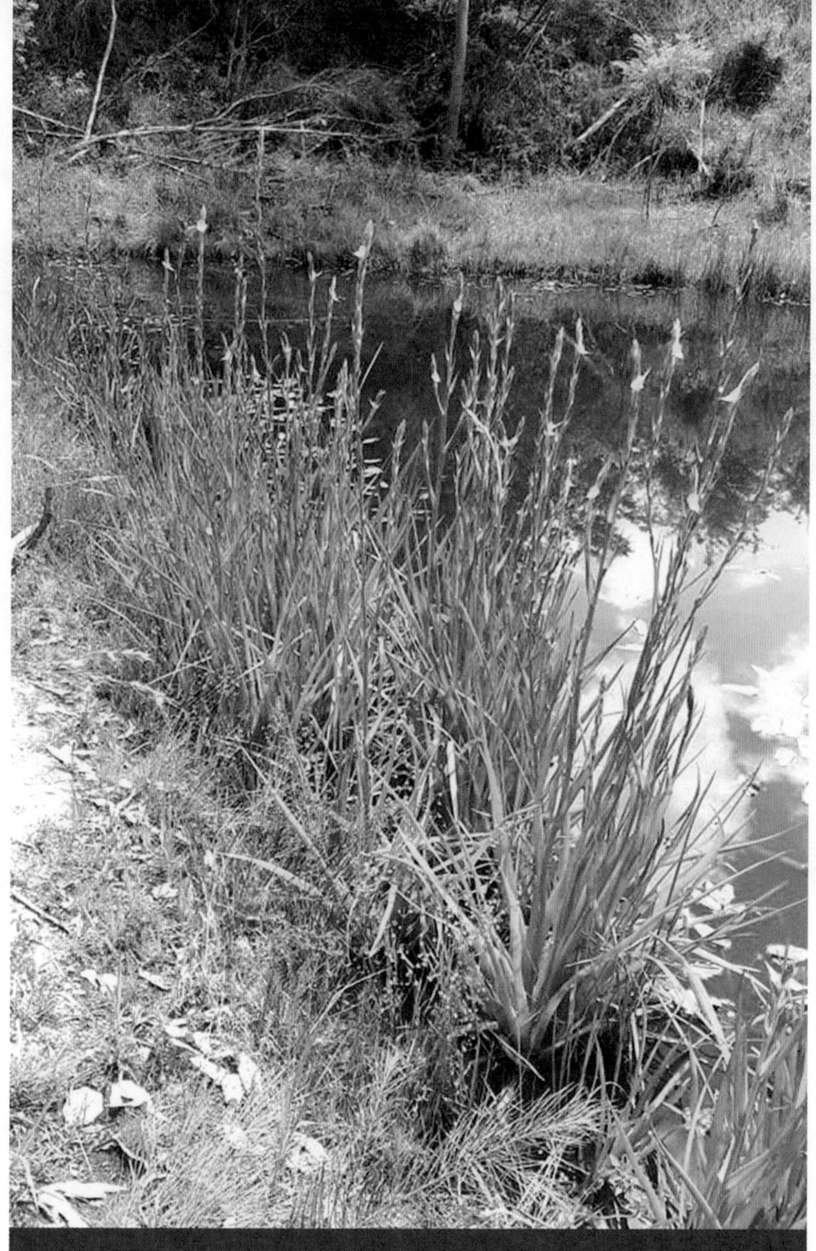

Medicinal Uses Decoctions of the whole plant were used as an antiseptic wash for skin sores and other skin conditions, such as scabies infestations and skin rashes due to allergies (Smith, 1991). The decoctions were also taken internally to treat diarrhoea (Yunupinu et al., 1995).

Gadji

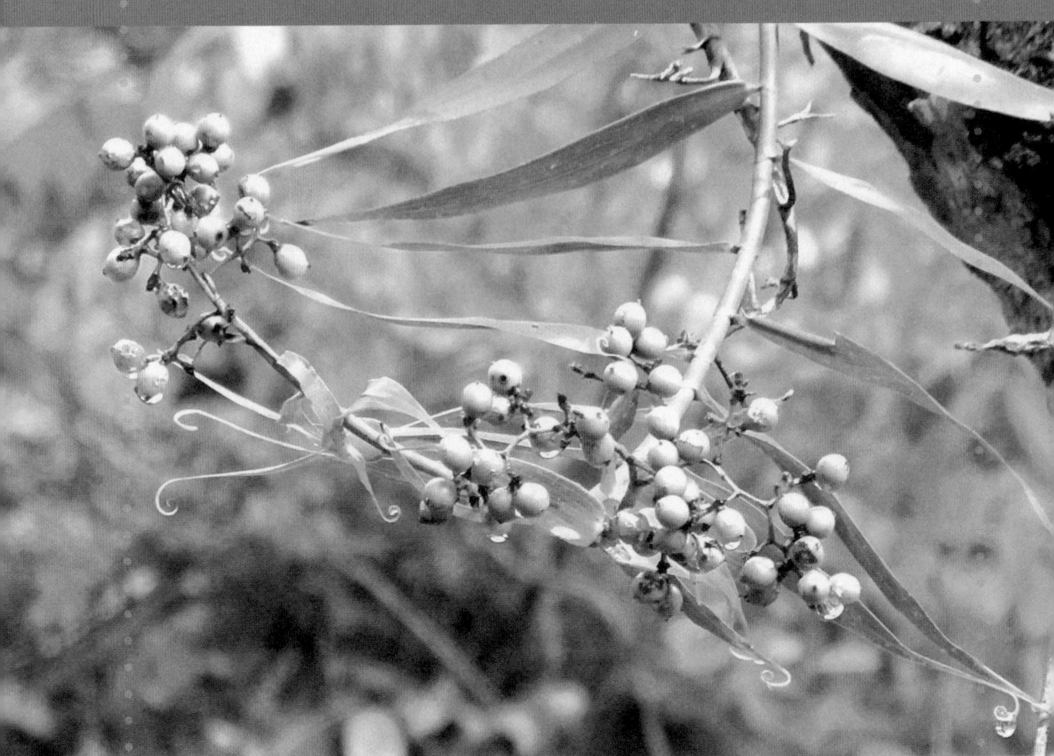

Scientific Name *Flagellaria indica* L.

Common Names Gadji, Supplejack, Supple Jack, False Rattan, Bangle Vine, Whip Vine.

Aboriginal Names Gaaji (Wunambal, Gaambera) (Karadada et al., 2011), Kaaji winya, Karral winya (Kwini) (Cheinmora et al., 2017), Balbal (Bardi) (Kenneally et al., 1996; Smith & Kalotas, 1985).

Field Notes Gadji is a rhizomatous, perennial climber or herb that grows to around 600 mm in height. The stems can be more than 15 mm in diameter. The leaves are lanceolate and up to 400 mm long. The curled tips of the leaves help the plant climb. Its fragrant white to cream flowers form in panicles and appear from April to December. Gadji occurs in sand, sandy clay and sandstone in coastal or riverine areas and vine thickets in the Kimberley region of Western Australia, the Northern Territory and Queensland, and down the east coast as far south as Newcastle in New South

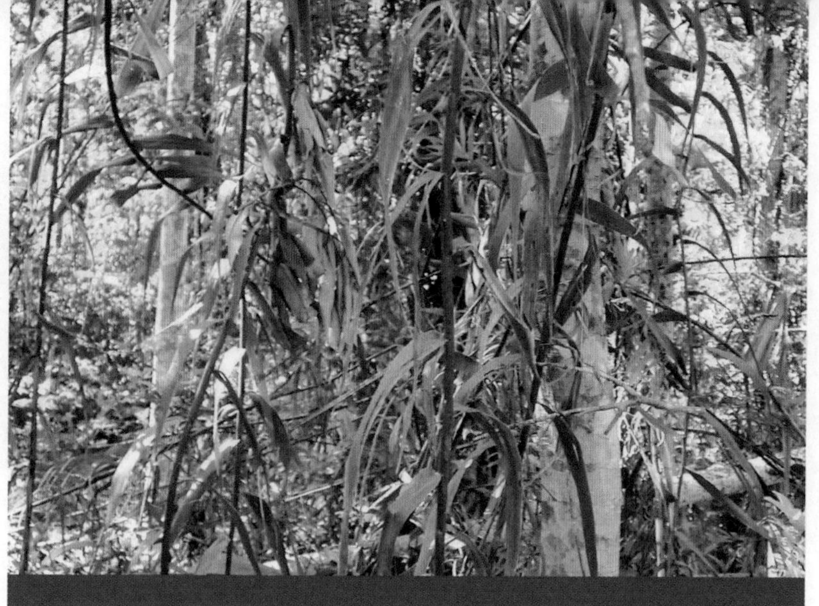

Wales. It also occurs in East Africa, through tropical and subtropical Asia to the western Pacific (ALA, 2022; ATRP, 2020; Fern, 2021; WAH, 2022).

Medicinal Uses The stems of the Gadji were chewed to relieve toothache (Low, 1990; Hiddins, 2001; Western Australia Now and Then, 2020). Decoctions of the root were drunk by some Aboriginal groups as a health tonic. Infusions or decoctions of the stems were drunk to relieve stomach ache, dysentery and diarrhoea (Cock, 2011; Smith, 1991). Decoctions of the leaves were drunk to treat asthma, general shortness of breath and fever (Fern, 2021; Hiddins, 2001; Lassak & McCarthy, 2001). Infusions of the 'young sappy tips' were applied externally as an eyewash to treat conjunctivitis (Webb, 1959). In Far North Queensland, Aboriginal groups chewed the leaves slowly and swallowed them to treat certain venereal diseases (efficacy unknown) (Edwards, 2005).

Other uses The young leafy shoots and buds were cooked and eaten as a vegetable. The pink fruit (apart from the seeds) are also edible, as are the stems, which contain a sweet sap and were chewed like sugarcane (Cribb & Cribb, 1981; Fern, 2021; Fox & Garde, 2018; MRCCC, n.d.; RFCA, 1993). The hard, flexible stems were traditionally used to make frames for small fish nets (Cheinmora et al., 2017).

Gandungai

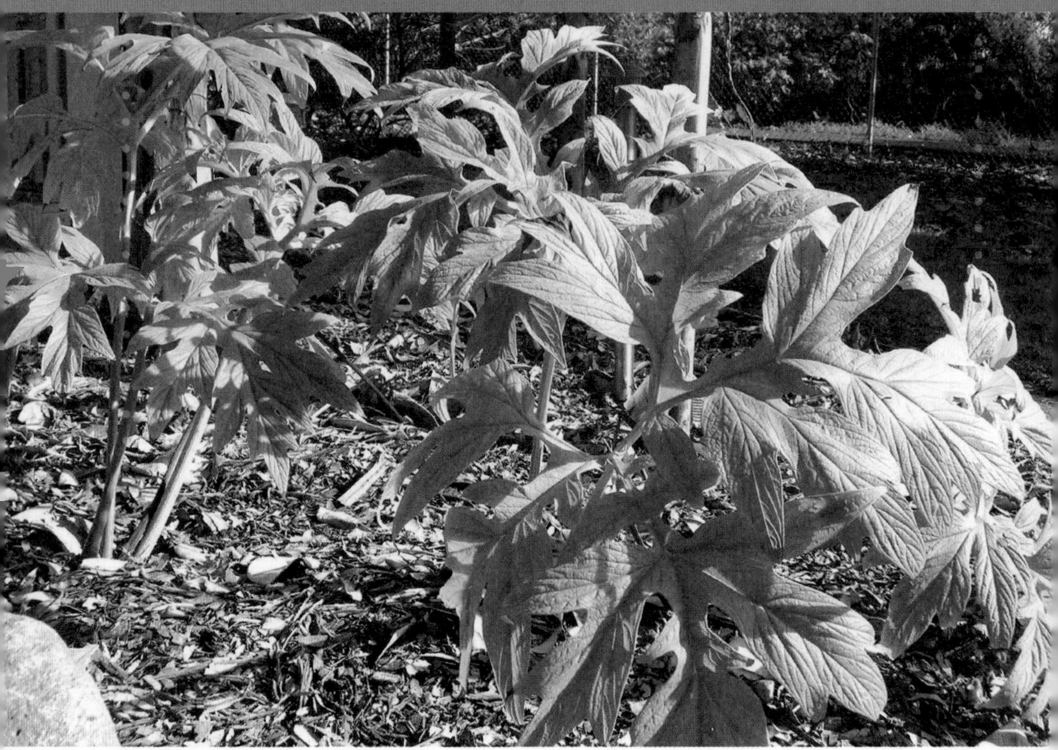

Scientific Name *Tacca leontopetaloides* (L.) Kuntze.

Common Names Gandungai, Bush Yam, Polynesian Arrowroot, Fiji Arrowroot, East Indies Arrowroot, Pia.

Aboriginal Names Langangu (Wunambal, Gaambera) (Karadada et al., 2011), Gandungai (Kwini) (Crawford, 1982), Pikirniny (Gija) (Wightman, 2003), K-manya, Jilji manya (Kwini) (Cheinmora et al., 2017).

Field Notes Gandungai is a tuberous, perennial plant that grows to around 1 m in height on a single stem. It has large leaves and greenish-purple flowers with long trailing bracts that appear in clusters from January to April. Its fruit are ovoid, ribbed and up to 30 mm in length. Gandungai occurs in basalt loam and sandy soils across the far north of Australia. It is also found, either naturally or as an introduced species, in parts of Africa, Asia and the Pacific (ALA, 2022; PFAF, 2022; WAH, 2022).

Medicinal Uses Gandungai is used in traditional medicine on some Pacific islands. The pulp of the root is squeezed in water and applied as a rinse to treat conjunctivitis. The starch from the tubers was used to treat diarrhoea and dysentery. The starch from the root was rubbed onto sores and burns to aid healing. Crushed leaf stalks were rubbed onto bee and wasp stings. The stem was roasted and the sap squeezed out and used as ear drops to treat earache (PFAF, 2022).

Other Uses The tubers of Gandungai are edible when prepared properly to leach out an irritating toxin (Cheinmora et al., 2017; Crawford, 1982; Edwards, 2005; Fox & Garde, 2018; Isaacs, 1987; Karadada et al., 2011; Low, 1991; Wightman, 2003). The tubers are harvested between May and November. They are prepared in many ways depending on the location and culture but must be cooked before they are eaten. Crawford (1982) describes how they are prepared in the Kimberley:

> *The tuber is split into quarters resembling orange segments (that is, it is split longitudinally). A hole is prepared with stones in the bottom. Over these, a fierce fire is lit, and this is left burning for about 40 minutes after which the burning wood is removed leaving a layer of coals above the stones. Three or four handfuls of wet soil are put on the coals. The tuber segments are liberally coated with very wet yulan ashes. The hole is then covered with paperbark and sand and left for eight hours. After this length of time, the pieces of Gandungai are still too hot to hold. On the following day, the Aborigines wash the segments of tuber, recoat them with fresh ashes and replace them in the 'bush oven'. On the next morning, they are taken out, and after washing, are ready for eating.*

A damper can be made from the tuber that can keep for months (Cheinmora et al., 2017; Crawford, 1982). In the Kimberley, there were age restrictions on who could eat the Gandungai tuber. According to Crawford (1982), only those who had reached middle age were allowed to eat it. The fruit or seed pods are also edible and are eaten raw when ripe (just after the wet season), and the seeds can be eaten or discarded (Fox & Garde, 2018; Kenneally et al., 1996; RFCA, 1993).

CAUTION: Hiddins (2001) advises that no more than two fruit with the seeds should be eaten at any one time as the fruit can be toxic if too many are eaten.

Ganmanggu

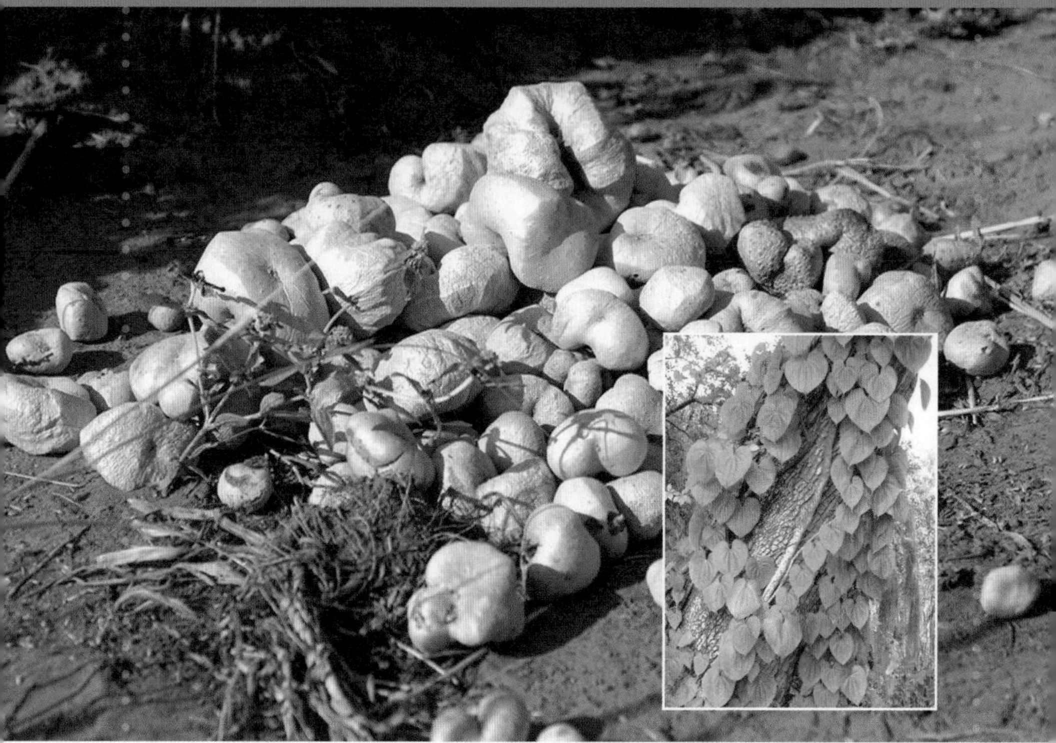

Scientific Name *Dioscorea bulbifera* L.

Common Names Ganmanggu, Water Yam, Cheeky Yam, Aerial Yam, Round Yam.

Aboriginal Names Mijad (Miriwoong) (Leonard et al., 2013), Ganmanggu (Kwini) (Crawford, 1982), Mardelang, Gulngariny (Bardi) (Smith & Kalotas, 1985), Garnawoony, Karnawuny (Gija) (Purdie et al., 2018; Wightman, 2003), Gunu (Wunambal, Gaambera) (Karadada et al., 2011), Kunu minya, Kurnu minya, Jungki minya (Kwini) (Cheinmora et al., 2017).

Field Notes Ganmanggu is a perennial, tuberous climber that grows up to 5 m in height. It has broad, ovate leaves and white-purple-brown flowers that appear between December and February. Its seed pods are small, light brown and butterfly shaped. Ganmanggu occurs in laterite and clay soils along rivers and on breakaways in the Kimberley region of Western Australia, the

Northern Territory, Queensland and down the east coast as far as Brisbane. It also occurs in parts of Africa and Asia (ALA, 2022; Fern, 2021; WAH, 2022).

Medicinal Uses On the Tiwi Islands, the flesh of the yam was rubbed directly and vigorously onto swollen and misshapen limbs to relieve the discomfort (Tiwi Land Council, 2001). The plant is used in folk medicine in other countries as well. The crushed tubers were applied as a poultice to treat wounds, sores, boils, inflammation and fungal infections, or crushed and mixed with palm oil and massaged into areas of rheumatic pain. Sap expressed from the vine stems was applied to the eyes to treat eye infections, such as conjunctivitis and trachoma (Fern, 2021). Aboriginal groups in north Queensland used decoctions of the yams externally to treat skin cancer (Williams, 2013).

Other Uses The parsnip-shaped tubers of Ganmanggu are edible and are eaten boiled, roasted in hot ashes or sand, or cooked in a ground oven with meat (Cheinmora et al., 2017; Crawford, 1982; Fox & Garde, 2018; Hiddins, 2001; Karadada et al., 2011; Purdie et al., 2018; Vigilante et al., 2013; Wightman, 2003). Sometimes the tubers are sliced and seasoned with the ash of the burnt bark of River Gum (*Eucalyptus camaldulensis*) before they are cooked in a ground oven. The ash is washed off before the tubers are eaten (Karadada et al., 2011). The name 'Cheeky Yam' refers to its irritant nature when eaten raw (Williams, 2012). The tubers are harvested between May and November (Crawford, 1982). The flowers are also edible (Fern, 2021).

Garuga

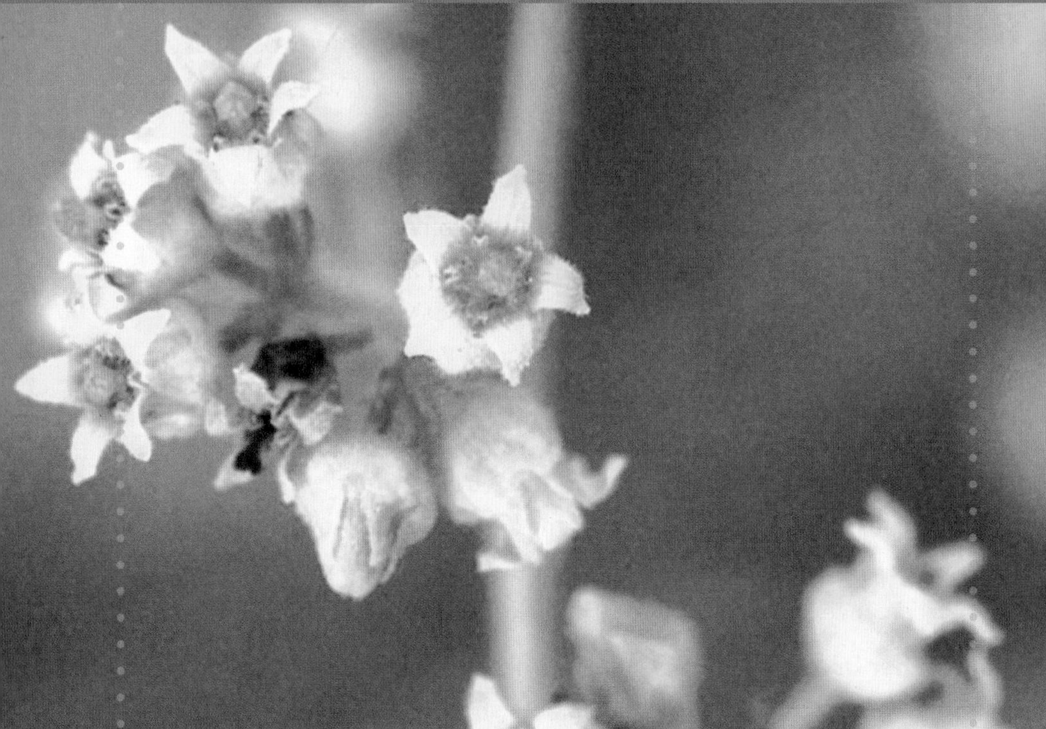

Scientific Name *Garuga floribunda* Decne.

Common Name Garuga.

Field Notes Garuga is a deciduous tree that grows up to 25 m in height. It has flaky bark and imparipinnate leaves up to 300 mm long with oblong-lanceolate leaflets. The leaves turn red before falling. Its small, white-cream-yellow flowers with five petals are present from September to October. Its fruit are dark green to blue, ovoid, rough drupes that are up to 17 mm long and 15 mm in diameter. In Australia, Garuga occurs in basalt and sandstone, on stony rises and rocky scree slopes in a variety of forest habitats in the Kimberley region of Western Australia, the Cape York Peninsula and north-east Queensland as far south as Townsville. It also occurs in Asia from India to western China, to the islands of South-east Asia and the Pacific islands (ALA, 2022; SMIP, 2022; WAH, 2022).

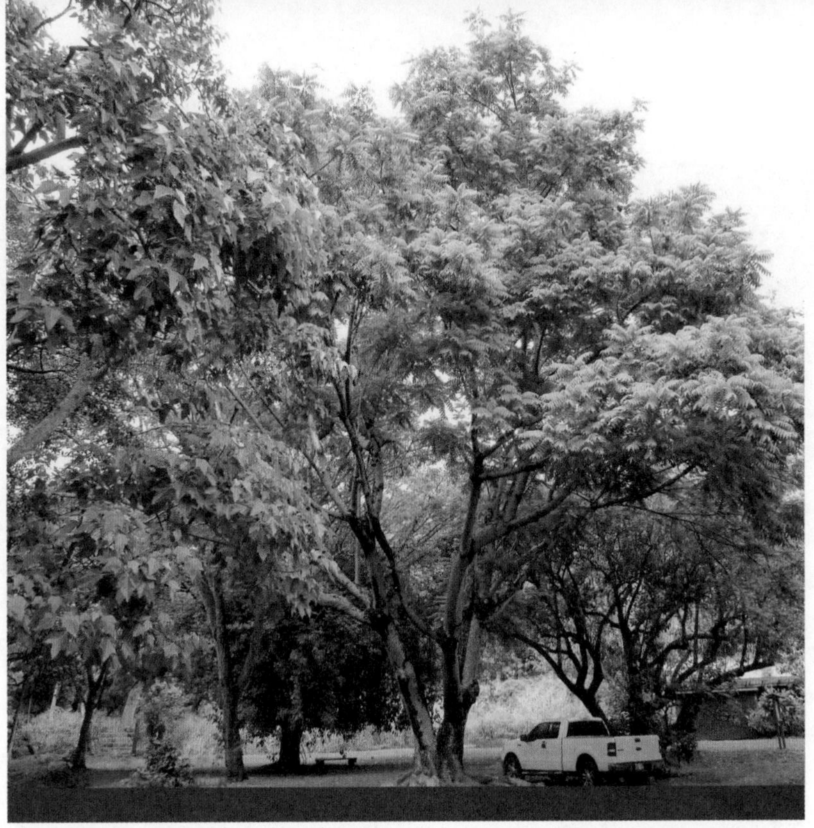

Medicinal Uses Although no medicinal use of the tree by Australian Aboriginals has been recorded, it has been used in folk medicine in Asian countries. In India, decoctions of the leaf were used in the treatment of asthma. The fruit were used to treat dysentery. Decoctions of the bark were applied to the eye to treat eye disorders and to wounds to aid healing. Decoctions of the roots were used as a wash for skin disorders. In the Philippines decoctions of the roots were used to treat tuberculosis (Philippine Medicinal Plants, 2022; Williams, 2011). The fruit are 'said to be an aid to digestion, to remove the discomfort of wind in the digestive tract, and to be an effective treatment for roundworm' (SMIP, 2022).

Other Uses The fruit of Garuga are edible when ripe (Williams, 2011).

Gawar

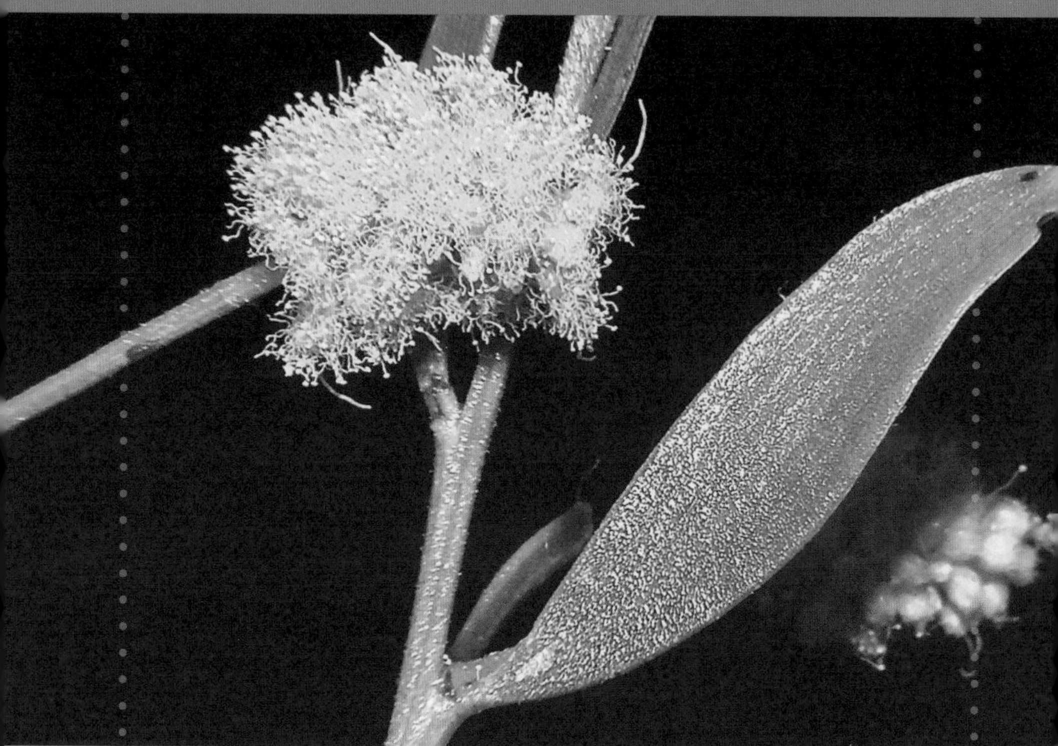

Scientific Name *Acacia monticola* J.M.Black.

Common Names Gawar, Curley-bark Wattle, Red Wattle, Curly-bark Tree, Hill Turpentine.

Aboriginal Names Galarrajen (Nyul Nyul), Warraka (Yawuru) (Kenneally et al., 1996), Gawar (Nyikina), Lirrwardi (Nyikina) (Young et al., 2012), Waroorr (Nyikina) (Smith & Smith, 2009), Burduwayi (Yindjibarndi and Ngarluma), Kawarr (Nyangumarta), Mangkalangu (Kurrama), Lingmidi, Galeran (Bardi) (Smith & Kalotas, 1985), Burrundu (Bunuba) (Moss et al., 2021).

Field Notes Gawar, as it is known in Western Australia, is a wattle that grows as a viscid shrub or tree up to 5 m in height. It has 'minni-ritchi' (curly) bark and elliptic to obovate phyllodes up to 32 mm long and 15 mm wide. Its yellow, globular flower heads are present between April and August. Small purple fruit appear in August. Gawar occurs in red sand, ironstone or lateritic soils over

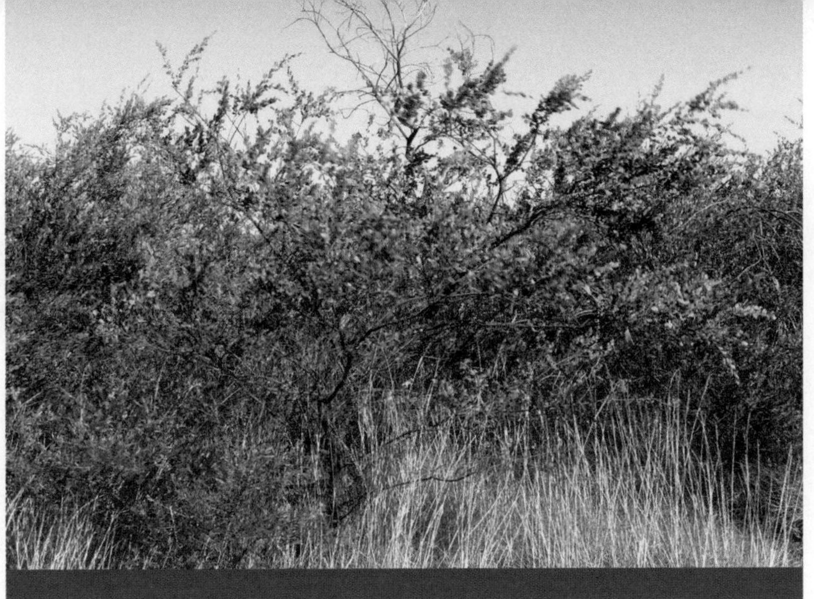

sandstone, on pindan plains, stony plains and low rocky ridges in the Pilbara and Kimberley regions of Western Australia, the Northern Territory and Queensland (ALA, 2022; Maslin et al., 2010; WAH, 2022).

Medicinal Uses Infusions or decoctions of the roots, or decoctions of the branchlets were taken internally to relieve coughs and colds (Lassak & McCarthy, 2001; Native Tastes of Australia, 2022; Williams, 2011). Infusions or decoctions of the crushed phyllodes were used externally as a liniment to treat bruised and painful areas of the body (Kenneally et al., 1996; Maslin et al., 2010) or as an external wash for headache, the symptoms of influenza and mumps (Williams, 2011). Heated leaves were used as a poultice to treat painful areas, such as joints and backs. Some Aboriginal groups used the foliage for smoke medicine (Morse, 2005).

Other Uses The seeds of Gawar are edible and were ground to flour to make damper or Johnny cakes, which were cooked in hot ashes (Bindon, 2014). The leaves and roots were burnt in campfires to repel mosquitoes (Reid, 1986). The wood was also used to make digging and clapping sticks, boomerangs and raft pegs (Kenneally et al., 1996; Maslin, 2010).

Gidgee

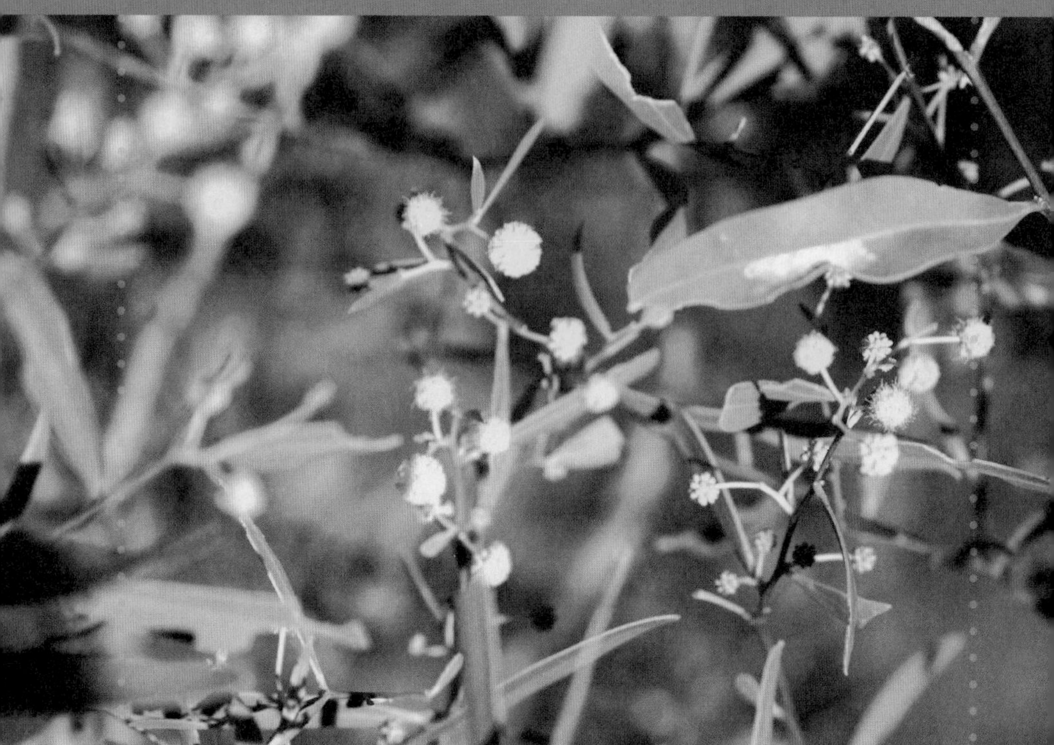

Scientific Name *Acacia pruinocarpa* Tindale.

Common Names Gidgee, Black Gidgee, Black Wattle, Tawu.

Aboriginal Names Muyurrpa, Ngurilpi, Nyurrilypi, Nyurilpa, Tjantjurru, Tjawu, Tjawilpa (Kukatja) (Valiquette, 1993), Janjuru, Marntarla or Marntirla (Ngardi) (Cataldi, 2004).

Field Notes Gidgee is a wattle that grows as a shrub or tree up to 12 m in height. It has rough, dark grey bark and grey-green phyllodes that are up to 170 mm long and 30 mm wide. Its yellow flowers are held in cylindrical clusters in spherical flower heads that have a diameter of 7–8 mm. Flowering is from October to December. The seed pods are narrowly oblong, pale brown and papery, and up to 120 mm long. Gidgee occurs in red sand or loam, often stony soils in the Pilbara and Kimberley regions of Western Australia, the western half of the Northern Territory and the Mann Range in South Australia (ALA, 2022; WAH, 2022).

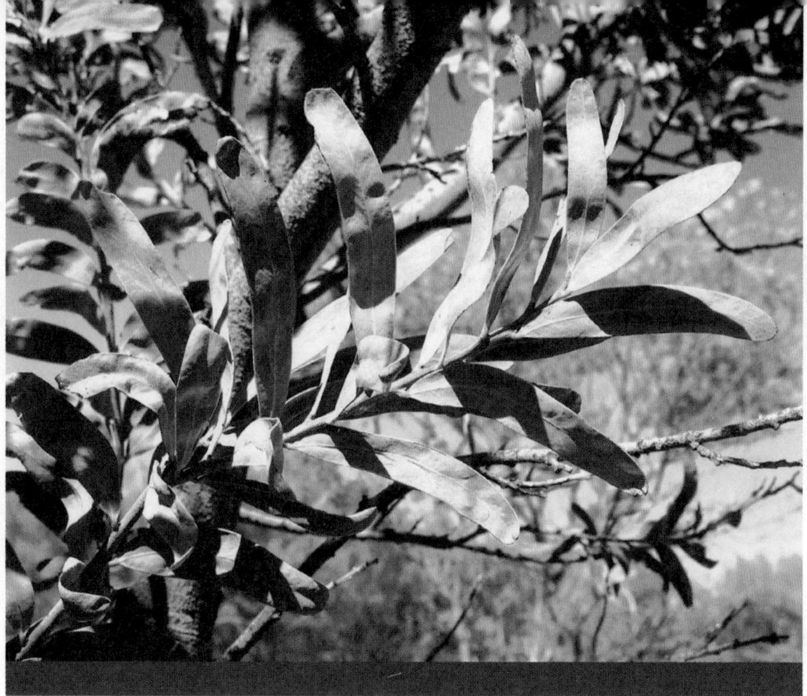

Medicinal Uses Some Aboriginal groups across the top end of Australia used the phyllodes for 'smoke medicine' to strengthen mothers and newborn babies (Morse, 2005).

Other Uses The gum that oozes from wounds in the tree of Gidgee is edible. Some Aboriginal groups mixed the ash from the tree with tobacco for chewing (Cancilla & Wingfield, 2017). The ground seeds are reported to 'produce a high quality, caffeine-free coffee-like beverage' when roasted (Fern, 2021).

Goat's Foot Vine

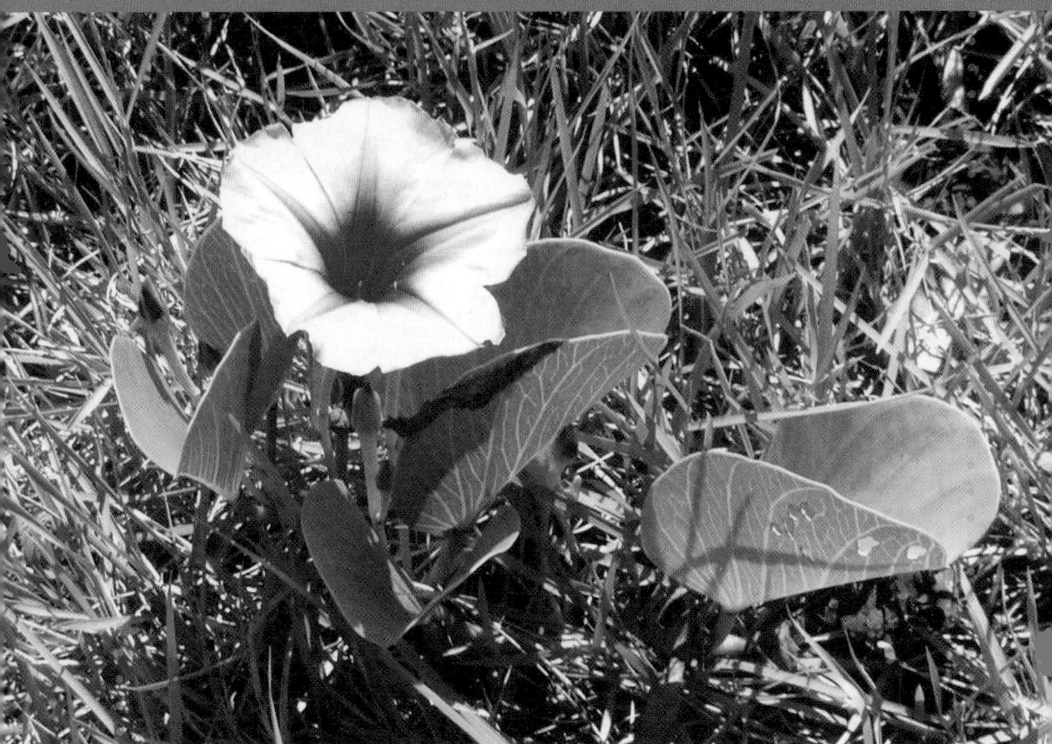

Scientific Name *Ipomoea pes-caprae* (L.) R.Br.

Common Names Goat's Foot Vine, Beach Morning Glory.

Aboriginal Names Wanbardarwou (Wunambal, Gaambera) (Karadada et al., 2011), Goordayoon (Bardi) (Kenneally et al., 2018), Yingka winya (Kwini) (Cheinmora et al., 2017), Waljaru (Karajarri) (Willing, 2014).

Field Notes Goat's Foot Vine is a very vigorous, creeping or scrambling, evergreen perennial plant of the morning glory family with large, thick roots that can be up to 3 m long and 50 mm in diameter. The plant spreads very quickly forming a dense mat. It has green, heart-shaped leaves, and pink to purple round flowers that can be present most of the year. Goat's Foot Vine occurs along the coastline in beach sand or clay loam in coastal or near-coastal areas of the tropical Atlantic, Pacific and Indian Oceans. In Australia, it occurs along the coast across the top half of the country from

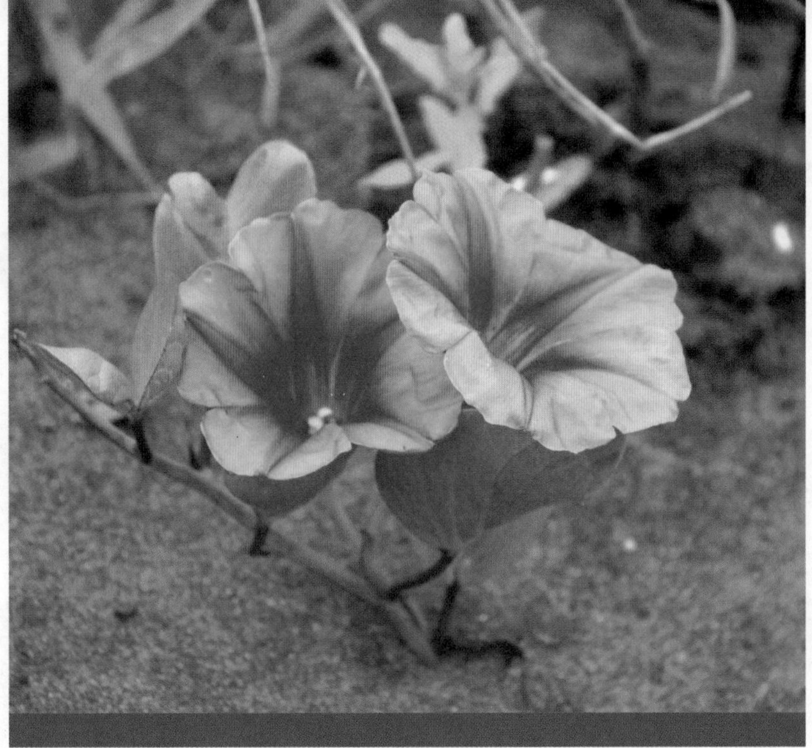

around Cervantes north of Perth to Sydney on the east coast (ALA, 2022; Fern, 2021; Lassak & McCarthy, 2001; WAH, 2022).

Medicinal Uses Crushed leaves of the Goat's Foot Vine were heated and applied to the skin as a poultice for pain relief from stingray and stonefish stings, and to treat skin sores, skin disorders and scabies infestations (CMKB, 2019; Kamenev, 2011; Smith, 1991; Webb, 1959). Decoctions of the leaves were also used for the same purposes. Small amounts of the decoction were also drunk to relieve the symptoms of colds and influenza (Smith, 1991). Aboriginal groups around the coast treated boils and sores by rubbing kino (gum) from eucalypts into the wounds then applying a bandage soaked with a decoction of Goat's Foot Vine. Bruised parts of the vine were often tied around the head to relieve headaches, especially migraines (Arrawarra Culture, n.d.). Decoctions of the vine were also drunk to treat venereal disease (efficacy not recorded) (Lassak & McCarthy, 2001; Webb, 1959).

Other Uses The swollen roots of Goat's Foot Vine are edible after they are roasted in hot ashes or boiled, and the bark scraped off (Cheinmora et al., 2017; Hiddins, 2001).

Gobin

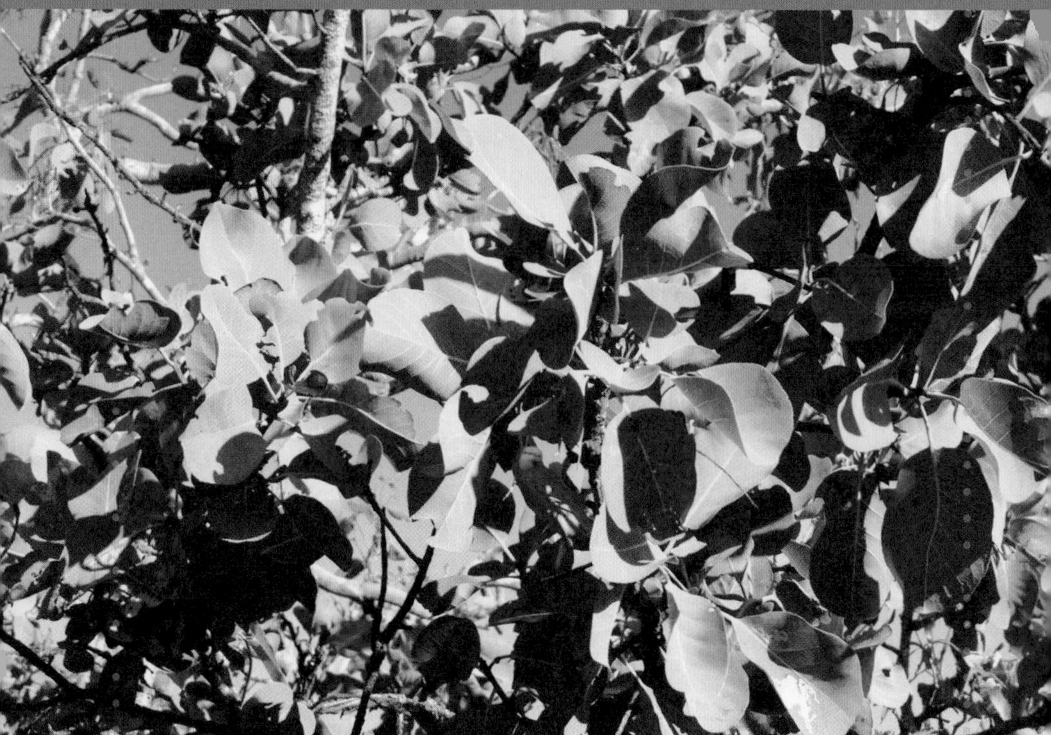

Scientific Name *Terminalia latipes* Benth.

Common Names Gobin, Kangaroo Plum, Salty Plum.

Aboriginal Name Guma (Wunambal, Gaambera) (Karadada et al., 2011).

Field Notes Gobin is a deciduous shrub or tree that grows up to 10 m in height. It has ovate leaves, and white flowers that are present between October and February. Its fruit are almond-shaped, similar to Gubinge, soft and yellow-green. Fruiting occurs at the end of the wet season from March to June. Gobin occurs in sand, loam and clay over sandstone, on rocky outcrops and hills, on floodplains and on coastal dunes in the Kimberley region of Western Australia and the Northern Territory (ALA, 2022; WAH, 2022).

Medicinal Uses Decoctions of the inner bark of Gobin are used as an antiseptic wash and applied to sores and wounds to aid the healing process (Wiynjorrotj et al., 2005).

Other Uses The fruit and nut of Gobin are edible and are usually eaten raw. The central stone was discarded (Bindon, 2014; Glasby, 2018; Hiddins, 2001). The fruit has a high ascorbic acid (vitamin C) content of 1800 mg per 100 g (Flavel, 2018). The fruit are available at the end of the wet season from March to May (Wiynjorrotj et al., 2005).

Golden Beard Grass

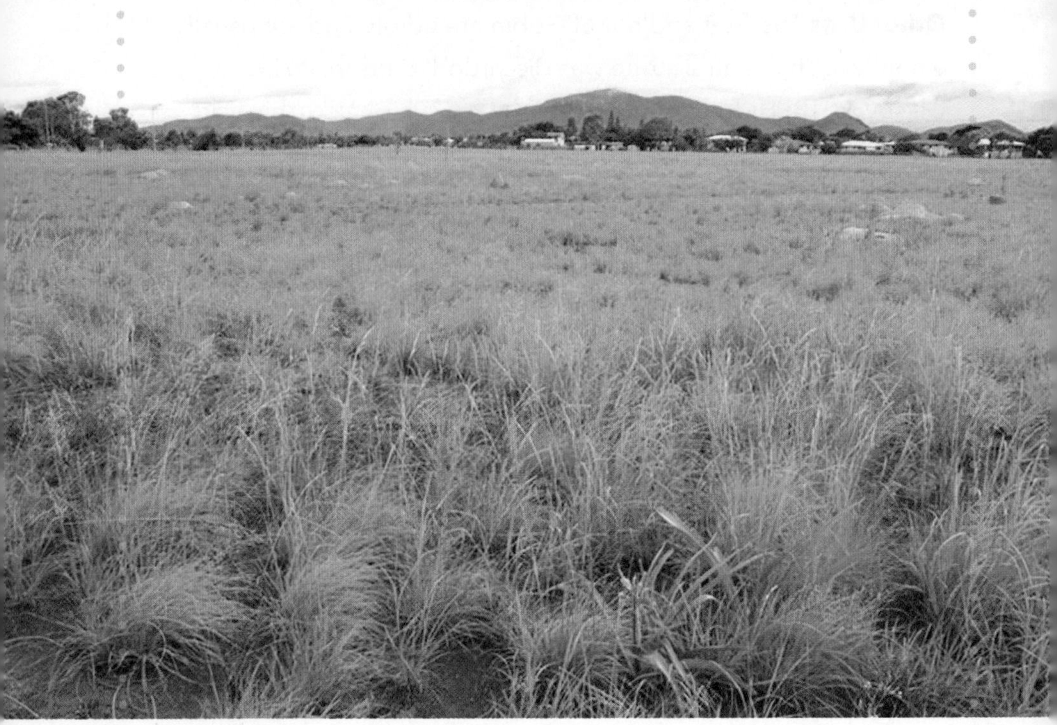

Scientific Name *Chrysopogon fallax* S.T.Blake

Common Names Golden Beard Grass, Ribbon Grass.

Aboriginal Names Tjipilpa (Kukatja) (Valiquette, 1993), Parlku (Walmajarri) (Richards & Hudson, 2012), Jajil, Janjal (Jaru) (Wightman, 2003).

Field Notes Golden Beard Grass is a rhizomatous, densely tufted perennial grass with culms (stems) that can reach up to 1.5 m in height. Its narrow, linear leaves are mostly basal. Its flowering units or spikelets are arranged in clusters in open inflorescences or flowering heads that are arranged in several whorls along a central stem. The green flower heads are present between January and June. Its spikelets, which contain the awns or seeds, are arranged in clusters of three along each branch, with each branch being up to 60 mm long with two or three spikelet clusters per branch. Its awns or seeds can be up to 45 mm long. Golden Beard Grass occurs in

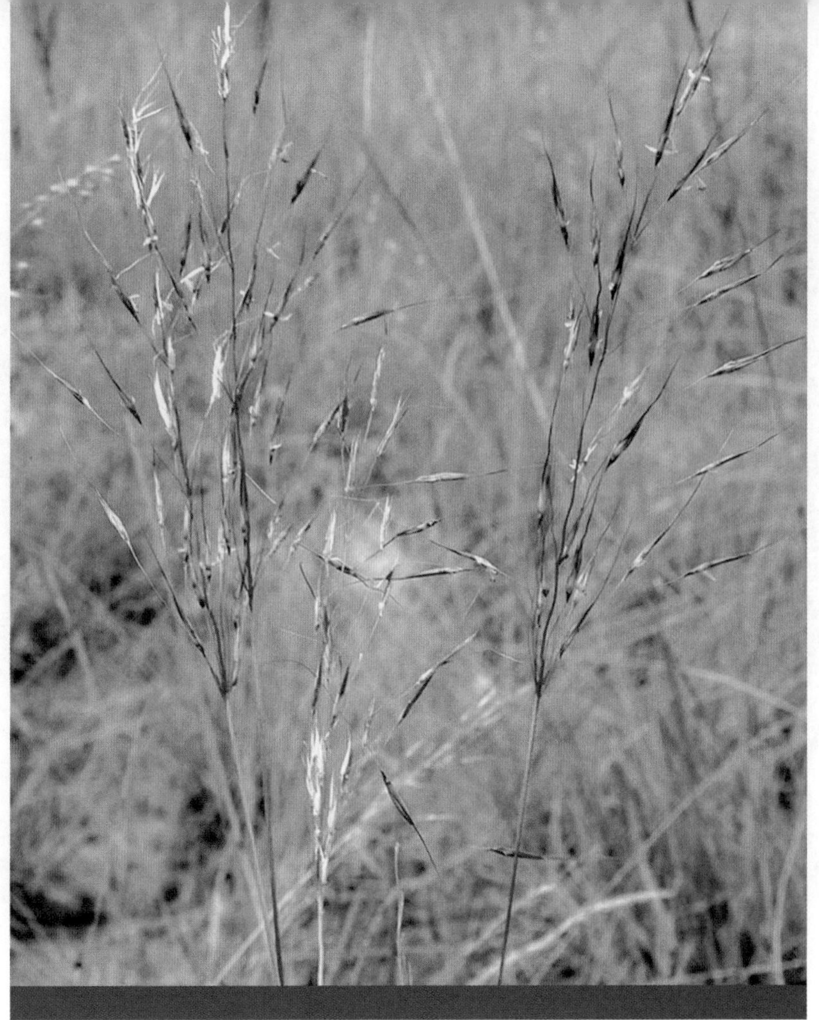

white sand, red clay or lateritic loam right across the top half of Australia, including the Pilbara and Kimberley regions of Western Australia (ALA, 2022; AusGrass2, 2022; WAH, 2022).

Medicinal Uses Decoctions of the swollen roots of Golden Beard Grass were used externally as a body wash to treat general malaise and were taken internally to treat diarrhoea (Morse, 2005; Thompson, 2020).

Other Uses The seeds of Golden Beard Grass are edible (Cancilla & Wingfield, 2017). Fibre from the roots of Golden Beard Grass was used to make fire using firesticks (Richards & Hudson, 2012).

Goolyi Bush

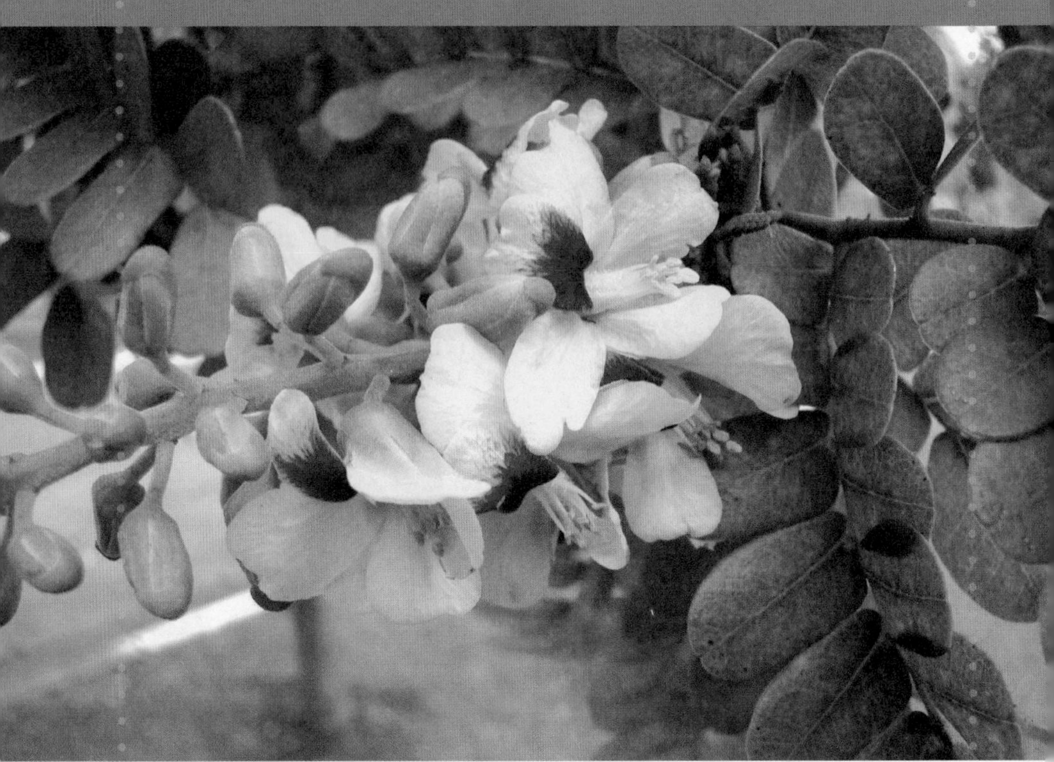

Scientific Name *Caesalpinia major* (Medik.) Dandy & Exell.

Common Names Goolyi Bush, Mato Amarillo.

Aboriginal Name Goolyi (Bardi) (Environs Kimberley, n.d.)

Field Notes Goolyi Bush is a vigorous, climbing or scrambling prickly shrub that grows to a height of 4 m. It has large, green, ovate leaves. The attractive yellow flowers, with flowers of both sexes on the same plant, have five petals and appear on long axillary clusters any time from November to June in Australia. Its fruit are very prickly oval pods that are up to 130 mm by 60 mm. Goolyi Bush is native to the Kimberley region of Western Australia where it occurs in sand and red pindan soils. It is also native to the Americas, India, Indonesia, Madagascar, Malaysia, New Guinea, Sri Lanka, the Pacific islands and the Philippines (ATRP, 2020; Fern, 2021; SKIPA, 2022; WAH, 2022).

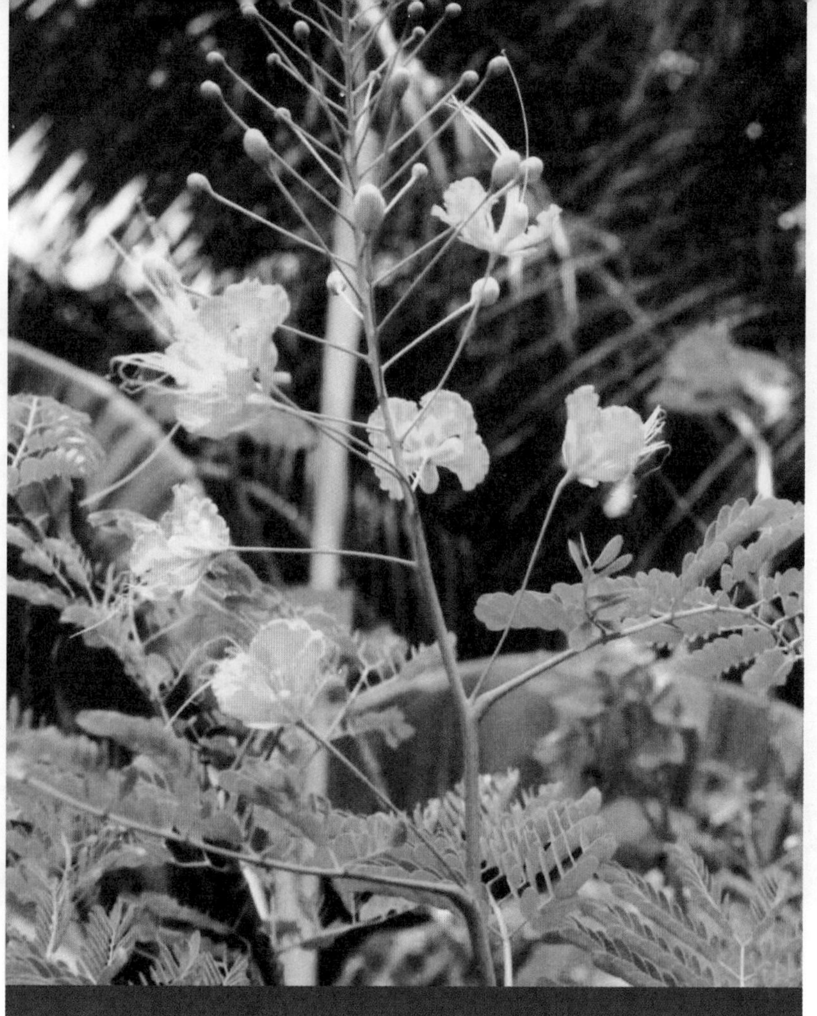

Medicinal Uses Goolyi Bush, being pantropical, is used in traditional medicine in many countries, especially in Ayurvedic medicine in India and Sri Lanka. The roots are anthelmintic and tonic. Decoctions of the roots were taken internally to rid the body of intestinal parasites. They were also drunk to treat rheumatic pain and backache. Decoctions of the roasted and ground seeds were drunk to treat respiratory illnesses (Fern, 2021).

Gooramurra

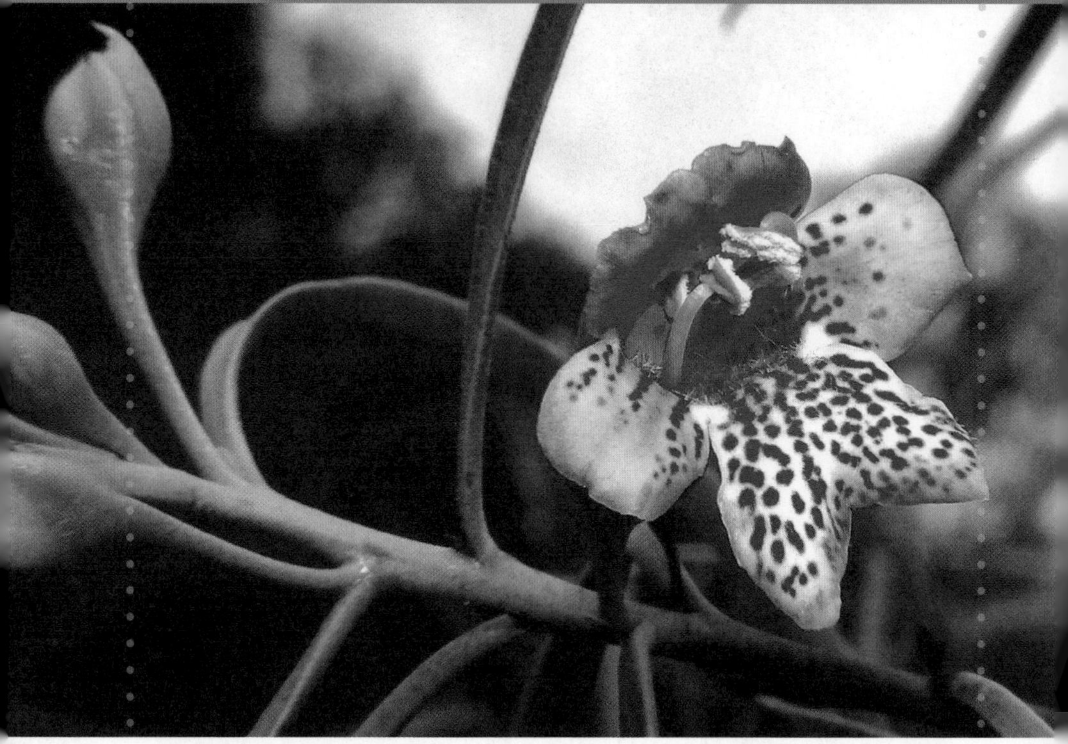

Scientific Name *Eremophila bignoniiflora* (Benth.) F.Muell.

Common Names Gooramurra, Dogwood, Bignonia Emu-Bush, Creek Wilga.

Field Notes Gooramurra is a shrub or tree that grows to 8 m in height. Its lanceolate leaves grow to 200 mm long and are tapered at both ends. Its creamy-yellow flowers are tubular with five lobes with pink, green or brown spots on the petals. The flowers are present from May to August. Its fruit are green, oval-shaped berries around 20 mm long. Gooramurra occurs in clay, alluvial soil and sand over clay on floodplains and along drainage lines in the Kimberley region of Western Australia, the Northern Territory, Queensland, New South Wales and in the north-east of South Australia (ALA, 2022; ANPSA, 2022; NSW Government Local Land Services, n.d.; WAH, 2022).

Medicinal Uses The smoke of Gooramurra was used by some Aboriginal groups as smoke medicine to treat coughs and general aches and pains. Infusions of the crushed pale green leaves were used as a laxative and to aid digestion. Decoctions of the leaves were used as an antiseptic wash for healing skin diseases, such as boils, rashes, itchy skin, sores and scabies infestations (Lassak & McCarthy, 2001; NSW Government Local Land Services, n.d.; Williams & Sides, 2008). Decoctions of the fruit were also used as a laxative (Williams, 2013). Decoctions of the leaves were used externally as a wash to treat the symptoms of colds and influenza, fever and headaches. Sometimes the boiled leaves were tied around the head to relieve headaches (Smith, 1991; Williams, 2013).

Great Morinda

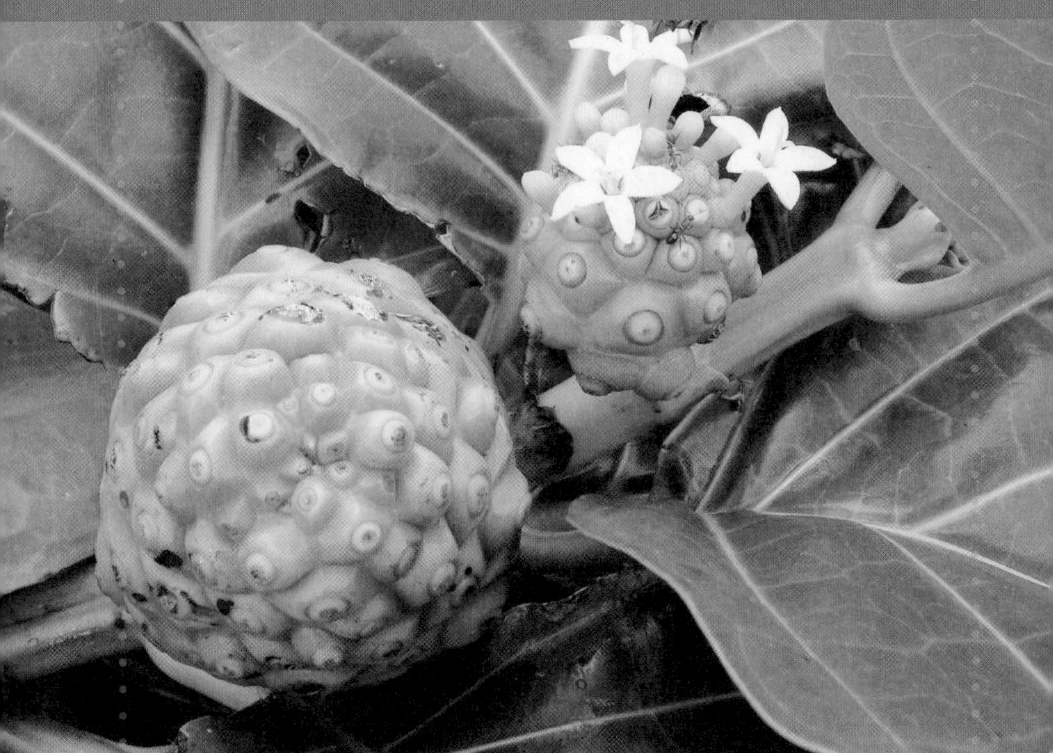

Scientific Name *Morinda citrifolia* L.

Common Names Great Morinda, Cheesefruit, Rotten Cheesefruit, Stinking Cheesefruit, Noni.

Field Notes Great Morinda grows as a large shrub or tree up to 12 m in height. It has ovate leaves up to 300 mm long and 150 mm wide. Its white flowers occur in clusters and are present mainly in summer and autumn. The flowers are followed by succulent fruit, which fuse into a large, compound, knobbly structure as they ripen from June to September in Australia. Great Morinda occurs in shallow skeletal soils in rocky crevices, on coastal sandstone, hillsides, cliffs and outcrops in coastal and near-coastal tropical Australia from the Kimberley region of Western Australia around to Rockhampton in Queensland. It also occurs in parts of Asia and Polynesia (ALA, 2022; ANPSA, 2022; Lassak & McCarthy, 2001; WAH, 2022).

Medicinal Uses Infusions of the root bark were used as an antiseptic wash to bathe wounds and sores to aid healing. Infusions of the roots and trunk are thought to have antihypertensive properties (Native Tastes of Australia, 2022). A poultice made from crushed leaves was applied to wounds to aid healing or to the head to treat headaches (Fern, 2021). Crushed fruit pulp was also applied to wounds and sores to aid healing (Low, 1990). The fruit were also eaten to treat an asthma attack and to ease a sore throat and bad coughs (Edwards, 2005; Fox & Garde, 2018; Smith, 1991). In Far North Queensland, decoctions of the fruit were taken internally to treat cancer (Edwards, 2005). Juice from the fruit is mixed with coconut milk or water in the Torres Strait Islands and given to patients as an effective cure for the painful disease ciguatera, a type of food poisoning from toxins found in some reef fish (Calvert, 2018).

Other Uses The ripe fruit are reported to smell like 'putrid cheese' but were only eaten raw or cooked in a ground oven by Aboriginal groups when food was scarce. The fruit has high levels of ascorbic acid (vitamin C) (Bindon, 2014; Edwards, 2005; Fern, 2021; Fox & Garde, 2018; Jackes, 2010; Maiden, 1889; RFCA, 1993; Vigilante et al., 2013). The flavour of the fruit is said to be like 'combining camembert cheese with Custard Apple' (Low, 1991). In Australia, Asia and New Guinea, the leaves are cooked and eaten as a vegetable (Calvert, 2018; Cribb & Cribb, 1981; Low, 1991).

Green Birdflower

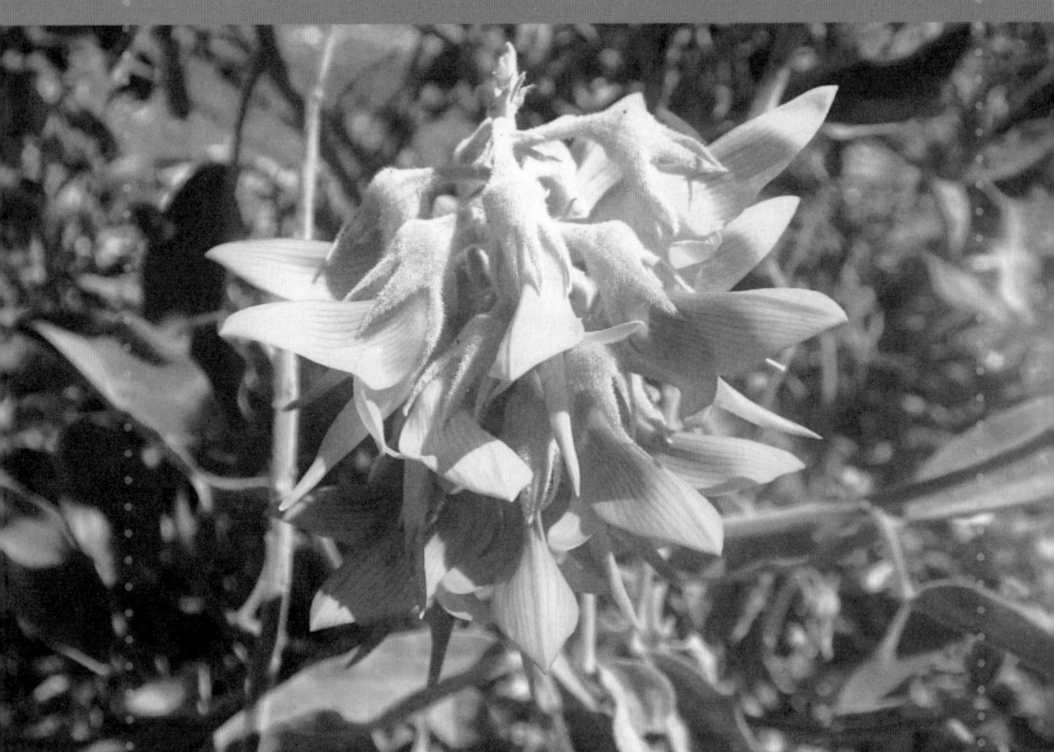

Scientific Name *Crotalaria cunninghamii* R.Br.

Common Names Green Birdflower, Parrot Pea, Rattlepod.

Aboriginal Names Barnar (Wunambal, Gaambera) (Karadada et al., 2011), Minmin (Yawuru) (Kenneally et al., 1996), Oolgoo, Urlga (Bardi) (Smith & Kalotas, 1985; Kenneally et al., 2018), Banarr (Kwini) (Cheinmora,et al., 2017), Ngalilirrki, Ngalyipi, Ngatjapiri, Purtpiri, Taliwanti (Kukatja) (Valiquette, 1993), Palykan, Yakapiri (Walmajarri) (Richards & Hudson, 2012), Palnga, Mangarr (Karajarri) (Willing, 2014).

Field Notes Green Birdflower grows as a short-lived erect shrub to 4 m in height. It has large, ovate, velvety, grey-green leaves and bird-like green-and-yellow flowers that can be present at any time of the year. Flowering is followed by velvety, club-shaped seed pods up to 50 mm in length. Green Birdflower occurs in sandy soils, on sand dunes, sandplains and along drainage lines all over the

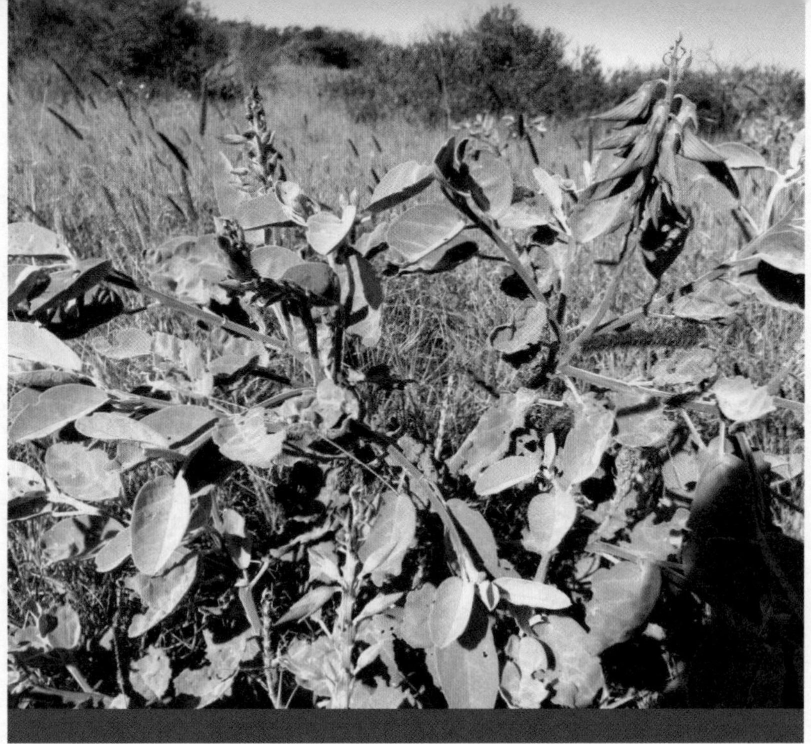

northern part of Western Australia, the eastern part of the Northern Territory, central Australia and south-west Queensland (ALA, 2022; Fern, 2021; WAH, 2022).

Medicinal Uses Decoctions of the leaves were used to bathe sore eyes due to conjunctivitis and were poured over the head to relieve headaches, as well as the symptoms of colds and influenza. Juice from the crushed leaves was used as eardrops to treat earache. Decoctions of the bark were used externally as a liniment for swellings of the body and legs (Cock, 2011; Lassak & McCarthy, 2001; Low, 1990; Reid, 1986; Webb, 1959; Wheatstone Project, n.d.; Willing, 2014).

Other Uses Aboriginal People in the Kimberley sucked the nectar straight from the flowers of the Green Birdflower. They also ate the flowers, which are reported to taste a bit like celery (Kane, 2022). Fibre from the stems of Green Birdflower was used traditionally for cordage and to make sandals to protect feet from the hot desert sand (Fern, 2021; Richards & Hudson, 2012; Willing, 2014).

Green Crumbweed

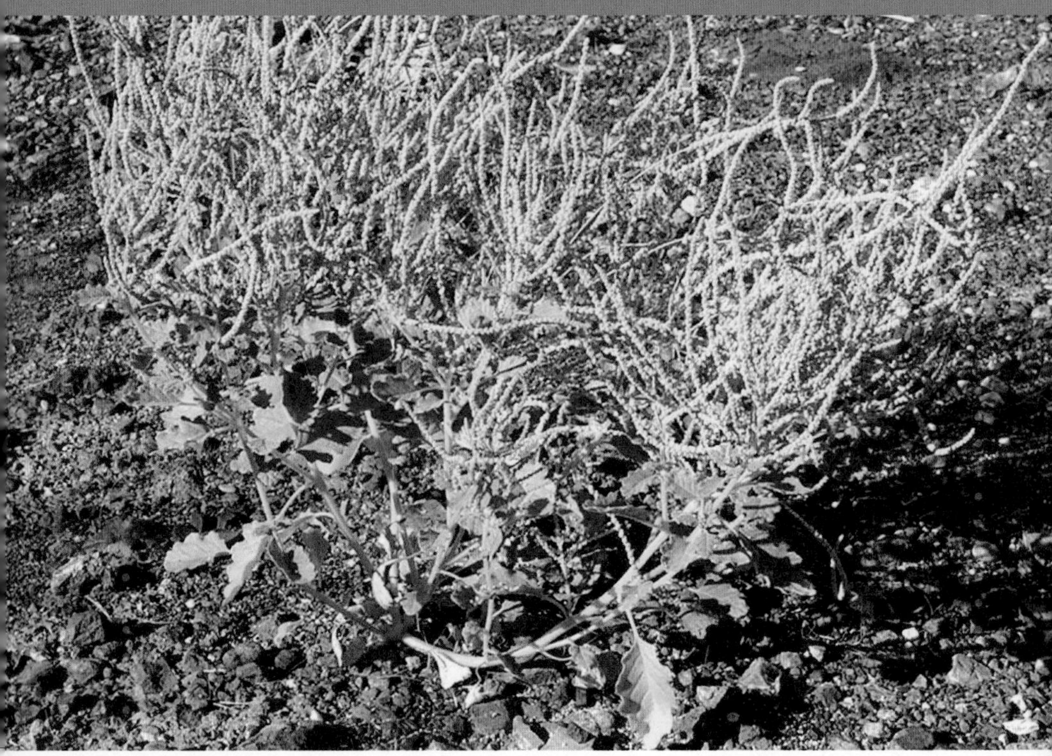

Scientific Name *Dysphania rhadinostachya* (F.Muell.) A.J.Scott, previously known as *Chenopodium rhadinostachyum* F.Muell.

Common Name Green Crumbweed.

Aboriginal Name Kalpari (Kulkatja) (Valiquette, 1993).

Field Notes Green Crumbweed is an erect, aromatic, annual herb that reaches 500 mm in height. It has small, ovate leaves up to 25 mm long, and small, white flowers that are arranged in a globular cluster on a spike that can be up to 120 mm long. Flowering is from August to November. Its red-black, globular fruit are up to 1.5 mm in diameter with downy hairs. Green Crumbweed occurs on stony sand or loam, clay or alluvium from Exmouth to the southern Kimberley region in Western Australia, through central Australia and into southern Queensland and northern New South Wales (ALA, 2022; Herbiguide, 2022; WAH, 2022).

Medicinal Uses Infusions of crushed Green Crumbweed leaves were used to bathe the head to relieve the symptoms of colds and influenza, and headaches (Cock, 2011; Low, 1990; Reid, 1986).

Other Uses The seeds of Green Crumbweed are edible. The seeds were ground on a stone and made into cakes, which were baked in hot ashes (Brand-Miller & Holt, 1998; Cancilla & Wingfield, 2017).

Green Tree Ants

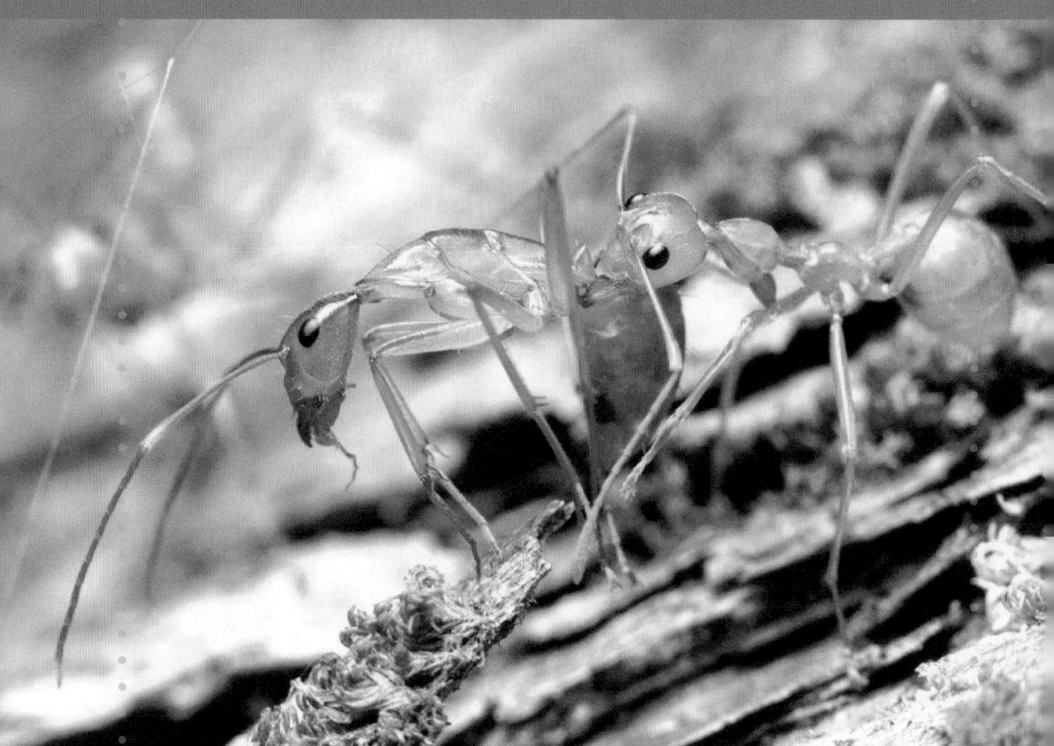

Scientific Name *Oecophylla smaragdina* (Fabricius, 1775).

Common Names Green Tree Ants, Green Ants, Weaver Ants.

Aboriginal Names Wawalji, Wawalel, Wawale, Minyal (Gija) Purdie et al., 2018), Yuulway, Yulwe (Wunambal, Gaambera) Karadada et al., 2011), Walurru (Jaru) (Deegan et al., 2010), Yilwei manya, Yilweyi manya (Kwini) (Cheinmora et al.,2017).

Field Notes Green Tree Ants are worth a mention in this book as they have been used in traditional Aboriginal medicine and as a traditional food source across the top end of Australia for centuries. Despite their name, only their abdomens are green. Green Tree Ants are squirters rather than stingers. After they bite you, they squirt formic acid into the wound to break down the flesh. This is what produces the pain. Green Tree Ant nests are made of leaves pulled together and expertly stitched or woven with silk, and the ants are easily collected by shaking the nest into a coolamon. The City of Townsville (n.d.) reports that:

> *A mature colony of green tree ants can hold as many as 100,000 to 500,000 workers and may span as many as 12 trees and contain as many as 150 nests. Green ant colonies have one queen and a colony can live for up to eight years. Minor workers usually remain within the egg chambers of the nest tending the larvae, whereas major workers defend the colony territory, assist with the care of the queen, and forage.*

Green Tree Ants are found in the tropical coastal areas in Australia as far south as Rockhampton in Queensland and across the coastal tropics of the Northern Territory down to Broome in the Kimberley region of Western Australia. They are also found in Bangladesh, Bhutan, Brunei, Cambodia, China, India, Indonesia, Laos, Malaysia, Myanmar, Nepal, Palau, Papua New Guinea, the Philippines, Singapore, Solomon Islands, Sri Lanka, Thailand, Timor and Vietnam (City of Townsville, n.d.; Outback Joe, 2018).

Medicinal Uses Green Tree Ants and larvae were pounded and mixed with water to produce a lime-flavoured drink to relieve the symptoms of colds, influenza, headaches and sore throats. In Far North Queensland, the whole nest was boiled and the strained liquid drunk for the same purpose (Edwards, 2005; Northern Territory Department of Health, 1983).

Other Uses Aboriginal people ate the white larvae found inside the leafy nests. They are reported to have a citrus flavour. In the Kimberley region of Western Australia, Green Tree Ants are added to some bland foods to give them a citrus flavour and make them more palatable (Isaacs, 1987; Northern Territory Department of Health, 1983). Aboriginal people across the top end also ate the abdomens of Green Tree Ants by holding the ant between their fingertips and biting off the green abdomen, which gave them a powerful lemon-flavoured burst (Outback Joe, 2018).

Grey-leaf Heliotrope

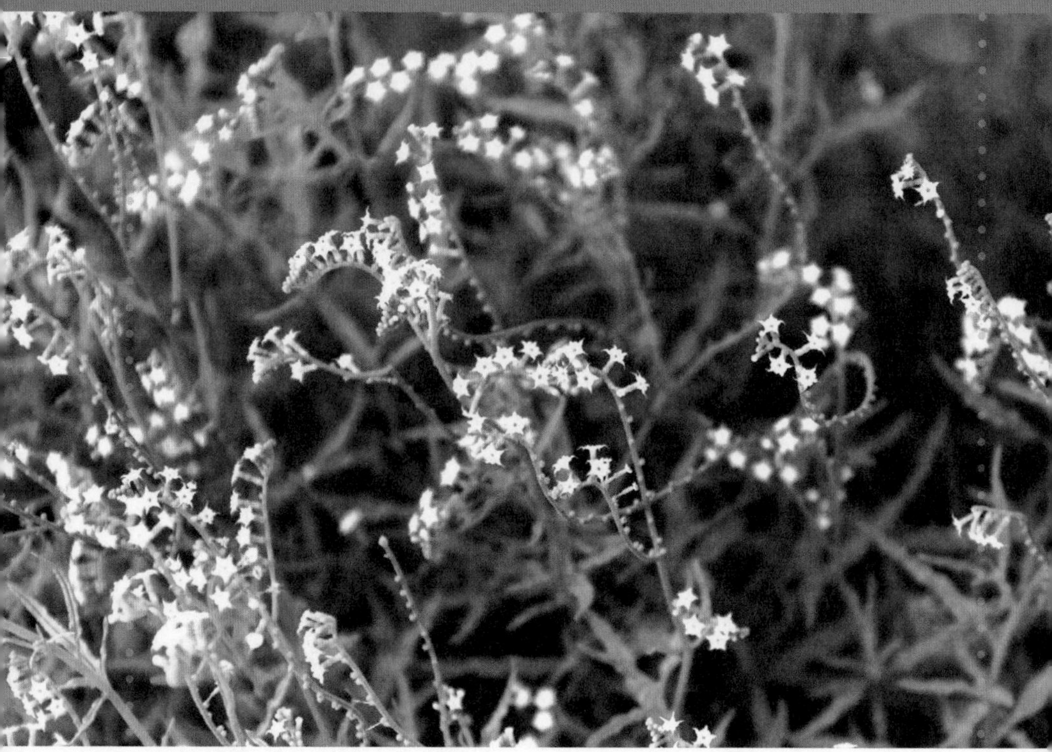

Scientific Name *Heliotropium ovalifolium* Forssk.

Common Name Grey-leaf Heliotrope.

Field Notes Grey-leaf Heliotrope grows as an ascending to spreading perennial or annual (in adverse conditions) herb to 800 mm in height. It has green to grey, multilobed leaves and tiny, white, star-shaped flowers with five petals that can be present all year round. Grey-leaf Heliotrope occurs in sand, clay, saline soils and pebbly loam on coastal plains and dunes, seasonally wet areas, rocky hills and river levees across the top half of Australia. It also occurs across tropical and subtropical Africa, including Madagascar and tropical Asia (ALA, 2022; WAH, 2022).

Medicinal Uses This plant is used in folk medicine in Australia and some African and Asian countries. Decoctions of the leaves were drunk or used as a wash applied over the head to treat the symptoms of colds and influenza (Reid, 1986). Decoctions of

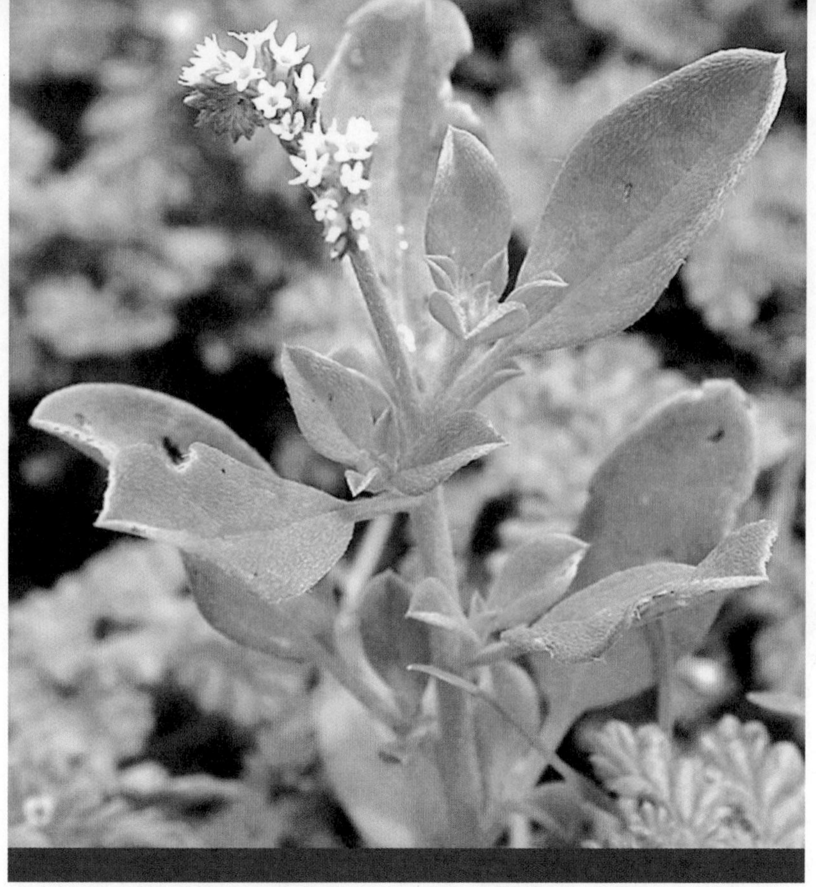

the whole plant were taken internally in small amounts to treat thrush, diarrhoea, diabetes, venereal diseases and frequency of micturition, and were also applied externally for heat rash. Infusions of the whole plant were also used in small amounts internally to treat asthma, ulcers, dysentery, bronchitis, and externally as a wash to treat red eyes, conjunctivitis and boils. Poultices made from the crushed leaves were applied to areas of rheumatic pain, wounds and insect bites (Fern, 2021).

CAUTION: This plant is thought to be carcinogenic if taken internally so its use internally these days is not recommended (Reid, 1986).

Gubinge

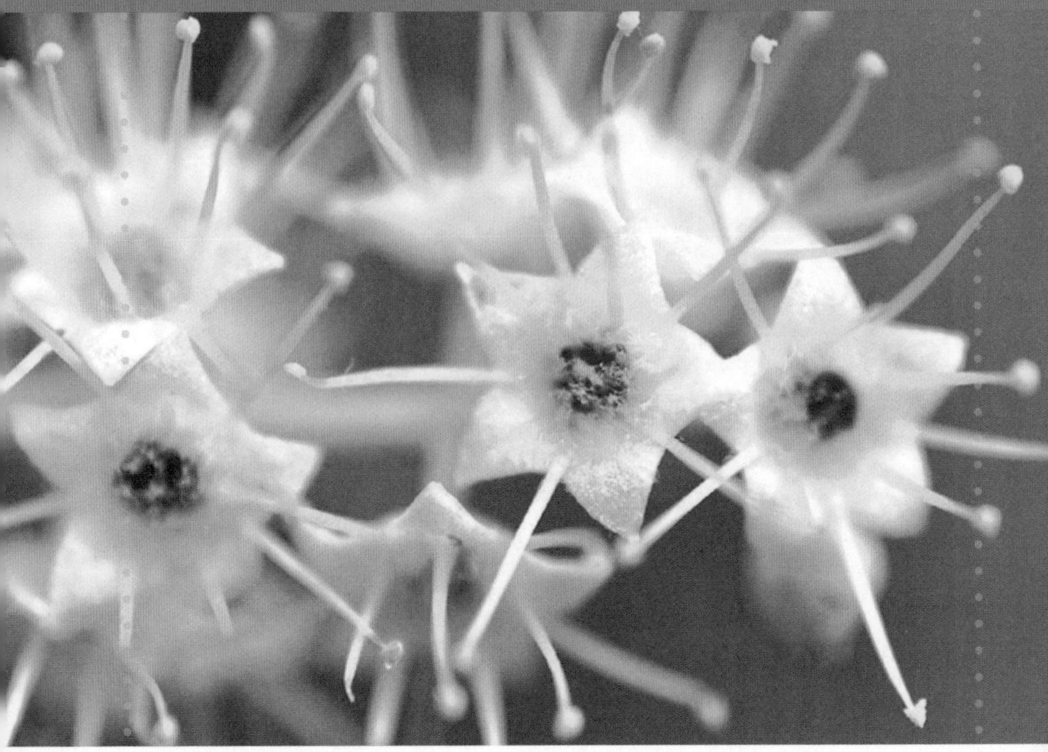

Scientific Name *Terminalia ferdinandiana* Exell., previously known as *Terminalia latipes* subsp. *psilocarpa* Pedley.

Common Names Gubinge, Mador, Billygoat Plum, Kakadu Plum, Green Plum, Salty Plum, Murunga.

Aboriginal Names Yaminyarri, Gabiny (Yawuru, Nyangumarta, Karajarri), Kabiny (Nyul Nyul), Gubinge or Gabindj (Bardi) (SKIPA, 2022; Lands, 1997), Arungul, Madoor (Bardi) (Smith & Kalotas, 1985), Arrangoor (Jawi), Nyaminyari (Karajarri) (Willing, 2014), Yaminyarri (Yawuru) (Moss et al., 2021).

Field Notes Gubinge grows as a small to medium-sized deciduous tree up to 14 m in height. Its bark is mottled grey, green, cream, orange, yellow and fissured. Its large ovate leaves are smooth and leathery. They occur in spirals near the ends of small branches. Its flowers are small, cream, fragrant spikes that are present from October to February. Its fruit are almond-shaped, soft and yellow-

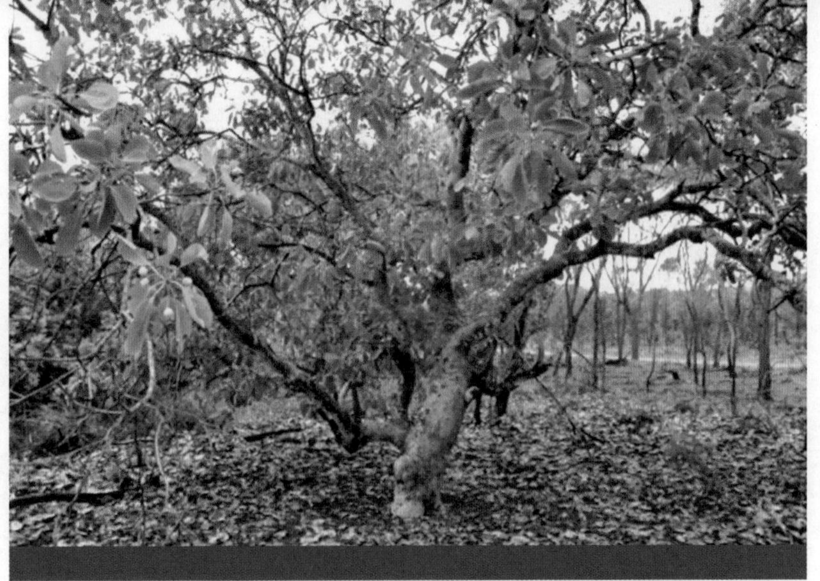

green. Fruiting is at the end of the wet season from March to June. Gubinge occurs in red sand, sandy clay and black peat over sandstone, ironstone and granite on sandplains behind beaches, dry creek beds, flood plains, cliff tops, ridges, coastal vine thickets and mangrove edges. Its range extends from the Kimberley region of Western Australia through the top end of the Northern Territory and the tip of Cape York Peninsula in Queensland (ALA, 2022; Fern, 2021; PFAF, 2022; WAH, 2022).

Medicinal Uses Gubinge fruit are thought to be the world's richest source of ascorbic acid (vitamin C; 5320mg per 100g) so would have helped protect the Aboriginal tribes across the north of Australia from getting scurvy (Kamenev, 2011). Infusions of the inner bark were used by some Aboriginal groups to bathe wounds and sores, and as a liniment to ease arthritic and rheumatic pain (Low, 1990; Paddy et al., 1993; Smith & Kalotas, 1985).

Other Uses Gubinge fruit is edible and was a major source of food for tribes in the areas where it grew (Bindon, 2014; Hiddins, 2001; Kamenev, 2011; Low, 1990; McMahon, 2006; Vigilante et al., 2013). The kernel of the fruit is also edible (Bindon, 2014; Fox & Garde, 2018; Smith & Kalotas, 1985). The gum that oozes from wounds in the tree is reported to be edible as well (Vigilante et al., 2013; Williams, 2011).

Gummy Spinifex

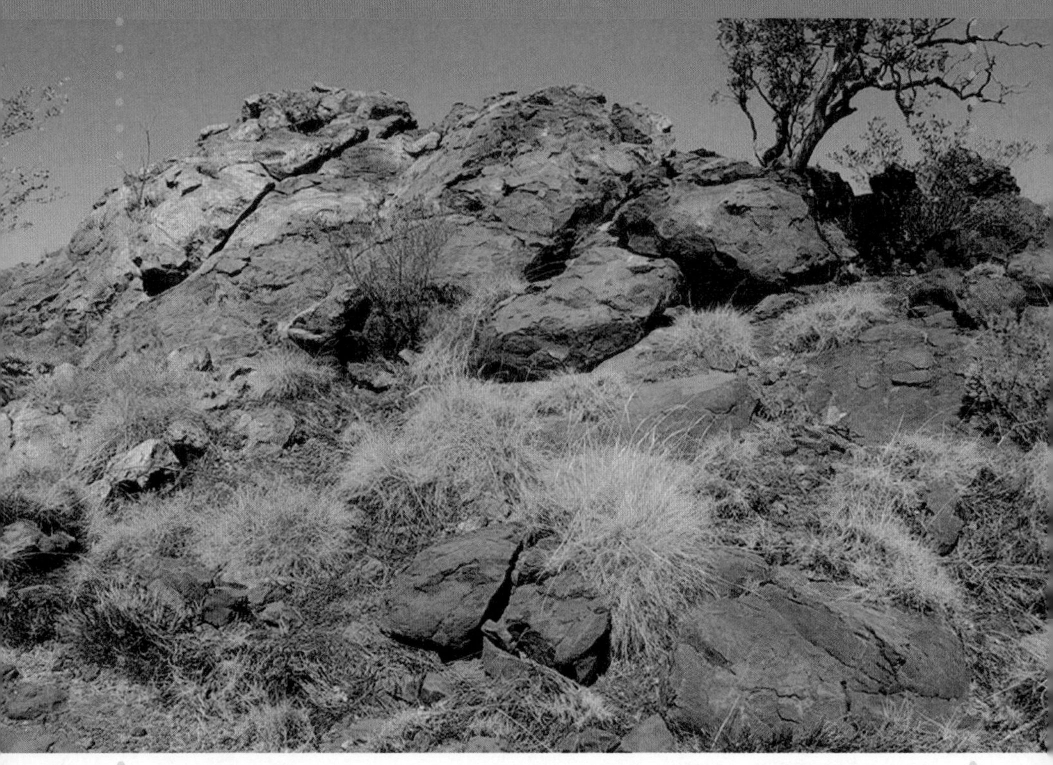

Scientific Name *Triodia pungens* R.Br.

Common Names Gummy Spinifex, Soft Spinifex.

Aboriginal Names Jawal, Nyanmi (Walmajarri) (Richards & Hudson, 2012), Gerlerneny (Gija) (Purdie et al., 2018), Tarl-tarlpanu (Ngardi) (Cataldi, 2004), Marnkalpa (Kukatja) (Valiquette, 1993), Kalajirdi (Walpiri) (Northern Tanami IPA, 2015).

Field Notes Gummy Spinifex is a tussock-forming, perennial grass that grows to around 2.3 m high, with resinous foliage that is sparsely hairy. The slender leaf blades are rolled, up to 300 mm long and have pointed ends. The spear-shaped seed heads form on single spikes. Its green-purple flowers can be present at any time of the year. Gummy Spinifex is found in a variety of soils and habitats right across the top half of Australia, including the Gascoyne, Pilbara and Kimberley regions of Western Australia (ALA,

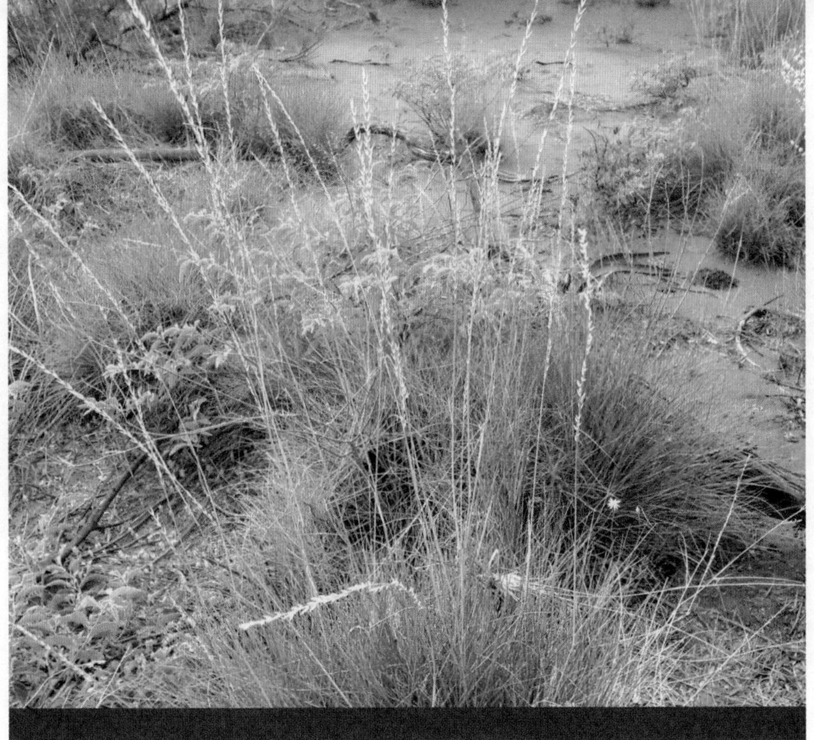

2022; AusGrass2, 2022; Department of Primary Industries and Regional Development, 2019; WAH, 2022).

Medicinal Uses Decoctions of the whole Gummy Spinifex plant were used as a medicinal body wash to relieve the symptoms of colds and influenza. Smith (1991) witnessed an interesting ritual with Soft Spinifex in the Northern Territory:

> *The whole plant is crushed in a coolamon with an axe or stone, mixing with a little termitaria (the clay casing of termite nests) and a little water. The coolamon is placed over a bed of hot coals whilst crushing. The dark coloured liquid is then poured off and drunk by the mother and newborn baby as a health promoter. This is carried out as soon as possible after childbirth to ensure that the child will grow up to be healthy and strong. It also helps in the mother's recovery after the trauma of childbirth.*

Other Uses Clumps of the Gummy Spinifex grass were burned on the campfires at night to repel mosquitoes from around the camp site. The crushed leaves were used as a fish poison to stun fish to make them easier to catch (Purdie et al., 2018).

Guttapercha

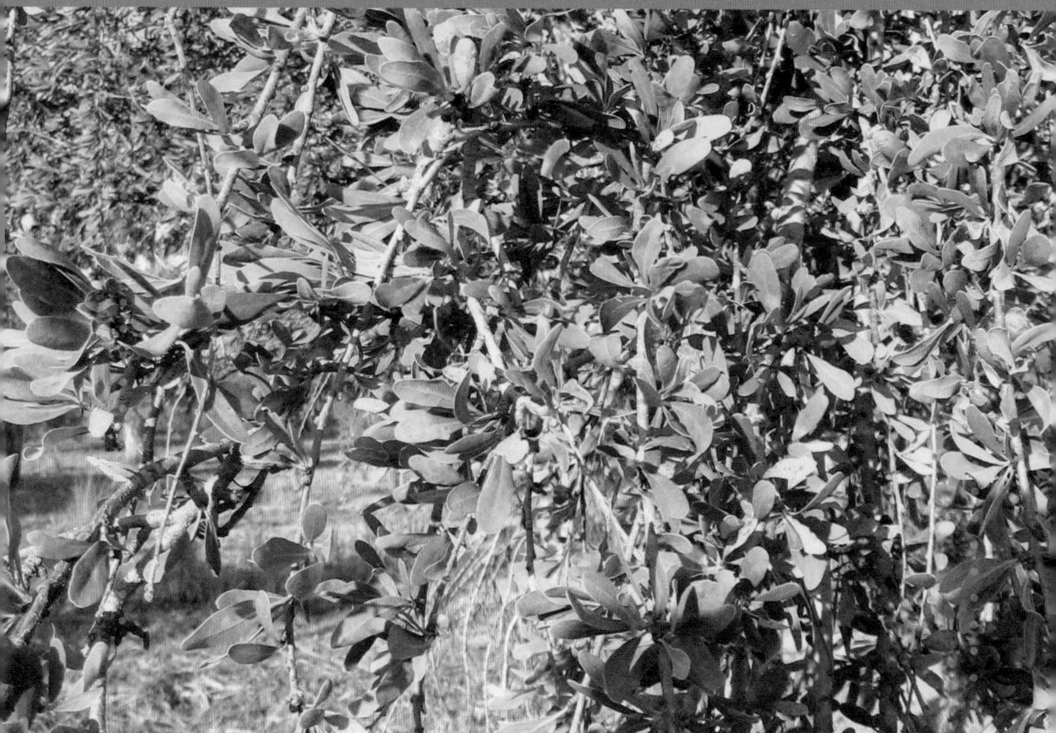

Scientific Name *Excoecaria parvifolia* Müll.Arg.

Common Names Guttapercha, Gutta Percha Tree, Northern Brown Birch.

Aboriginal Name Gutta Percha (Miwa) (Kimberley Specialists, 2020).

Field Notes Guttapercha grows as a shrub or tree to 6 m in height. Its leaves are alternate, narrow ovate, blunt tipped and up to 25 mm long. Its flower spikes are up to 25 mm long. The flowers are present in November. Its fruit is a capsule. Guttapercha is found in clay soils on the edges of lagoons and on river plains across the top end of Australia from the eastern Kimberley to northern Queensland (ALA, 2022; Inner Path Herbal Materia Medica, 2019; WAH, 2022).

Medicinal Uses Infusions or decoctions of mashed bark were heated and rubbed into parts of the body for rheumatic pain

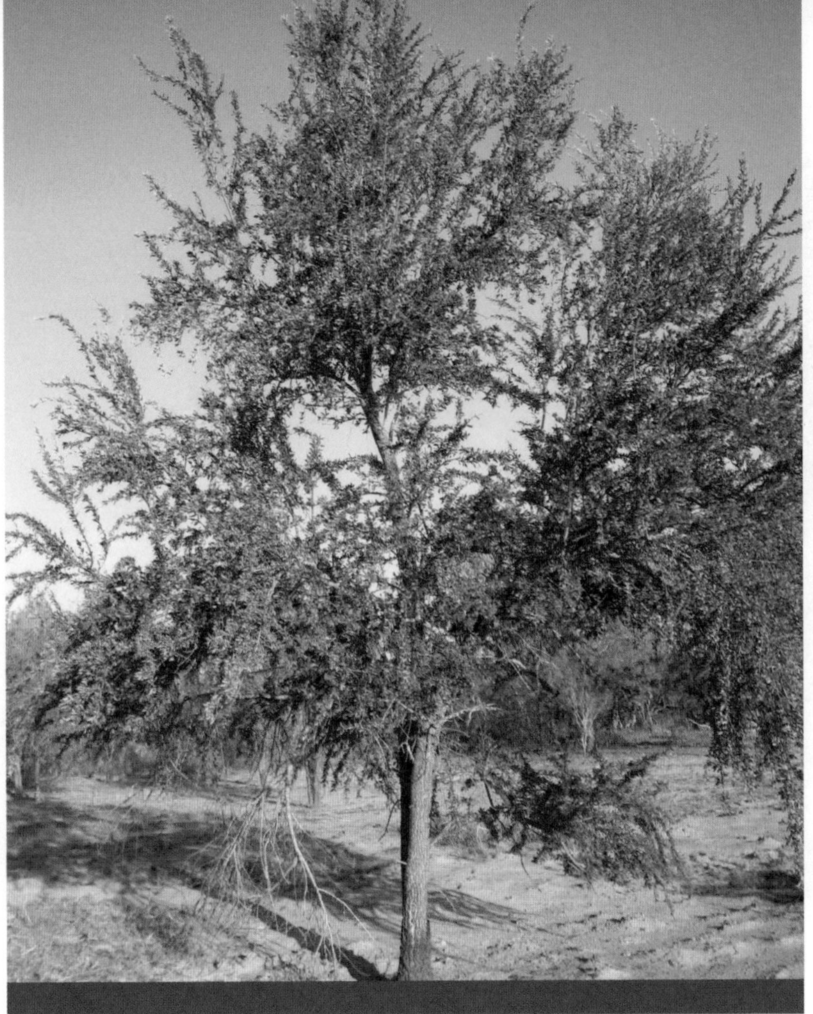

and general malaise (Cock, 2011; Devanesen, 2000; Lassak & McCarthy, 2001; Smith, 1991; Williams, 2012). Decoctions of the bark or leaves were rubbed on injuries to reduce pain and swelling, and used as a wash for cuts, sores, boils, scabies infestations, chickenpox rash and other skin disorders (Cock, 2011; Devanesen, 2000; Smith, 1991; Williams, 2013).

Other Uses The hard wood of the Guttapercha tree was good for making boomerangs (Kimberley Specialists, 2020) and nulla nullas (Williams, 2012).

CAUTION: Smith (1991) warns that one 'should not get the latex into the eyes as it will cause blindness'.

Hairy Lolly Bush

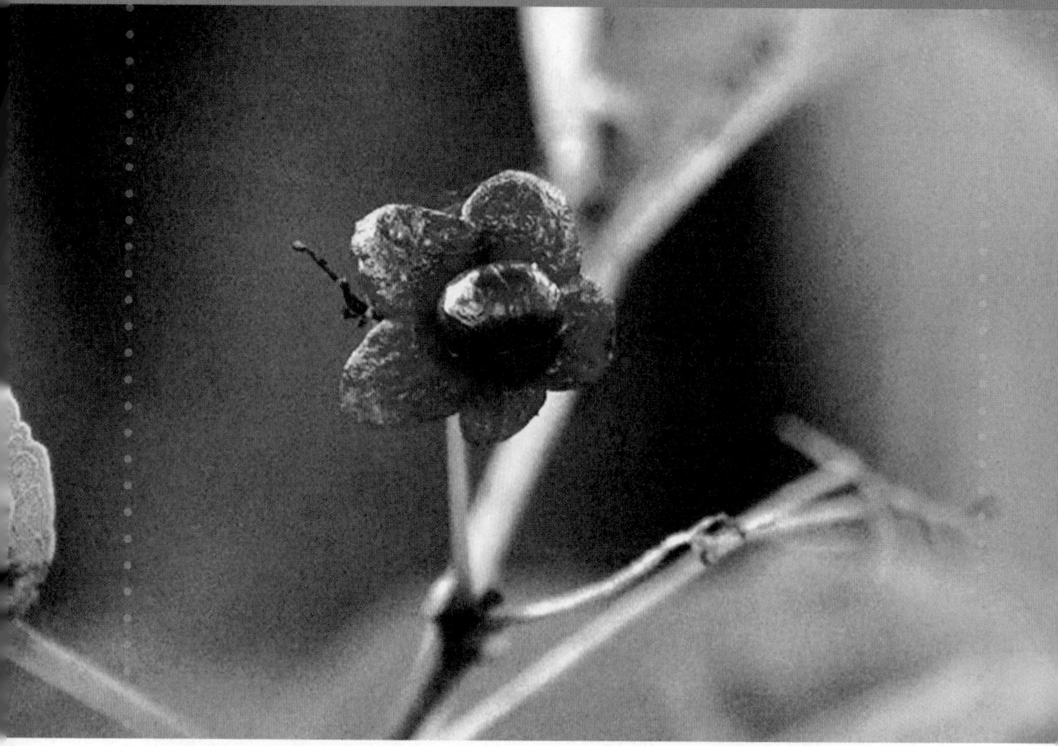

Scientific Name *Clerodendrum tomentosum* (Vent.) R.Br.

Common Names Hairy Lolly Bush, Hairy Clairy, Hairy Clerodendrum, Hairy Clerodendron, Downy Chance, Flowers of Magic, Downy Chance Tree, Witches Tongues.

Field Notes Hairy Lolly Bush grows as a shrub or tree up to 15 m in height in good conditions. It has grey or fawn bark that can be scaly or corky on larger plants, and large ovate, opposite, veiny leaves with fine hairs that are up to 140 mm long and 45 mm wide. Showy white flowers with five petals and long stamens form in clusters between October and January. Its fruit are black, shiny or navy-blue drupes with four lobes. The fruit are surrounded by fleshy red calyxes. Hairy Lolly Bush occurs in rocky and sandy soils and limestone on sandhills, plains, dunes, rocky outcrops, rainforest margins and in gullies in wet sclerophyll forests in the Pilbara and Kimberley regions of Western Australia, the Northern Territory,

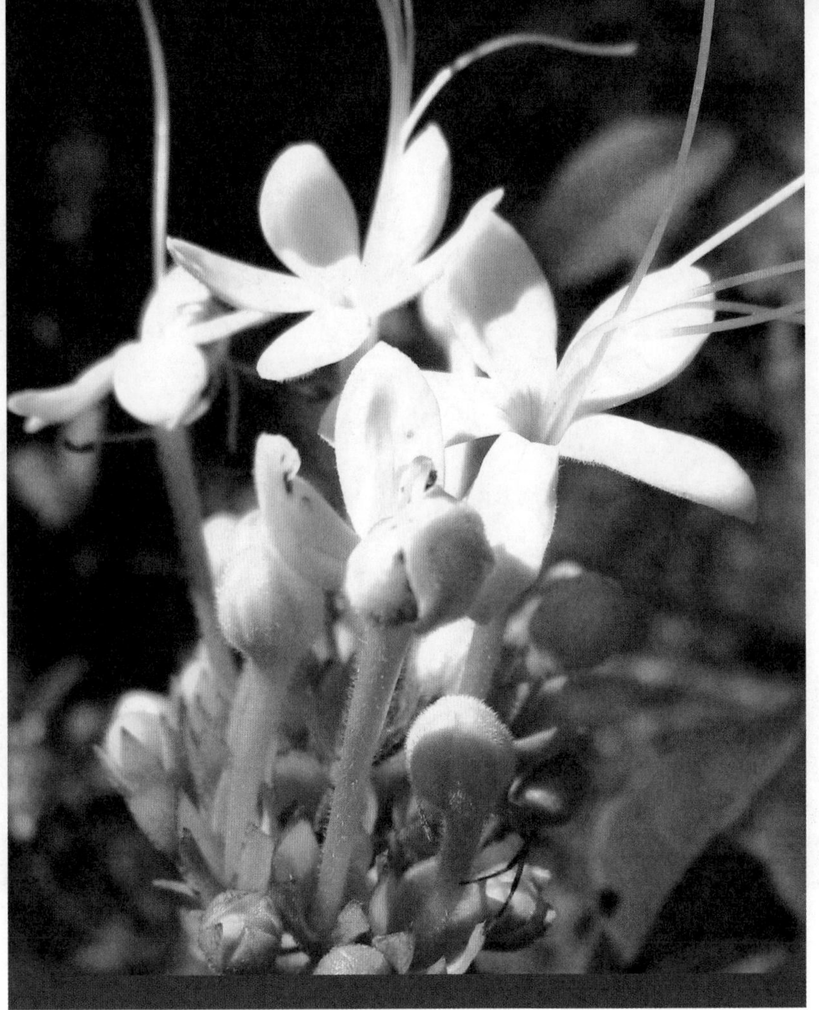

Queensland, and coastal regions of New South Wales. It also occurs in New Guinea (ALA, 2022; WAH, 2022).

Medicinal Uses Decoctions of the wood of Hairy Lolly Bush were drunk by some Aboriginal groups as an analgesic to ease aches and pains (BRAIN, 2022).

Other Uses The tuberous roots of the Hairy Lolly Bush are eaten by some Aboriginal groups. The roots are roasted in hot ashes before they are eaten or cooked in a ground oven with other vegetables and meat (Spearritt, 2016).

Hard Cascarilla

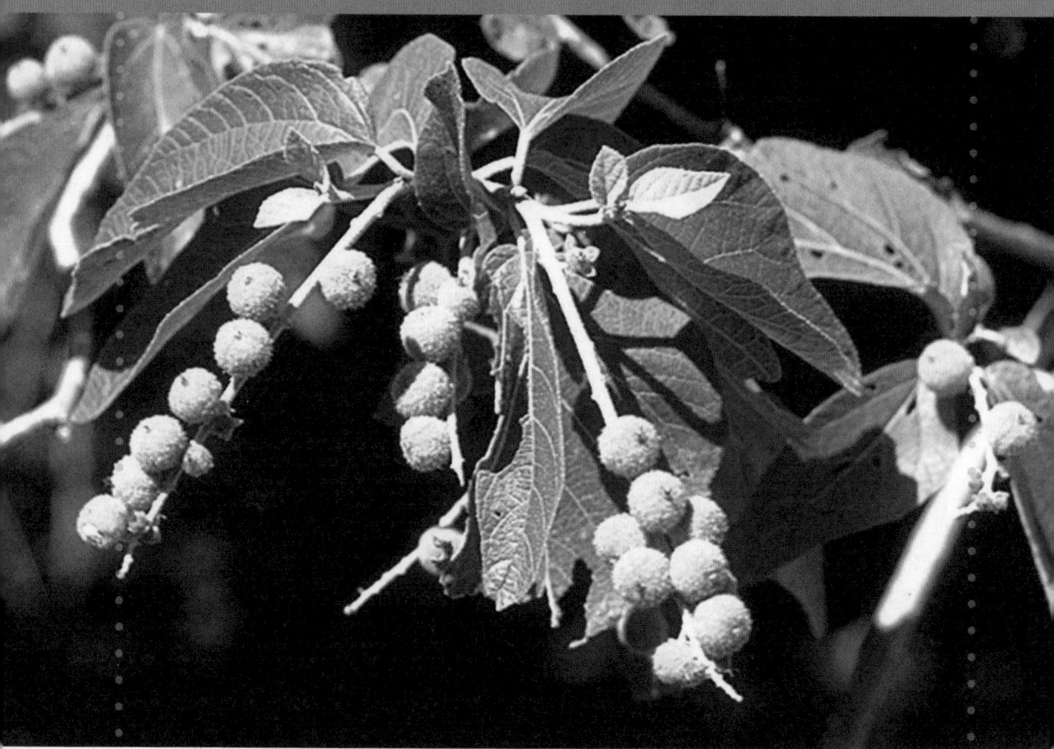

Scientific Name *Croton arnhemicus* Müll.Arg.

Common Names Hard Cascarilla, Croton.

Field Notes Hard Cascarilla is a deciduous shrub or small tree that grows up to 12 m in height. It has pale bark and ovate, lanceolate or broadly lanceolate leaves that are up to 380 mm long and 280 mm wide. They turn red before falling. Its small, white male flowers are about 4 mm in diameter and have long stamens. Its fruit are globular capsules about 10 mm diameter. Hard Cascarilla is found in the northern part of the Kimberley in Western Australia, the Northern Territory and northern Queensland (ALA, 2022; ATRP, 2020; FloraNT, 2022).

Medicinal Uses Infusions or decoctions of the inner bark of Hard Cascarilla were used as an antiseptic wash for sores and cuts, to relieve headaches and applied externally as a liniment to the joints to treat rheumatic and arthritic pain (Smith, 1991).

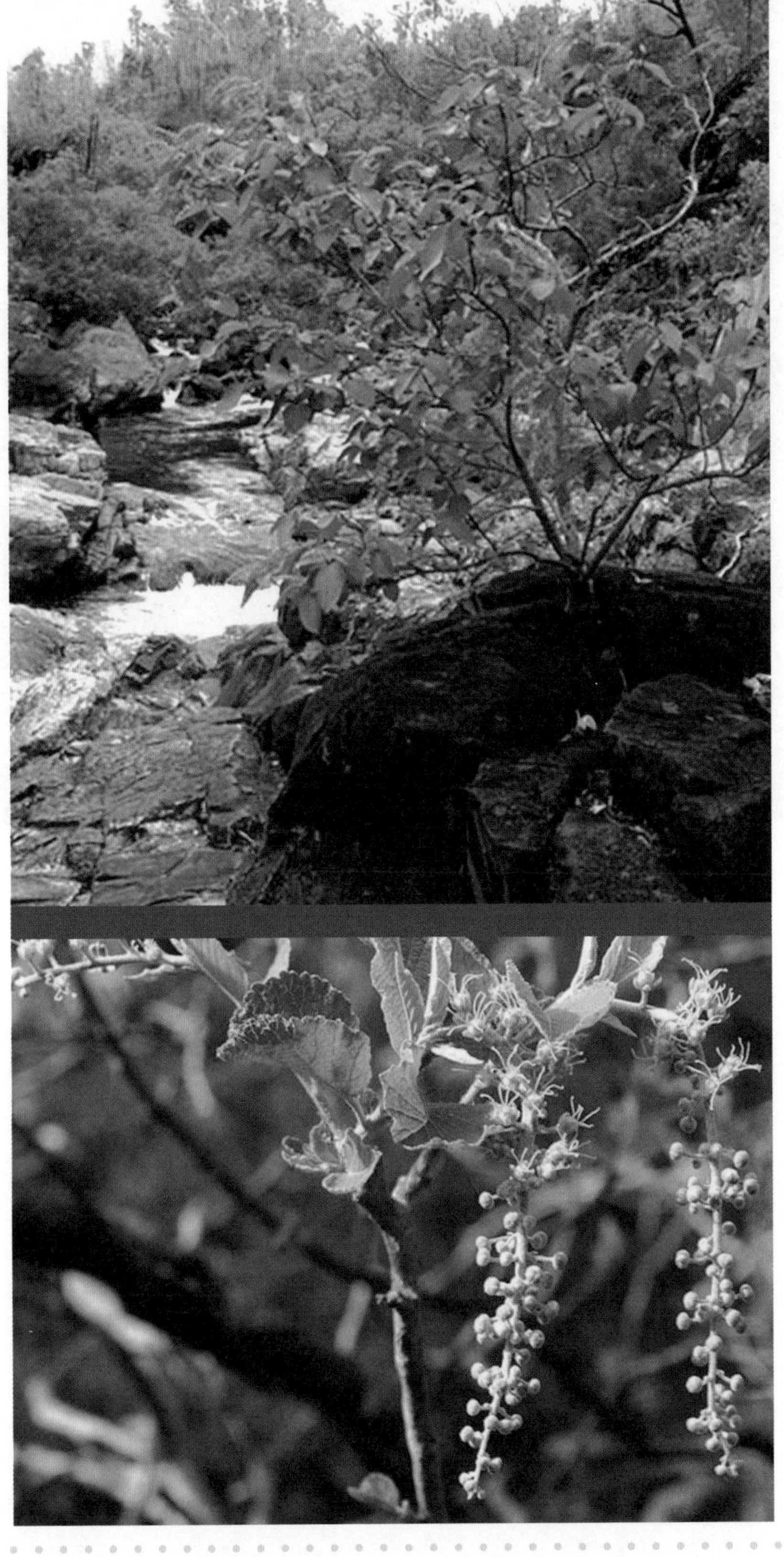

Harpoon Bud

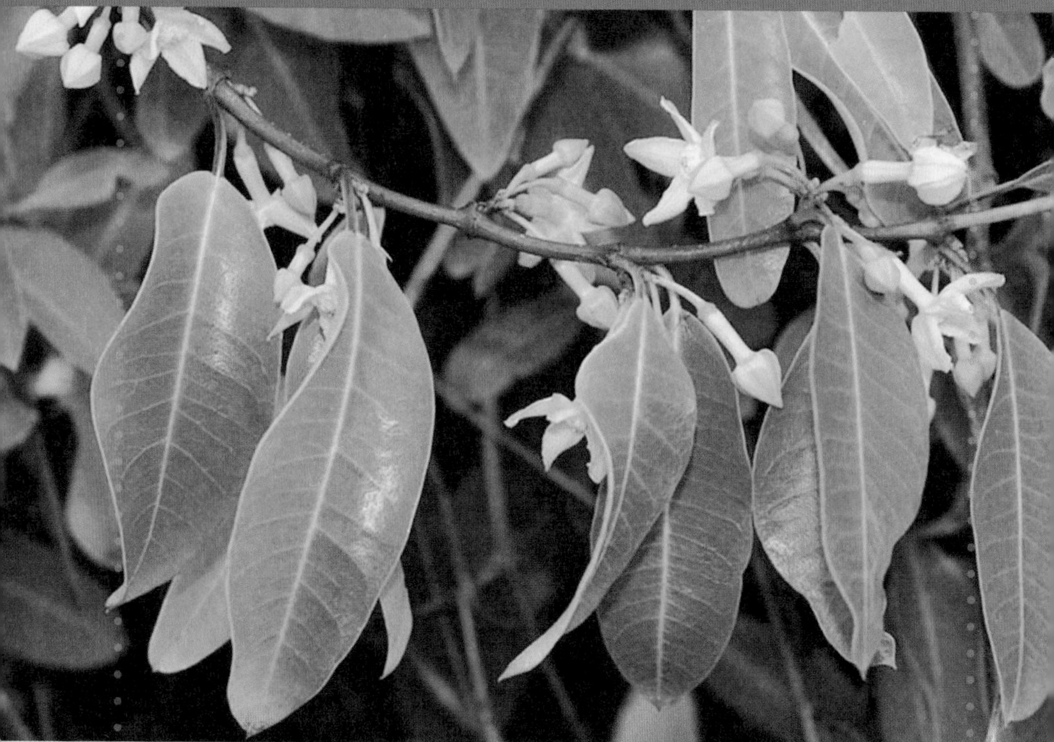

Scientific Name *Gymnanthera oblonga* (Burm.f.) P.S.Green, previously known as *Gymnanthera nitida* R.Br.

Common Name Harpoon Bud.

Aboriginal Names Gargar (Bardi) (Kenneally et al., 1996; Smith & Kalotas, 1985), Garrgarr (Bardi) (Paddy et al., 1993).

Field Notes Harpoon Bud is a scrambling or twining shrub or climber that has been seen up to 6 m in height. Its oblong or elliptic leaves are up to 55 mm long and 25 mm wide. Its small white or cream-yellow-green, star-shaped flowers with five petals appear from March to August or from October to December. Its fruit are about 85 mm long by 5 mm wide with numerous seeds. Harpoon Bud occurs in a variety of habitats in the Kimberley region of Western Australia, the top half of the Northern Territory, the Cape York Peninsula and down the east coast of Queensland as far as Townsville. It also occurs in Cambodia, southern China, Indonesia,

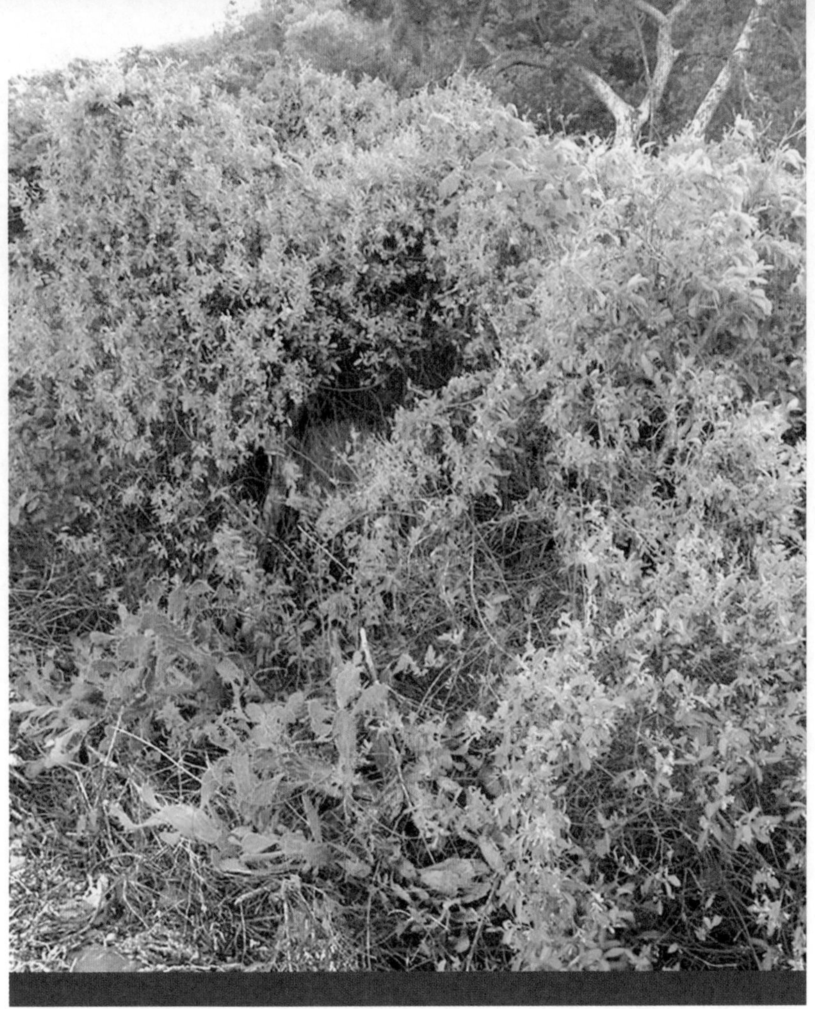

Malaysia, New Guinea, the Philippines, Thailand and Vietnam (ALA, 2022; ATRP, 2020; WAH, 2022).

Medicinal Uses Crushed leaves of Harpoon Bud were warmed and applied as a poultice to affected areas of the body to treat arthritic and rheumatic pain (Kenneally et al., 1996; Smith & Kalotas, 1985).

Other Uses Cordage was made from the vine of Harpoon Bud (Kenneally et al., 1996; Smith & Kalotas, 1985).

Helicopter Tree

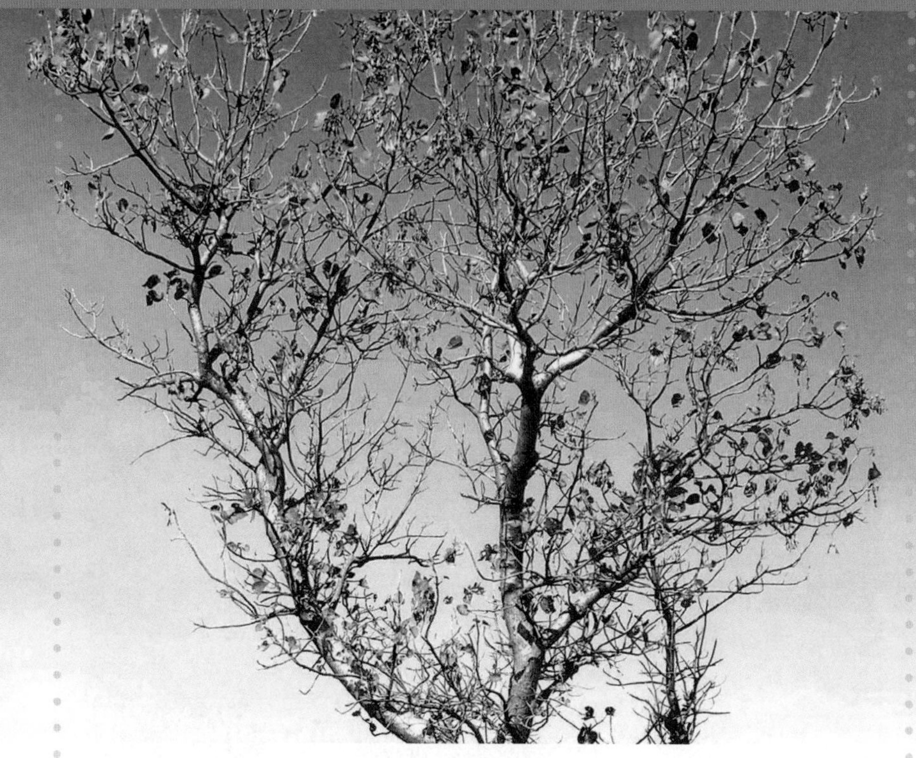

Scientific Name *Gyrocarpus americanus* Jacq.

Common Names Helicopter Tree, Propeller Tree, Coolaman Tree, Shitwood.

Aboriginal Names Jalaloong (Miriwoong) (Leonard et al., 2013), Thalaji (Bunuba) (Oscar et al., 2019), Mirda (Yawuru) (Kenneally et al., 1996), Mida, Dyiwididiny (Nyikina), Bilanggamar (Bardi) (Smith & Kalotas, 1985), Jarlarloony, Jalaloony (Gija) (Purdie et al., 2018), Jarlarloo (Gooniyandi) (Dilkes-Hall et al., 2019), Jardalu, Jadalu (Jaru) (Wightman, 2003), Karlbi (Kwini) (Cheinmora et al., 2017), Yanganyja (Walmajarri) (Richards & Hudson, 2012), Mirta (Karajarri) (Willing, 2014) Joowadidiny (female), Mirda (male) (Nyikina) (Smith & Smith, 2009).

Field Notes The Helicopter Tree grows to 12 m in height. Its leaves are long and ovate and up to 150 mm long by 120 mm wide. Its flowers are cream to yellow and form in compact heads. They are present from January to March. The fruit is a woody capsule with two long thin wings that help the wind to disperse it. The Helicopter Tree occurs in sandy, skeletal soils on alluvial plains, sandplains and rocky outcrops over limestone. In Australia it is found across the top end from the Kimberley region in Western Australia through the Northern Territory and into northern Queensland (ALA, 2022; Fern, 2021; Lassak & McCarthy, 2001; WAH, 2022).

Medicinal Uses Infusions or decoctions of the roots and young shoots were rubbed on cuts (old cuts rather than fresh ones) to aid healing. They were also used as a liniment for areas of rheumatic pain. The wood of the tree was burnt and the charcoal was then crushed and applied to wounds and sores to aid healing (Cock, 2011; Kenneally et al., 1996; Lassak & McCarthy, 2001; Reid, 1986; Webb, 1959). Decoctions of the inner bark were used as an antiseptic wash to treat dermatophytosis (ringworm and tinea), skin sores and itchy skin (Kenneally et al., 1996; Purdie et al., 2018; Smith, 1991; Wightman, 2003). Poultices of warmed leaves were applied to areas of rheumatic pain (Paddy et al., 1993).

Other Uses The bark of the Helicopter Tree has been used by Aboriginal people in the Kimberley to make shields (Kane, 2022). The soft wood was used to carve coolamons (Cheinmora et al., 2017; Kimberley Specialists, 2020; Oscar et al., 2019).

Honey or Sugarbag

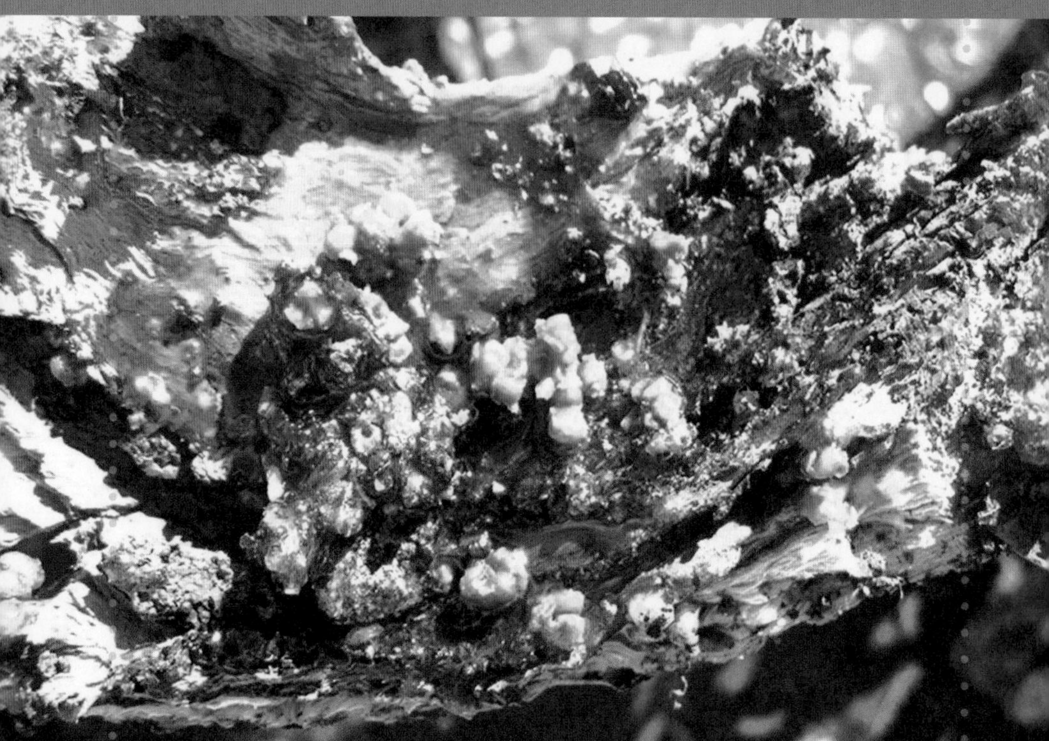

Common Names Honey, Wild Honey, Sugarbag.

Aboriginal Names (Honey) Moonga (Bardi, Nyul Nyul), Ngareng (Miriwoong), Walaja or Kirpaju (Karajarri), Walaja (Nyangumarta), Girrbaju or Nulu (Yawuru), Nhaa or Jimani (Bunuba), Karangu (Ngardi), Karlaka (Nyikina), Ngeenya nyina (Worroorra), Ngarem (Gija), Ngarlu (Walpiri).

Aboriginal Names (Native Bees or Honey Flies) Biyarrimbin (Yawuru), Munukuyu (Kukatja), Angaburra inja (Worrorra), Ngalinya, (Gooniyandi), Ngurriny, Purrmuru, Mawukarra (Walmajarri), Jurlarda (Walpiri),

Field Notes Sugarbag or honey produced by native bees, primarily *Tetragonula hockingsi* and *Austroplebeia essingtoni* (often called Honey Flies), is an important food and medicine source for Aboriginal people in the Kimberley, so is worth a mention in this book as the nectar that the bees make Sugarbag from is, of course, from flowers. Isaacs (1987) talks about three *Trigona* (now *Tetragonula*) and *Austroplebeia* species of native bee that are the main producers of Sugarbag in the Kimberley and have been identified by anthropologist Kim Akerman and recognised by the Ngarinjin and Worora people. They call them *Namiri*, *Narra* and *Wanangka*. The *Namiri* have thick honey and build their hives in the ground under rocks, in ant beds and hollow trees, usually eucalypts. *Wanangka* make a runnier honey, whilst *Narra* honey is even more fluid.

Medicinal Uses Sugarbag was used to soothe sore throats and was smeared on wounds and skin rashes to aid the healing process (Martin, 2014; Williams, 2010). Sugarbag honey is noted for its antimicrobial activity and antioxidant properties and is on par with regular honey from the introduced European bees (Williams, 2020).

Other Uses Sugarbag is prized as a food and is either eaten straight from the hive or mixed with water to make a sweet drink (Bates, 1985). Yellow bee cake is also taken from the hives and eaten. Small amounts of Sugarbag are now being produced commercially in the Kimberley (Dollin & Dollin, 2021). The dark brown wax obtained from Sugarbag hives was used to coat the mouthpieces of didgeridoos and was used to attach axe heads and spear tips. The wax was heated and moulded accordingly and twine was used as a binding to finish the attachments (Martin, 2014).

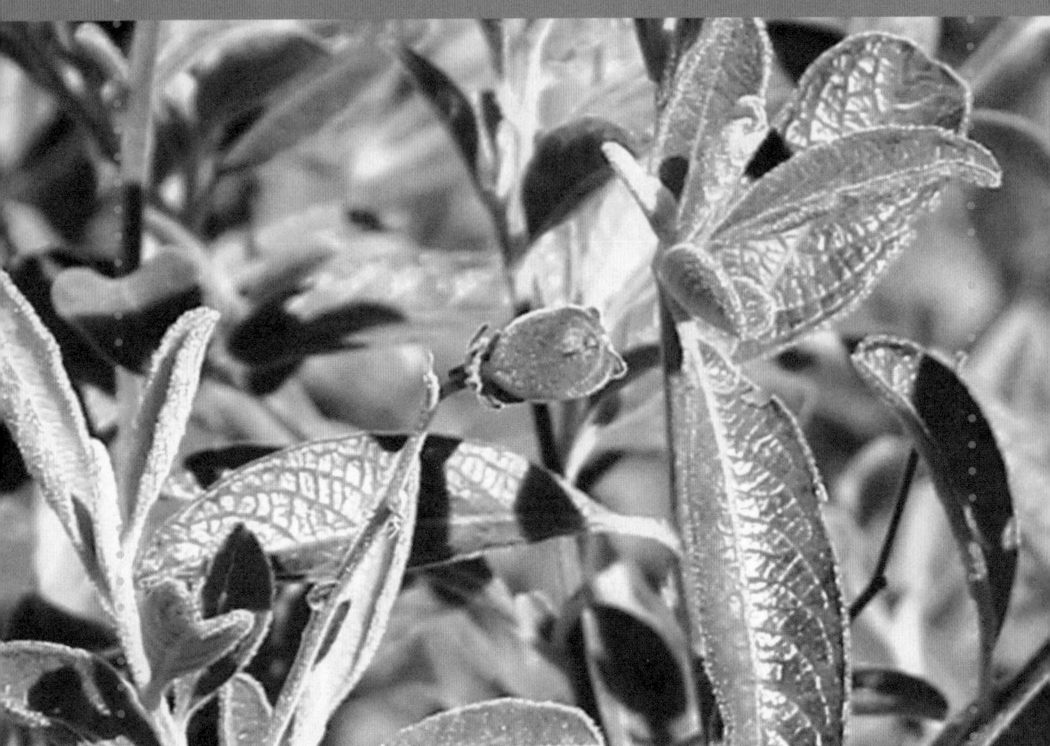

Scientific Name *Dodonaea hispidula* var. *arida* (S.T.Reynolds) M.G.Harr.

Common Name Hopbush.

Aboriginal Name Boorrboon (Nyikina) (Young et al., 2012).

Field Notes This Hopbush is a multi-stemmed shrub that grows up to 1.5 m in height. It has bright green ovate leaves that are tapered at the base. It has separate male and female pinkish-white flowers that form in clusters. Its pinkish-purple-red, ovoid fruit capsules have four narrow wings. Hopbush is endemic to the Kimberley region of Western Australia and the Northern Territory (ALA, 2022; Young et al., 2012).

Medicinal Uses The Hopbush leaves were rubbed into the feet to protect them from coral cuts and stonefish stings when the men were fishing (Kenneally et al., 1996).

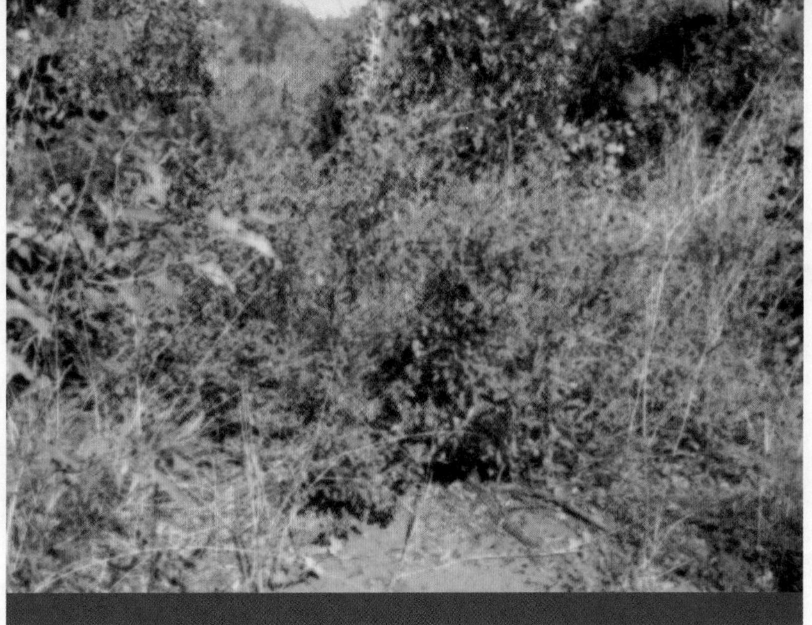

Other Uses The leaves of this Hopbush are edible (Young et al., 2012).

Hopbush (*Dodonaea physocarpa*)

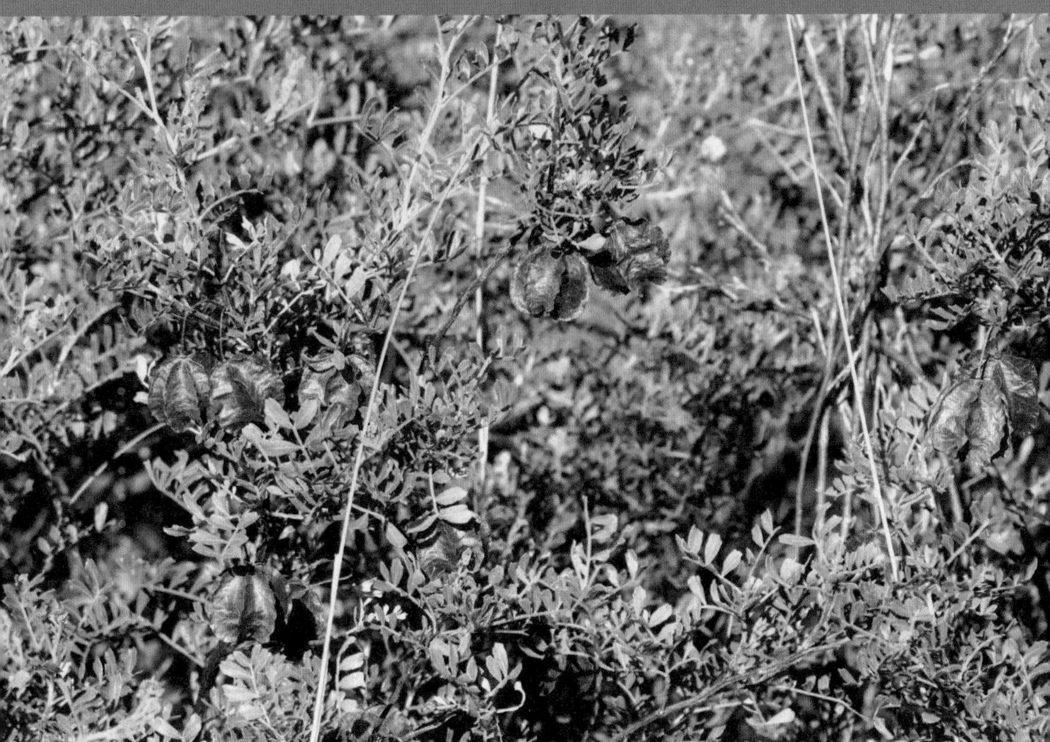

Scientific Name *Dodonaea physocarpa* F.Muell.

Common Name Hopbush.

Field Notes This Hopbush grows as a shrub to approximately 2 m in height. Its light green, ovate leaves have a slightly pointed end. Its flowers are usually in axillary, few-flowered cymes, sometimes solitary, with pedicels up to 13 mm long and four to six lanceolate to ovate sepals up to 3.6 mm long. Its fruit are red or white, winged ellipsoidal, greatly inflated capsules that are up to 26 mm long and 25 mm wide. Hopbush occurs across the tropical north of Australia from the Kimberley region of Western Australia to Far North Queensland (ALA, 2022; WAH, 2022).

Medicinal Uses Decoctions of the branches and leaves of this Hopbush were used as a wash to bathe the head and chest to relieve the symptoms colds and influenza (Smith, 1991).

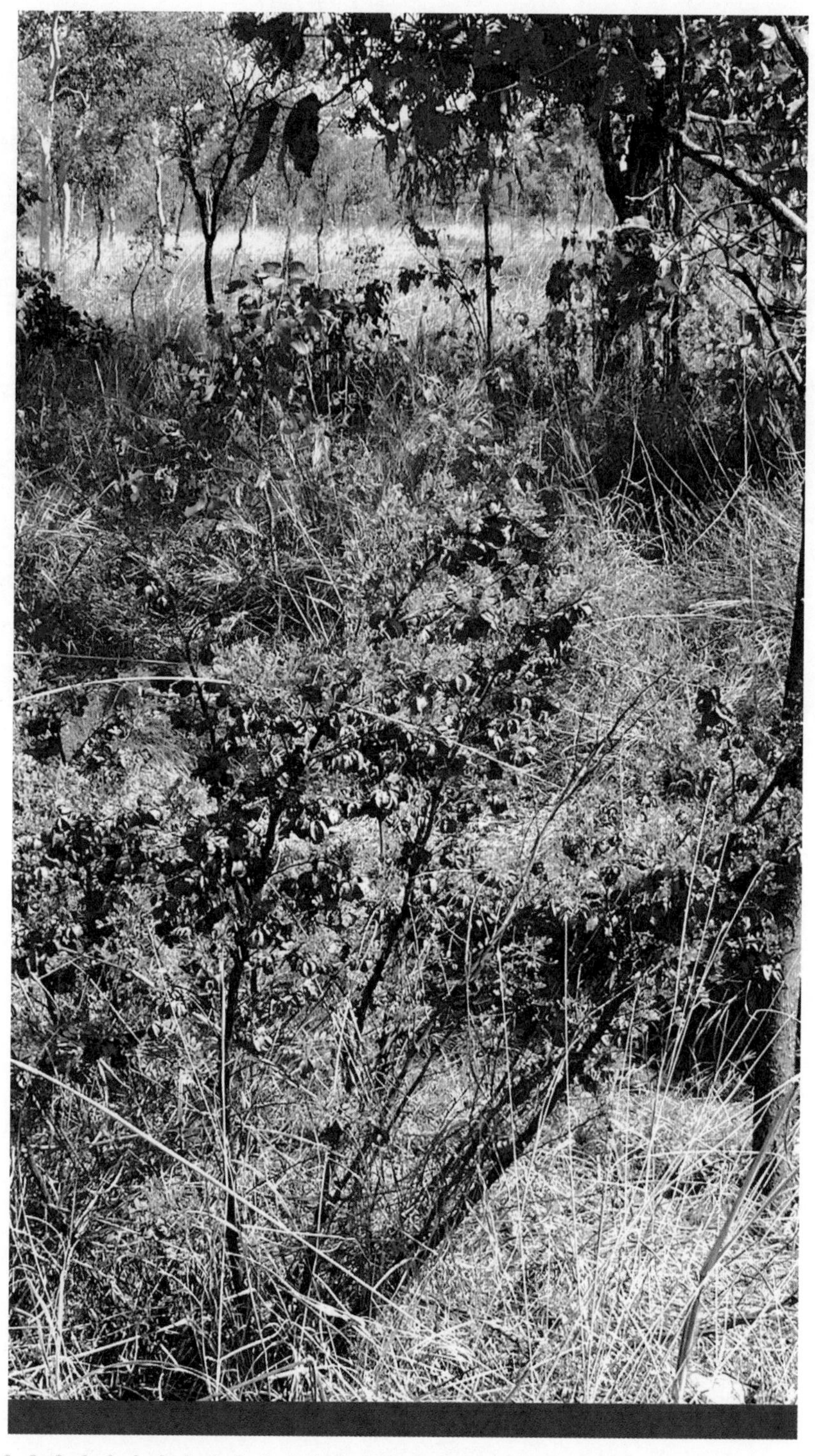

Ironwood

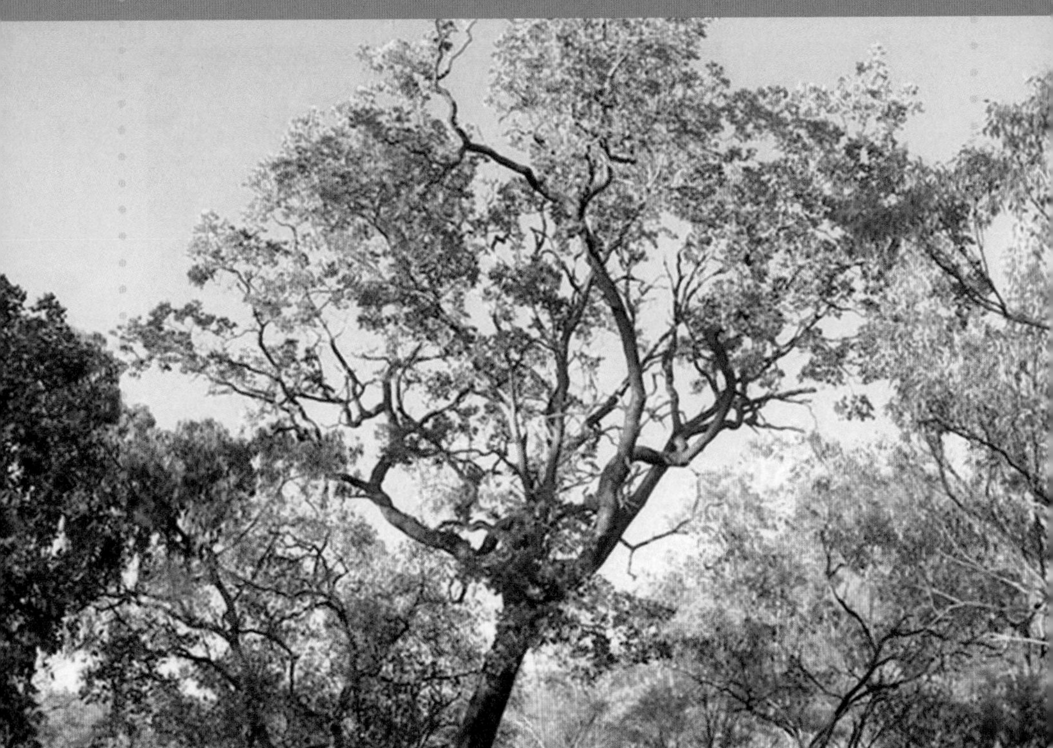

Scientific Name *Erythrophleum chlorostachys* (F.Muell.) Baill.

Common Names Ironwood, Cooktown Ironwood, Poison Tree, Camel Poison.

Aboriginal Names Remerreng (Miriwoong) (Leonard et al., 2013), Bandarrawu (Bunuba) (Oscar et al., 2019), Birmana or Dyundyu (Nyikina), Djungumara (Bardi) (Smith & Kalotas, 1985), Joonggorrmarr (Bardi), Jun'ju, Bilamana (Yawuru) (Kenneally et al., 1996), Berawooroony, Perawuruny (Gija) (Purdie et al., 2018; Wightman, 2003), Winjabarr minya, Winjibarr minya (Kwini) (Cheinmora et al., 2017), Junju (Karajarri) (Willing, 2014), Joonyjoo (Nyikina) (Smith & Smith, 2009).

Field Notes Ironwood grows as a semi-deciduous shrub or tree up to 15 m in height depending on conditions. It has tessellated bark, large ovate leaves, large flat pods and white to yellow-green bottlebrush-type flowers that are present from July to November.

Ironwood occurs in a variety of habitats all over tropical Australia from the Kimberley region in Western Australia through the Northern Territory to northern Queensland (ALA, 2022; Fern, 2021; Flora of Australia Online, 2022; WAH, 2022).

Medicinal Uses Infusions or decoctions of the bark and roots of Ironwood were used externally as an antiseptic wash to treat spear wounds, cuts and sores, and were rubbed all over the body for general malaise (Cock, 2011; Lassak & McCarthy, 2001; Reid, 1986; Webb, 1959). They were also used as a liniment for areas of rheumatic pain (Cock, 2011; Devanesen, 2000; Smith, 1991; Tiwi Land Council, 2001), and to treat scabies infestations (Wiynjorrotj et al., 2005).

Other Uses The gum of Ironwood is edible and is reported to taste like commercial toffee (Fox & Garde, 2018; Wiynjorrotj et al., 2005). The Gija used the wood of the Ironwood tree to make digging sticks and 'fighting sticks' (Purdie et al., 2018; Wightman, 2003).

CAUTION: The leaves and sucker shoots of Ironwood are very toxic and should not be eaten (Kenneally et al., 1996).

Jalkay

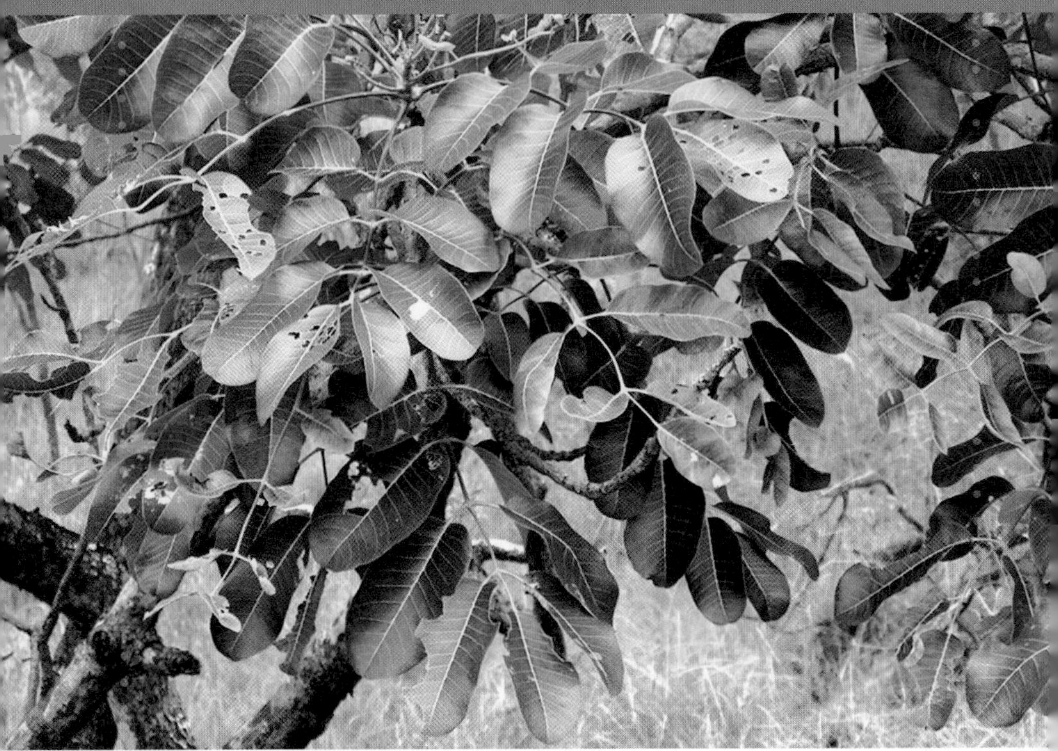

Scientific Name *Canarium australianum* F.Muell.

Common Names Jalkay, White Beech, Mango Bark, Scrub Turpentine, Turpentine Tree, Carrot Wood, Parsnip Wood, Melville Island White Beech, Styptic Tree, Brown Cudgerie.

Aboriginal Names Diiwal (Wunambal, Gaambera) (Karadada et al., 2011), Jalkay (Kwini) (Crawford, 1982), Djalgay (Bardi) (Smith & Kalotas, 1985), Jalgir (Bardi) (Paddy et al., 1993), Wûrndûr manya (Kwini) (Cheinmora et al., 2017).

Field Notes Jalkay is a tree that grows up to 20 m in height. Its ovate leaflet blades are glabrous and up to 190 mm long by 80 mm wide. Its small flowers are white and are present between November and April. Its fruit are ellipsoid, smooth drupes that are blue in colour and about 20 mm long. The fruit are available between May and November. Jalkay occurs in sand, clay and shallow skeletal soils over basalt, on lateritic scree and sandstone

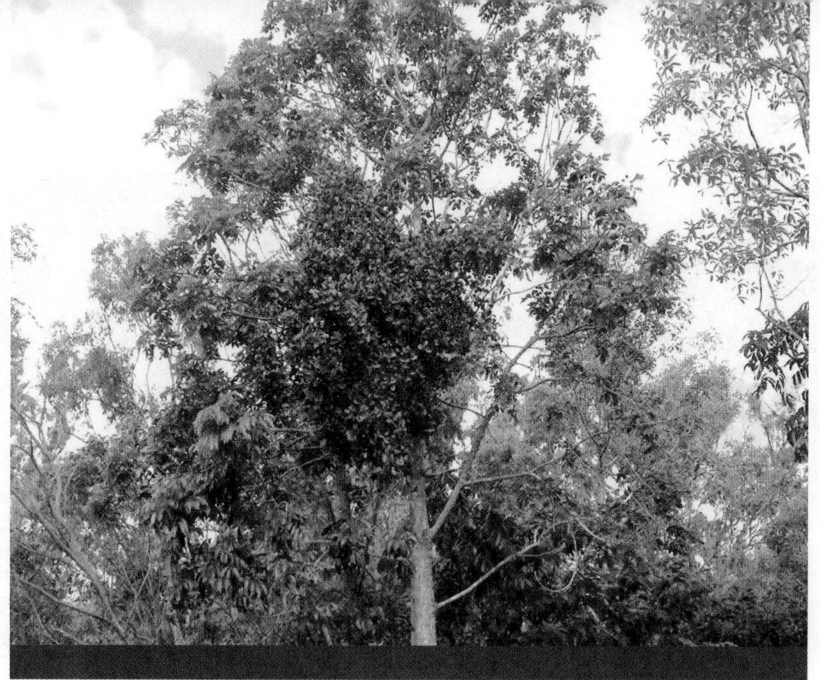

ridges, in open forest, rainforest and near the sea north of Kununurra in the Kimberley region of Western Australia, the Northern Territory, northern Queensland and New Guinea (ALA, 2022; Fern, 2021; WAH, 2022).

Medicinal Uses Infusions of the bark, made by breaking the bark up and rubbing it in water until a milky substance is produced, were drunk, after straining the liquid, to treat diarrhoea and stomach cramps (Lassak & McCarthy, 2001), although this was regarded by some Aboriginal groups in the Northern Territory as a 'hazardous undertaking and was avoided' (Williams, 2011). The sappy inner bark was applied to cuts to stop the bleeding, but not to larger wounds (Williams, 2011).

Other Uses The seeds of Jalkay are edible. The fruit are usually collected from the ground. The seeds are cracked open and the kernel is eaten raw (Cheinmora et al., 2017; Crawford, 1982; DBCA, 2019; Fox & Garde, 2018; Isaacs, 1987; Karadada et al., 2011; RFCA, 1993; Territory Native Plants, 2021). The fruit flesh is also edible but the fruit is usually roasted before eating (Fern, 2021; Smith & Kalotas, 1985). The trunks of these trees have been used traditionally to make dugout canoes (Cheinmora et al., 2017; Crawford, 1982).

Java Brucei

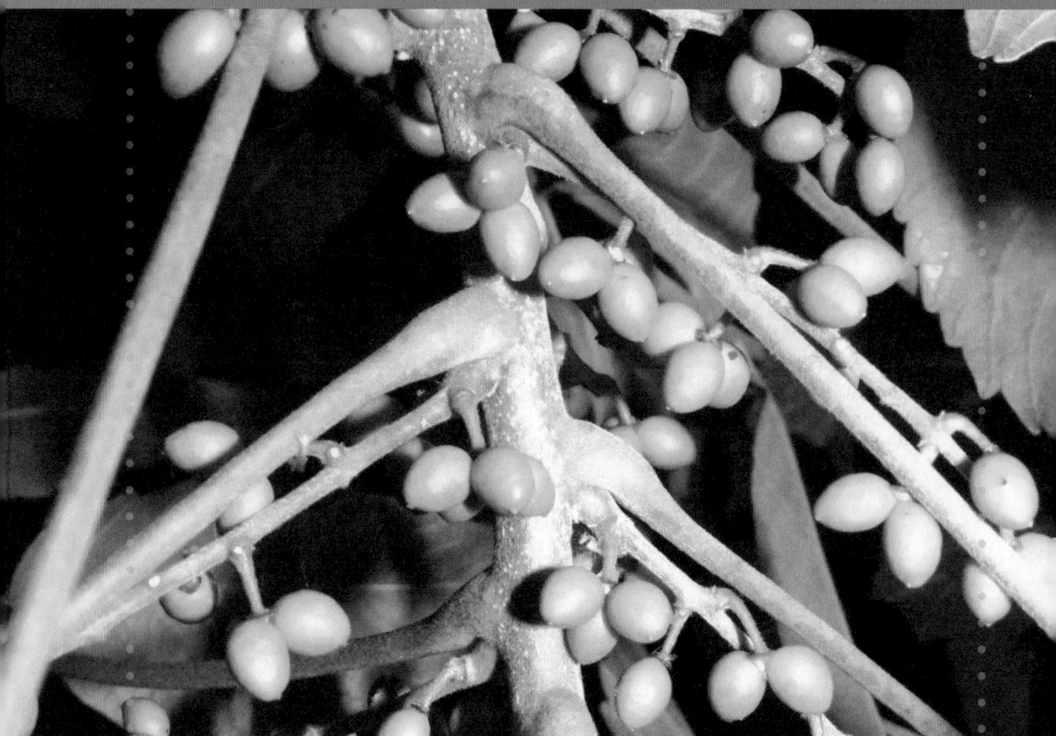

Scientific Name *Brucea javanica* (L.) Merr.

Common Names Java Brucei, Kosam, Macassar Kernels.

Field Notes Java Brucei grows as a shrub or tree to 6 m in height in Australia and up to 10 m elsewhere. It has large, ovate, serrated, dark green leaf blades, which are pointed at the distal end and are up to 110 mm long by 55 mm wide. The leaves have hairs on both the upper and lower surfaces. Its flowers are green-white with red anthers. Flowering is in November in Australia. Its fruit are drupes that look like black olives when mature. Java Brucei occurs in sand over sandstone, on hills and amongst boulders in the tropics from the Kimberly region of Western Australia through the Northern Territory and into northern Queensland. It is also found in China, India, Indonesia, Malaysia, New Guinea and Sri Lanka (ALA, 2022; Fern, 2021; GBIF, 2022; WAH, 2022).

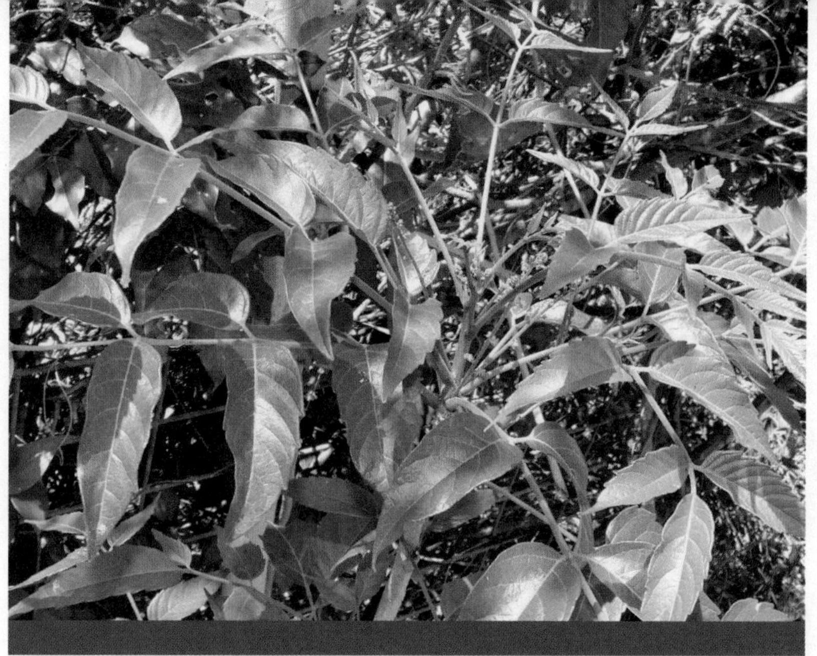

Medicinal Uses The bitter seed can be eaten to stop diarrhoea. The Chinese used Java Brucei to treat the symptoms of malaria. Aboriginal groups use the leaves and roots as an analgesic (ATRP, 2020; Lassak & McCarthy, 2001). The plant has also been used in the treatment of abdominal pain, coughs, haemorrhoids, corns, warts, ulcers and cancer. Poultices of the crushed leaves were applied externally to treat enlarged spleens, scurf (scaly or shredded dry skin, such as that which occurs as dandruff), dermatophytosis (ringworm and tinea), boils and centipede bites. The bark and roots have been used to treat toothache (Fern, 2021).

Jersey Cudweed

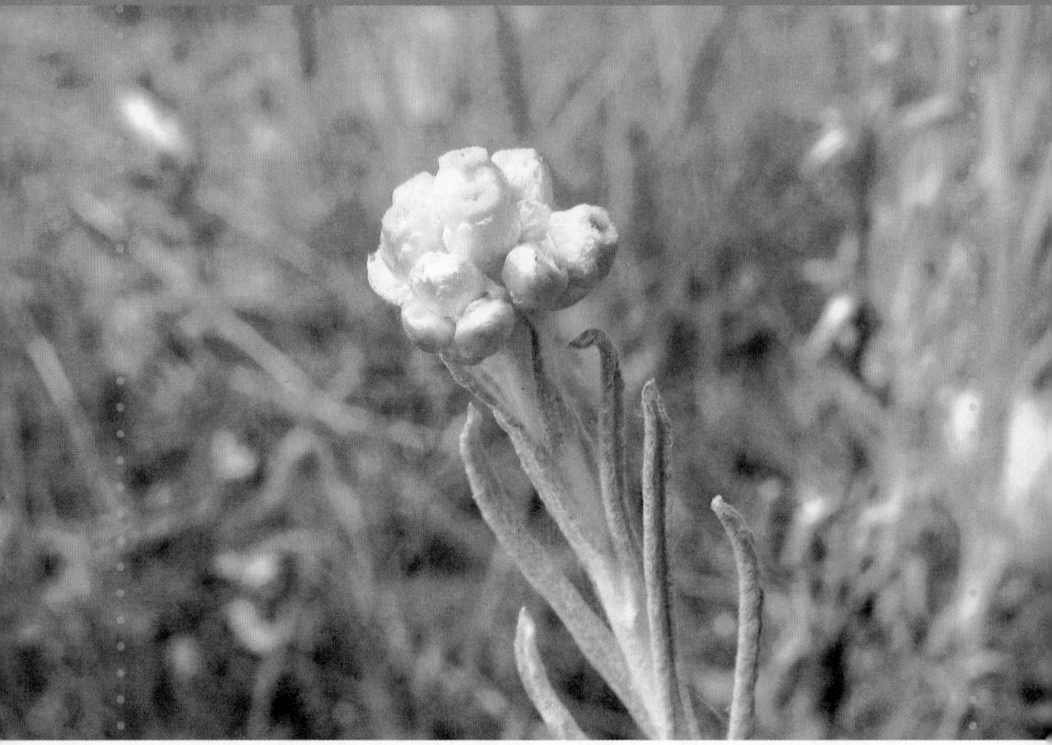

Scientific Name *Pseudognaphalium luteoalbum* (L.) Hilliard & B.L.Burtt, previously known as *Helichrysum luteoalbum* (L.) Rchb.

Common Names Jersey Cudweed, Cudweed, Flannel-leaf.

Field Notes Jersey Cudweed is a greyish-white, woolly, annual herb that grows up to 500 mm in height. Its leaves are narrow to lanceolate and up to 65 mm long by 8 mm wide, with margins wavy and rolled under. The leaves become smaller and narrower up the stem. Its small, creamy-white flowers appear in terminal clusters of up to 20 tiny button flower heads from September to March. Jersey Cudweed occurs in many habitats and soils over most of mainland Australia and Tasmania. It also occurs in most of Europe, including Britain, and most other warm temperate regions of the world (ALA, 2022; VicFlora, 2022; WAH, 2022).

Medicinal Uses The leaves of Jersey Cudweed have astringent, cholagogue, diuretic, febrifuge, haemostatic and vulnerary

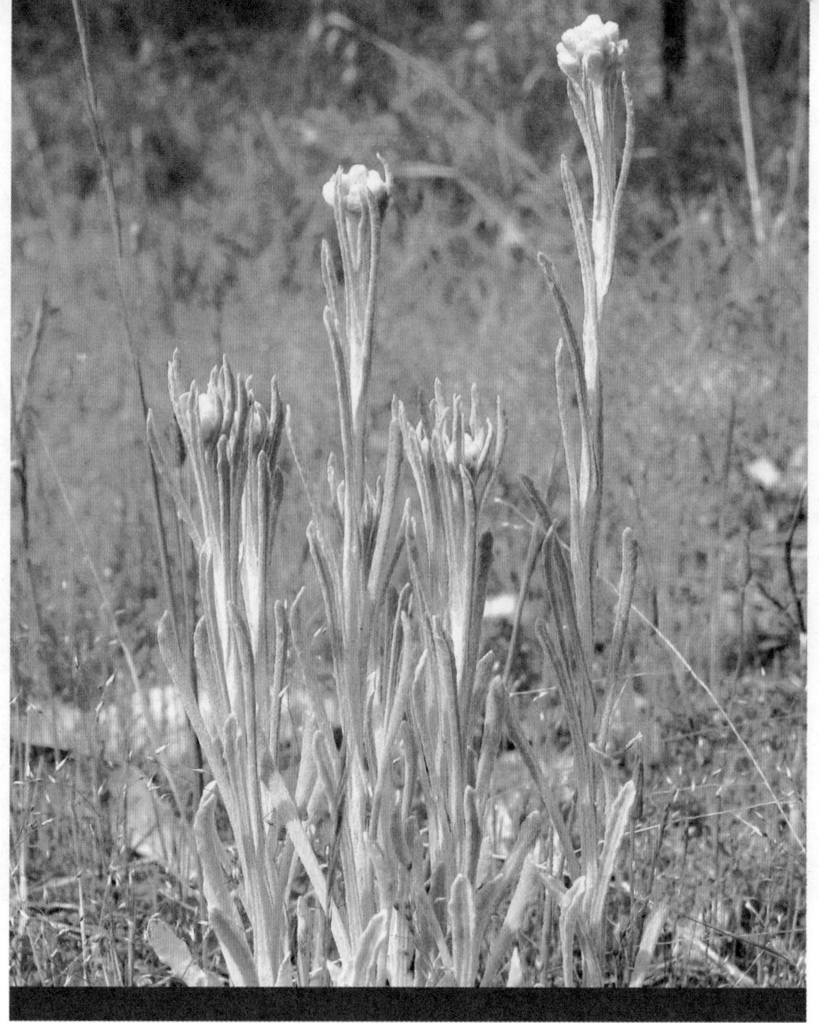

properties and have been used medicinally by some Aboriginal groups around Australia. Decoctions of the leaves were taken internally by Aboriginal Australians to treat general malaise. The plant is used in the treatment of breast cancer in Belgium (Fern, 2021; Herbiguide, 2022; PFAF, 2022).

Other Uses The leaves of Jersey Cudweed are edible raw or cooked (Fern, 2021; PFAF, 2022).

Jigal Tree

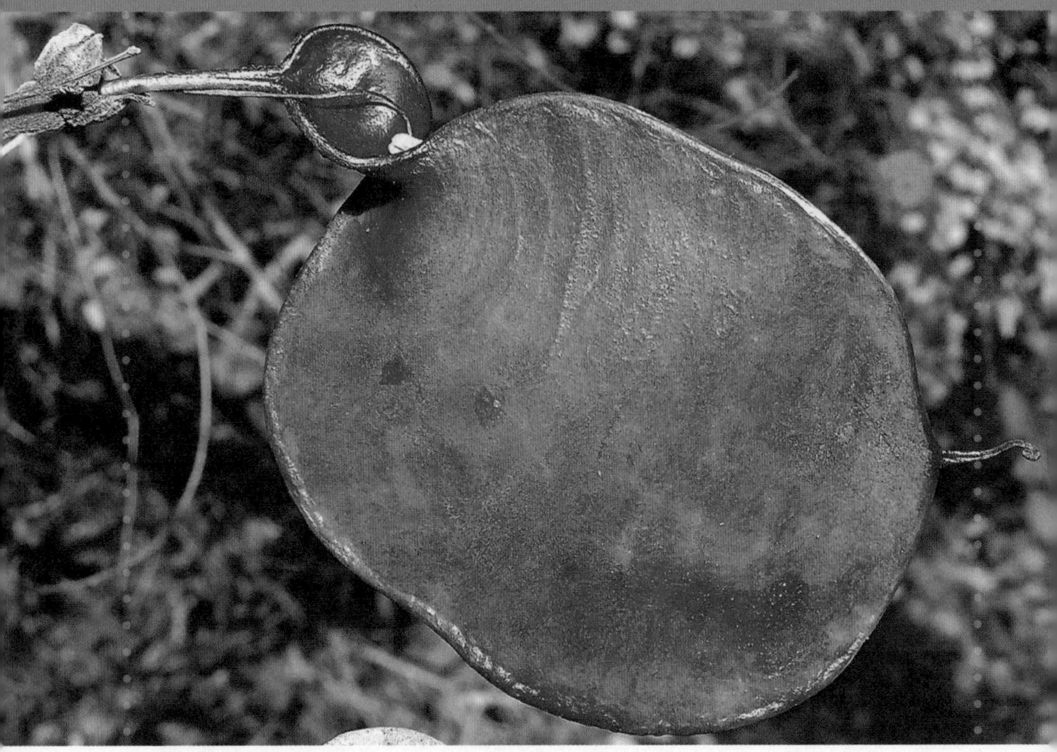

Scientific Name *Bauhinia cunninghamii* (Benth.) Benth., previously known as *Lysiphyllum cunninghamii* (Benth.) de Wit.

Common Names Jigal Tree, Jiggle Tree, Mother-in-Law Tree, Bauhinia, Kimberley Bauhinia.

Aboriginal Names Wanyarring (Miriwoong) (Leonard et al., 2013), Ngiyali (Bunuba) (Oscar et al., 2019), Gundulu (Wunambal, Gaambera) (Karadada et al., 2011), Warimba (Nyikina) (Young et al., 2012), Joomoo (Bardi) (Paddy et al.,1993), Djuuma, Jooma, Jigal (Bardi) (DAWE, n.d.; Smith & Kalotas, 1985), Pirral, Karliwarn (Walmajarri) (Richards & Hudson, 2012), Jikaly (Nyangumarta), Kunjiny or Goonjiny, Wanyarriny, Wanjarriny (Gija) (Purdie et al., 2018; Wightman, 2003), Wanyari (Miwa) (Kimberley Specialists, 2020), Joowoorljidi (Gooniyandi) (Dilkes-Hall et al., 2019), Gunji (Jaru) (Wightman, 2003), Burrari (Kwini) (Cheinmora et al., 2017), Jikily (Karajarri) (Willing, 2014).

Field Notes The Jigal Tree grows as a shrub or tree to 12 m in height depending on conditions. It has rough, tessellated to fissured bark and small ovate leaves that form in pairs which face back-to-back. The Jigal is so called because its leaves face back-to-back as in the term 'Jigal', 'used to describe the (avoidance) relationship between son-in-law and mother-in-law in Kimberley Aboriginal culture. According to Aboriginal Law, mother-in-law and son-in-law must not directly face each other' (SKIPA, 2022). Its stunning red flowers with long staminal filaments appear from April to October. The Jigal Tree occurs in red alluvial sand, red-brown sandy loam, sandstone scree over basalt, in creek beds and on levees at the edge of monsoonal forests and floodplains in the Kimberley region of Western Australia, the Northern Territory and parts of northern Queensland (ALA, 2022; ATRP, 2020; SKIPA, 2022; WAH, 2022).

Medicinal Uses Decoctions of the inner bark were drunk to treat fever, headache, bronchitis, coughs and sore throats. They were also used externally as a wash for sores, cuts, boils, to treat scabies infestations and to bathe the head to treat fever (Devanesen, 2000; El Questro, n.d.; Purdie et al., 2018; Smith, 1991).

Other Uses Aboriginal people in the Pilbara and Kimberley regions of Western Australia and the Northern Territory are known to suck the sweet nectar straight from the flowers, and to eat the sweet gum that oozes from wounds in the tree (Cheinmora et al., 2017; Karadada et al., 2011; Purdie et al., 2018; Smith, 1991; Smith & Kalotas, 1985; Wightman, 2003; Young et al., 2012). Native beehives (Sugarbag) are often found in the trunk of this tree (Oscar et al., 2019; Smith, 1991). The dry sap is often mixed with nectar, forming a sweet, chewy gum (Kane, 2022).

Joolal

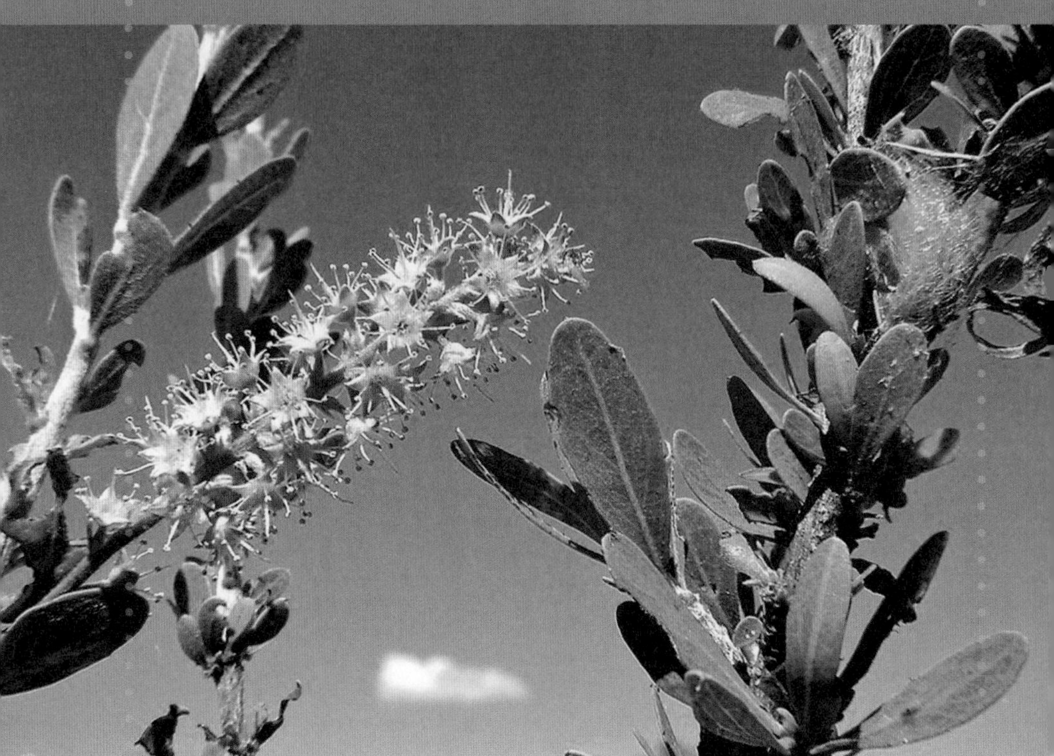

Scientific Name *Terminalia canescens* (DC.) T.Durand.

Common Names Joolal, Winged Nut Tree, Bush Gum Tree, Yellow Jacket.

Aboriginal Names Walula (Wunambal, Gaambera) (Karadada et al., 2011), Djulal, Joolal (Bardi) (Smith & Kalotas, 1985), Jilungin, Jilangen, Joolangen (Nyul Nyul) (DAWE, n.d.), Yirriyarriny, Biriwooriny, Berewereny (Gija) (Purdie et al., 2018), Biriwiri, Biyiwiri (Jaru) (Wightman, 2003), Nyallung (Mirriwong) (Kimberley Specialists, 2020), Warlula minya (Kwini) (Cheinmora, et al., 2017; Crawford, 1982), Jirarl (Nyikina) (Smith & Smith, 2009).

Field Notes Joolal is a deciduous shrub or tree that is often found up to 10 m in height in good conditions. Its bark is grey to brown in colour and flaky. Its leaves are narrowly elliptic to oblanceolate in shape and up to 75 mm long. Its small, cream-white or white-green flowers form in clusters at the end of branchlets and can be present at any time of the year. Its dry, winged fruit have a flattened, elliptic to obovate shape and can be up to 40 mm long. Joolal occurs in stony soils, red sand, sandstone or laterite in a variety of habitats in the Kimberley region of Western Australia and the Northern Territory (ALA, 2022; WAH, 2022).

Medicinal Uses Infusions or decoctions of the bark and leaves of Joolal were taken internally by the Nyul Nyul people of the Dampier Peninsula to treat anxiety and promote a restful sleep. The herb is also reported to improve digestion, mental focus and one's libido. Joolal tea is reported by researchers to contain more antioxidants than green tea (Allen, 2019).

Other Uses The gum that oozes from the tree is edible. If the gum is too hard it can be softened in hot ashes (Cheinmora, et al., 2017; Karadada et al., 2011; Purdie et al., 2018; Vigilante et al., 2013; Wightman, 2003). The Gija call the gum 'nyaarnte' (Wightman, 2003) and the Bardi call it 'gim' (Kenneally et al., 1996). The gum was also used to glue spearheads to the shafts (Karadada et al., 2011).

Kankulang

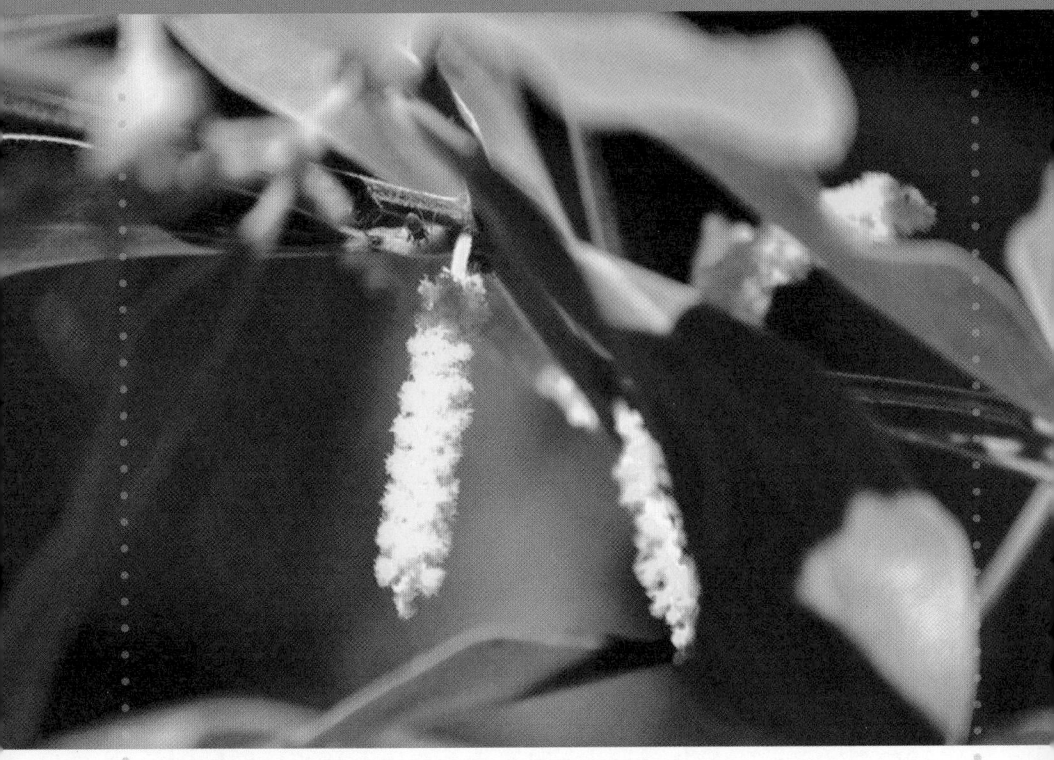

Scientific Name *Acacia pellita* O.Schwarz

Common Names Kankulang, Silver Wattle.

Field Notes Kankulang is a wattle that grows as a shrub or tree up to 6 m in height. It has slightly fibrous, brown or grey bark and narrowly elliptic to elliptic phyllodes that are up to 195 mm long and 100 mm wide with prominent veins. Its cylindrical flower-spikes are up to 70 mm in length and are packed with golden coloured flowers from May to August. Its seed pods are densely haired, up to 70 mm long and 5 mm wide, and are tightly coiled in masses. Kankulang occurs in sandy loam and alluvium in damp situations in the Kimberley region of Western Australia and the Northern Territory (ALA, 2022; WAH, 2022).

Medicinal Uses Decoctions or infusions of the twigs and leaves of Kankulang were used as a medicinal wash to treat itching from a number of skin conditions, such as allergies (hives) and rashes,

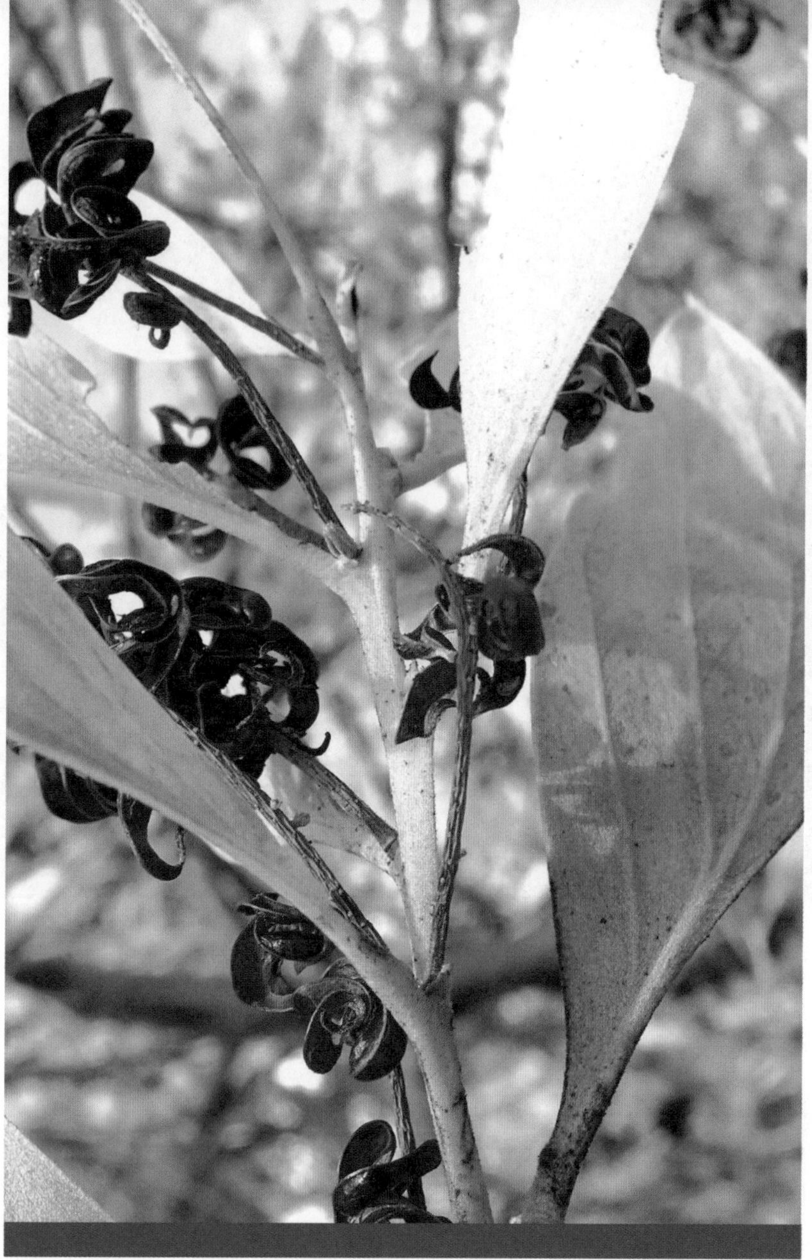

including those caused by hairy stinging caterpillars (itchy grubs) (Searle, 2020).

Other Uses The clear gum that oozes from wounds in the tree is edible. Edible grubs can be found in the roots of this tree (Wiynjorrotj et al., 2005).

Kapok Bush

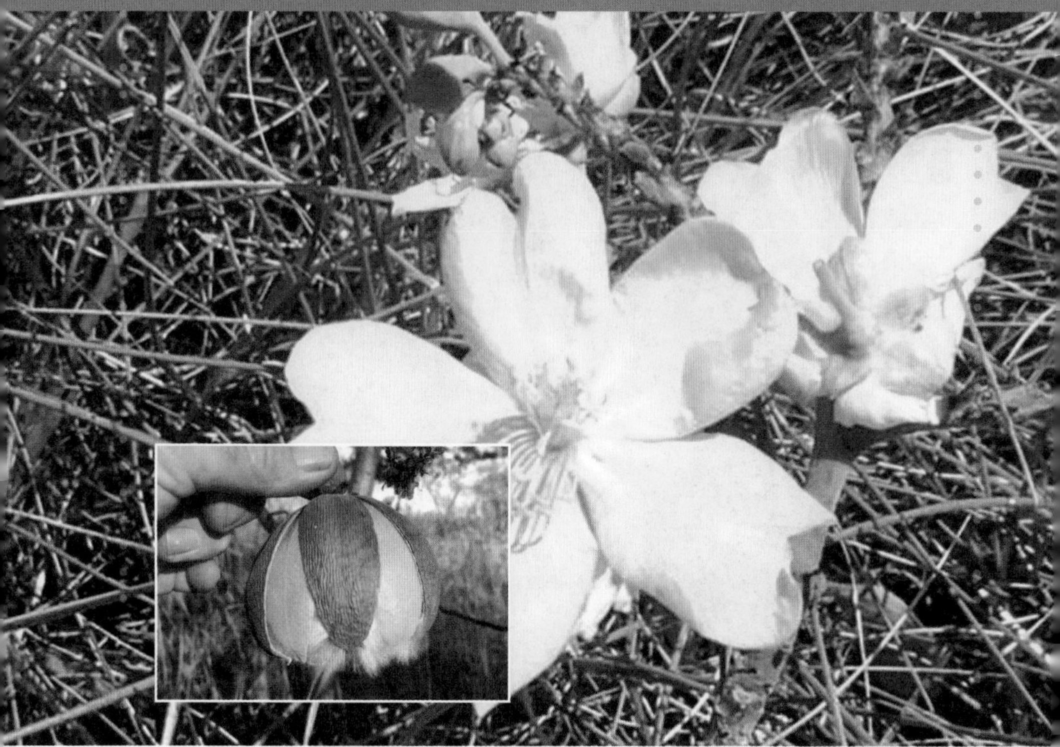

Scientific Name *Cochlospermum fraseri* Planch.

Common Names Kapok Bush, Kapok Tree, Cotton Tree, Yellow Kapok.

Aboriginal Names Wanggu (Bunuba) (Oscar et al., 2019), Goonjang (Miriwoong) (Leonard et al., 2013), Gulun (Bardi) (Smith & Kalotas, 1985), Goonjal or Kunjal (Gija) (Purdie et al., 2018), Wanggoo (Gooniyandi) (Dilkes-Hall et al., 2019), Wayina, Gunyjali, Juwa (Jaru) (Wightman, 2003), Yaarla, Malinja (Wunambal, Gaambera) (Karadada et al., 2011), Marlinjarr minya, Wiyana minya (Kwini) (Cheinmora et al., 2017; Crawford, 1982), Karlwarl (Nyikina) (Smith & Smith, 2009).

Field Notes The Kapok Bush grows as a deciduous shrub or tree up to 6 m in height. It has smooth grey bark, light green, large-lobed leaves and big yellow flowers that appear after the leaves have dropped from March to August. The large kidney-shaped fruit

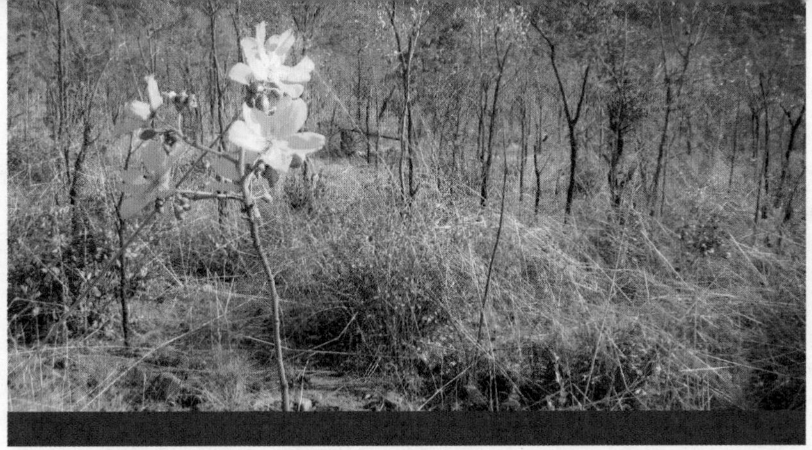

or seed pods have long cotton-like hairs inside. Kapok Bush occurs in a variety of soils and habitats in the Kimberley region of Western Australia and in the top half of the Northern Territory (ALA, 2022; SKIPA, 2022; WAH, 2022).

Medicinal Uses The seeds of Kapok Bush were crushed and applied to boils and carbuncles to ripen them and draw them out (Low, 1990). The mucilage surrounding the seeds was used for the same purpose. Decoctions of the inner bark and flowers, when available, were taken internally to treat fever (Smith, 1991).

Other Uses The young roots of Kapok Bush can be eaten raw but are usually roasted. The flowers are also edible (Crawford, 1982; El Questro, n.d.; Fern, 2021; Fox & Garde, 2018; Karadada et al., 2011; Low, 1991; Native Tastes of Australia, 2020; Purdie et al., 2018; Smith, 1991; Wightman, 2003). The gum that oozes from wounds in the tree is edible and was eaten like toffee (Cheinmora et al., 2017). The cottony fibres in the seed pods have recently been used as a stuffing for pillows and cushions (Cheinmora et al., 2017; Smith, 1991). In the past, Kimberley women used this cotton wool material as sanitary pads when menstruating (Wightman, 2003). The wood was used to make fire sticks (Purdie et al., 2018). The Gija and Kwini used the bark to make cordage or string that was sometimes made into baby harnesses (Wightman, 2003).

Kapok Mangrove

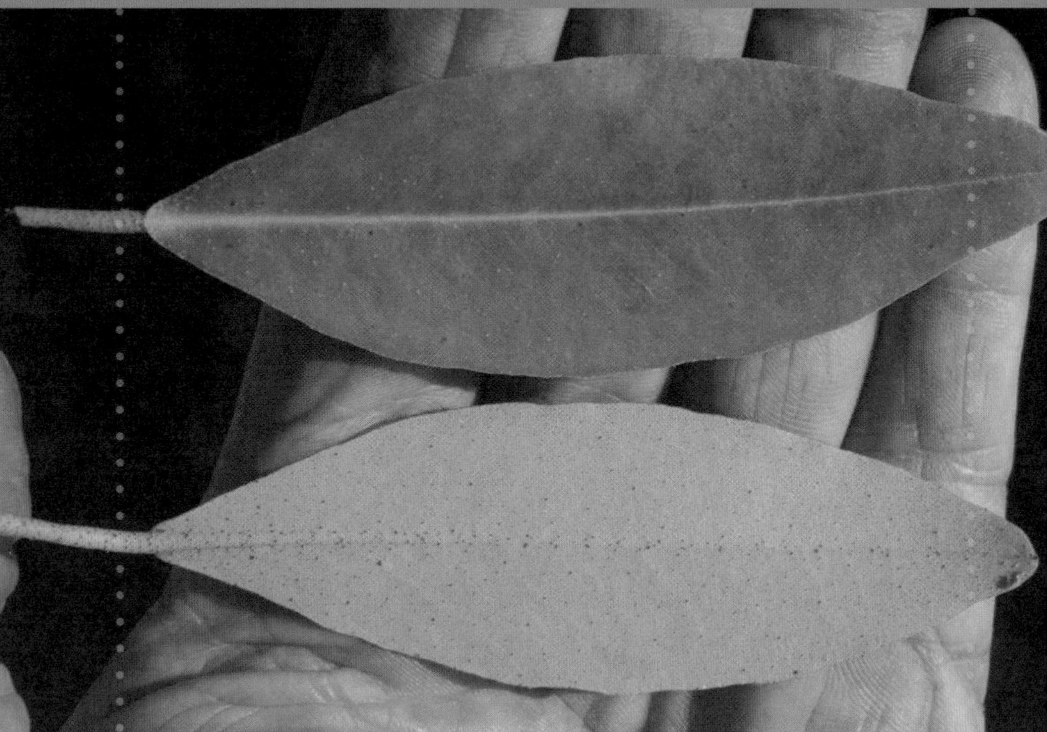

Scientific Name *Camptostemon schultzii* Mast.

Common Name Kapok Mangrove.

Aboriginal Names Djulba, Choolboor (Bardi) (Smith & Kalotas, 1985), Joolboo (Bardi) (Kenneally et al., 1996), Biyal Biyal (Yawuru) (Kenneally et al., 1996), Wurndala (Wunambal, Gaambera) (Karadada et al., 2011), Wundala minya (Kwini) (Cheinmora et al., 2017).

Field Notes Kapok Mangrove grows as a shrub or tree to 20 m in height. It has smooth silver-grey bark, narrow elliptic leaves and small white flowers that smell like champagne. The flowers appear between November and April. The silvery, scaly fruit open to reveal the seeds, which are covered in long, slender white hairs. Kapok Mangrove is found on tidal flats and along creeks around the coast in the Pilbara and Kimberley regions of Western Australia, the Northern Territory and the Cape York Peninsula in Queensland's far north (ALA, 2022; Foulkes, n.d.; WAH, 2022).

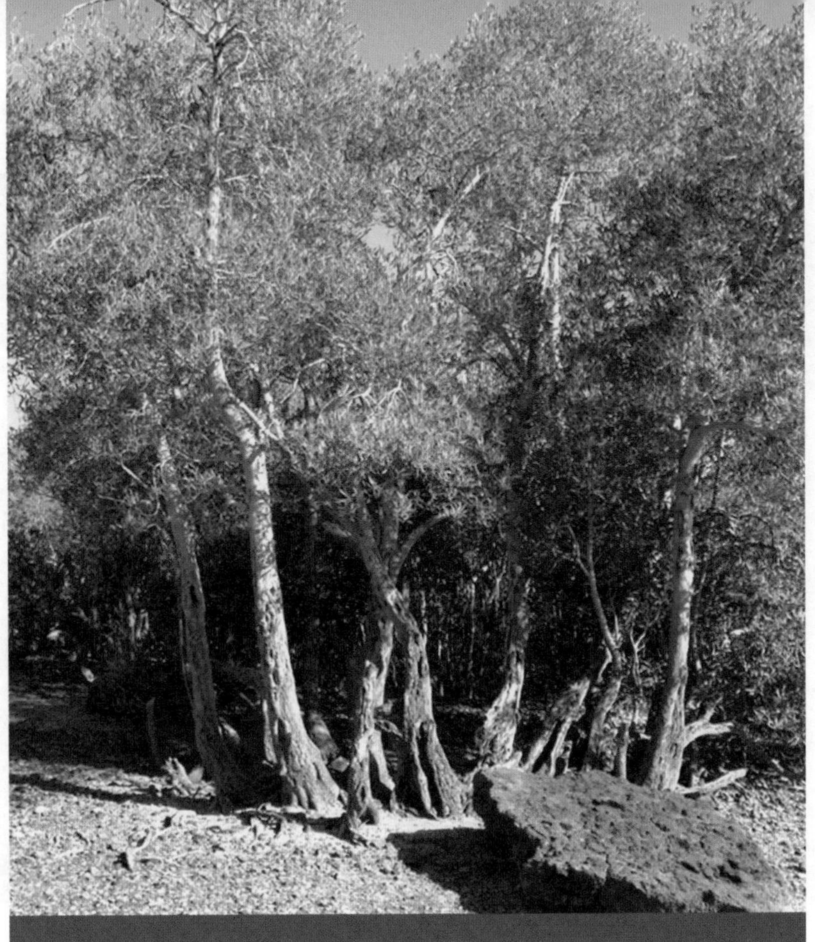

Medicinal Uses Decoctions or infusions of old Kapok Mangrove wood were used as an antiseptic wash applied to the skin to treat sores, boils, cuts, wounds, scabies infestations and leprosy (Devanesen, 2000; Foulkes, n.d.; Mitchie, 1993). The wood was burnt and the ashes were rubbed onto the skin to treat blotchy skin, fungal infections, scabies infestations and leprosy (Smith, 1991).

Other Uses The Kwini use the leaves of Kapok Mangrove to improve the flavour of dugong and saltwater turtles and to help keep the meat moist (Cheinmora et al., 2017). The Bardi, Djawi, Worora and other people of the Kimberley used the wood from the Kapok Mangrove to build rafts to hunt turtle and dugong. Larger rafts were made of up to seven tree trunks (Foulkes, n.d.; Karadada et al., 2011; Kenneally et al., 1996).

Karnboor

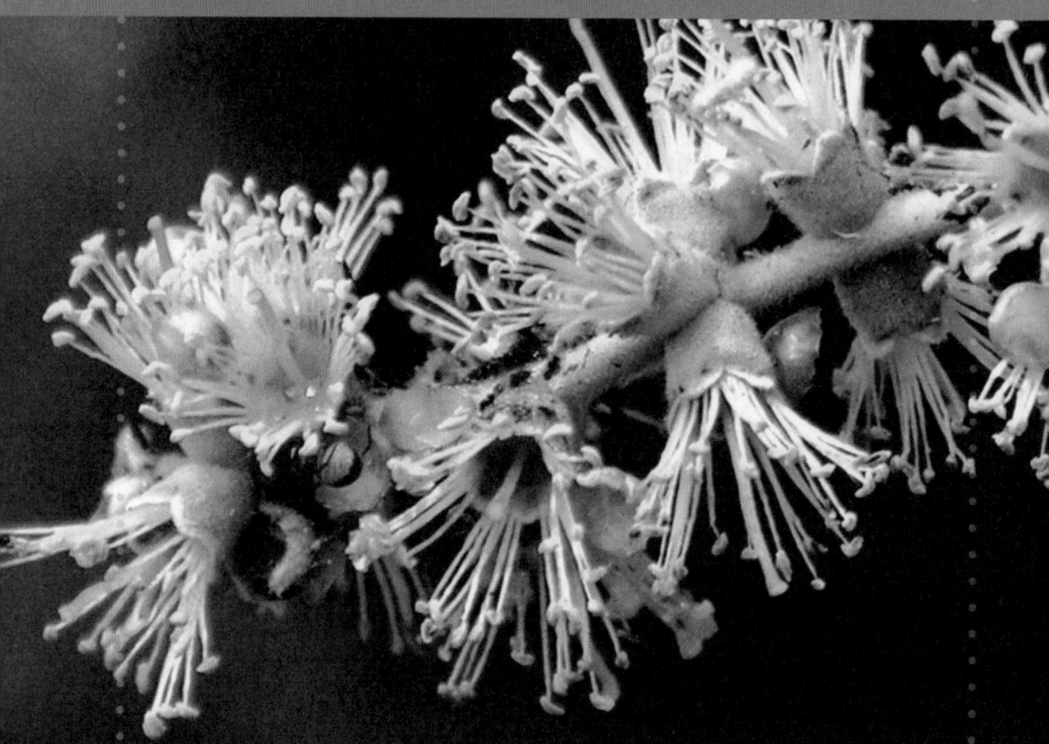

Scientific Name *Melaleuca dealbata* S.T.Blake.

Common Names Karnboor, Blue Paperbark, Soapy Tea Tree, Cloudy Tea Tree, Honey Tree, White Leaf Melaleuca.

Aboriginal Names Karnboor (Nyul Nyul) (Dobbs et al., 2015; Paddy et al., 1993), Garnburu (Bardi) (Smith & Kalotas, 1985), Karnpurr (Karajarri) (Willing, 2014)

Field Notes Karnboor is a paperbark tree that grows up to 15 m in height. It has pale, papery bark and narrowly elliptic leaf blades up to 120 mm long, with three to five longitudinal veins. Its cream, bottlebrush-type inflorescences are up to 20 mm wide and usually occur in threes. Flowering is from August to November. Its seed capsules are sessile, up to 3 mm in diameter and densely clothed in short, silver hairs when young. Karnboor occurs in sand or sandy soils, on coastal dunes, seasonally wet depressions and along small watercourses in the Kimberley region of Western Australia, the

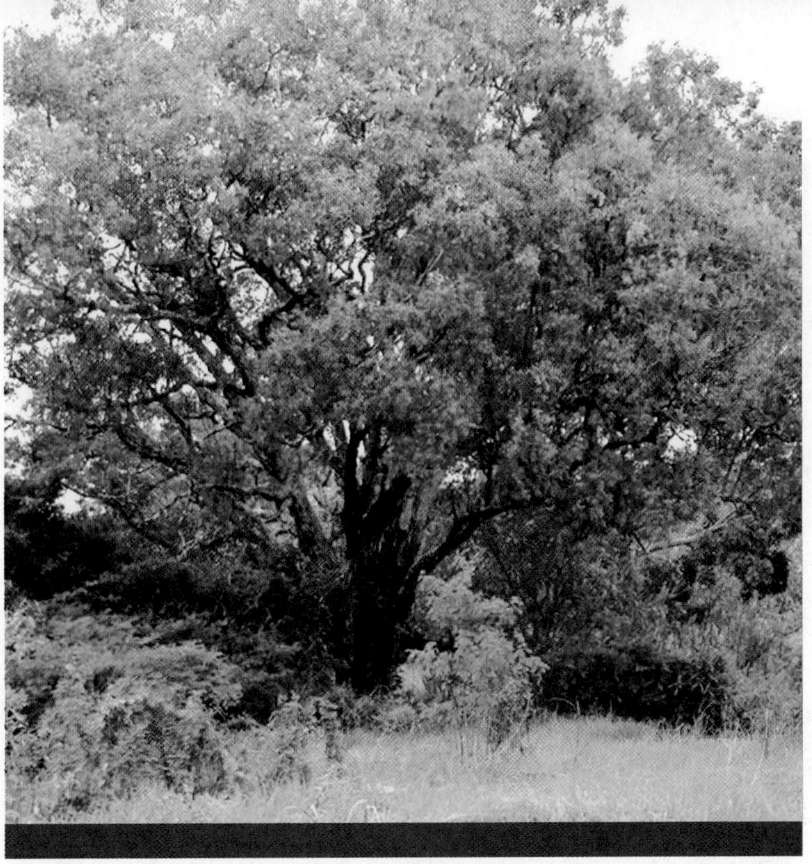

Northern Territory and Queensland. It also occurs in New Guinea and Indonesia (ALA, 2022; ATRP, 2020; WAH, 2022).

Medicinal Uses Infusions of crushed leaves of Karnboor were used as an antiseptic wash to bathe skin sores and wounds, and the head to relieve 'cold sick', the symptoms of colds and influenza (Edwards, 2005; Willing, 2014). Crushed leaves were held under the nose and the vapours inhaled to relieve the symptoms of colds and influenza (Edwards, 2005; Williams, 2011). Alternatively, the leaves were boiled and the steam inhaled for the same purpose (Williams, 2011).

Other Uses Nectar was either sucked directly from the flowers of Karnboor, or the flowers were soaked in water to make a sweet drink. Sugarbag honey is often found in this tree (Willing, 2014). Sheets of Karnboor bark were used as 'bush plates' for food or for creating roofs for small huts (Kenneally et al., 1996; Willing, 2014).

Kimberley Heather

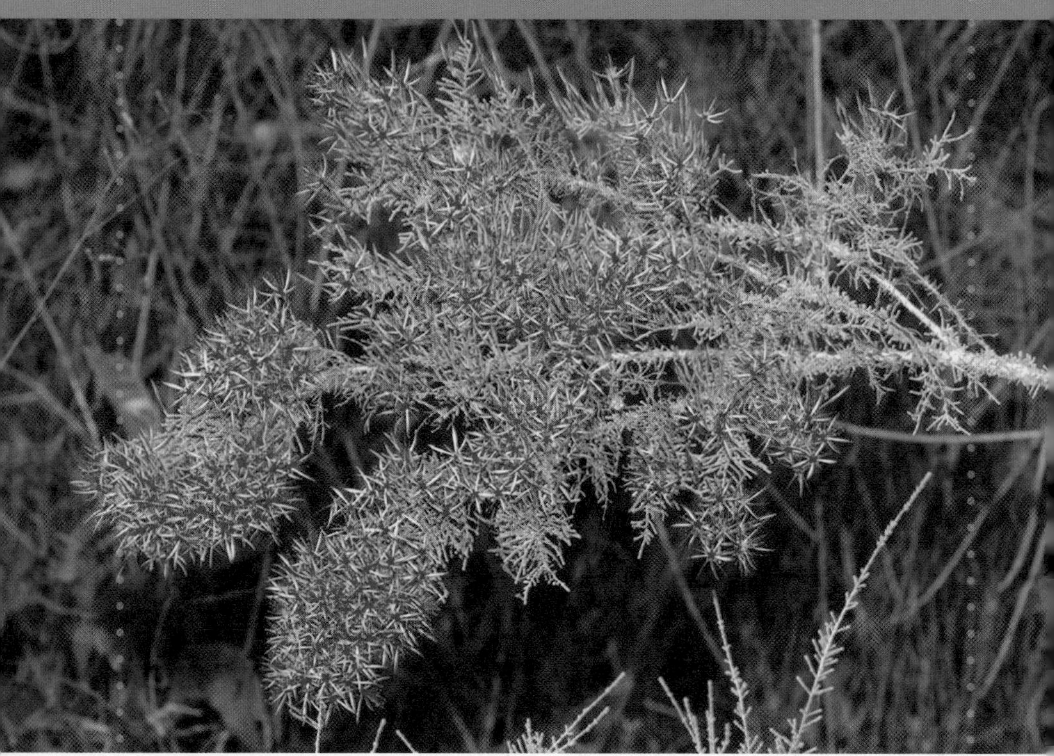

Scientific Name *Calytrix exstipulata* DC.

Common Names Kimberley Heather, Pink Turkey Bush, Turkey Bush. (The common name Turkey Bush is because the Plains Turkey (*Ardeotis australis*) hides amongst its foliage when being chased by hunters.)

Aboriginal Names Mangadang (Miriwoong) (Leonard et al., 2013), Liyarndu, Mada, Marda, Girra (Wunambal, Gaambera) (Karadada et al., 2011), Gidigid (Bardi) (Kenneally et al., 2018), Lindij (Nyikina) (Young et al., 2012), Ngarrwarnji (Nyikina) (Smith & Smith, 2009), Wiyurr (Walmajarri) (Richards & Hudson, 2012), Mangadany (Gija) (Purdie et al., 2018), Kurntili-kurntili, Wurntili-wurntili (Kukatja) (Valiquette, 1993), Wunggun (Jaru) (Wightman, 2003), Marda, Nangurra, Mangkada ninya, Liija (Kwini) (Cheinmora et al., 2017).

Field Notes Kimberley Heather grows as a shrub or tree to 4.5 m in height depending on conditions. It has densely packed pine-like

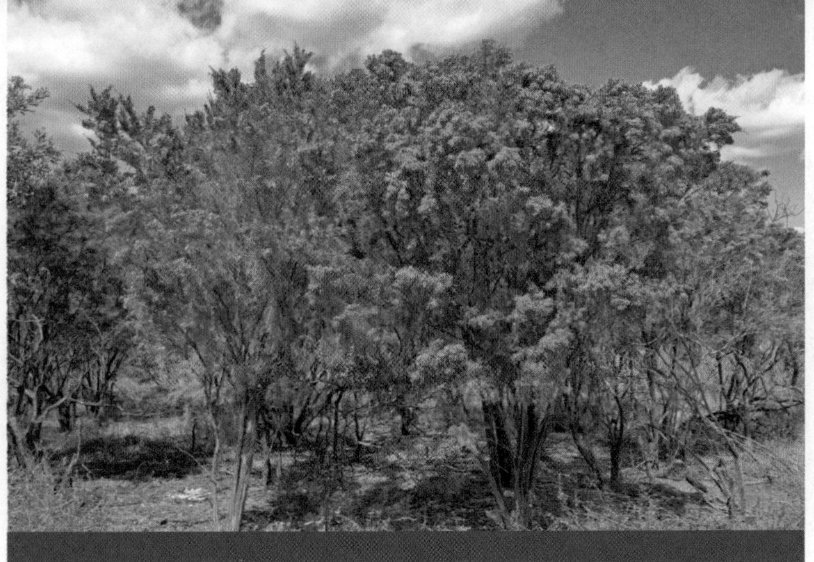

leaves and fine-haired pink and white, star-shaped flowers that have five long petals and long stamens. Fine hairs extend from the calyx lobes beyond the petals. The flowers cover the shrub from May to August. Its fruit are very small nuts that are fully enclosed in the old flower tubes. Kimberley Heather occurs in sand and clayey soils, on sandstone or limestone plateaus or outcrops and along watercourses in the Kimberley region of Western Australia, the Northern Territory and North Queensland (ALA, 2022; ANPSA, 2022; SKIPA, 2022; WAH, 2022).

Medicinal Uses The leaves of Kimberley Heather were crushed and applied as a liniment poultice for rheumatic pain, and as an antiseptic wash to treat wounds to aid healing. Decoctions or infusions of the leaves and flowers were used externally as a liniment for sore muscles and arthritic pain. Decoctions of the bark and flowers were drunk to treat fever (Low, 1990; SKIPA, 2022; Valiquette, 1993). The leaves are reported to contain an antiseptic substance called alpha-pinene (Low, 1990).

Other Uses The flowers and leaves of Kimberley Heather can be crushed and rubbed on the skin to repel insects (Kakadu National Park, 2016). The hard wood was used to make spear points and digging sticks (Karadada et al., 2011).

Kunai Grass

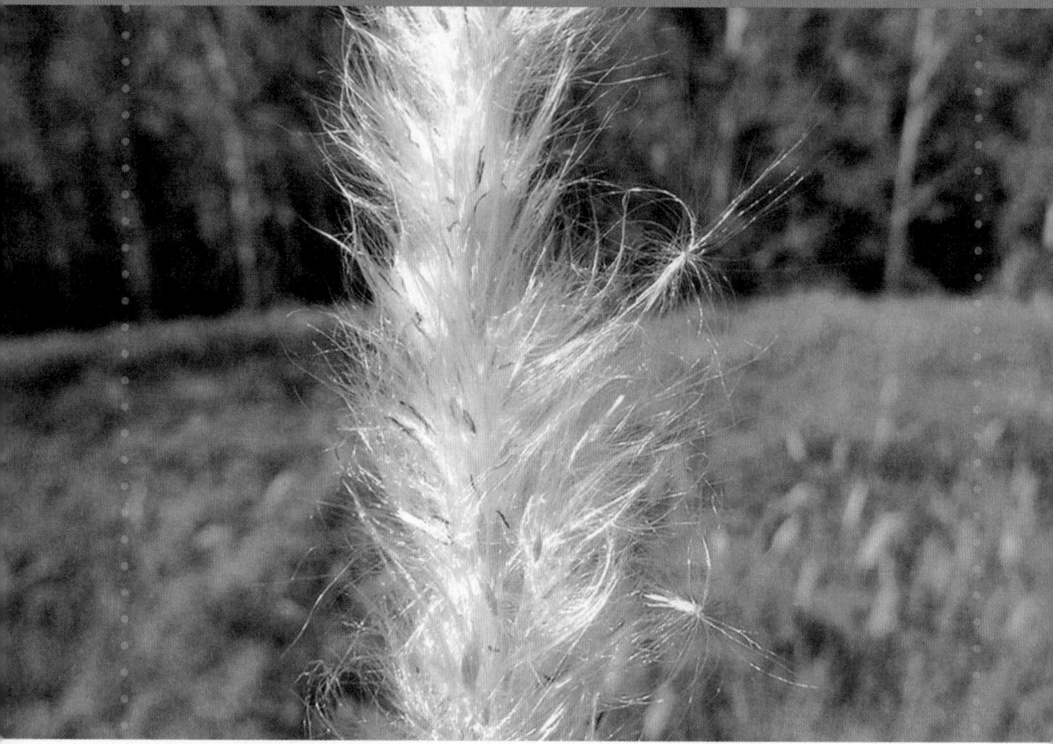

Scientific Name *Imperata cylindrica* (L.) P.Beauv.

Common Names Kunai Grass, Blady Grass, Cogon Grass, Cotton Wool Grass, Silver Spike, Sword Grass.

Field Notes Kunai Grass is a rhizomatous, densely tufted, perennial grass-like plant that grows up to 3 m in height. It is spread by its creeping rhizomes. Its leaves are khaki green during the year with red tones over winter, and are about 20 mm wide near the base, narrowing to a sharp point at the top. Its small flowers are white, appearing between May and September. These are followed by white fluffy seed heads. Kunai Grass occurs in the Kimberley region of Western Australia, the Northern Territory, the Torres Strait Islands, the Cape York Peninsula and down the east coast and around into the south-east corner of South Australia (ALA, 2022; WAH, 2022). It is also found in other warm temperate to tropical areas of the world (Fern, 2021).

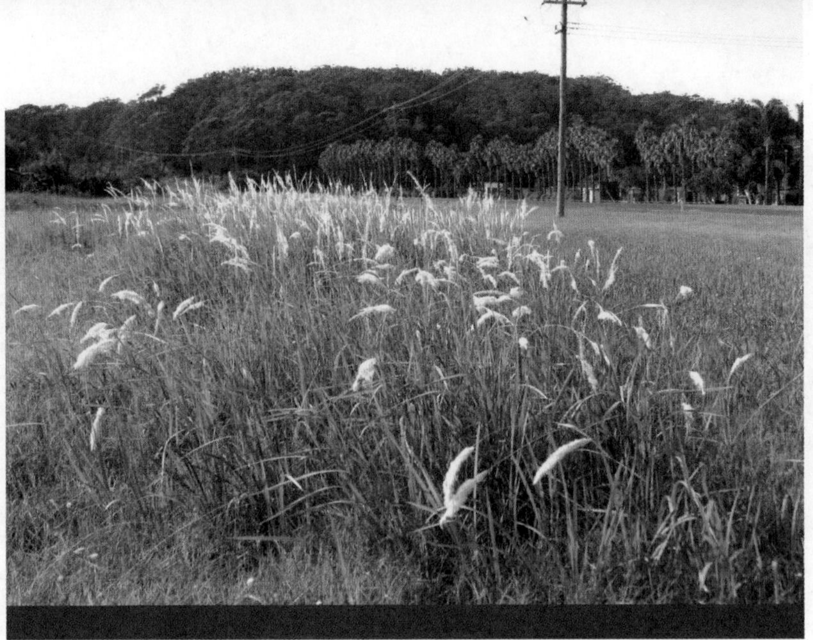

Medicinal Uses The flowers and the roots are used in folk medicine in some countries and are reported to have antibacterial, diuretic, febrifuge, sialagogue, styptic and tonic properties. The flowers were applied as a poultice used in the treatment of wounds to stem bleeding. Decoctions of the flowers were taken internally to treat urinary tract infections and fevers. In Nepal, decoctions of the root were used to treat intestinal parasites and digestive disorders such as indigestion, diarrhoea and dysentery. Research has shown that the plant has viricidal and anti-cancer properties (Fern, 2021).

Other Uses The young flowers and young shoots of Kunai Grass are edible and are usually cooked before eating (BushcraftOz, 2022; Fern, 2021). The fibrous roots and stems are reported to be pleasant to chew raw or after roasting them in hot ashes. They contain starch and sugar (Cicada Woman Tours, 2013; Fern, 2021; Glasby, 2018). Fern (2021) advises that 'the taste is sweetest in the wet season in Australia and the worst from plants growing in sand'.

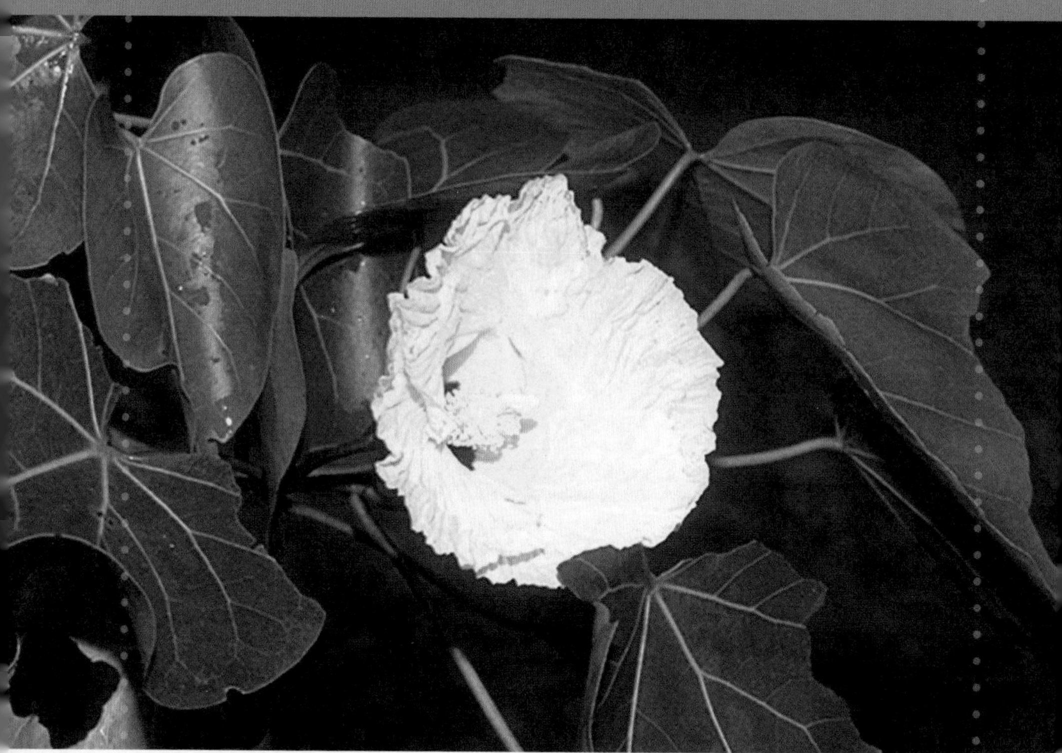

Scientific Name *Thespesia populneoides* (Roxb.) Kostel.

Common Names Laba, Tulip Tree, Indian Tulip Tree, Beach Yellow Hibiscus, Portia Tree, Pacific Rosewood.

Aboriginal Names Laba (Wunambal, Gaambera) (Karadada et al., 2011), Luruda (Bardi) (Smith & Kalotas, 1985), Loorrood (Bardi) (Kenneally et al., 1996), Laba manya, Laaba manya (Kwini) (Cheinmora et al., 2017).

Field Notes Laba grows as a shrub or tree to 12 m in height. It has large, green, heart-shaped leaves and large, drooping, yellow, hibiscus-type flowers that are up to 120 mm long. In Australia, flowering is between February and August. Its fruit are depressed globular to broadly ovoid and up to 45 mm in diameter. Laba occurs in coastal regions, often on the landward side of mangroves or tidal creeks around the top end of Australia from the Kimberley region of Western Australia to the southern coast of Queensland.

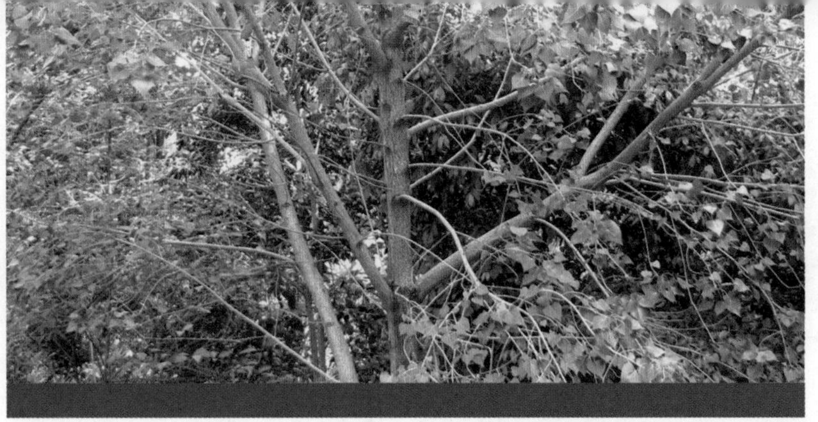

It is also found in the coastal regions of the other countries of the Indian Ocean from Africa to India and Sri Lanka (ALA, 2022; ATRP, 2020; Fern, 2021; WAH, 2022).

Medicinal Uses Laba is valued in traditional medicine around the Indian Ocean region. Decoctions of the wood have been found useful in treating pleurisy, cholera, colic and high fever. The juice of the fruit was used externally to treat herpes outbreaks. Infusions of the crushed fruit were used internally to treat urinary tract infections and abdominal swellings. The cooked fruit, when crushed and mixed with coconut oil and applied to the hair, kills lice. An extract of the fruit was applied to swollen testicles to reduce the swelling and pain. Decoctions of the leaves were taken internally to treat rheumatic pain, urinary retention, coughs, influenza and headaches. Decoctions of most parts of the plant were used externally to treat various skin diseases. The juice from the pounded fruit was mixed with pounded leaves and used externally as a poultice to treat headaches and itchy skin. Decoctions of the bark and fruit, when mixed with oil, provided a good treatment for scabies infestations. Decoctions of the astringent bark were taken internally to treat dysentery, haemorrhoids and intestinal parasites. Decoctions of the leaves and bark were taken internally to treat hypertension (Fern, 2021; PFAF, 2022).

Other Uses The fruit of Laba are edible and were eaten raw or preserved for later use (Fern, 2021). The flowers, flower buds and young leaves are also edible (Hiddins, 2001; Plants for a Future, 2020). The wood of Laba was used by some Aboriginal groups to make fire sticks and spears (Hiddins, 2001; Karadada et al., 2011).

Lather Leaf

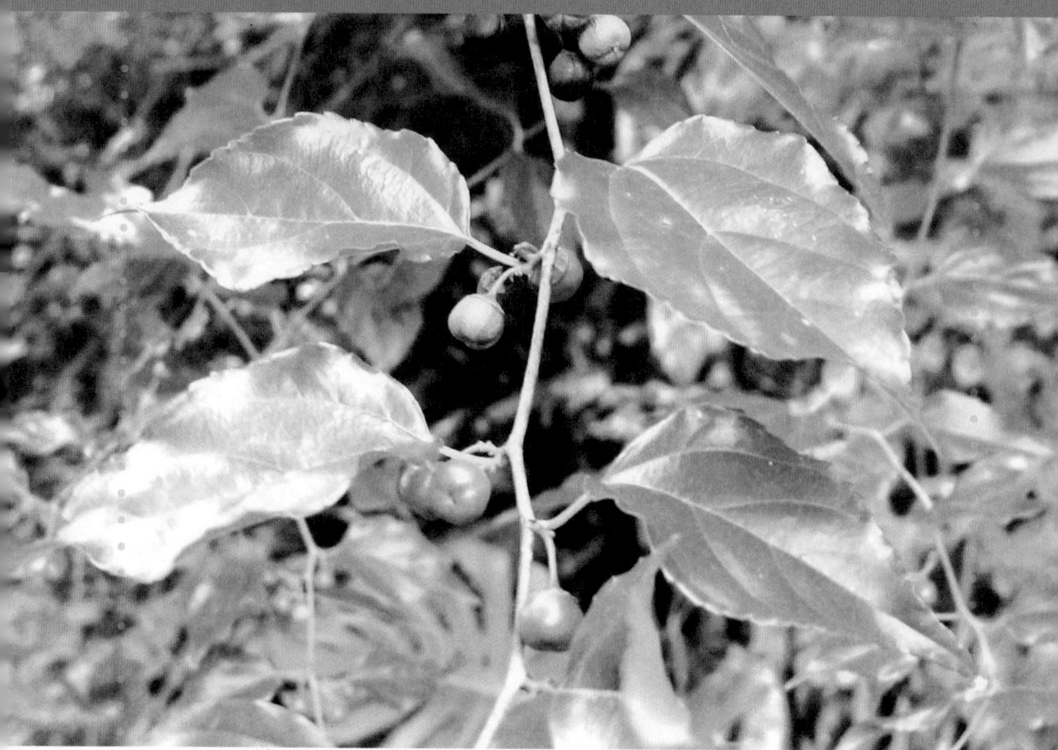

Scientific Name *Colubrina asiatica* (L.) Brongn.

Common Names Lather Leaf, Asian Nakedwood, Asiatic Colubrina, Asian Snakewood.

Field Notes Lather Leaf is a vine-like shrub that sends out multiple stems that can reach 9 m in length. Its leaves are simple, alternate, glossy, ovate, up to 130 mm long, have several prominent veins and are pointed at the apex. Its small greenish flowers appear in clusters in leaf axils all year round. Its fruit are berry-like capsules with small grey seeds. Its seeds float and are tolerant of salt water, which allows the species to spread across oceans. Lather Leaf occurs along the coast in the Kimberley region of Western Australia, the Northern Territory and Queensland. It is also native to other tropical and sub-tropical regions of the Old World, including eastern Africa, India, South-east Asia and the Pacific islands, including Hawaii (ALA, 2022; Fern, 2021).

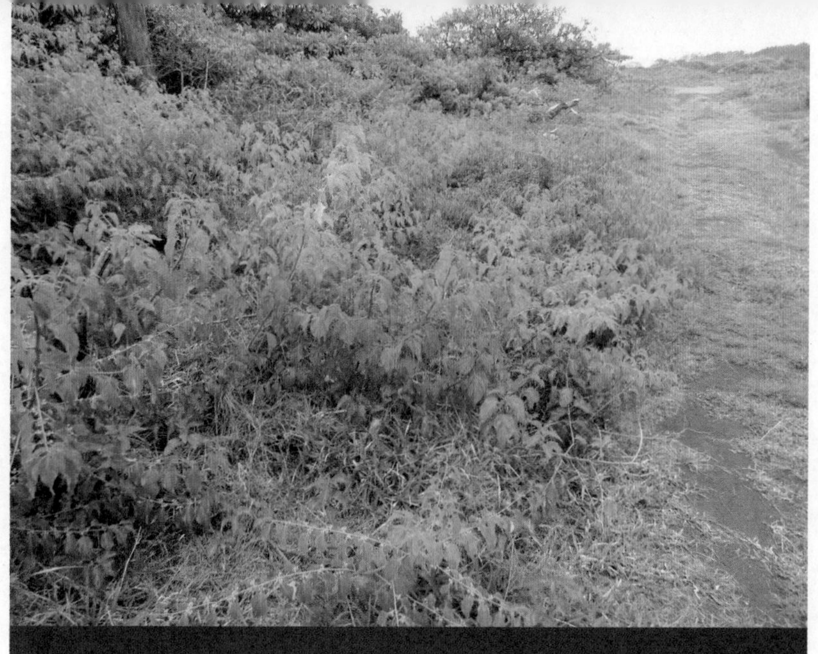

Medicinal Uses Lather Leaf is used in folk medicine throughout the tropics. Decoctions of the leaves are used externally to alleviate skin irritation and to treat a variety of skin diseases. Decoctions of the fruit are applied externally as a wash to hasten the healing of sores and wounds (Fern, 2021).

Other Uses The leaves of Lather Leaf are reported to be edible (Jones, 1996). The fruit have been used as 'fish poison' in some countries. The bark, roots and leaves can be used as a soap substitute (Jones, 1996).

Lawyer Vine

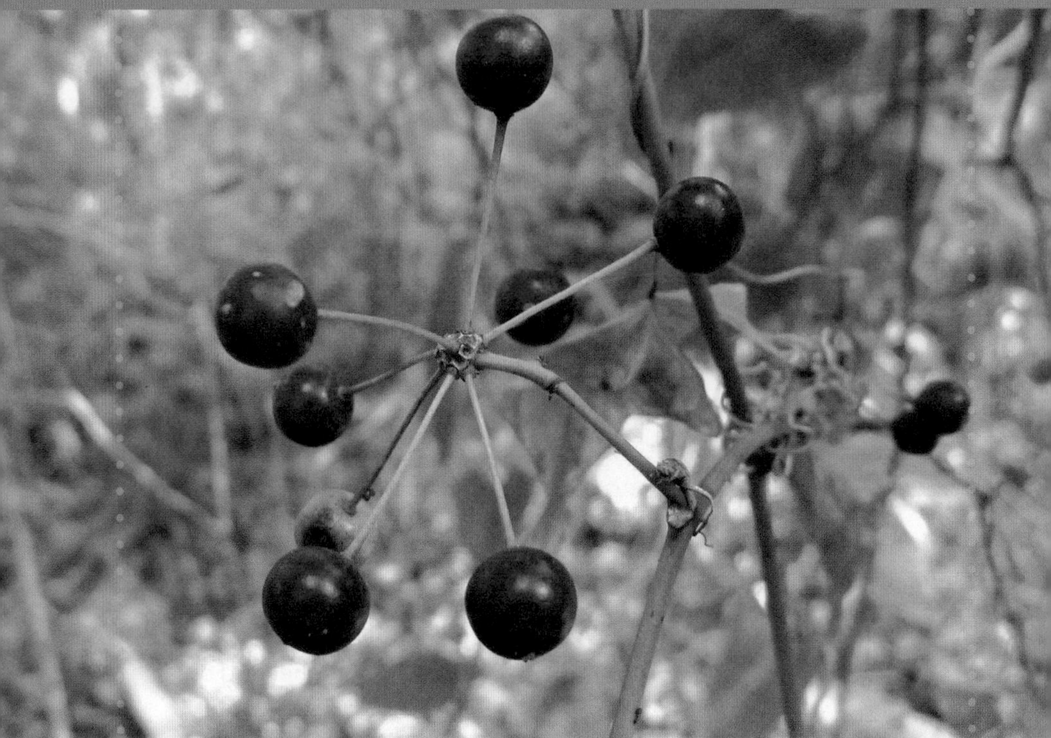

Scientific Name *Smilax australis* R.Br.

Common Names Lawyer Vine, Austral Sarsaparilla, Native Sarsaparilla, Wide Leaf Sarsaparilla, Barbed Wire Vine, Barbwire Vine, Wait-a-while.

Field Notes Lawyer Vine is a twining, perennial herb or climber. Its prickly stems with curled tendrils climb up to 8 m high. Its dark green, ovate to broadly elliptic leaves are pointed at the apex and are up to 150 mm long and 90 mm wide. Its small, green-white flowers form on many flowered umbels from February to May. Its fruit are ovoid berries that are up to 10 mm in diameter and are black when ripe. Lawyer Vine occurs in white sand and sandstone in the far north of the Kimberley region of Western Australia, the top end of the Northern Territory, through Far North Queensland and down the east coast into Victoria (ALA, 2022; ATRP, 2020; WAH, 2022).

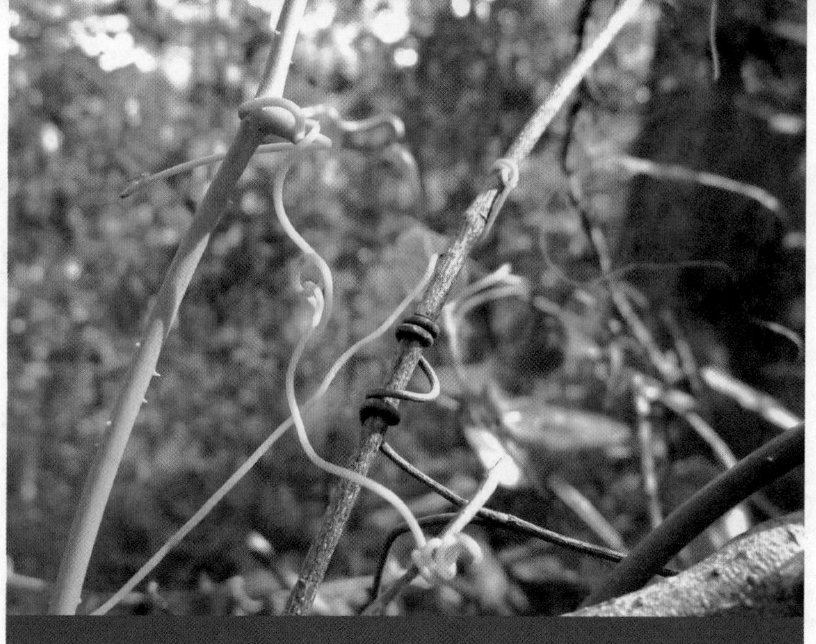

Medicinal Uses Infusions of crushed leaves are taken internally as a blood cleanser. Young leaves can also be sucked or chewed for the same purpose (Macquarie University, 2020). The rhizomes are said to be a remarkably effective treatment for diabetes (Edwards, 2005). Decoctions of the leaves have been used for chest complaints such as bronchitis, and the symptoms of colds and influenza. Juice from the leaves has been used as eyedrops to treat conjunctivitis. In Far North Queensland, poultices made from ground-up roots have been used to treat snakebite, with the bitten part cut open and the poultice applied to the wound (efficacy not recorded) (Williams, 2010; Williams, 2020).

Other Uses The fruit of Lawyer Vine are edible and are eaten raw when black and ripe (Fox & Garde, 2018; MRCCC, n.d.; RFCA, 1993; Williams, 2010). The fruit are reported to have a 'hot, peppery flavour' (Williams, 2010). The young leaves can be eaten raw (Macquarie University, 2020). The stem of Lawyer Vine was used to make tough fibre rope and fish traps (Williams, 2010).

Leafy Nineawn

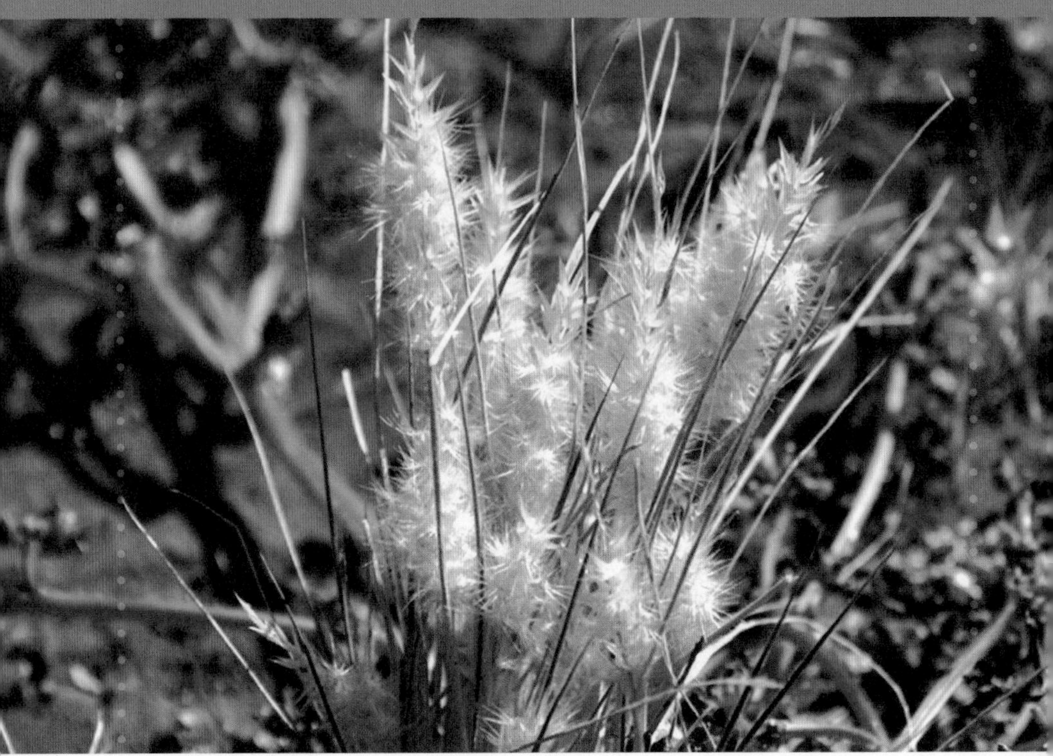

Scientific Name *Enneapogon polyphyllus* (Domin) N.T.Burb.

Common Names Leafy Nineawn, Woolly Oat Grass, Limestone Grass.

Aboriginal Names Ngirriliis (Jaru) (Wightman, 2003), Yawila, Yikatiri (Kukatja) (Valiquette, 1993).

Field Notes Leafy Nineawn is an annual or perennial, tufted grass growing up to 400 mm in height. Several stems grow from the base and each plant spreads to 150 mm wide. The leaves are 150 mm long, bright green and covered in soft, fine hairs. Its flower heads are straw-coloured and fluffy. Its seed heads are compact and narrow, and up to 90 mm in length. Leafy Nineawn is endemic to most of Western Australia (except the south-west), the Northern Territory, Queensland, South Australia and New South Wales (ALA, 2022; AusGrass2, 2022).

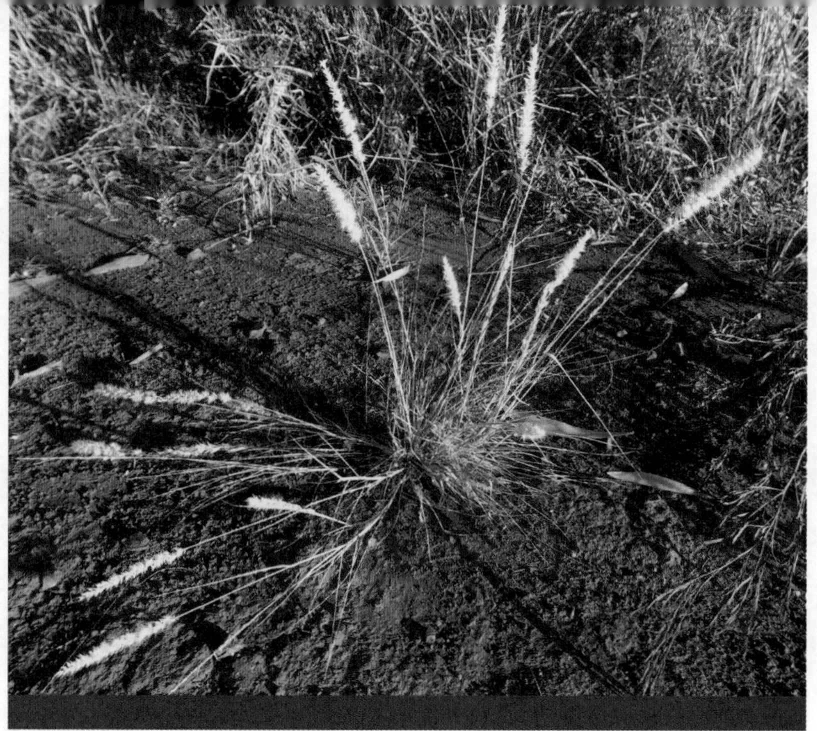

Medicinal Uses The dry stems and leaves of Leafy Nineawn are burnt and the black soot-like ash rubbed onto the sore gums of babies who are teething. This is reported to stop the pain and help the gums heal, thus ensuring the parents a good night's sleep (Wightman, 2003).

Other Uses The seeds of Leafy Nineawn are edible and were eaten raw (Valiquette, 1993).

Leichardt Tree

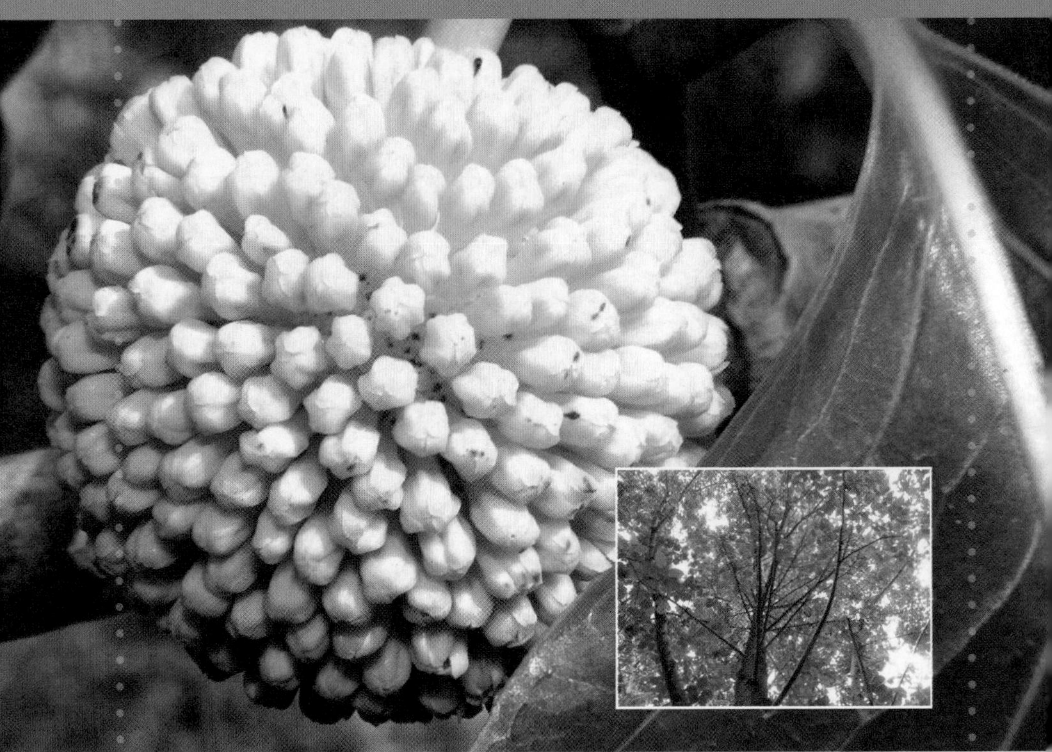

Scientific Name *Nauclea orientalis* (L.) L.

Common Names Leichardt Tree, Leichardt Pine, Bur Tree, Yellow Cheesewood, Canary Cheesewood.

Aboriginal Names Jambeng (Miriwoong) (Leonard et al., 2013), Murrura (Bunuba) (Oscar et al., 2019), Marr, Barrawar (Wunambal, Gaambera) (Karadada et al., 2011), Marrkurta (Walmajarri) (Richards & Hudson, 2012), Ngimilil, Ngimirlil, Marroorool, Marrooral (Gija) (Purdie et al., 2018), Marroora (Gooniyandi) (Dilkes-Hall et al., 2019), Ngimili (Jaru) (Wightman, 2003), Maar minya, Kûlau-ngei minya (Kwini) (Cheinmora et al., 2017; Crawford, 1982), Marrgurda (Yawuru) (Moss et al., 2021).

Field Notes Leichardt Trees grow to 21 m in height. They have large, glossy, ovate leaves and spherical clusters of fragrant flowers that develop into golf ball-sized, knobbly, edible but bitter fruit. Their flowers are present between May and November. In Australia,

Leichardt Trees occur in peaty soils, along creeks and rivers across the northernmost parts of Western Australia, the Northern Territory and Queensland, where it is found in coastal regions as far south as Brisbane. It is also found in Cambodia, Indonesia, Sri Lanka, Myanmar, the Philippines, Thailand and Vietnam (ALA, 2022; BushcraftOz, 2022; Fern, 2021; WAH, 2022).

Medicinal Uses Infusions of the bark of Leichardt Trees that were left to ferment were taken internally as a bitter tonic. Infusions of the bark were used as an emetic to induce vomiting and to treat certain snakebites. Decoctions of the bark were used externally as a liniment for rheumatic pain and internally to treat diarrhoea and toothache (Cribb & Cribb, 1981; Lassak & McCarthy, 2001). Crushed leaves of Leichardt Trees were applied externally as a poultice to draw out boils and carbuncles (BushcraftOz, 2022; Fern, 2021). Eating the fruit is supposed to be a good treatment for general malaise (Edwards, 2005).

Other Uses The fruit of Leichardt Trees, though a little bitter, were eaten by some Aboriginal groups when the fruit was brown and ripe. Unripe fruit were heated in hot ashes or hot sand to make them edible. The young leaves and tender shoots are also edible and were usually steamed before eating (Cheinmora et al., 2017; Fox & Garde, 2018; Karadada et al., 2011; Purdie et al., 2018; Wightman, 2003). The larger Leichardt Trees were used by some Aboriginal groups to make rafts and canoes. The bark was used to make 'fish poison' to make fish float to the surface so they were easier to catch by hand (Cheinmora et al., 2017; Karadada et al., 2011; Oscar et al., 2019). The Gija used the wood to make coolamons and clap sticks (Purdie et al., 2018). In the past the logs from this tree 'were used as floats when swimming across large rivers' (Wightman, 2003).

Lemon Grass

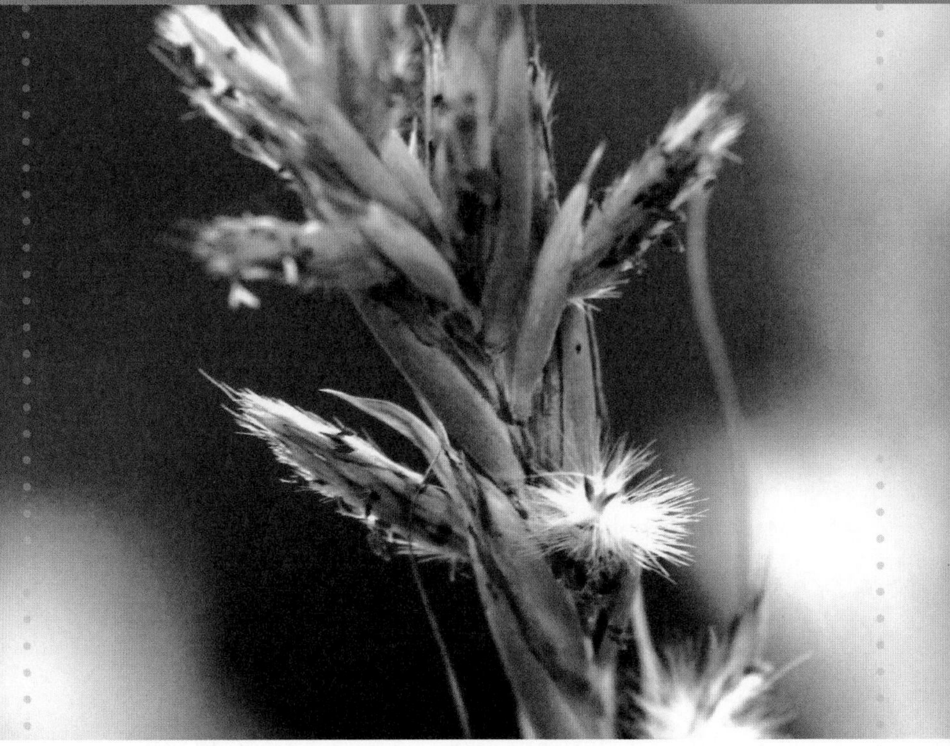

Scientific Name *Cymbopogon procerus* (R.Br.) Domin.

Common Names Lemon Grass, Scent Grass, Citronella Grass, Scented Grass.

Aboriginal Names Janjani (Bunuba) (Oscar et al., 2019), Lomelomel (Wunambal, Gaambera) (Karadada et al., 2011), Marrankangu (Jindjiparndi) (Clark, 1986), Ngarrngarrji, Malmalji (Gija) (Purdie et al., 2018), Giwiri, Guwuru (Jaru) (Wightman, 2003), Majal (Kwini) (Cheinmora et al., 2017).

Field Notes Lemon Grass is an aromatic, tufted perennial grass whose culms can reach 2.2 m high. Its flowers are green, compound racemes that are usually present from March to September. Lemon Grass occurs in red or brown loam, sand, sandstone or laterite in the Kimberley region of Western Australia and the Northern Territory (ALA, 2022; AusGrass2, 2022; WAH, 2022).

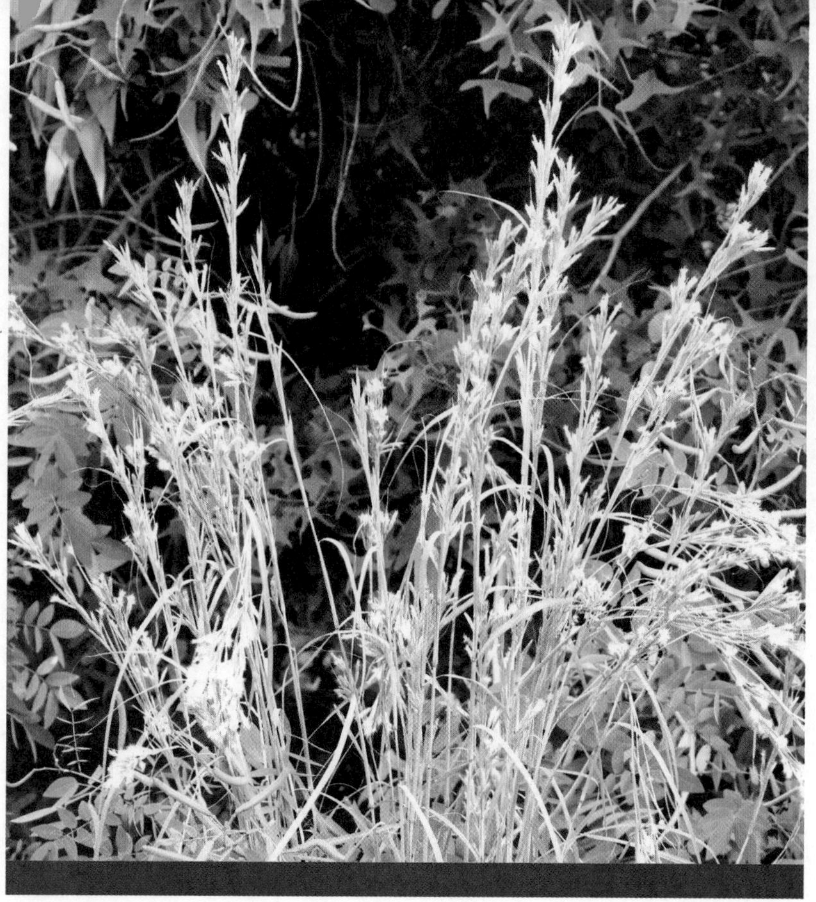

Medicinal Uses The leaves of Lemon Grass were chewed slowly to relieve the symptoms of colds and influenza. Decoctions of the leaves were taken internally or used as a wash to relieve the symptoms of colds and influenza (Lassak & McCarthy, 2008; Purdie et al., 2018; Reid, 1986; Smith, 1991; Webb, 1959; Wightman, 2003). Leaves, softened by boiling or soaking them, were inserted and left in the nasal cavity to provide relief from sinusitis. Decoctions of the whole plant left for two to three days were used as a wash to treat sores and cuts. Strong decoctions of the crushed leaves and stems were applied externally to the head to relieve headaches (Smith, 1991) and in the ears to treat earache due to infection of the auditory canal (Edwards, 2005). Weak decoctions of the plant were used externally as eyedrops to treat sore eyes due to conjunctivitis (Wightman, 2003).

Other Uses Lemon Grass can be used to give fish a citrus flavour when cooking it (Karadada et al., 2011).

Lemon-scented Grass

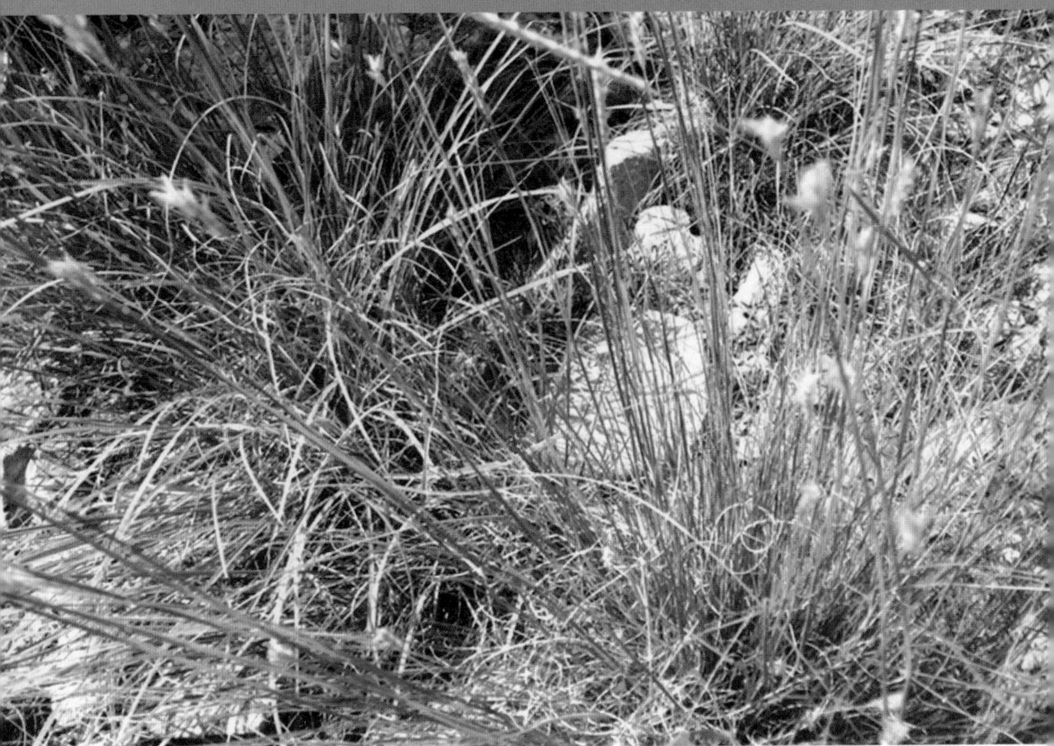

Scientific Name *Elionurus citreus* (R.Br.) Benth.

Common Name Lemon-scented Grass.

Field Notes Lemon-scented Grass is a tufted perennial, grass-like herb that grows up to 1 m in height. The leaves roll inwards, are 2–3 mm wide, and are often hairy on the upper surface of the blade. The leaves have a distinct lemon smell when crushed. The flower spikes are up to 120 mm long and the spikelets overlap in two rows. Its flowers occur as a panicle of racemes up to 120 mm long. In Western Australia, the plant flowers in June and towards summer elsewhere. Lemon-scented Grass occurs in white sand sporadically around Broome in the Kimberley region of Western Australia but is more common in the Northern Territory, Queensland and parts of New South Wales. It also occurs in New Guinea (ALA, 2022; AusGrass2, 2022; NSW Government Office of the Environment & Heritage, 2020; WAH, 2022).

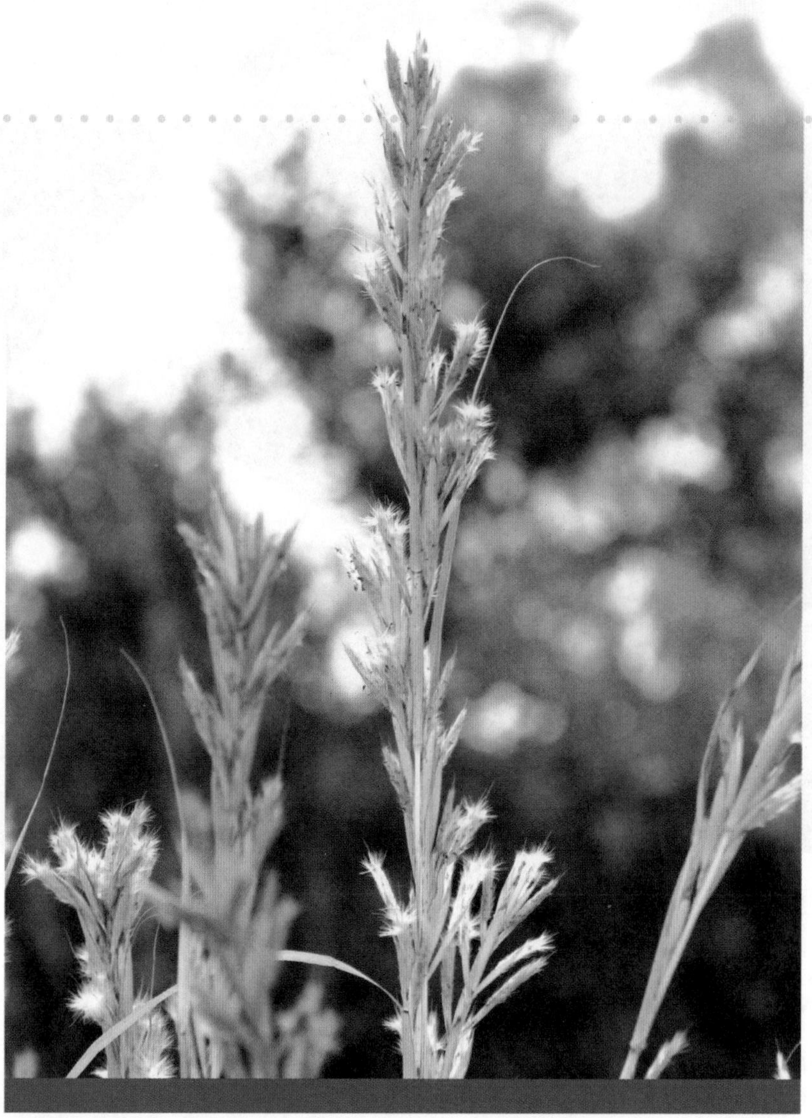

Medicinal Uses Decoctions of the whole Lemon-scented Grass plant were used externally as eardrops to treat earache due to infection of the auditory canal. The decoctions were also used to bathe the whole body as a treatment for general malaise. The whole plant is crushed and held under the nose and the vapours inhaled to ease the symptoms of colds and influenza. The roots were crushed and a portion stuffed into a tooth cavity to ease the pain of toothache (Edwards, 2005).

Lemonwood

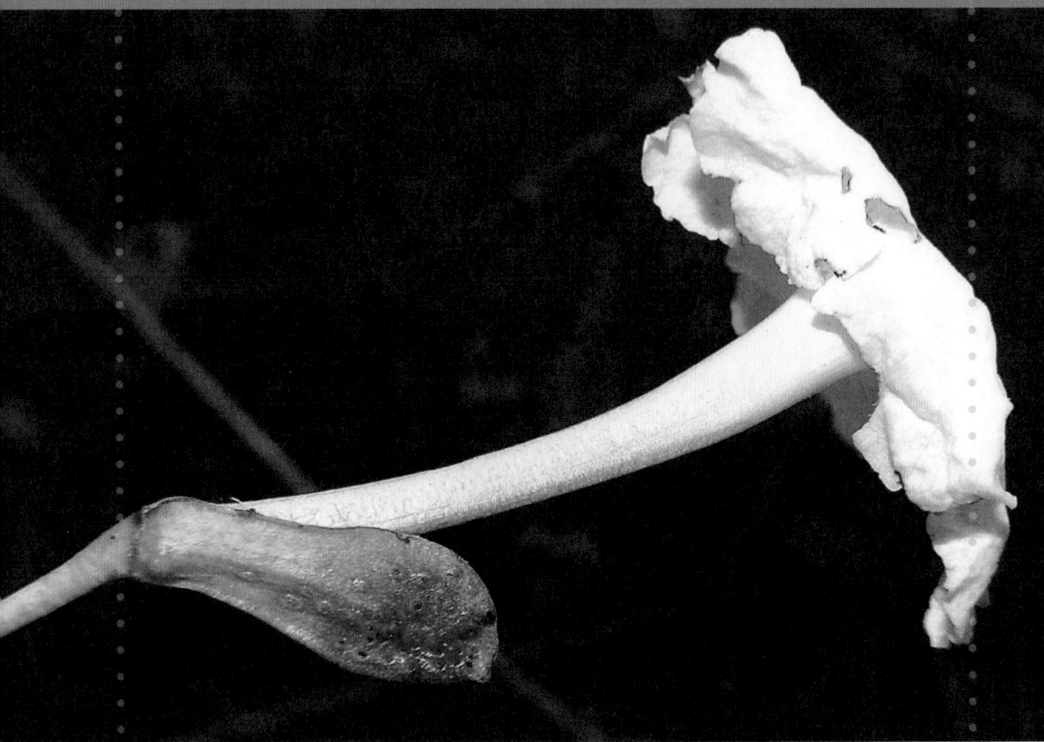

Scientific Name *Dolichandrone occidentalis* Jackes, previously known as *Dolichandrone heterophylla* (R.Br.) F.Muell.

Common Name Lemonwood.

Aboriginal Names Laweng (Miriwoong) (Leonard et al., 2013), Lawu (Bunuba) (Oscar et al., 2019), Jumburru (Yawuru) (Kenneally et al., 1996), Jumpurru (Karajarri) (Willing, 2014), Lawiny, Lawoony, Lawuny (Gija) (Purdie et al., 2018), Lowoo (Miwa) (Kimberley Specialists, 2020), Lawa (Walmajarri) (Richards & Hudson, 2012), Gara, Lawa (Jaru) (Wightman, 2003), Joomboorroo (Nyikina) (Smith & Smith, 2009).

Field Notes Lemonwood is a small tree that grows to around 4 m in height. It has ovate leaves with prominent white veins and large, white, trumpet-shaped flowers. Its seed pods are long and thin. Lemonwood is endemic to the Pilbara and Kimberley regions of

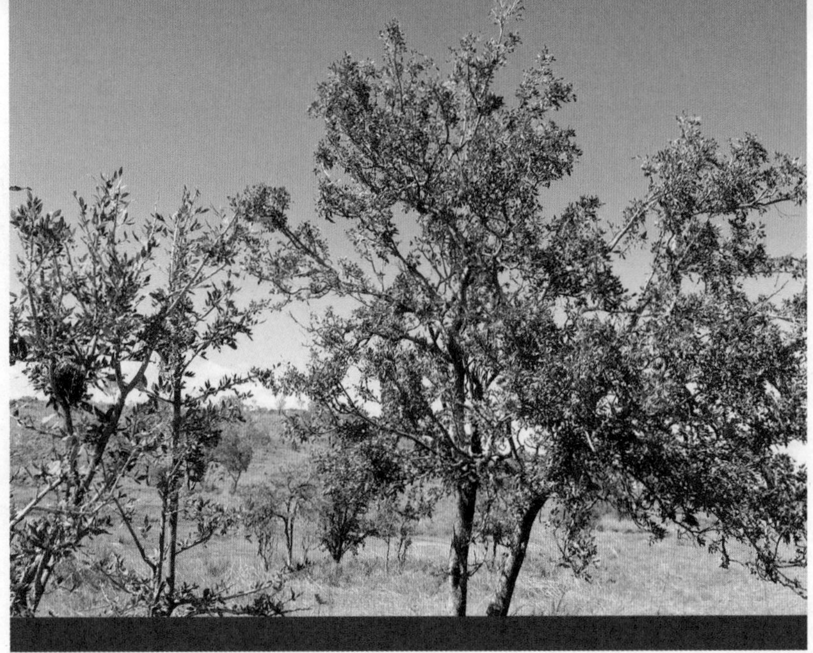

Western Australia and the western part of the Northern Territory (ALA, 2022; WAH, 2022).

Medicinal Uses Decoctions of the leaves and bark were used as a wash, or a small amount was taken internally to treat sunburn, measles, anaemia, coughs, sores, skin lesions, boils, scabies infestations, osteoarthritis and to ease the symptoms of colds and influenza (Kimberley Specialists, 2020; Purdie et al., 2018; Wightman, 2003; Wilson et al., n.d.).

Little Gooseberry Tree

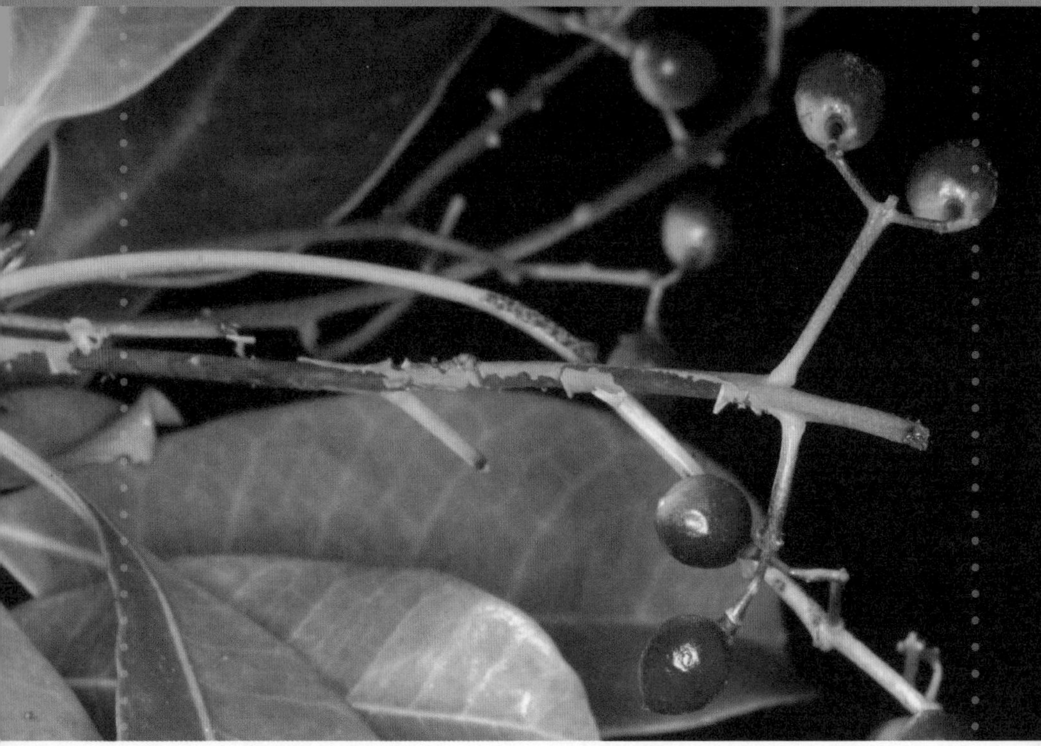

Scientific Name *Buchanania arborescens* (Blume) Blume.

Common Names Little Gooseberry Tree, Jam Jam, Buchanania, Green Plum, Lightwood, Sparrow's Mango, Satinwood.

Field Notes The Little Gooseberry Tree is a slender, evergreen, medium-sized tree that grows up to 12 m in height. Its smooth, leathery, elongated oblong leaves are up to 240 mm long and 70 mm wide. Its small, cream to yellow-white, star-shaped flowers are roughly 6 mm in diameter. Its fruit are about 10 mm in diameter and are black when ripe. The Little Gooseberry Tree occurs in seasonal tropical forests in the Kimberley region of Western Australia, the Northern Territory, the Cape York Peninsula and as far south in Queensland as the Paluma Range. It also occurs in parts of South-east Asia and on some Pacific islands (ALA, 2022; ATRP, 2020).

Medicinal Uses Infusions of the inner bark and sapwood or the roots were used as a mouthwash to treat toothache, but the liquid

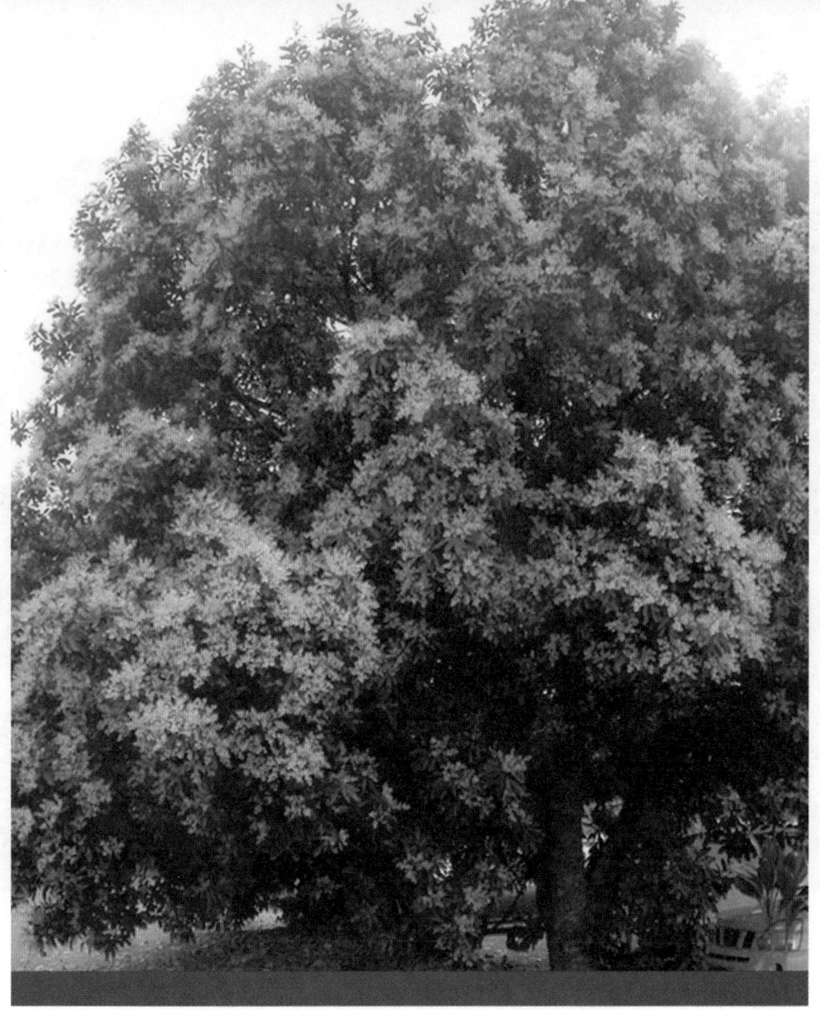

was not swallowed (Cribb & Cribb, 1981; Webb, 1959). Infusions of the inner bark were used as an antiseptic wash to bathe cuts and wounds, and as an eyewash to treat conjunctivitis (Hiddins, 2001; Northern Territory Department of Health, 1981).

Other Uses The fruit of the Little Gooseberry Tree are edible and are usually eaten raw (ALA, 2022; Cribb & Cribb, 1981; Fox & Garde, 2018; Hiddins, 2001; Maiden, 1889; Territory Native Plants, 2022). Unripe fruit can be boiled in water to make a tangy drink (Hiddins, 2001).

Lollybush

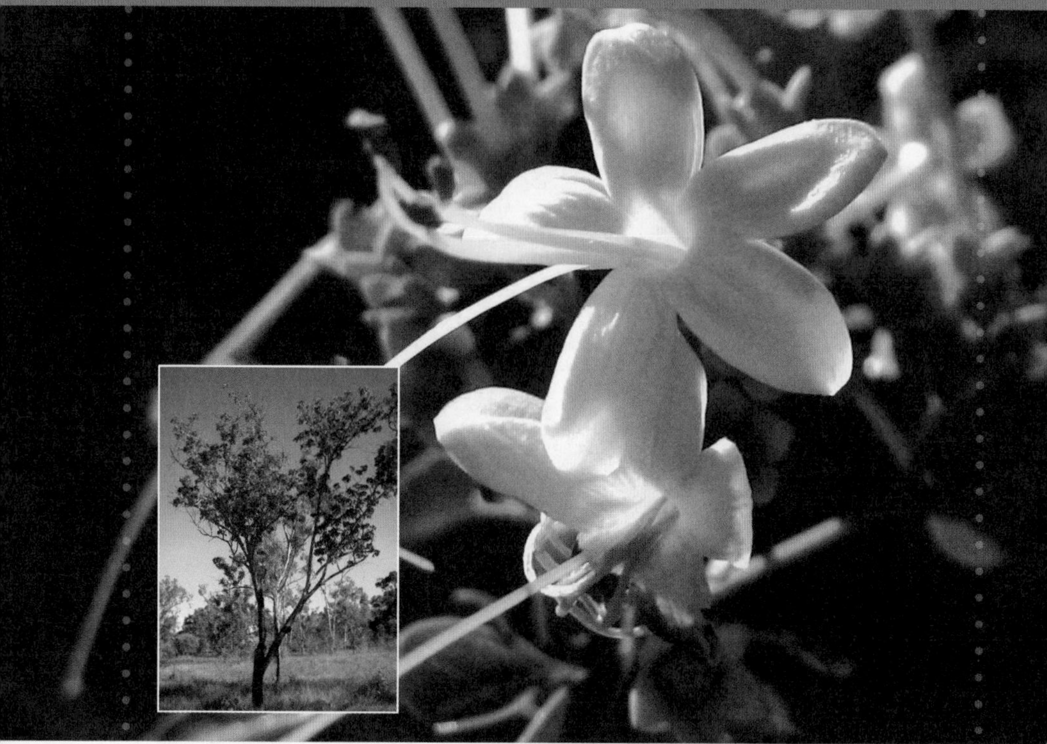

Scientific Name *Clerodendrum floribundum* R.Br.

Common Names Lollybush, Lottery Tree, Fire-stick Tree, Smooth Clerodendrum.

Aboriginal Names Goonggalany, Kungkalany, Birrindilinyji, Pirrintilinyji, Gerlarriny, Kerlarriny (Gija) (Purdie et al., 2018), Gunggala (Jaru) (Wightman, 2003), Kantunpa, Marnakara, Pirrintjiri Tatupitji, Witiluru, Wiituka, Yarrnginyi (Kukatja) (Valiquette, 1993), Wirtipi, (Kukatja, Ngardi) (Cataldi, 2004), Kungkala (Walmajarri) (Richards & Hudson, 2012), Ngula (Kwini) (Cheinmora et al., 2017; Crawford, 1982).

Field Notes Lollybush grows as a shrub or tree to 8 m high depending on conditions. It has light grey, rough, deeply furrowed bark and large, ovate leaves that are rounded at the base and are up to 170 mm long by 130 mm wide. Its white-cream flowers are 80 mm in diameter, tubular with the tube about 30 mm long, branching into five petals with long stamens in the centre. Flowering occurs any time from January to November. The fruit are black and shiny, about 10 mm across, and are surrounded by a red calyx. Despite looking like a lolly, the fruit are not edible. Lollybush is found in stony skeletal soils, sandy and loamy soils over sandstone and basalt, on rocky sites, in gorges, on cliffs, floodplains and creek beds over most of the top half of Australia and down the east coast as far south as Taree in New South Wales (ALA, 2022; Native Plants Queensland, 2022; Noosa's Native Plants, 2022; WAH, 2022).

Medicinal Uses Decoctions of the wood were taken internally for aches and pains, gastrointestinal disorders and the relief of the symptoms of colds and influenza. Decoctions of the wood and leaves were also applied externally for sores, cuts, skin rashes and itchy skin. A small amount of the decoctions were sipped to treat diarrhoea. The leaves were mixed with ash and chewed for their stimulant effect (Devanesen, 2000; Lassak & McCarthy, 2001; Noosa's Native Plants, 2022; Smith, 1991; Webb, 1959). The leaves were boiled and the vapours inhaled to relieve sinusitis. Decoctions of the leaves were also sipped to relieve the symptoms of colds and influenza, especially the associated aches and pain in the joints and muscles, and as an expectorant to make breathing easier (Morse, 2005; Smith, 1991).

Other Uses The roots are edible and were usually boiled before eating (Glasby, 2018; Isaacs, 1987; Native Tastes of Australia, 2019; Smith, 1991). This was an important plant for some Aboriginal groups who knew that they could find water wherever this tree grew. The fruit are inedible and poisonous (Noosa's Native Plants, 2021). The Gija used the wood from this tree to make fire sticks (Purdie et al., 2018). The Kwini mixed the leaves with ash and used the mixture as chewing tobacco when there was no regular chewing tobacco available (Cheinmora et al., 2017; Crawford, 1982).

Lotus

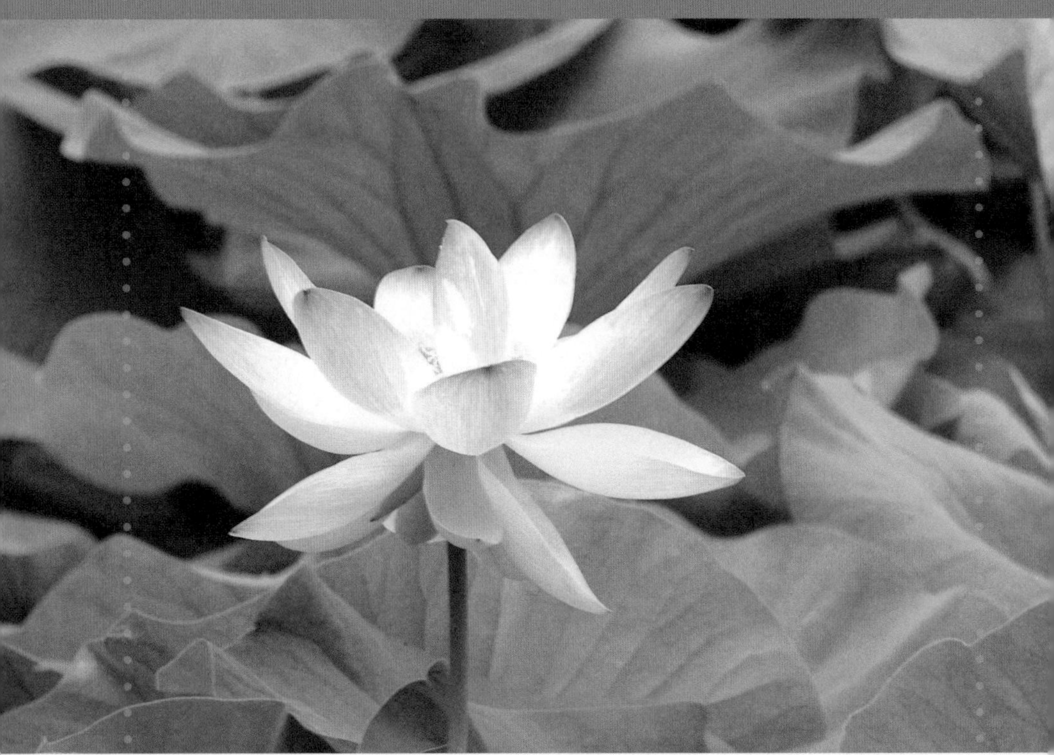

Scientific Name *Nelumbo nucifera* Gaertn.

Common Names Lotus, Pink Water Lily, Sacred Lotus, Nangram Lily.

Field Notes The Lotus is an aquatic, perennial plant that grows from a rhizome or tuber. They usually have multiple tubers that can be up to 250 mm long or larger. They have large round leaves that are held above the water, rather than floating, and tall flower stems with white to pink, spectacular scented flowers. Flowering occurs in summer in Australia. The flowers open in the morning and are finished by midday. Flowering is followed by the appearance of striking, spongy, flat-topped seed pods. The Lotus occurs in shallow water and mud, in permanent billabongs and lagoons, and in tropical and sub-tropical areas across the top end of Australia. It also occurs in Bhutan, India, Indonesia (Java), Japan, Korea, Malaysia, Myanmar, Nepal, New Guinea, Pakistan, the Philippines, Russia (far east), Sri Lanka, Thailand and Vietnam (ALA, 2022; Department of Primary Industries, 2022; Low, 1998).

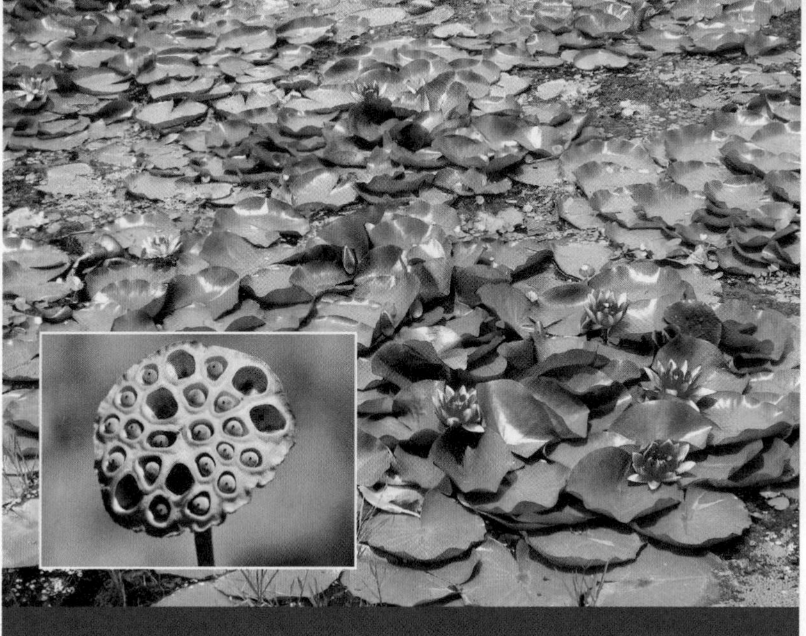

Medicinal Uses The Lotus is used medicinally in traditional Chinese, Indian, Japanese, Korean and Thai folk medicines, and in folk medicine in many other countries. The whole plant is used to treat diarrhoea, insomnia, fever, body heat imbalance and gastritis. The flowers and pedicels are used as both cardiac and hepatic tonics. The seeds are prepared to treat skin diseases. In China, the leaves are used to treat hyperlipidaemia, haematemesis (the vomiting of blood due to bleeding in the upper gut), metrorrhagia (abnormal bleeding from the uterus), fever and skin disorders. In Thailand, decoctions of the stamens are used to improve the circulatory system and to decrease blood glucose and blood lipid levels (Tungmunnithum et al., 2018).

Other Uses Aboriginal groups all over the top end of Australia ate Lotus tubers raw or roasted, the seeds raw or roasted and the inner leaf stalks. The seeds were often ground to a flour to make damper. The tubers are usually harvested at the end of summer. Early explorers thought the roasted seeds made an excellent coffee. In some Asian countries, the young leaves are eaten as a vegetable (Isaacs, 1992; Low, 1998). The flowers are also edible (Department of Primary Industries, 2022).

Love Vine

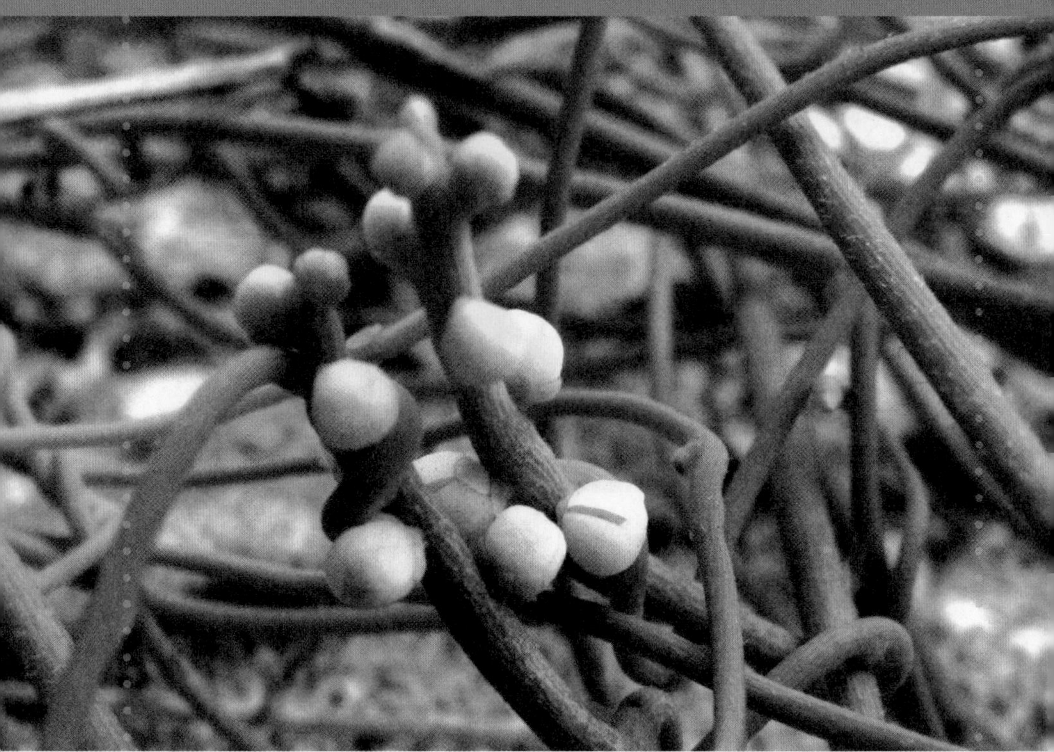

Scientific Name *Cassytha filiformis* L.

Common Names Love Vine, Devil's Twine, Creeping Dodder, Dodder Laurel.

Aboriginal Names Yangowi (Wunambal, Gaambera) (Karadada et al., 2011), Mawajawaja (Mangarrayi) (Wightman, 2017), Yugulu (Yawuru), Djirawan, Jirrawany (Bardi), Koodikoodi (Nyul Nyul), Yukuli (Nyangummarta), Yurrkulu (Karajarri) (Kane, 2022), Warirrinji (Gija) (Purdie et al., 2018), Yarda (Miwa) (Kimberley Specialists, 2020), Jilili, Dalunggurra, Mirdimirdi, Yinyjarlarra (Jaru) (Wightman, 2003), Yankeyi winya (Kwini) (Cheinmora et al., 2017), Jilili, Takurtakurta (Ngardi) (Cataldi, 2004), Taatu-taatu, Tjaakuta-kuta, Warla-warla (Kukatja) (Valiquette, 1993), Yukurlu (Karajarri) (Willing, 2014), Yookooloo (Nyikina) (Smith & Smith, 2009).

Field Notes Love Vine is a parasitic, perennial, twining herb with many branches. It usually forms a dense mat over the host plant,

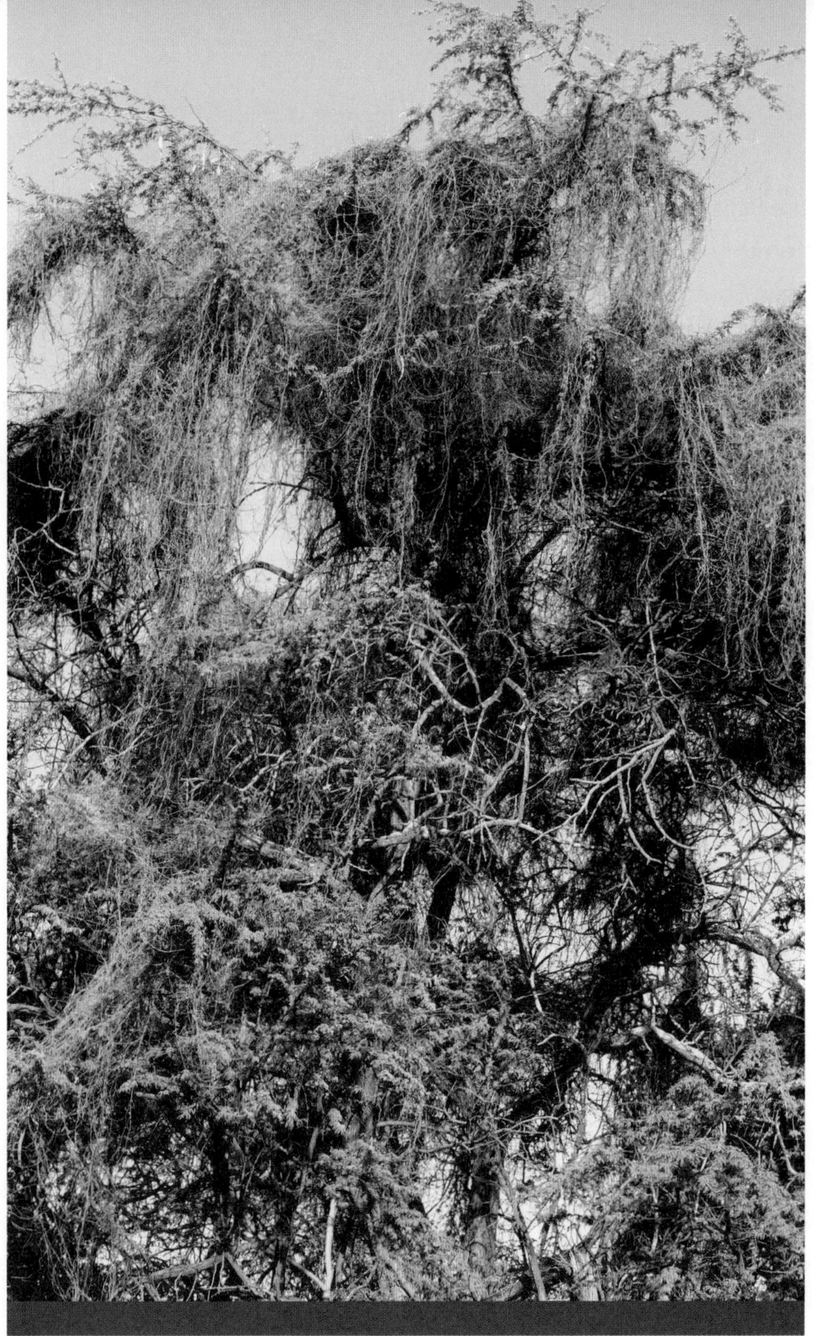

often killing it. Its leaves are scales about 1 mm long. Its flowers are borne either in spikes or solitary and are six tepals arranged in swirls. The flowers can be present all year round. The fruit are globular drupes about 7 mm in diameter. In Australia, Love Vine is usually found draped over Melaleuca and Acacia species on sandstone outcrops and plateaus, on mangrove swamps and coastal dunes in the Pilbara and Kimberley regions of Western Australia, the Northern Territory, northern Queensland, then down the coast as far as Taree in New South Wales. Love Vine is also found in the Americas, Indonesia, Malaysia, Polynesia and tropical Africa (ALA, 2022; ATRP, 2020; Noosa's Native Plants, 2022; WAH, 2022).

Medicinal Uses A poultice of the crushed Love Vine leaves was applied externally to ease joint and muscle pain (Kenneally et al., 1996; Webb, 1959; Western Australia Now and Then, 2020). Infusions of the crushed stems were taken internally for several complaints, including indigestion, biliousness, diarrhoea, fever, nephritis, oedema, headache, hepatitis, haemorrhoids, sinusitis, intestinal parasites and spermatorrhoea. The infusions were also given to women to stimulate menstruation, hasten parturition and to suppress lactation after a stillbirth. Infusions of the stems were used as a wash for skin conditions, including itchy skin, eczema, ulcers, as well as scabies and lice infestations (Edwards, 2005; Fern, 2021). The infusions were also used by the Gija as a wash to treat headaches and to make people feel strong. The plant is reported to have a 'good smell that makes people feel better' (Edwards, 2005; Purdie et al., 2018; Wightman, 2003).

Other Uses Love Vine leaves are edible and were generally steamed before eating (Fern, 2021). The fruit are also edible when ripe (translucent) in the early dry season, but should only be eaten in small amounts as they can have a laxative effect. The seeds should be discarded as they contain small quantities of poisonous alkaloids (Cheinmora et al., 2017; Fox & Garde, 2018; Hiddins, 2001; Karadada et al., 2011; Smith, 1991; Vigilante et al., 2013; Wightman, 2003). The Nyangummarta made their footwear (jinapuka) with small hanks of this plant (Kane, 2022). The Jaru of the East Kimberley burnt the stems of Love Vine on the campfire to keep mosquitoes away. They also boiled the stems in water for a long period and used the liquid as a wash 'to make hair become thick, healthy and dark' (Wightman, 2003).

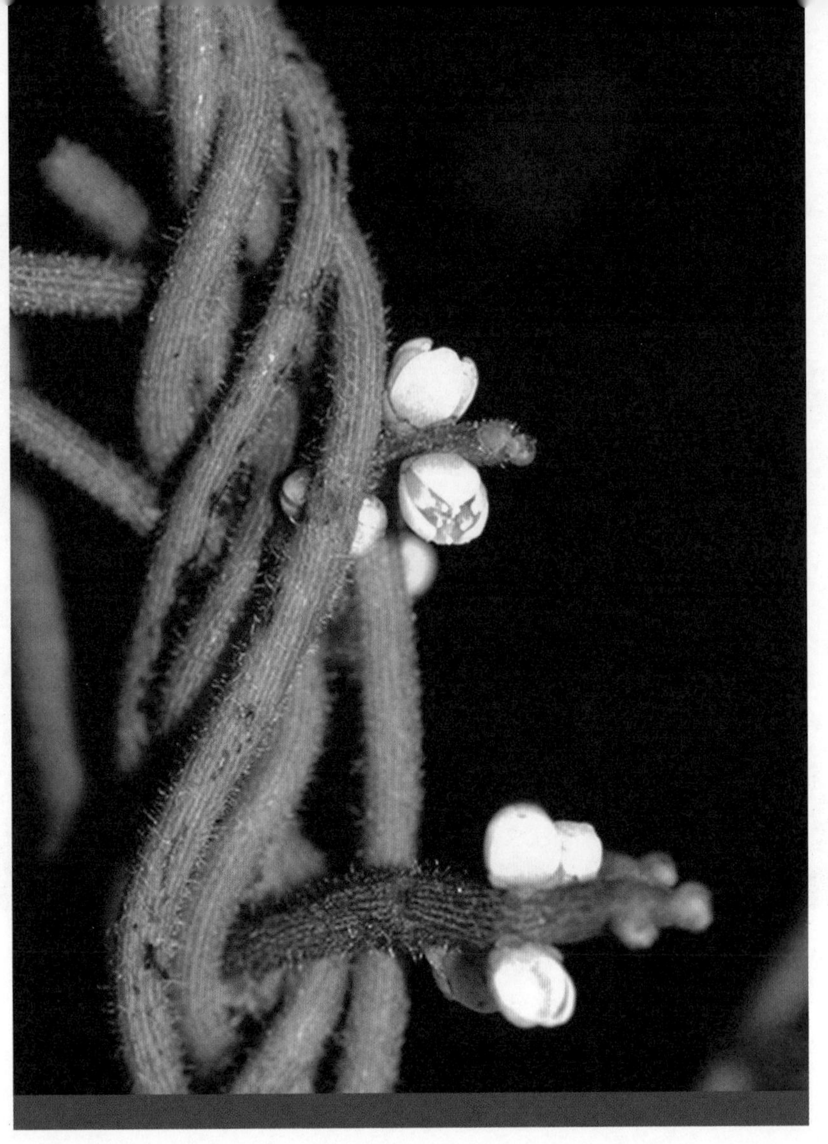

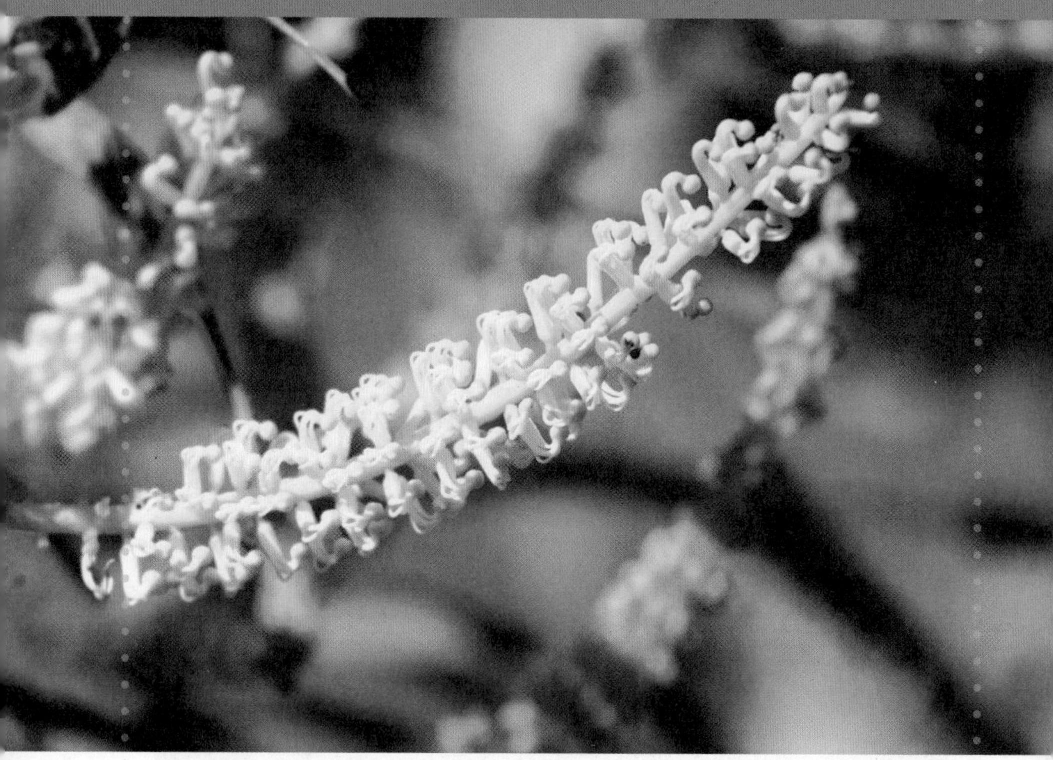

Scientific Name *Grevillea pyramidalis* R.Br., and *Grevillea pyramidalis* subsp. *leucadendron* (R.Br.) Makinson

Common Names Maangga, Willing, Caustic Tree, Blister Bush, Caustic Bush.

Aboriginal Names Wiling (Miriwoong) (Mirima Dawang Woorlab-gerring, 2013), Wilinyi (Bunuba) (Oscar et al., 2019), Wularmi (Wunambal, Gaambera) (Karadada et al., 2011), Willing) (Bardi (Clarke et al., 2012), Maangga (Bardi) (Kenneally et al., 1996), Wilinyji, Wilinyel (Gija) (Purdie et al., 2018), Wiliriny (Jaru) (Wightman, 2003), Wiliriny (Gooniyandi) (Dilkes et al., 2019), Kayala, (Ngardi), Yananti (Ngardi, Kukatja) (Cataldi, 2004), Bambûra manya (Kwini) (Cheinmora et al., 2017), Parntalpa (Kukatja (Valiquette, 1993), Wiliny (Walmajarri, Nyikina) (Smith & Smith, 2009).

Field Notes Maangga grows as a shrub or tree up to 6 m in height. Its leaves are simple, long, flat blades that are up to 410 mm long

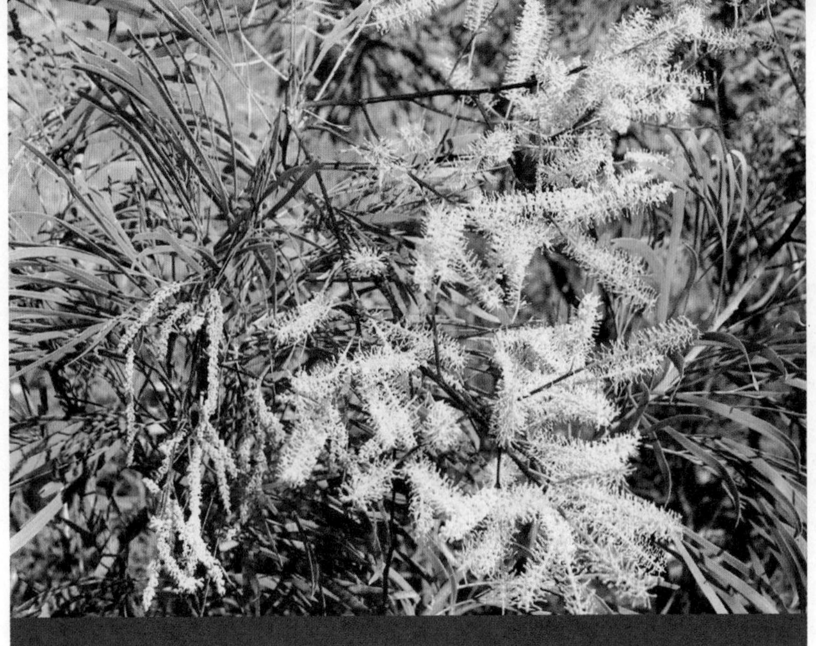

and 20 mm wide. Its flowers are exquisite white-cream-yellow racemes that appear from May to July. The sticky, obovoid, glabrous fruit are up to 23 mm long. Maangga occurs in sand, gravel, loam and skeletal sandy soils on sandstone, laterite and granite in the Pilbara and Kimberley regions of Western Australia and in the top end of the Northern Territory (ALA, 2022; WAH, 2022).

Medicinal Uses The greenish inner bark of the Maangga tree was crushed and mixed with water until a white solution was produced. This was then applied to the breasts of nursing mothers to stimulate milk production. The solution was also applied to sores to aid healing and used as ear drops to clean out ears and treat earache (Cock, 2011; Lassak & McCarthy, 2001; Reid, 1986; Webb, 1959; Williams, 2011).

Other Uses The sticky varnish that covers the fruit is an irritant and was used by the Gija and Bunuba to create ceremonial scars. The Gija used the timber for making boomerangs and slender shields (Oscar et al., 2019; Purdie et al., 2018; Wightman, 2003).

CAUTION: SKIPA (2022) warns that 'The resin on the seed pods is very sticky and caustic and can cause severe skin irritation', even being known to have caused second-degree burns.

Magabala

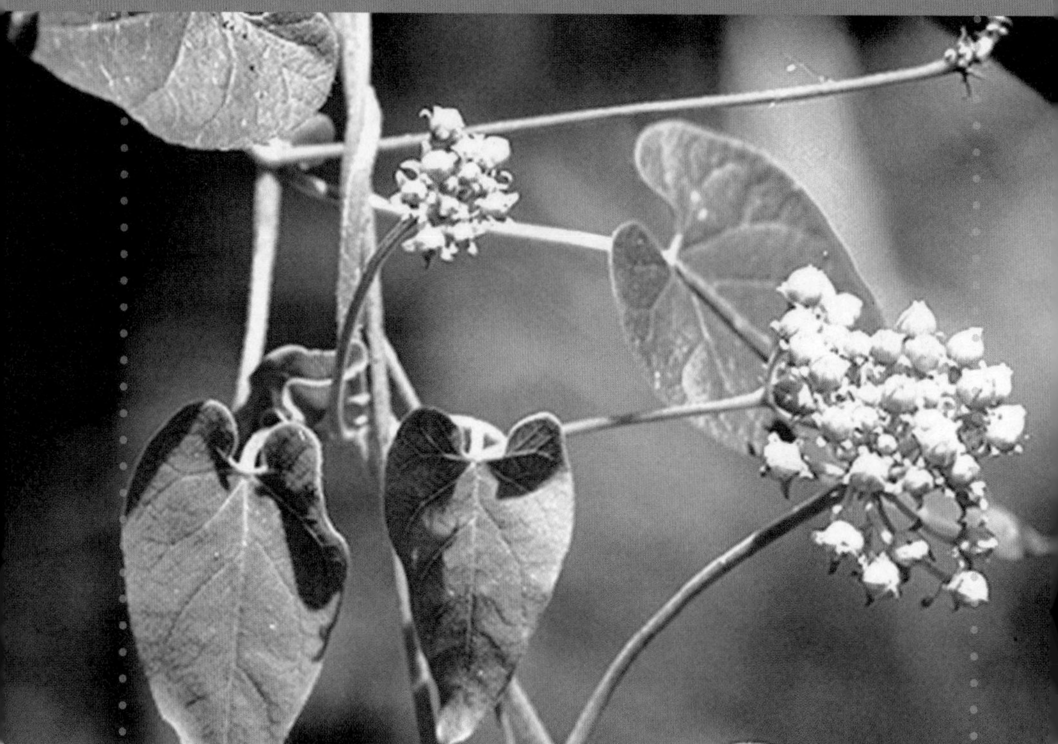

Scientific Name *Cynanchum pedunculatum* R.Br.

Common Names Magabala, Bush Banana.

Aboriginal Names Garlarla (Wunambal, Gaambera) (Karadada et al., 2011), Oonggannjoon (Bardi) (Kenneally et al., 1996), Unggandjun (Bardi) (Smith & Kalotas, 1985), Makabala (Yawuru), Koolookoonarr (Bardi), Makabala (Nyul Nyul), Makapala (Karajarri) (SKIPA, 2022), Jumbu manya (Kwini) (Cheinmora et al., 2017; Crawford, 1982), Magabala (Nyikina) (Milgin, 2009).

Field Notes Magabala is a prostrate or twinning perennial herb or climber. The vine is quite thin and does not exceed 20 mm in diameter. The leaves are elongated and heart-shaped. Its white-cream or red-purple umbelliform flowers appear between January and November. In the dry season, the vine sometimes dies back to the root stock, then springs forth again in the wet. Its fruit are often paired and are fluted, triangle-shaped carpels or seed pods that

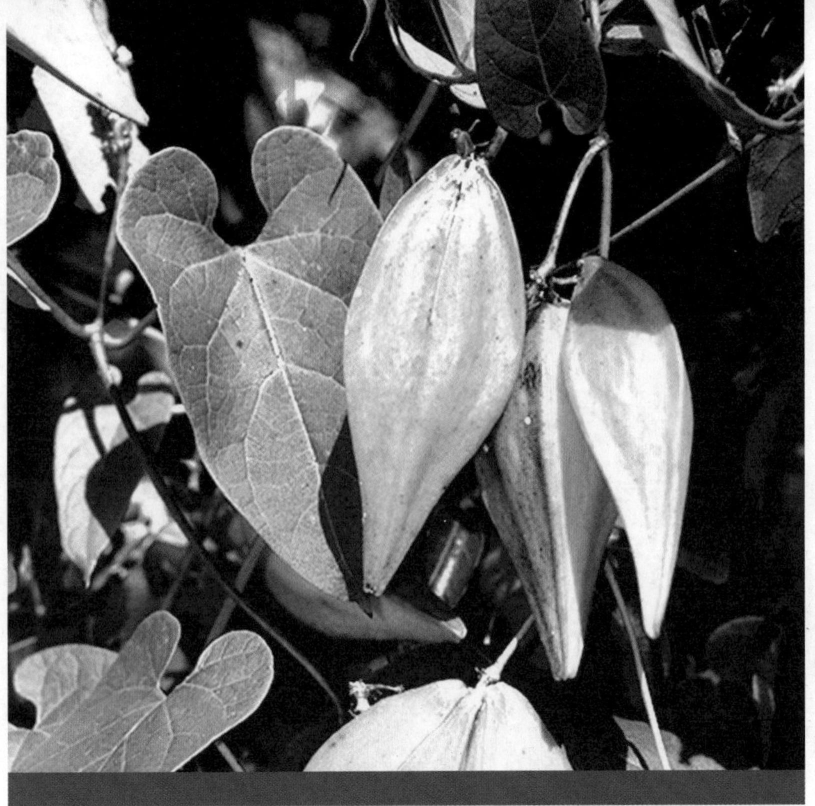

are up to 90 mm long and 35 mm in diameter. Magabala occurs on granite, sandstone or limestone substrates, often in rocky habitats, in the Pilbara and Kimberley regions of Western Australia, the Northern Territory and Queensland (ALA, 2022; ATRP, 2020; WAH, 2022; Young et al., 2012).

Medicinal Uses Crushed leaves of the Magabala vine were used as a poultice that was placed on the forehead to relieve headaches (Young et al., 2012).

Other Uses The fruit (seed pods) of Magabala are edible after they are roasted on hot coals, but not the woolly fibres and seeds inside. The pods are harvested from May to August (Cheinmora et al., 2017; Crawford, 1982; Fox & Garde, 2018; Karadada et al., 2011; Young et al., 2012). The roots are also edible and are usually baked in hot ashes before they are eaten (Fox & Garde, 2018).

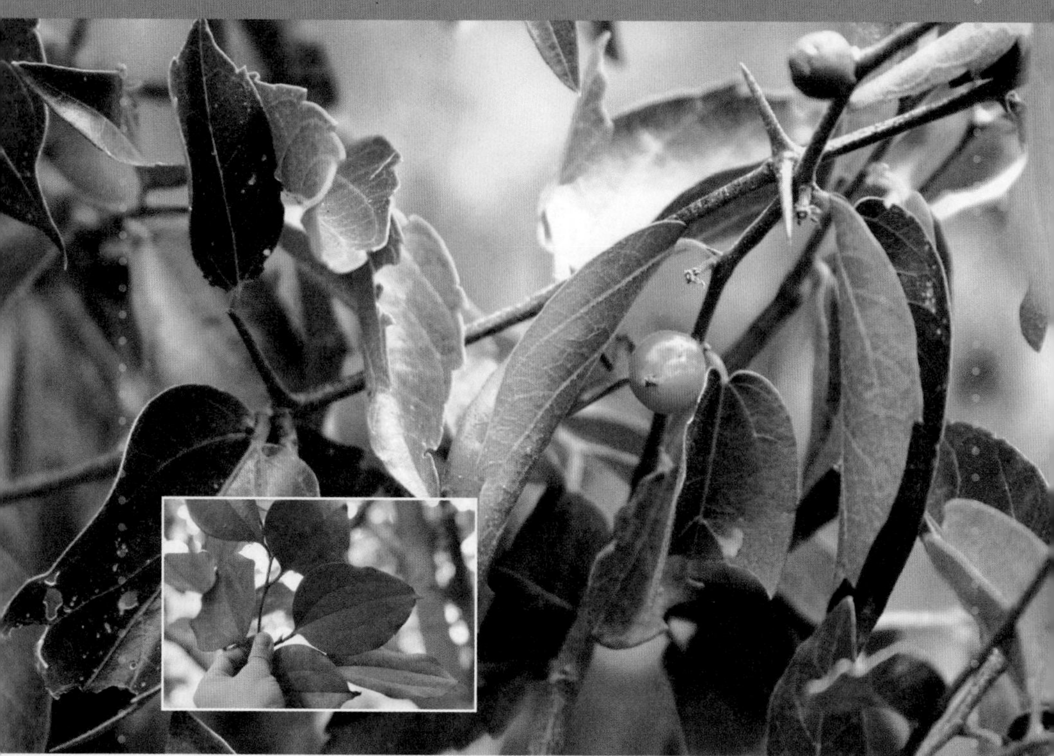

Scientific Names *Celtis strychnoides* Planch., also known as *Celtis australiensis* Sattarian, and *Celtis philippensis* Blanco (misapplied).

Common Names Malaiino, Celtis, Kaju Lulu.

Aboriginal Names Gunyjili (Bunuba) (Oscar et al., 2019), Gulyindji (Bardi) (Smith & Kalotas, 1985), Goolnji (bardi), Goonj (Nyul Nyul) (Kenneally et al., 1996), Thewengginy, Thewengkiny, Gooroorrji, Kururrji, Thoowoonggeny (Gija) (Purdie et al., 2018), Minthiwili (Gooniyandi) (Dilkes-Hall et al., 2019), Yimar (Jaru) (Wightman, 2003).

Field Notes Malaiino is a tree that grows up to 10 m in height but is usually smaller. Its bark is speckled, darkening to dark brown on exposure. Its green leaf blades are ovate and measure up to 70 mm long and 40 mm wide. Its small, insignificant white-and-green flowers appear in clusters of up to 40. Its orange fruit are globular or ovoid and up to 11 mm in diameter. The fruit are ripe between May and July. Malaiino occurs in monsoon forest and

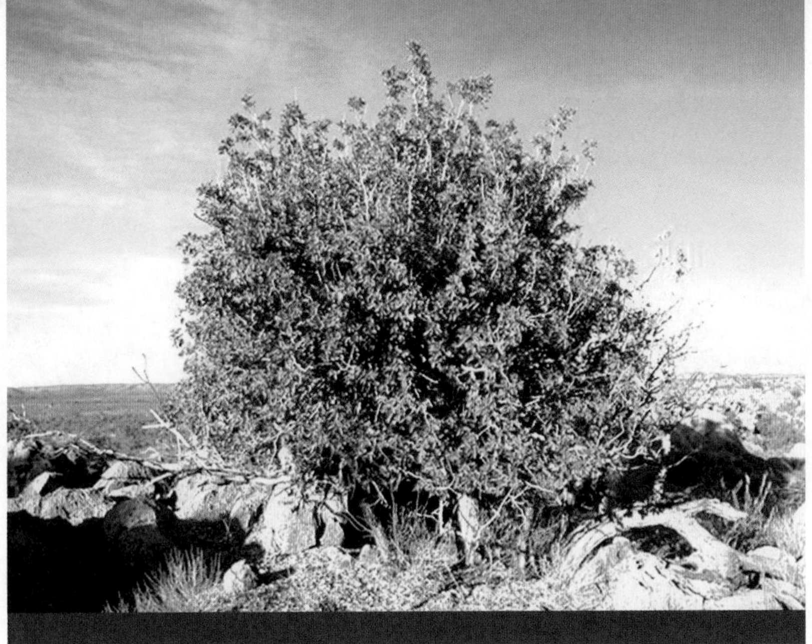

drier, more seasonal rainforest areas of the Kimberley region of Western Australia, the Northern Territory and Far North Queensland (ALA, 2022; ATRP, 2020). It also occurs in tropical Africa, India, Madagascar, southern China, India, the Solomon Islands and South-east Asia (Fern, 2021).

Medicinal Uses Decoctions of the inner bark were used as a medicinal wash to treat leprosy and to treat skin conditions such as sores, itchy skin and scabies infestations (Smith, 1991). The roots were eaten to treat diarrhoea (Fern, 2021).

Other Uses The fruit of the Malaiino tree are edible when they are red and ripe but are not very palatable (DBCA, 2019; Fox & Garde, 2018; Oscar et al., 2019; RFCA, 1993; Smith & Kalotas, 1985; Vigilante et al., 2013; Wightman, 2003).

Malara

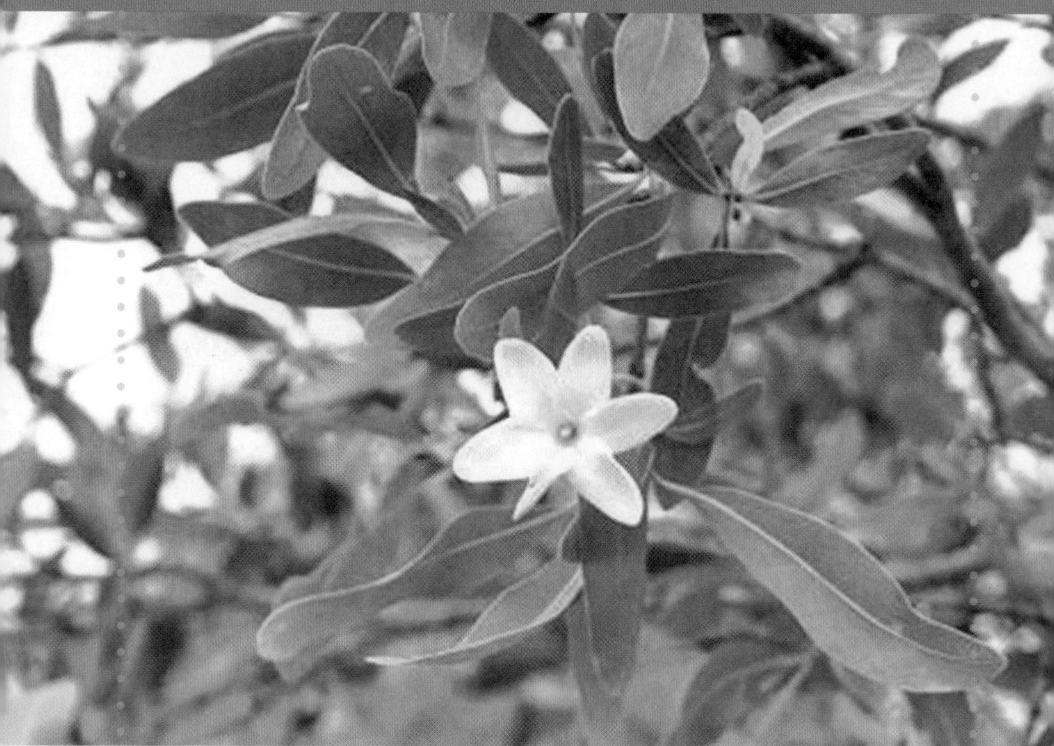

Scientific Names *Gardenia pyriformis* Benth., and *Gardenia pyriformis* subsp. *keartlandii* (Tate) Puttock, previously known as *Gardenia edulis* F.Muell.

Common Names Malara, Native Gardenia, Turpentine Tree.

Aboriginal Names Wudarr (Yawuru), Dalwarr (Bardi) (Smith & Kalotas, 1985), Daloorr (Nyul Nyul), Lirta (Nyangumarta), Wutarr (Karajarri) (Kane, 2022), Wurtarr (Walmajarri) (Richards & Hudson, 2012), Malarra winya (Kwini) (Cheinmora et al., 2017; Crawford, 1982).

Field Notes Malara grows as a shrub or tree to 6 m in height depending on conditions. It has smooth bark (sometimes with a slight orange tinge), green, leathery, obovate leaves, and large, white flowers that appear between February and May or July and December. Its green fruit are globular, hard and ribbed. Malara is found in red sandy soils over sandstone, on sandplains and dunes, stony ridges, cliffs and scree slopes in the Pilbara and Kimberley

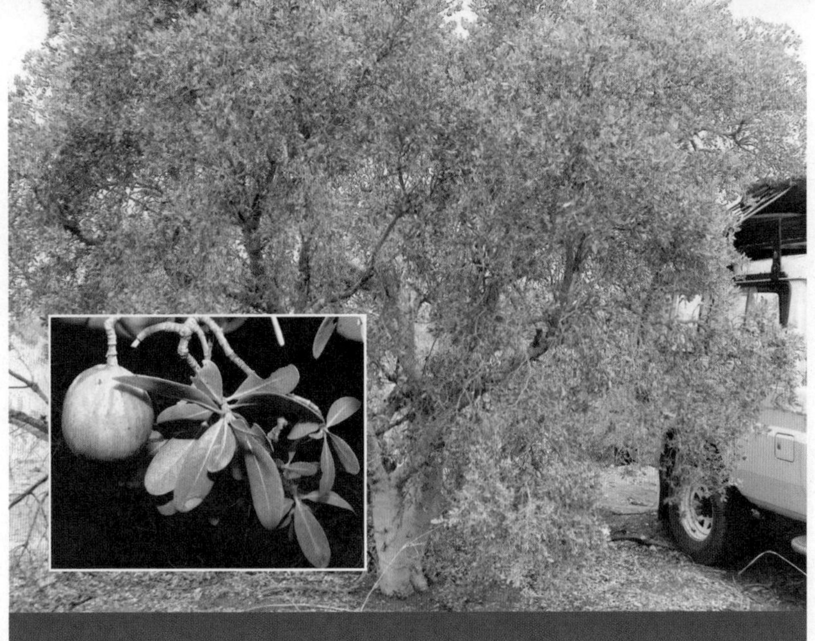

regions of Western Australia and the Northern Territory (ALA, 2022; SKIPA, 2022; WAH, 2022).

Medicinal Uses Infusions of the bark were taken internally for 'cold sick', presumably to relieve the symptoms of colds and influenza, and were also applied as a wash or liniment to ease arthritic and rheumatic pain, as well as sores and wounds to aid healing (Kane, 2022; Paddy et al., 1993; SKIPA, 2022). Crushed leaves were rubbed on feet to protect them against stonefish stings and coral cuts (Kane, 2022; Kenneally et al., 1996) and to protect feet from the heat of hot sand (Willing, 2014).

Other Uses The fruit of the Malara are edible when they are ripe and fall from the tree. The flesh is squeezed out of the fruit and eaten. The seeds are discarded. The fruit are available from May to August (Bindon, 2014; Crawford, 1982; Vigilante et al., 2013). The Kwini use the leaves to wrap food that is being cooked in a ground oven to keep it moist and give it some flavour (Cheinmora et al., 2017).

Mamukata

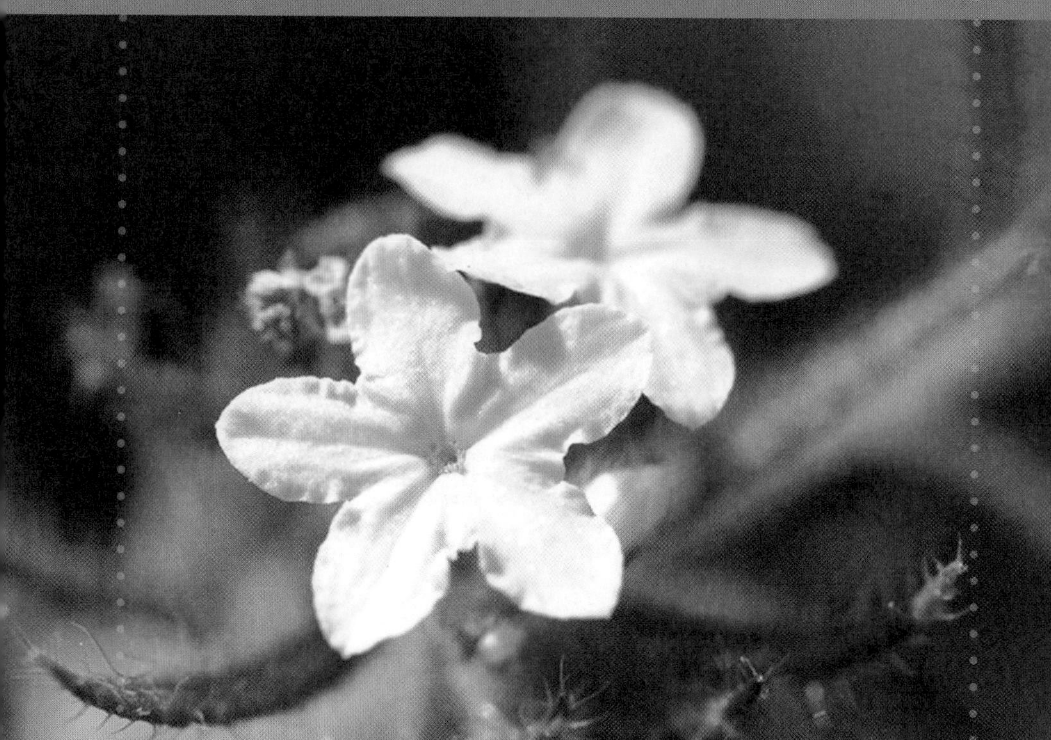

Scientific Name *Heliotropium tenuifolium* R.Br.

Common Names Mamukata, Bushy Heliotrope.

Aboriginal Names Mamanganpa, Tjaniwira, Mirra-mirra, Tulpa-tulpa, Yararra, Yara-yara (Kukatja) (Valiquette, 1993).

Field Notes Mamukata is an ascending to spreading annual or perennial that only grows to around 600 mm high. It has thin, hairy leaves and white flowers with five petals that are present between January and October. Its small seeds are broadly ovate to sub-oblong mericarps. Mamukata occurs in a variety of habitats across the top half of Australia, which includes the Pilbara and Kimberley regions of Western Australia (ALA, 2022; ATRP, 2020; WAH, 2022).

Medicinal Uses Decoctions of the leaves of Mamukata were used as a healing wash for skin conditions such as eczema and psoriasis (Morse, 2005).

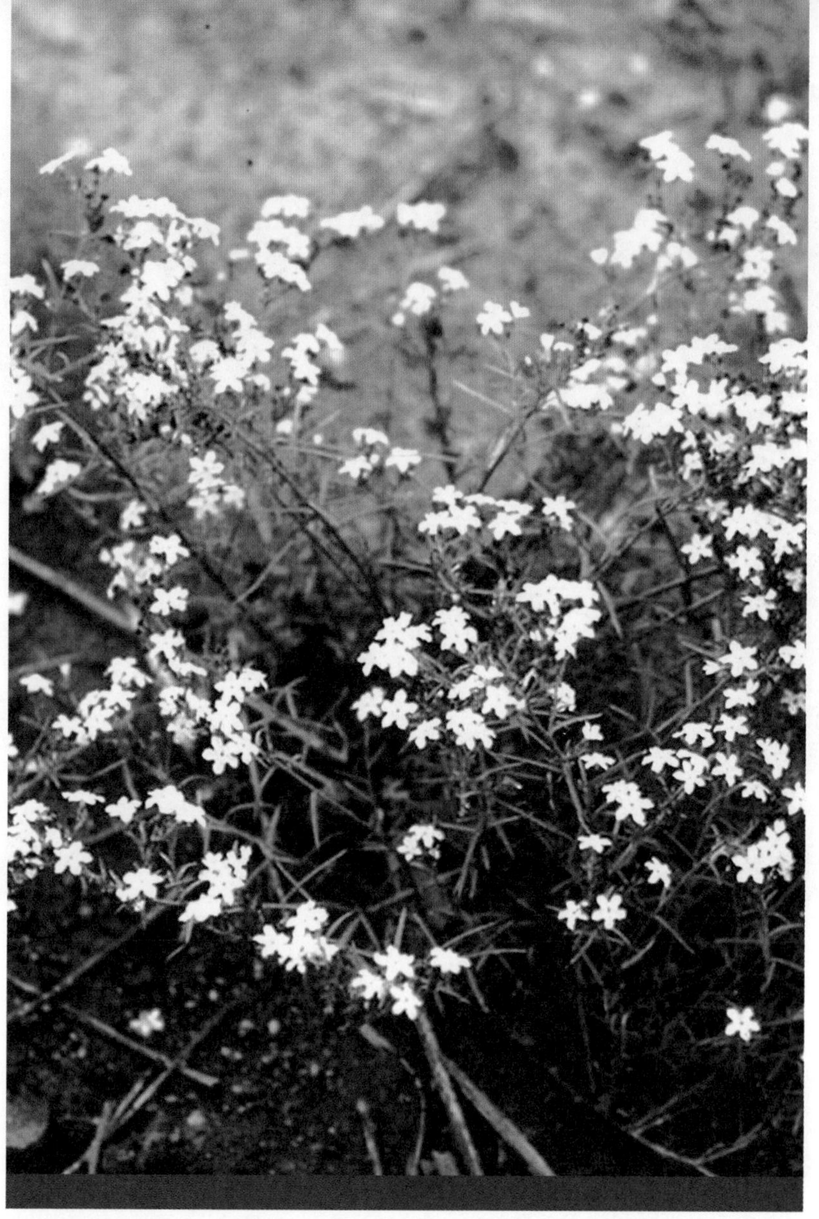

Other Uses The seeds of Mamukata are edible (Cancilla & Wingfield, 2017).

Mangaloo

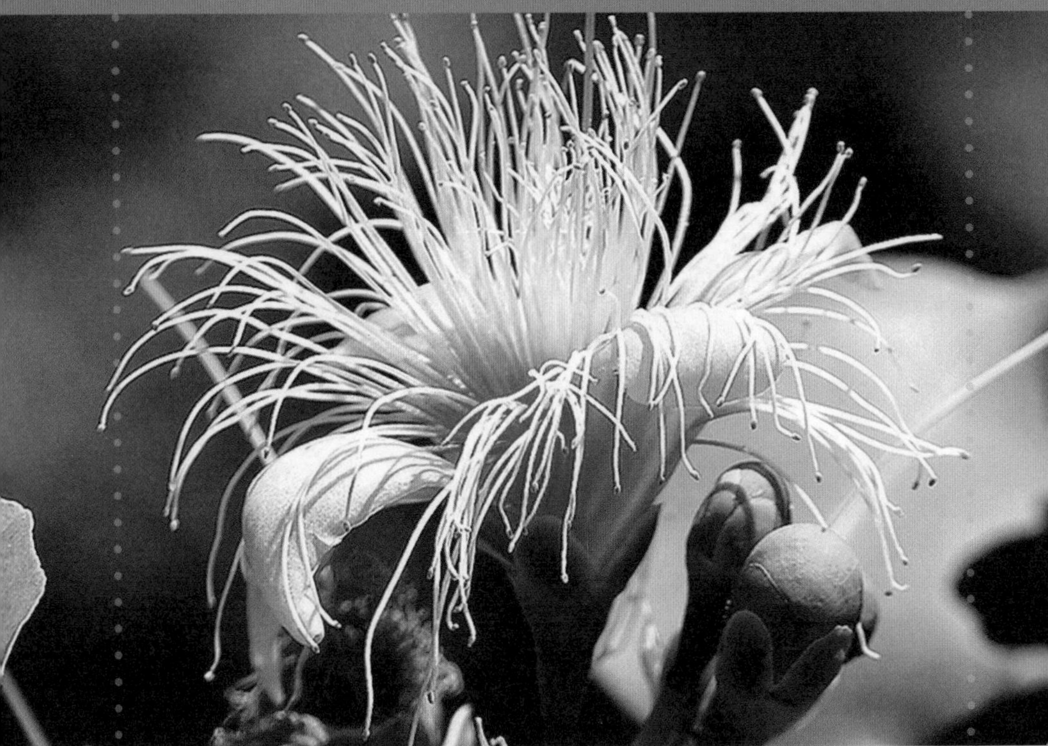

Scientific Names *Planchonia careya* (F.Muell.) R.Knuth., and *Planchonia rupestris* R.L.Barrett

Common Names Mangaloo, Billygoat Plum, Cocky Apple, Cockatoo Apple.

Aboriginal Names Guranbi (Bunuba) (Oscar et al., 2019), Mangala (Wunambal, Gaambera) (Karadada et al., 2011), Gwiyaroi (Nyikina) Gunthamurrah (Mitchell River), Kuiperi (Batavia River), Karoo (Dunk Island) Ootcho, Gwiyarbi, Gulay (Nyul Nyul), Gulayi, Goolay (Bardi) (Smith & Kalotas, 1985; Paddy et al., 1993), Banggiya (Kwini) (Crawford, 1982), Yundu minya, Yurndu minya (Kwini) (Cheinmora et al., 2017; Crawford, 1982).

Field Notes Mangaloo grows as a shrub or tree up to 15 m in height. The tree is briefly deciduous in the dry season. Its bark is grey, rough, slightly corky and fissured. Its leaves are spatula-shaped, tapering to the base and up to 100 mm long by 60 mm

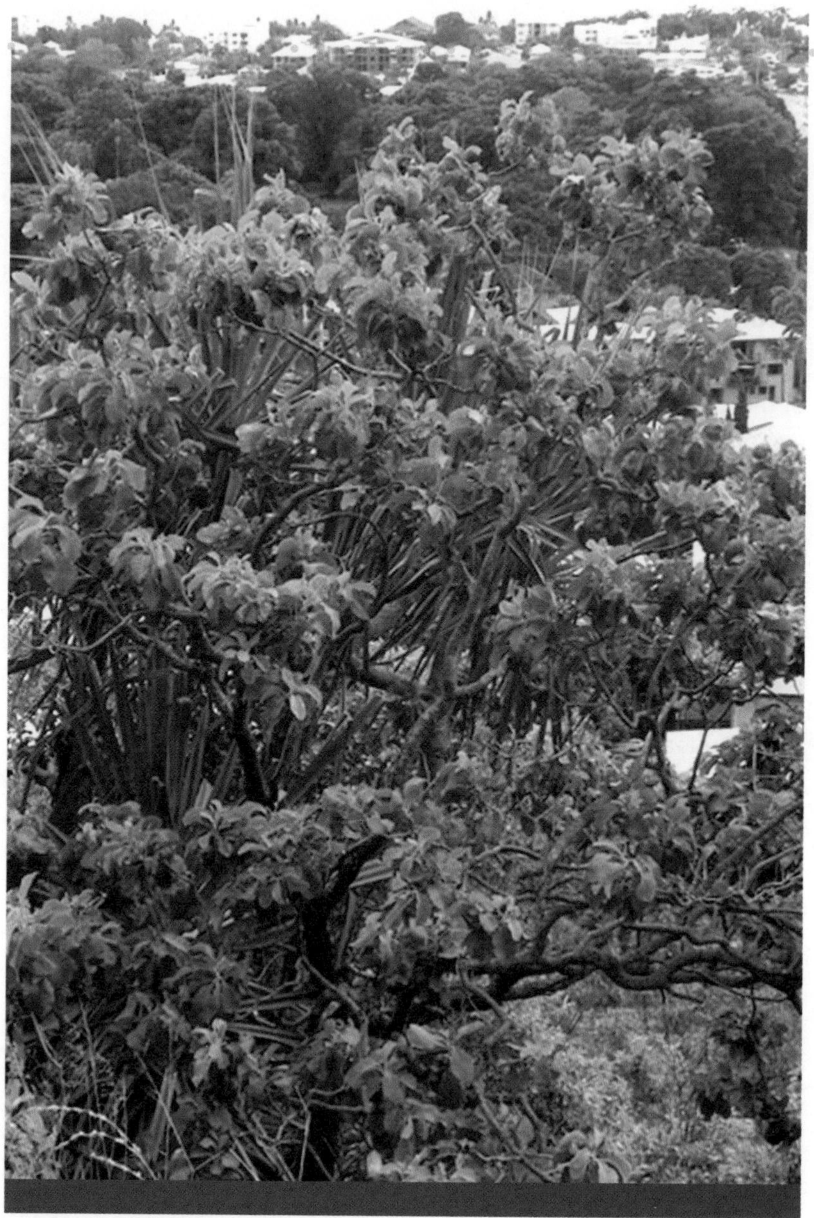

wide. Its large, white flowers have numerous pink and white stamens about 60 mm long. The flowers open in the evening and fall by morning. Flowering is more prolific between July and October. Its fruit are ovoid, green, smooth and approximately 90 mm long and 40 mm in diameter. Mangaloo is found in sand to clay soils over sandstone along the edges of creeks, swamps, screes and in open forests and woodlands. It is distributed across northern tropical Australia from the Kimberley region in Western Australia through the northern Territory and Northern Queensland and down the east coast to around Fraser Island. It also occurs in New Guinea (ALA, 2022; ANPSA, 2022; ATRP, 2020; WAH, 2022).

Medicinal Uses Infusions of the red inner bark of Mangaloo were used as an antiseptic wash to treat skin sores and wounds. Infusions of the crushed roots were used to treat prickly heat and chickenpox rash. Decoctions of the inner bark were used to treat scabies infestations (Cock, 2011; Edwards, 2005; Isaacs, 1987; Lassak & McCarthy, 2001; Reid, 1986; Smith, 1991), and as a mouthwash to ease the pain of toothache (Edwards, 2005). Infusions of the crushed roots were used as a wash to relieve itching due to insect bites (Low, 1990). Heated leaves were placed over mosquito and sandfly bites to relieve the soreness and itchiness (Smith, 1991). Warmed leaves were placed on the head to treat headaches (Isaacs, 1987). The juice from pulped roots was used to treat burns and sores. Infusions of the mashed small roots were applied externally for prickly heat rash, chickenpox and sores. Decoctions of the bark were rubbed on the body for general malaise and rheumatic pain. Crushed leaves and stems were applied to ulcers and sores to aid healing (Edwards, 2005; Isaacs, 1987; Lassak & McCarthy, 2001; Low, 1990; Paddy et al., 1993; Webb, 1959).

Other Uses Aboriginal groups across the top of Australia ate Mangaloo fruit pulp either raw or roasted. They are usually soft when ripe but still green. The fruit is peeled and only the outside flesh is edible, as the inside flesh is like whiskers and can irritate the throat. The fruit are available from mid-November to February. Sugarbag honey is often found in this tree (Bindon, 2014; Cheinmora et al., 2017; Crawford, 1982; Fox & Garde, 2018; Karadada et al., 2011; Jackes, 2010; Low, 1991; Oscar et al., 2019; Smith, 1991; Vigilante et al., 2013). The flower buds are also edible (Karadada et al., 2011). The roots and bark of Mangaloo were used

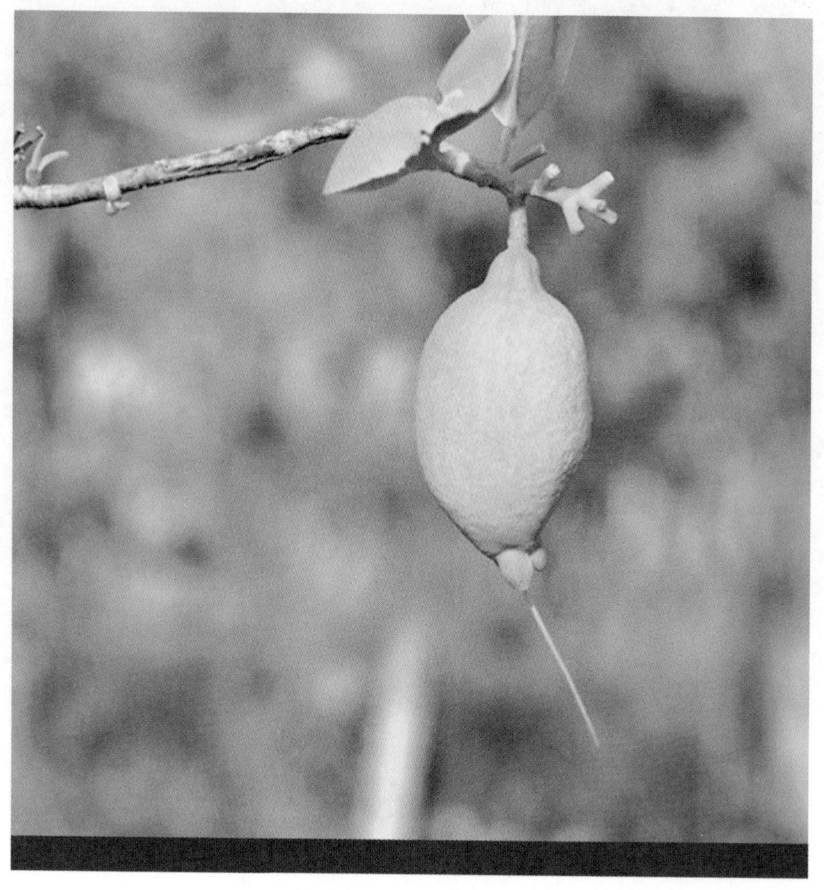

as a 'fish poison' in the late dry season (Cheinmora et al., 2017; Crawford, 1982; Low, 1991; Smith, 1991).

Maroon Bush

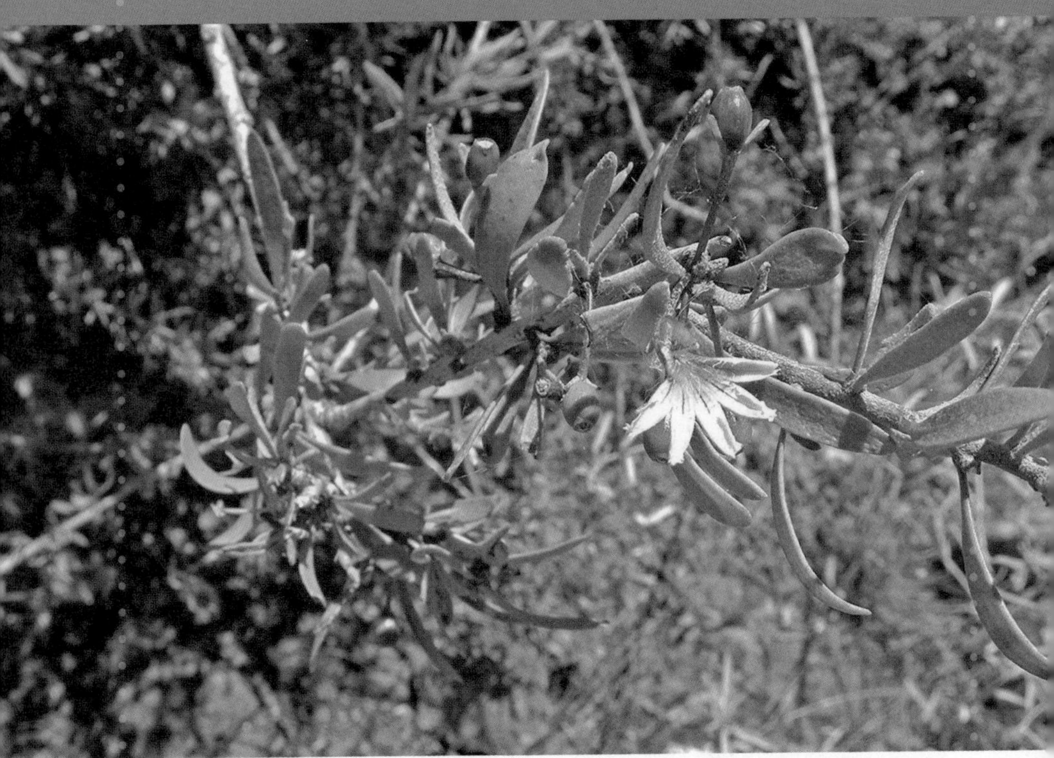

Scientific Name *Scaevola spinescens* R.Br.

Common Names Maroon Bush, Cancer Bush, Prickly Fanflower, Currant Bush.

Field Notes Maroon Bush is a medium-sized shrub that grows to around 2 m in height. Its leaves are flat, ovate and 6–40 mm long and 1–8 mm wide. The fan-like creamy-white to yellow flowers are present for most of the year. The fruit appear as small, purplish berries or currants. Maroon Bush occurs in sandy loam on hills in the drier inland regions of Western Australia, including the Gascoyne, Mid-West, Pilbara and the southern part of the Kimberley region around Halls Creek, as well as in Central Australia and New South Wales (ALA, 2022; Lassak & McCarthy, 2001; WAH, 2022).

Medicinal Uses Decoctions made from the whole plant were drunk to treat cancer, intestinal complaints, heart disease, urinary

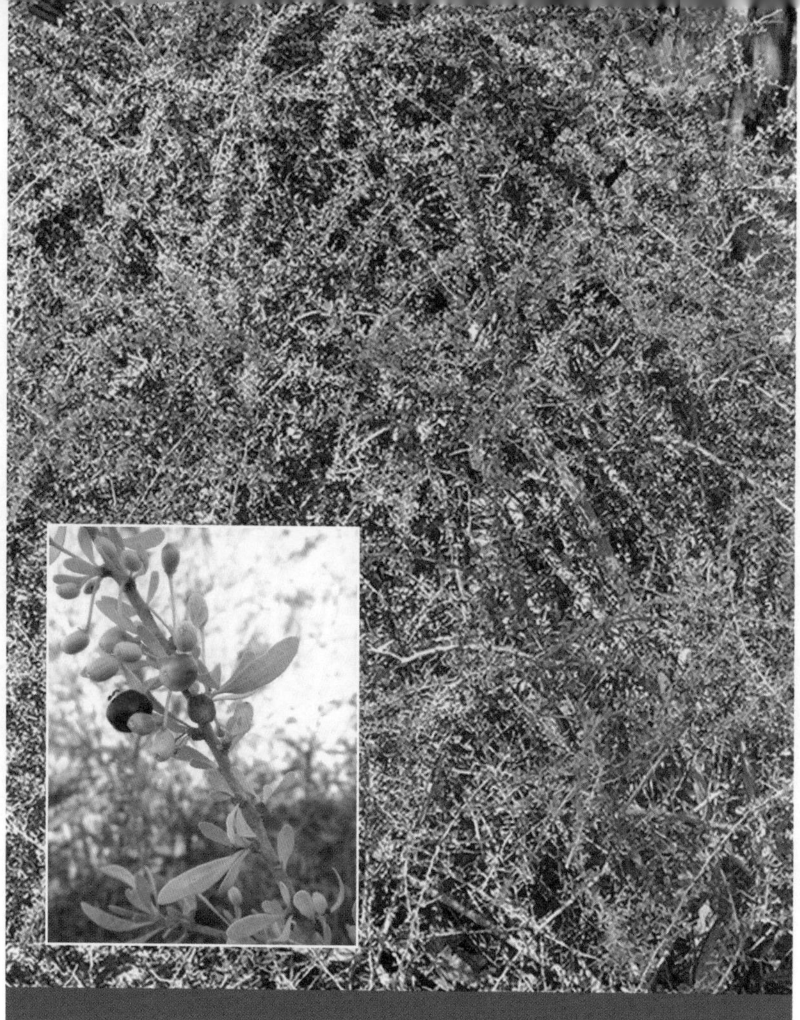

and kidney problems, and as an immune system stimulant (Cribb & Cribb, 1983; Lassak & McCarthy, 2001). Decoctions of the stems were taken internally to treat sores and boils. The entire plant was burnt and the smoke inhaled to relieve the symptoms of colds and influenza ().

Other Uses The purple berries of Maroon Bush are edible and made a good snack for Aboriginal people who lived in the drier areas of Western Australia (Hansen & Horsfall, 2016).

Marsh Stemodia

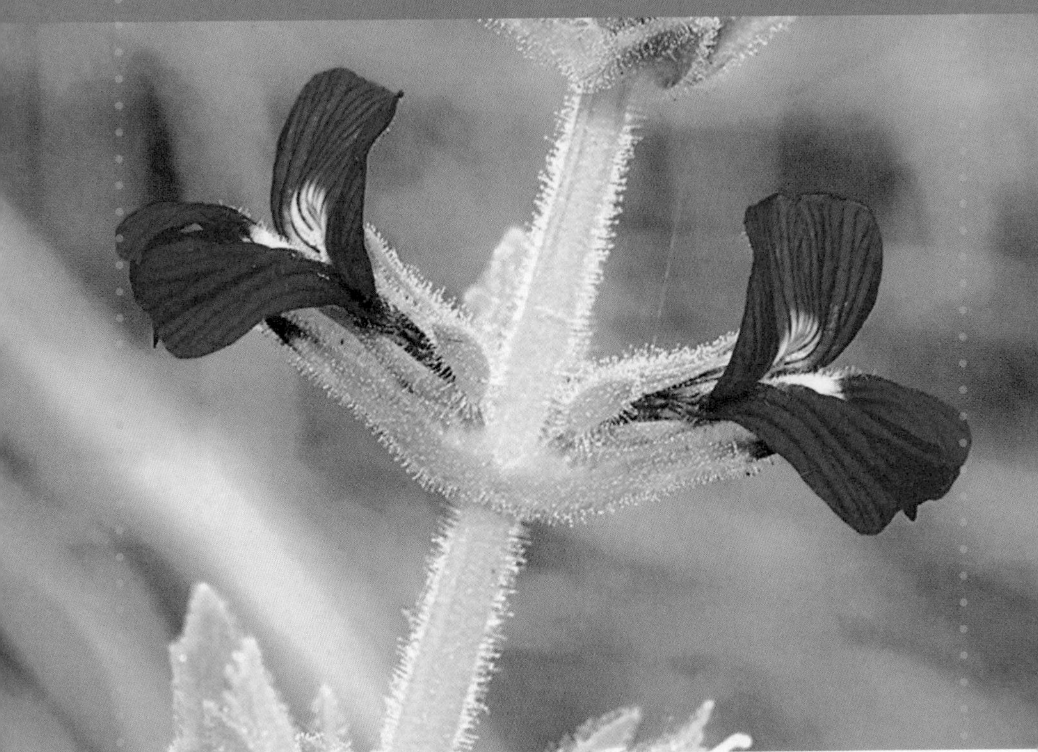

Scientific Name *Stemodia grossa* Benth.

Common Name Marsh Stemodia.

Aboriginal Name Ngunungunu (Bunuba) (Oscar et al., 2019).

Field Notes Marsh Stemodia is an erect or spreading, viscid, strongly aromatic perennial plant that grows to around 2.5 m in height. Its leaves are opposite and form in tight whorls, generally with shallow teeth along the edges. It has rich, blue flowers that are strongly scented, with the corollas twice as long as the calyxes. Flowering is from June to October. Marsh Stemodia occurs in alluvial soil and clayey sand, in river and creek beds and crabholes in the Pilbara and Kimberley regions of Western Australia and the Northern Territory (ALA, 2022; Lassak & McCarthy, 2001; WAH, 2022).

Medicinal Uses Infusions or decoctions of the crushed leaves of Marsh Stemodia were used as a liniment to ease arthritic and rheumatic pain or to bathe the head for the relief of colds

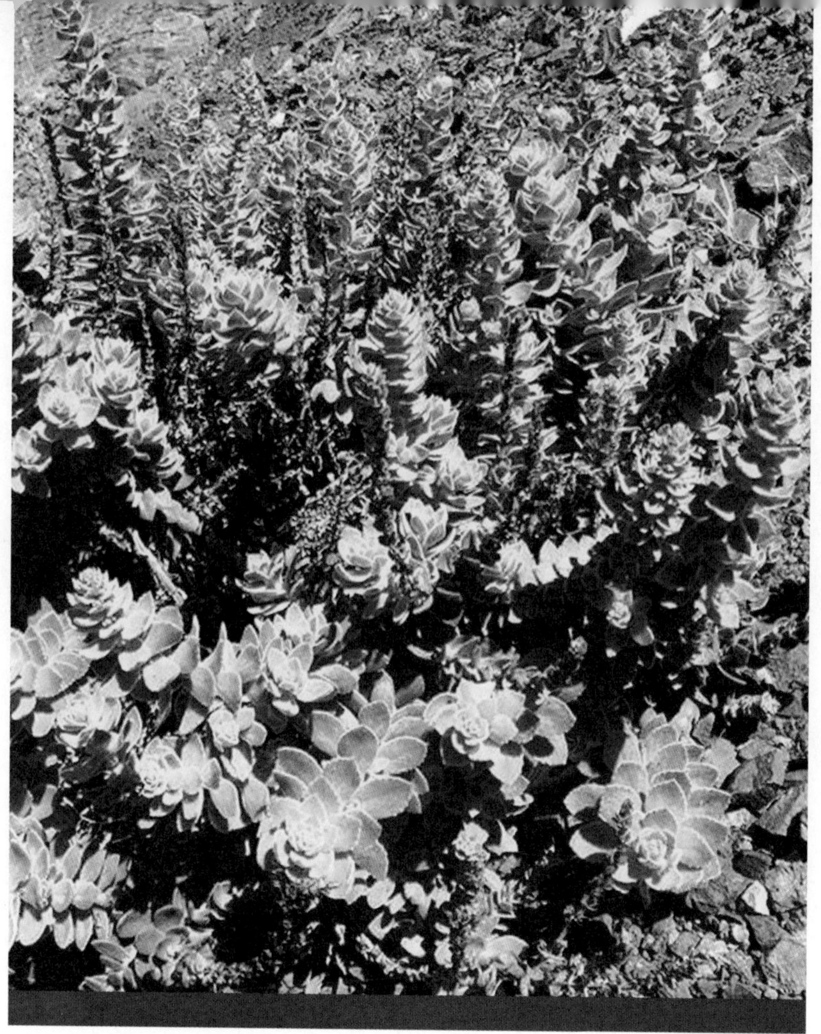

or headache. Sweetened decoctions of the leaves were taken internally for the relief of colds and influenza (Cock, 2011; Lassak & McCarthy, 2001; Oscar et al., 2019; Reid, 1986; Webb, 1959).

Milky Mangrove

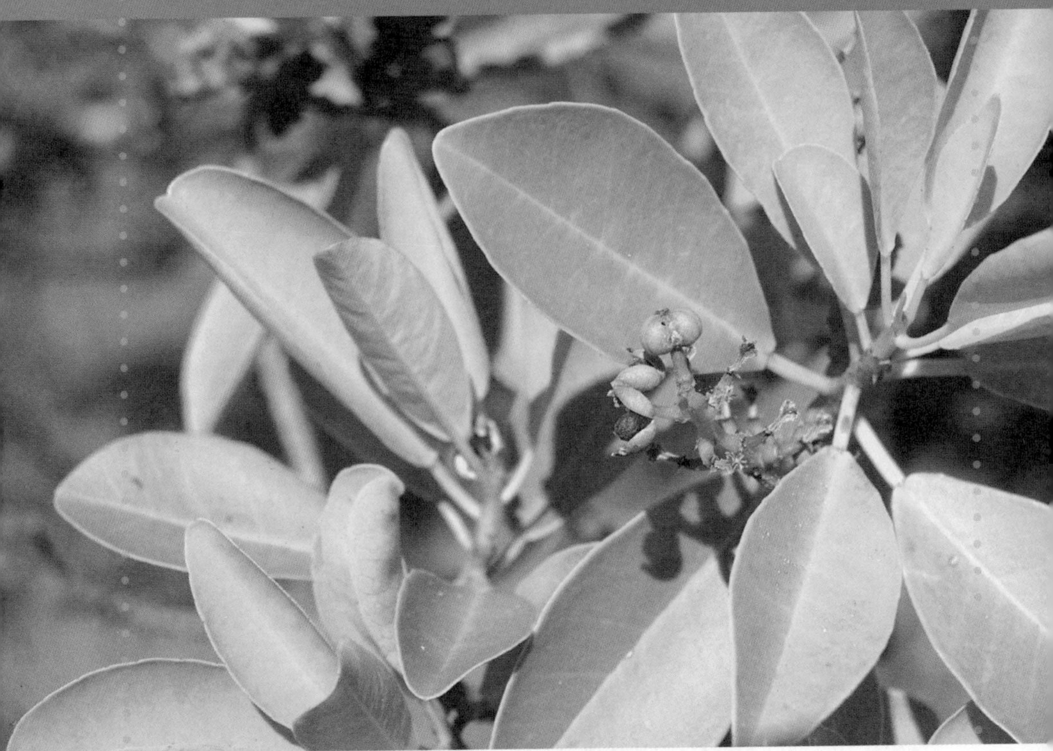

Scientific Name *Excoecaria agallocha* L.

Common Names Milky Mangrove, Blind-your-eye Mangrove, River Poison Tree, Balavola Karping.

Aboriginal Names Djolor (Bardi) (Smith & Kalotas, 1985), Jolorr (Bardi), Garl Garl (Yawuru) (Kenneally et al., 1996).

Field Notes Milky Mangrove is an evergreen or briefly deciduous shrub or tree with stilt roots that grows up to 30 m in height. It has large, heart-shaped leaves that are often variegated with flashes of red, pink, white or green. It has small flowers that are approximately 2 mm in diameter that appear on spikes 25–35 mm long from October to April. Male and female flowers are located on separate trees. Its fruit are small, three-lobed, fleshy green capsules that are approximately 5 mm in diameter and are arranged in clusters. Milky Mangrove is known as a back mangrove and is found at higher elevations back away from the ocean where salinity is lower.

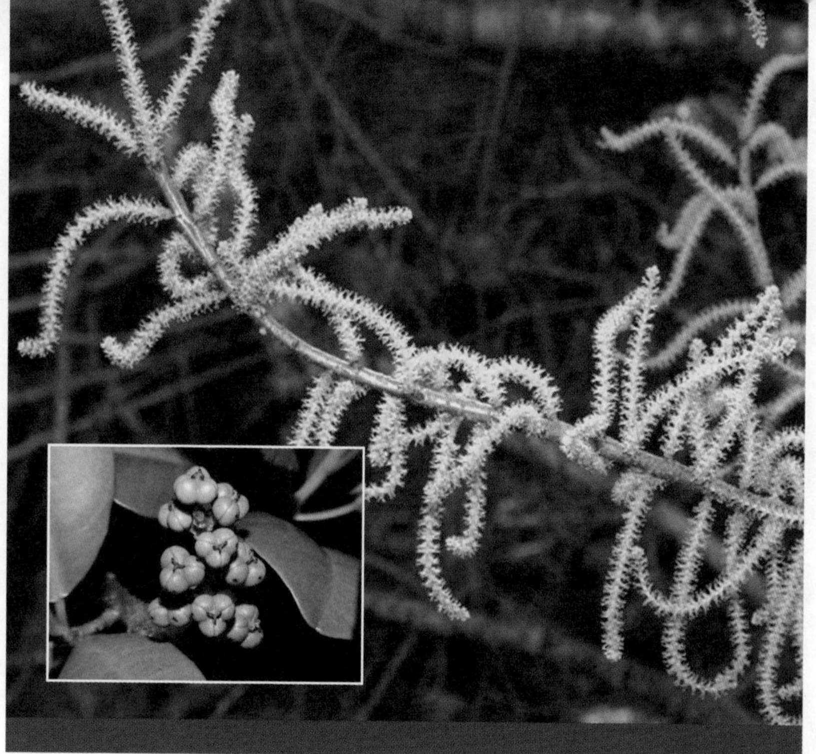

In Australia, it occurs in the Broome area of Western Australia and along the Northern Territory and Queensland coastlines to the northernmost part of New South Wales. It also occurs in southern China, the Indian subcontinent, Indonesia, Malaysia, Myanmar, New Guinea, the Philippines, Thailand, Vietnam and on some Pacific islands (ALA, 2022; Fern, 2021).

Medicinal Uses The poisonous juice or sap from the Milky Mangrove was used externally to treat chronic ulcerative conditions such as leprosy, as well as sores and wounds. It was also used to treat stings from marine animals, such as catfish and stingrays. Infusions of the mashed bark were applied externally to areas of rheumatic pain and for general malaise (Edwards, 2005; Lassak & McCarthy, 2001).

Other Uses The wood was used to make shields (Smith & Kalotas, 1985).

CAUTION: The milky sap can cause intense pain and blistering if it comes in to contact with good skin so its use today is not recommended. It can also cause intense pain and temporary blindness if it gets into the eyes (Children's Health Queensland, 2019).

Mimosa Bush

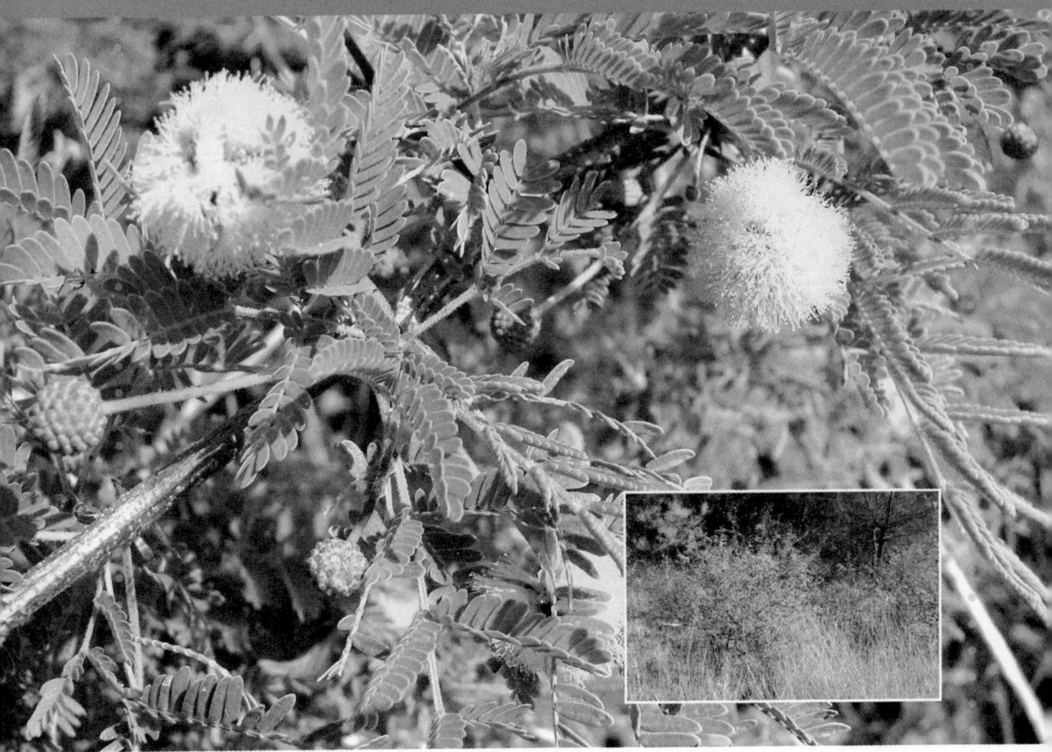

Scientific Name *Vachellia farnesiana* (L.) Wight & Arn., previously known as *Acacia farnesiana* (L.) Willd.

Common Names Mimosa Bush, Prickle Bush, Spiky Wattle, Thorn Bush.

Aboriginal Names Gulumarra (Bunuba) (Oscar et al., 2019), Bagawagany, Moorrooloomboony (Gija) (Purdie et al., 2018), Murrulumbu, Gulumarra, Pakawaka (Ngardi) (Cataldi, 2004), Kurlu, Kurlumarra, Pakaaka (Walmajarri) (Richards & Hudson, 2012), Bagawaga (Jaru) (Deegan et al., 2010).

Field Notes Mimosa Bush, thought to be originally from sub-tropical and tropical parts of America, was probably introduced to Australia before colonisation. It is now naturalised throughout the tropics and subtropics. It is an erect, spreading, thicket-forming thorny tree or shrub that grows only up to 4 m in height in Western Australia but can reach up to 9 m elsewhere. It has rough, dark grey bark and bipinnate leaves with leaflets that are narrowly oblong and up to 15 mm long and 3.5 mm wide. Its yellow, globular flower heads are present between June and August in Australia. Its fruit or seed pods are slightly constricted between the seeds and up to 85 mm long and 17 mm wide. Mimosa Bush occurs in a variety of soils in low-lying areas, on river and creek banks and disturbed sites in the Pilbara and Kimberley regions of Western Australia and in all other mainland states and territories except Victoria (ALA, 2022; WAH, 2022; World Wide Wattle, 2022).

Medicinal Uses Aboriginal groups in Australia have been known to poke the thorns of Mimosa Bush into warts to make them disappear. Decoctions or infusions of the bark are drunk as a cough suppressant. The wood (with bark removed) is burnt and the white ash is applied to open wounds to aid the healing process. The leaves were chewed to treat stomach ache and diarrhoea (World Wide Wattle, 2022). The Bunuba used the thorns to pierce gum abscesses (Oscar et al., 2019).

Other Uses The gum, green seed pods and seeds of Mimosa Bush are edible and were eaten by some Aboriginal groups in Australia (Fern, 2021, Isaacs, 1987). The green pods were roasted before eating (Cribb & Cribb, 1981). Wood from the Mimosa Bush was used to make boomerangs and punishment spears (World Wide Wattle, 2022). In Europe, a substance called 'cassie' is extracted from the flowers to make perfume (Cribb & Cribb, 1981).

Mistletoe

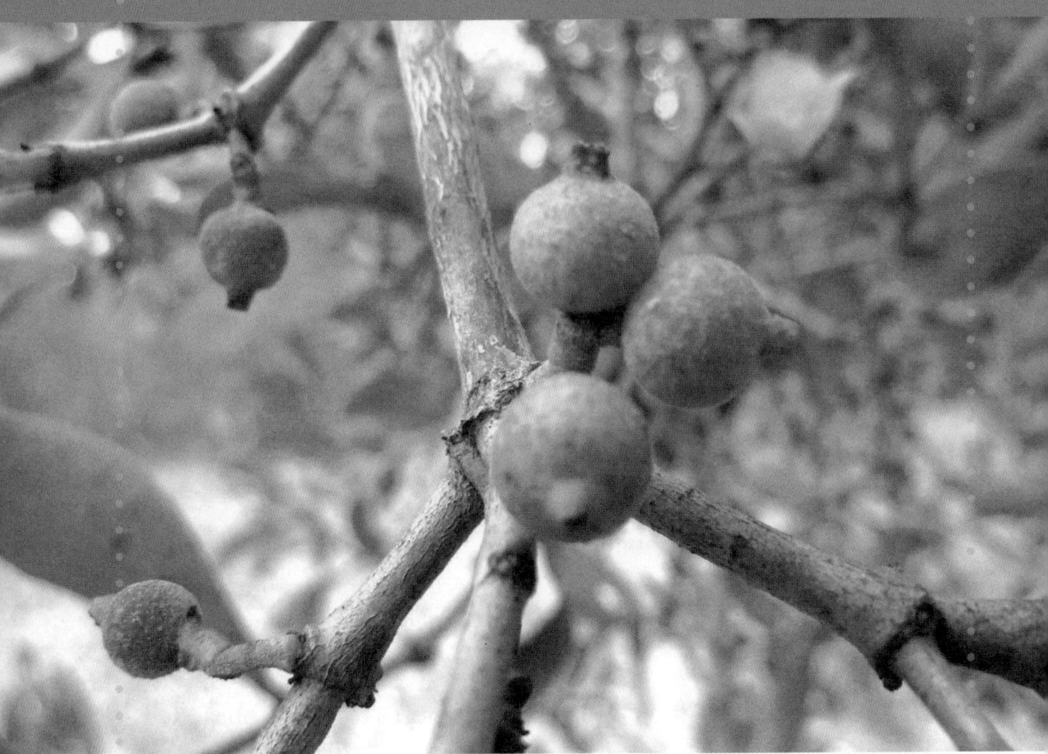

Scientific Name *Amyema villiflora* (Domin) Barlow, and *Amyema villiflora* (Domin) Barlow subsp. *villiflora*.

Common Name Mistletoe.

Aboriginal Name Nyil Nyil (Bardi) (Smith & Kalotas, 1985).

Field Notes This Mistletoe is a hemiparasitic, aerial shrub. It thick and fleshy, ovate leaf blades are up to 80 mm long and 40 mm wide, and sometimes pink to reddish on the upper surface. Its green-orange-red or yellow tubular flowers are borne in triads and are present between December and April. This mistletoe occurs on *Terminalia* and *Lysiphyllum* species in the Kimberley region of Western Australia, the Northern Territory and Queensland (ALA, 2022; ATRP, 2020; WAH, 2022).

Medicinal Uses Decoctions of the leaves of this Mistletoe are taken internally to treat the symptoms of colds and influenza (Wiynjorrotj et al., 2005).

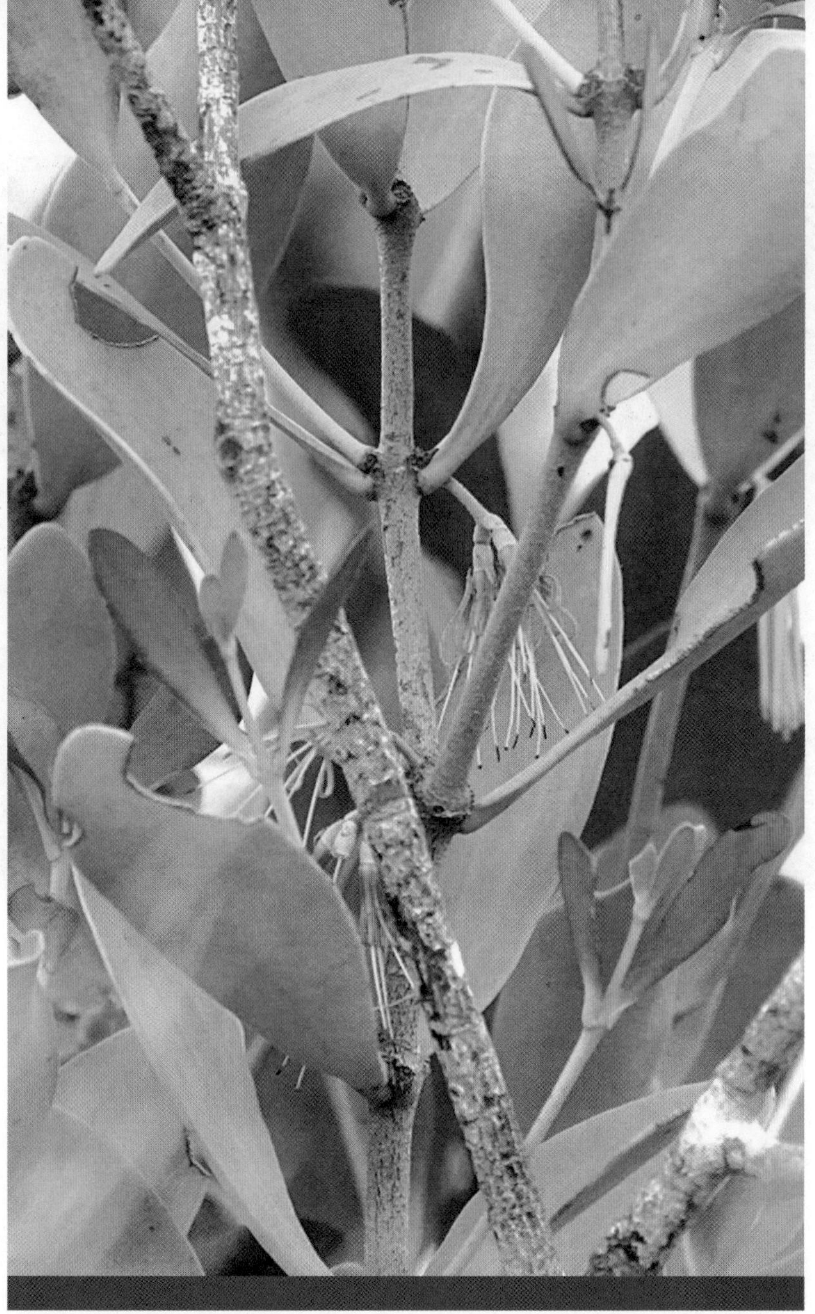

Other Uses The fruit of this mistletoe are edible when yellow and ripe (Wiynjorrotj et al., 2005).

Moonia

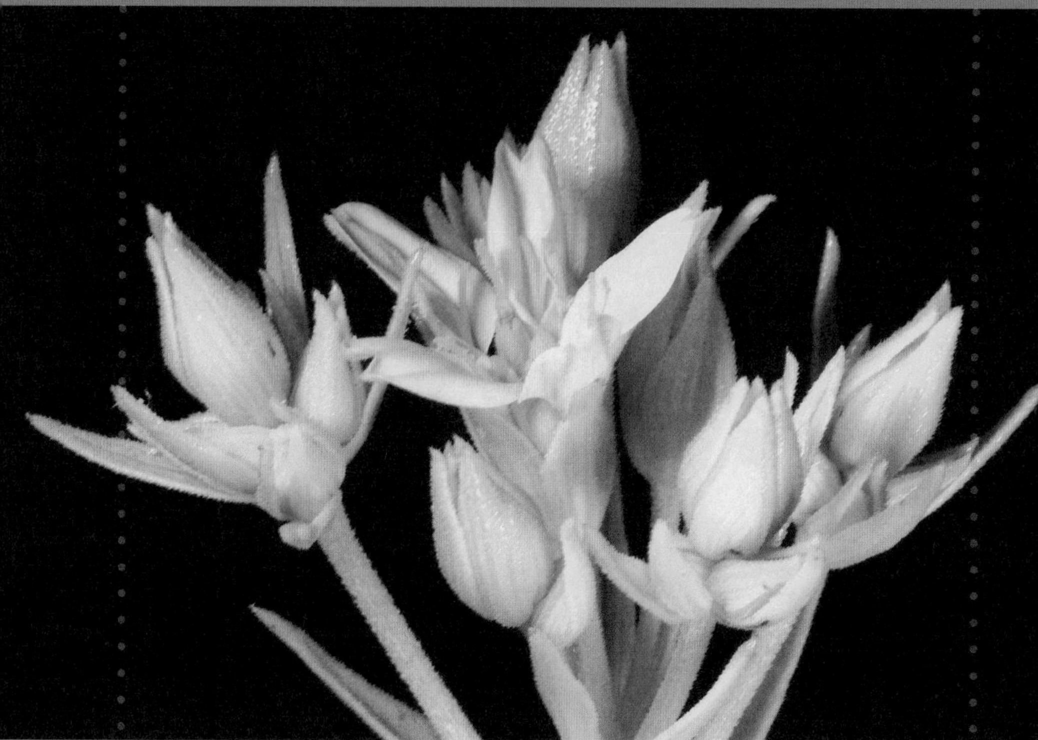

Scientific Name *Pentalepis trichodesmoides* F.Muell., also known as *Moonia trichodesmoides* (F.Muell.) Benth.

Common Name Moonia.

Aboriginal Name Walaaba (Bunuba) (Oscar et al., 2019).

Field Notes Moonia is an erect perennial herb or shrub that grows to around 1 m in height. It has short hairs on the upper stems and glossy, ovate leaves that are wider at the base. Its small, yellow flowers have five ovate petals. They appear in clusters between April and December. Moonia occurs in skeletal soils, sand and loam on stony grounds, along watercourses and near springs in the Pilbara and Kimberley regions of Western Australia and the western edge of the Northern Territory (ALA, 2022; Oscar et al., 2019; WAH, 2022).

Medicinal Uses Decoctions of the leaves and stems of Moonia were taken internally as a detoxifying drink. The same decoctions

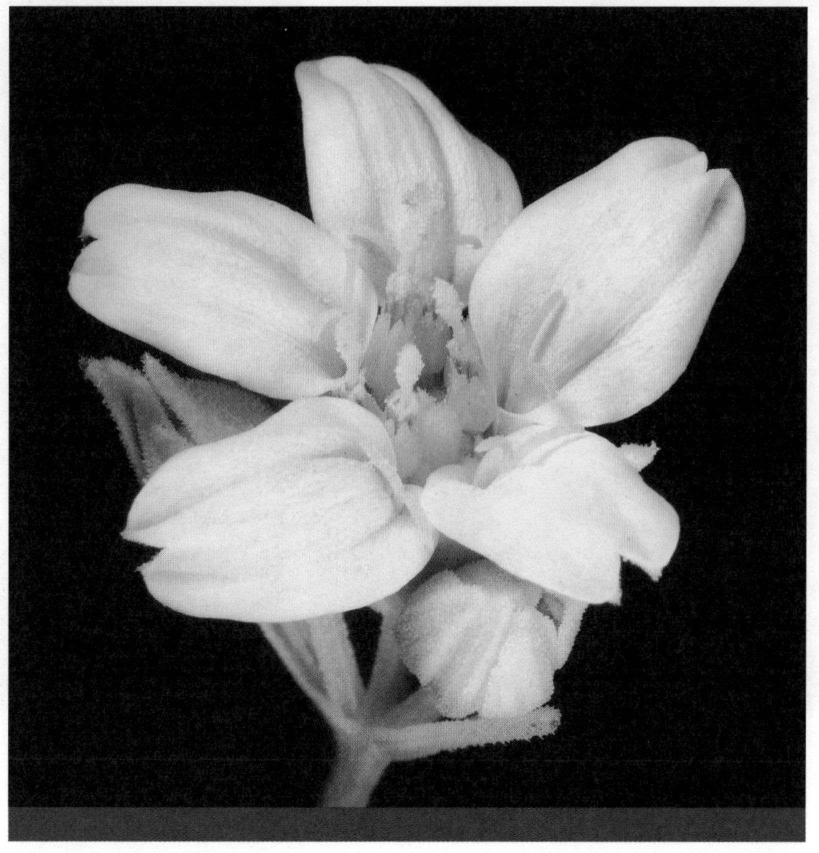

were also used externally as an antiseptic wash to treat skin sores and wounds (Oscar et al., 2019).

Musk Basil

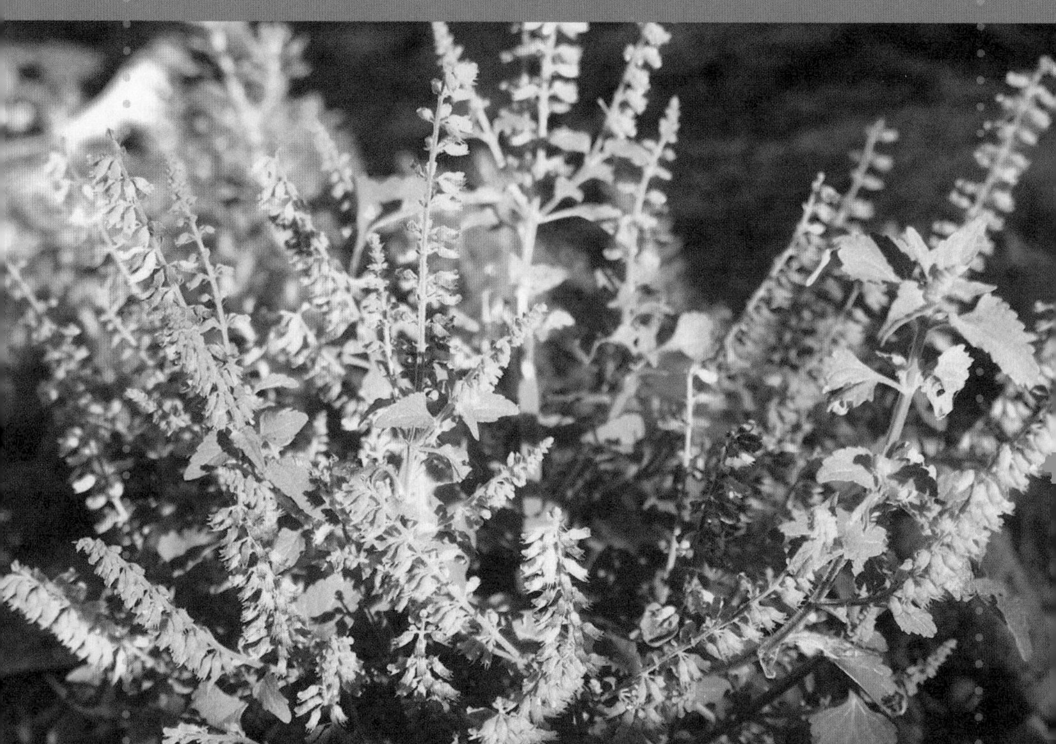

Scientific Name *Basilicum polystachyon* (L.) Moench.

Common Name Musk Basil.

Field Notes Musk Basil is an erect annual or perennial herb that grows up to 1.2 m in height. Its leaves are opposite, elliptic and up to 50 mm long. Its small, blue-purple or white flowers form in slender, loose, spike-like clusters from March to July in Western Australia. Its fruit are small, dry nuts. Musk Basil occurs in loam, sandy loam and clay on river and creek banks and in swampy areas across the top end of Australia from the Pilbara and Kimberley regions of Western Australia through to most of Queensland (Lassak & McCarthy, 2001; WAH, 2022). It also occurs in Africa, Borneo, China, India, Indochina, Madagascar, New Guinea, the Philippines, Saudi Arabia, southern Asia and various islands of the Pacific and Indian oceans (Fern, 2021).

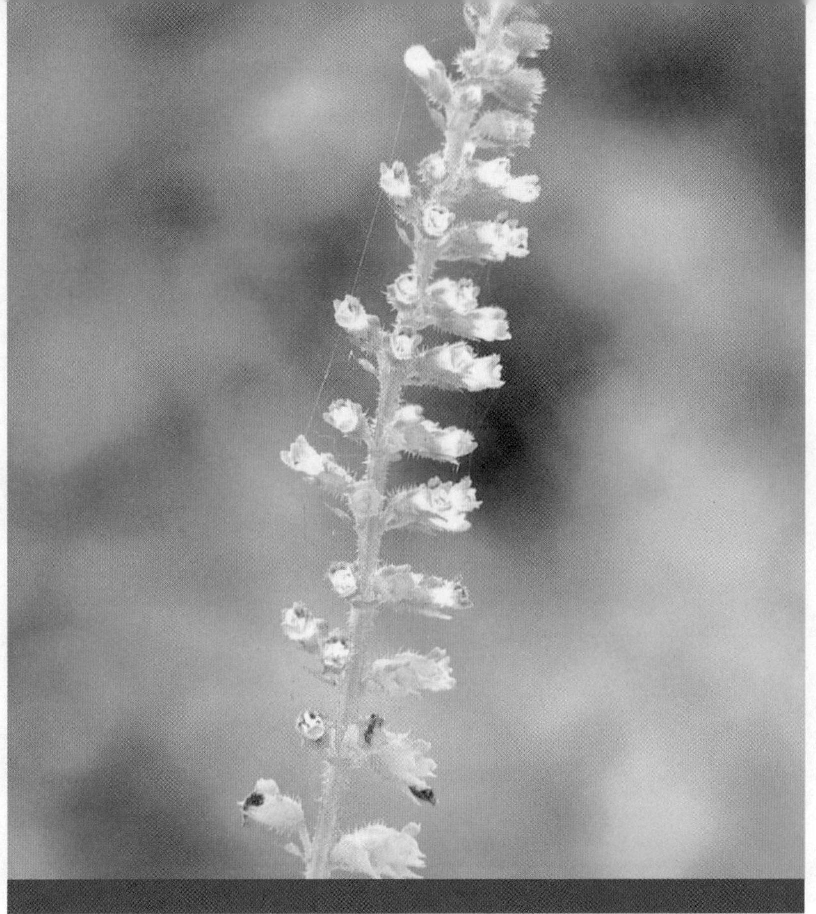

Medicinal Uses Infusions of the leaves, stems and flowers of Musk Basil were taken internally to treat fever (Cock, 2011; Lassak & McCarthy, 2001; Williams, 2010). In other countries, Musk Basil is used in folk medicine for a variety of complaints. Decoctions of the crushed leaves are taken internally as a sedative and used externally as a liniment to relieve painful sprains and limbs. Decoctions are also taken internally to treat epilepsy, palpitations, neuralgia, headaches, anxiety after childbirth and rheumatic pain. The fresh roots are chewed as a cough suppressant or cooked with food to reduce flatulence. Infusions of the fruit are taken internally for parturition in cases of delayed birth. Sap from the leaves is squeezed into the nostrils of children to cause sneezing in order to cure headache (Fern, 2021).

Other Uses Musk Basil is used in some Asian countries as a flavouring in food similar to Holy Basil (*Ocimum tenuiflorum*) (Fern, 2021).

Myrtle Mangrove

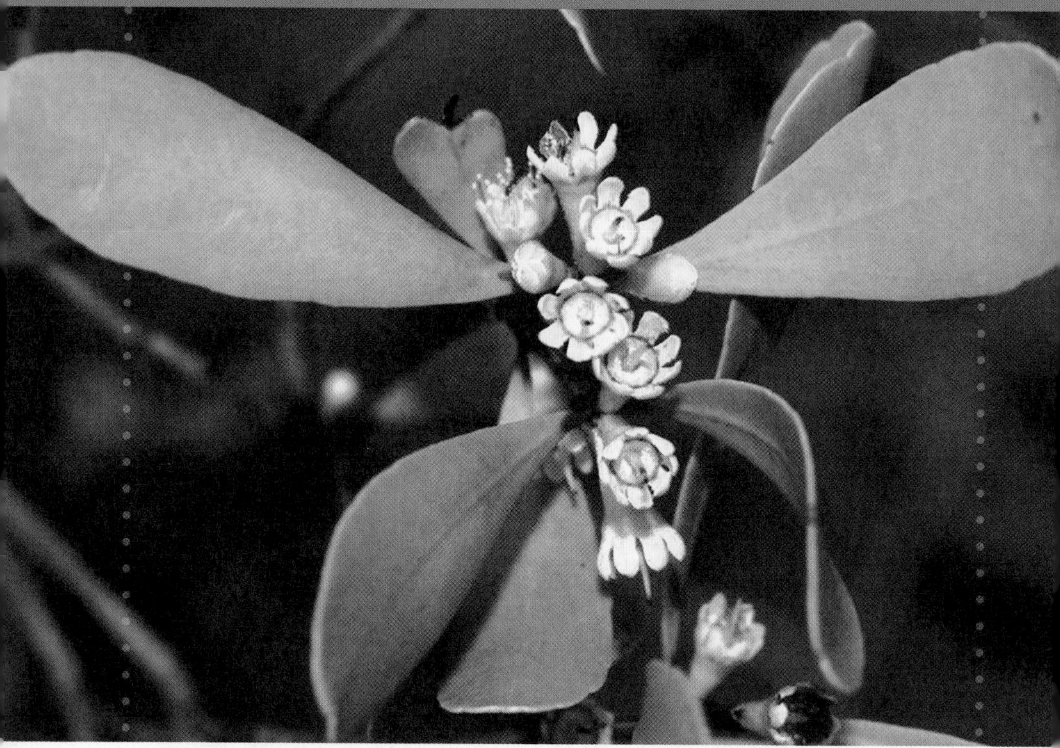

Scientific Name *Osbornia octodonta* F.Muell.

Common Name Myrtle Mangrove.

Aboriginal Names Darrngala (Wunambal, Gaambera) (Karadada et al., 2011), Alarga (Bardi) (Kenneally et al., 1996), Leiyini ninya, Limii ninya (Kwini) (Cheinmora et al., 2017).

Field Notes Myrtle Mangrove is a shrub or tree that grows up to 9 m in height. It has ovate leaves that are narrow at the base, and small, white, tubular flowers with eight tiny petals and long stamens that are present in Australia between December and April. Myrtle Mangrove occurs in sandy soils in coastal mangrove habitats around the northern coastline of Australia from the Pilbara and Kimberley regions of Western Australia almost to the Queensland border with New South Wales. It is also endemic to the island of Borneo, New Guinea and the Philippines (ALA, 2022; WAH, 2022).

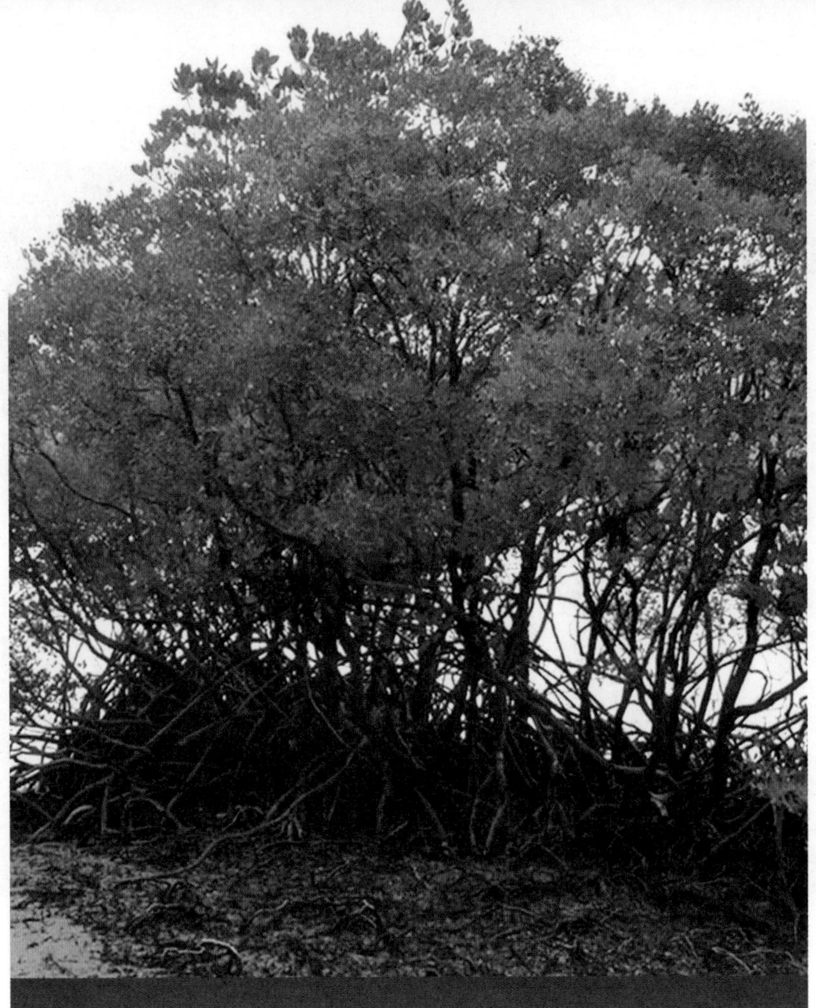

Medicinal Uses Decoctions of the leaves of Myrtle Mangrove were used as a body wash to treat general malaise and the symptoms of colds and influenza. The leaves were crushed and the vapours inhaled to clear the head. The leaves were boiled with ashes and the decoction applied externally to ease the pain of catfish stings (Edwards, 2005). The leaves were crushed and rubbed on the skin as an insect repellent. The leaves were chewed but not swallowed to ease the pain of toothache (Bancroft, n.d.).

Namana

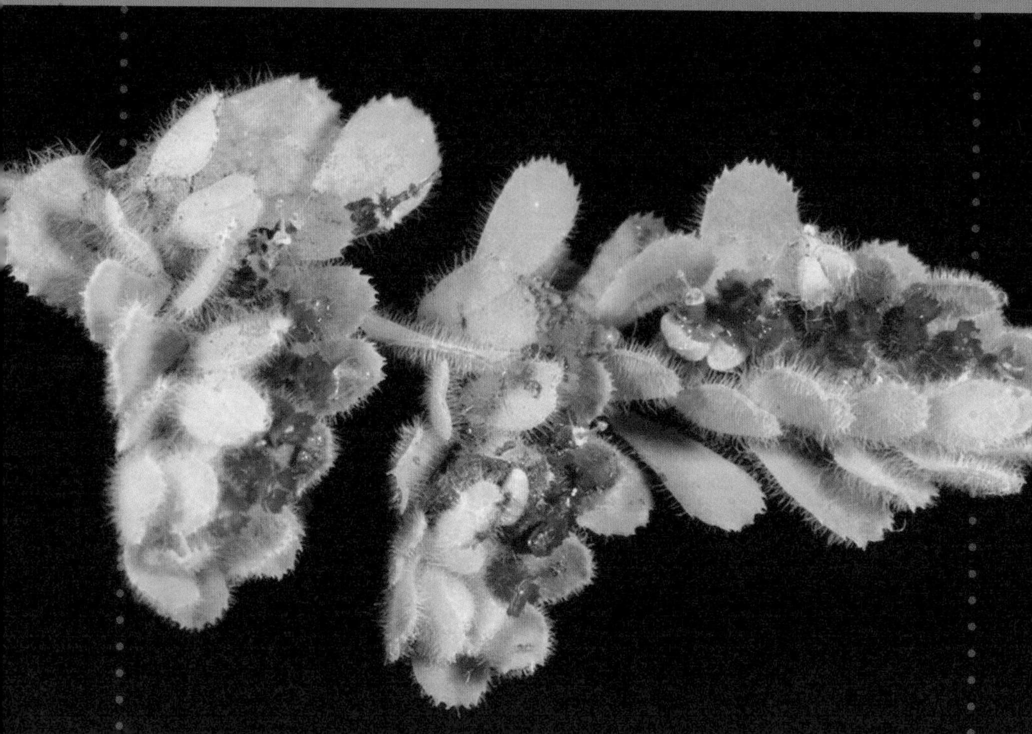

Scientific Name *Euphorbia australis* Boiss.

Common names Namana, Caustic Weed, Hairy Caustic Weed.

Aboriginal Name Puntipu (Kukatja) (Valiquette, 1993).

Field Notes Namana grows as a prostrate, annual or perennial herb with many woody, green or reddish branches up to 300 mm long and a woody tap root. Its small, ovate, hairy leaves have serrated edges. Its tiny red-pink flowers are present between April and November. Its fruit are hairy capsules. Namana is found in all mainland states of Australia except Victoria. In Western Australia, it is found mostly in the Gascoyne, Pilbara and Kimberley regions (ALA, 2022; eFlora.SA, 2022; Lassak & McCarthy, 2001; WAH, 2022).

Medicinal Uses Namana plants were crushed and the milky sap produced was rubbed into sores and wounds to aid healing. Alternatively, the sap was boiled with water and the decoction used as a wash for the same purpose. The sap was also used to treat

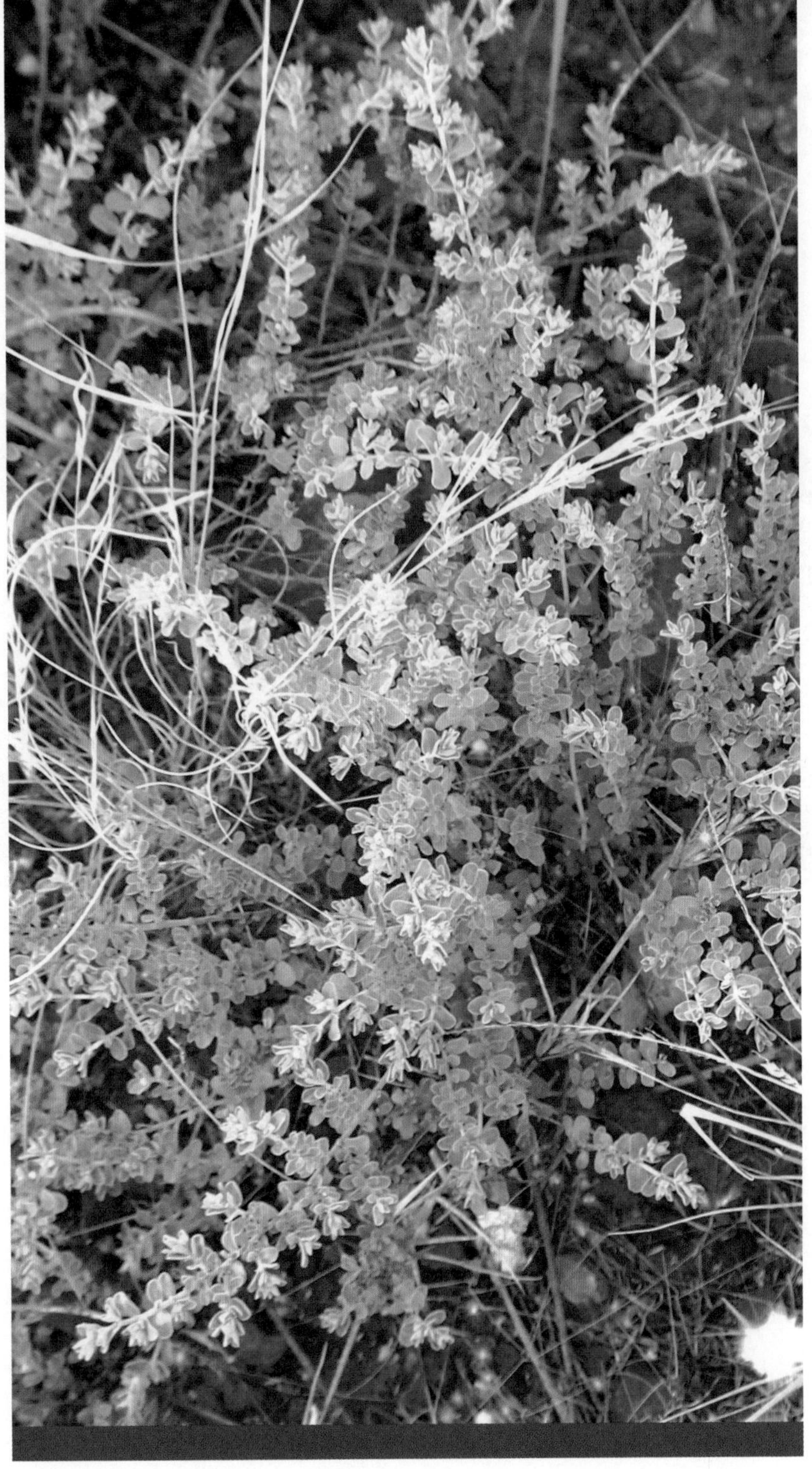

non-malignant skin cancers. The sap, when rubbed on the breast of nursing mothers, was thought to stimulate lactation (Cock, 2011; Lassak & McCarthy, 2001; Reid, 1986; YMAC, 2016).

Native Apple

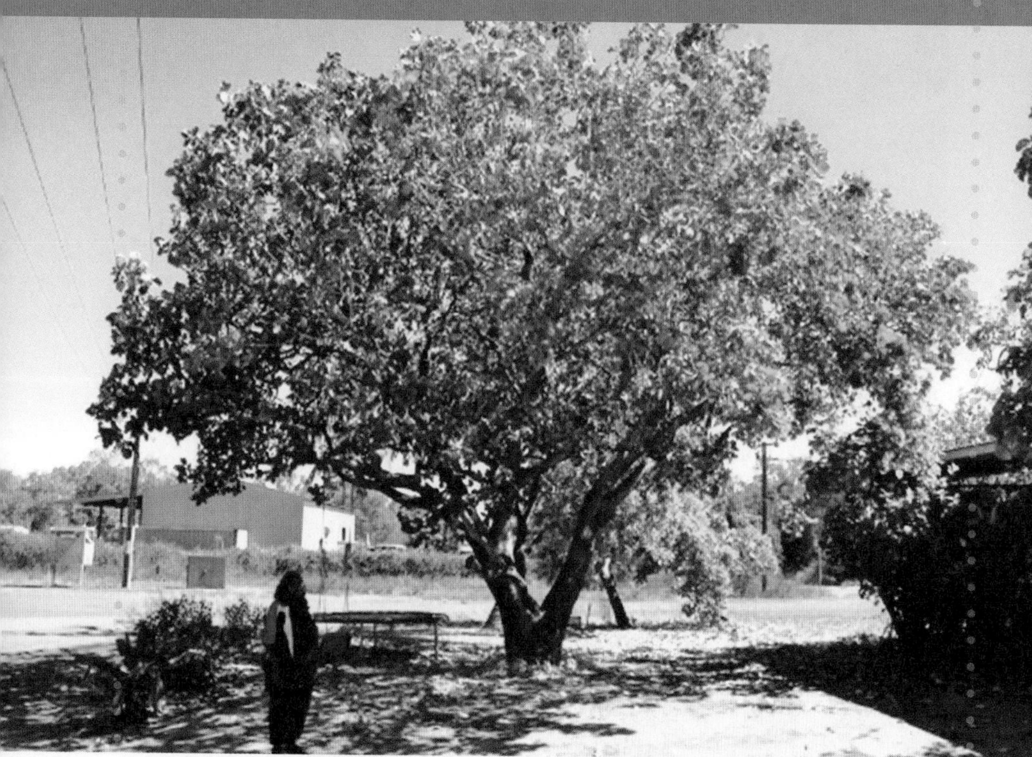

Scientific Name *Syzygium eucalyptoides* subsp. *bleeseri* (O.Schwarz) B.Hyland.

Common Names Native Apple, White Apple, White Bush Apple.

Aboriginal Names Ngarlirrgi (Wunambal, Gaambera) (Karadada et al., 2011), Lilarr (Bardi) (Vigilante et al., 2013), Dingarla minya (Kwini) (Cheinmora et al., 2017).

Field Notes Native Apple is an evergreen shrub or tree that grows up to 10 m in height. Its bark is usually smooth and grey to brown. Its leaves are circular to elliptic, ovate or obovate and up to 150 mm long by 23 mm wide. Its cream to white fluffy flowers appear from August to November. Its globular, reddish-cream fruit are approximately 40 mm in diameter. Fruiting occurs between November and February. Each fruit contains a single seed. Native Apple is found in alluvium or sand along watercourses in the northernmost part of the Kimberley region of Western Australia, the far north of the Northern Territory and the Cape York Peninsula in

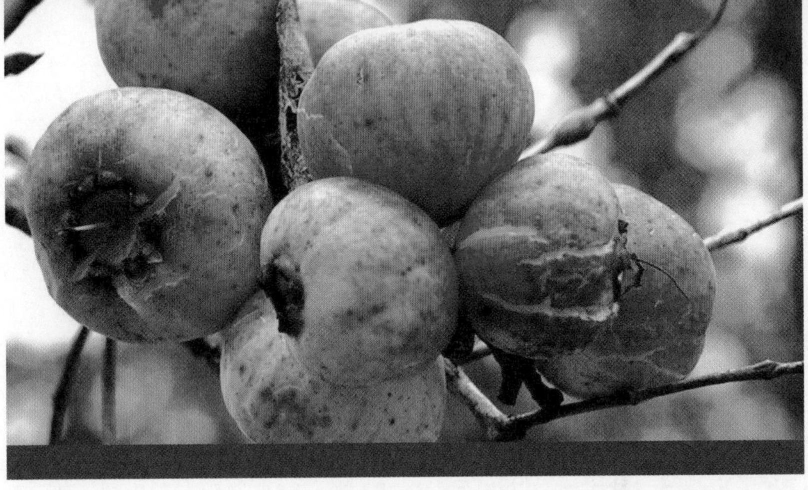

Far North Queensland (ALA, 2022; Fruitipedia, 2022; WAH, 2022).

Medicinal Uses The fruit of the Native Apple are high in ascorbic acid (vitamin C) and were chewed to cure a sore throat or as a cough suppressant (Edwards, 2005).

Other Uses The fruit of the Native Apple are edible and are eaten raw when white and ripe. The fruit are available between September and November and are usually collected from the ground (Cheinmora et al., 2017; Fox & Garde, 2018; Glasby, 2018; Karadada et al., 2011; Kenneally et al., 1996; Vigilante et al., 2013).

Native Bryony

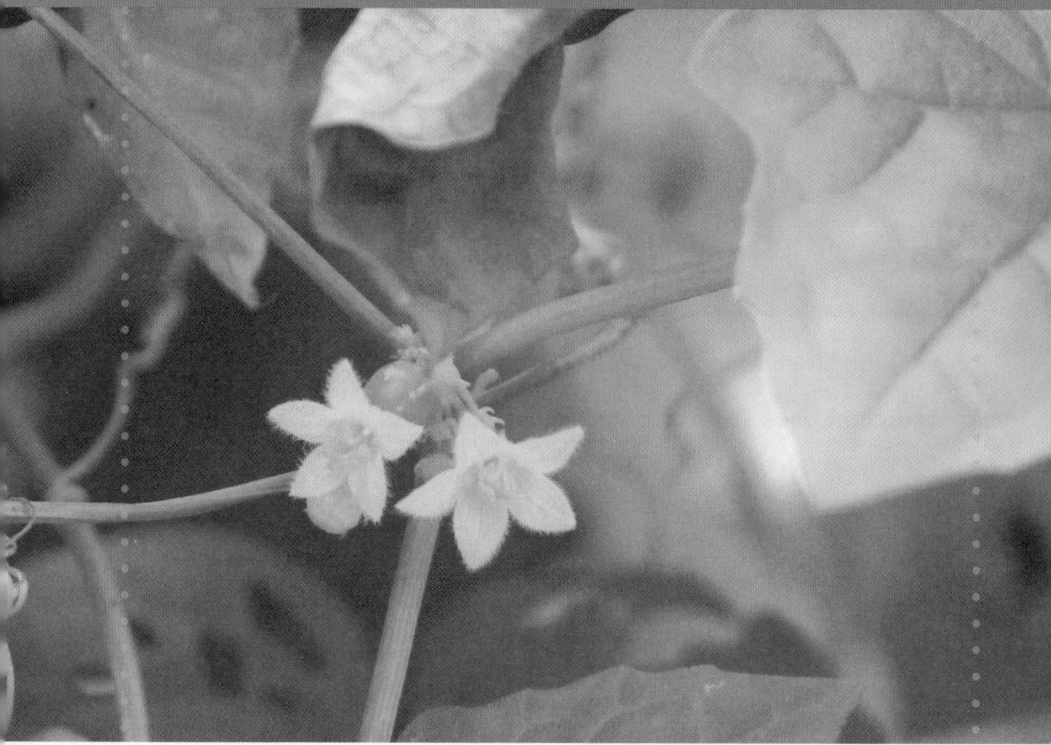

Scientific Name *Diplocyclos palmatus* (L.) C.Jeffrey.

Common Names Native Bryony, Red-striped Cucumber, Striped Cucumber, Snakeberry.

Field Notes Native Bryony is a perennial climbing vine with branches up to 5 m in length. Its leaves are mid-green and palmately lobed. Its yellow-cream, star-shaped flowers have five petals and are present in Australia from March to April. Its fruit are globose, red with white stripes when ripe and up to 50 mm in diameter. Native Bryony occurs on coastal flats in vine thickets in the northern Kimberley region of Western Australia, the Northern Territory, the Cape York Peninsula and down the east coast to the northern coast of New South Wales (ALA, 2022; WAH, 2022). It also occurs in the tropical areas of Africa, India and South-east Asia, including Indonesia and New Guinea (Fern, 2021).

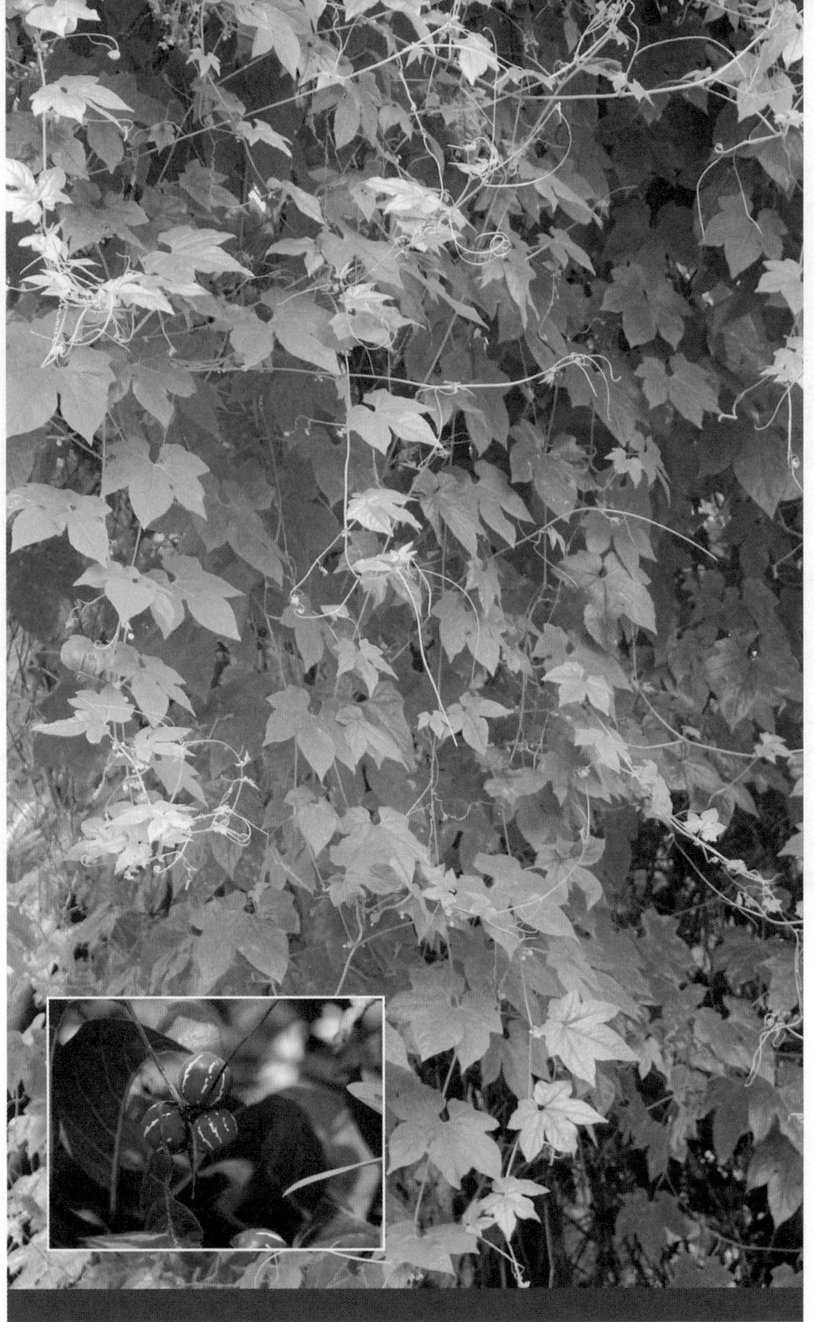

Medicinal Uses The fruit of Native Bryony were crushed and the pulp rubbed on the skin to treat fungal infections such as dermatophytosis (ringworm and athlete's foot) (Packer et al., 2012).

Native Coleus

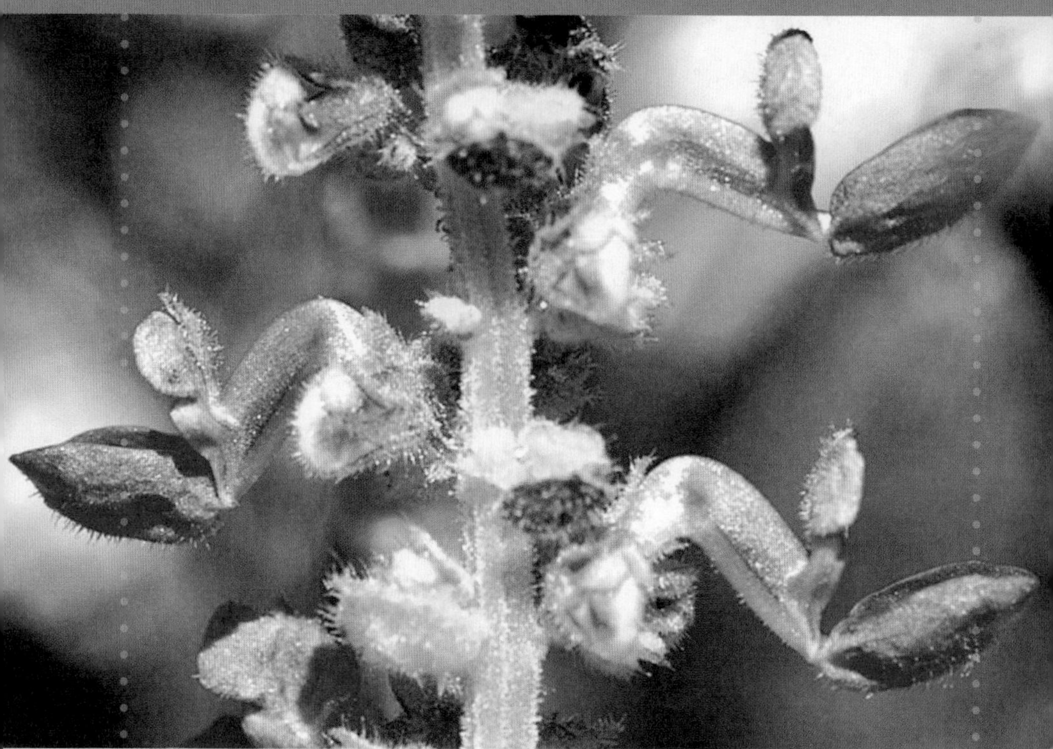

Scientific Name *Coleus congestus* (R.Br.) A.J.Paton, previously known as *Plectranthus congestus* R.Br.

Common Name Native Coleus.

Field Notes Native Coleus is an erect annual or perennial shrub that grows to 1.5 m in height. Its leaf blades are ovate and up to 80 mm long by 60 mm wide with hairs on both sides. Its blue flowers form in dense clusters, which form false spikes. Flowering in Australia is from April to July. Native Coleus occurs along watercourses in the Kimberley region of Western Australia and the east coast of northern Queensland. It also occurs in the Louisiade Islands, New Guinea and Timor (ALA, 2022; ATRP, 2020; Fern, 2021; WAH, 2022).

Medicinal Uses Crushed leaves of Native Coleus were applied to wounds as an antiseptic poultice. The sap from crushed leaves was

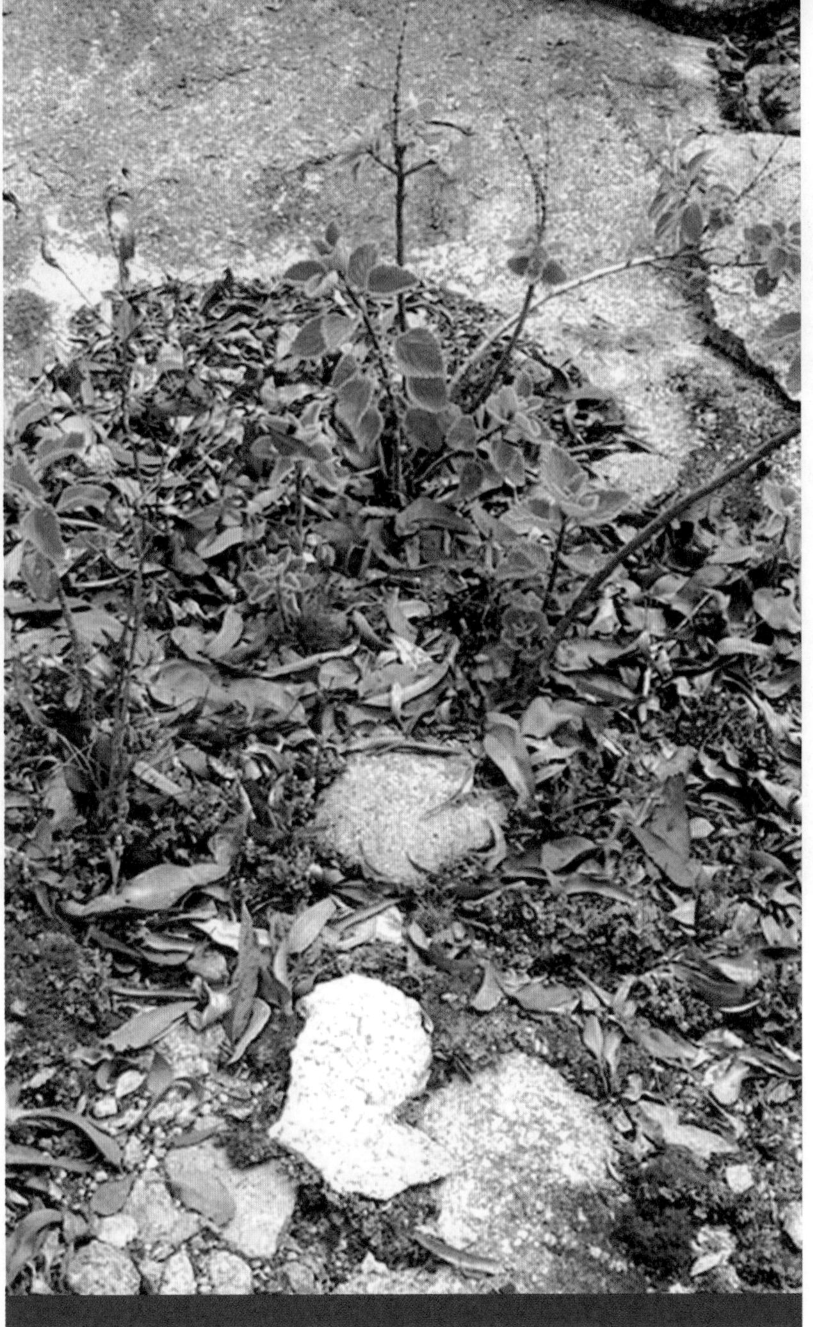

applied to wounds and sores to aid the healing process, and the skin to treat scabies infestations (Fern, 2021; Williams, 2013).

Native Cowpea

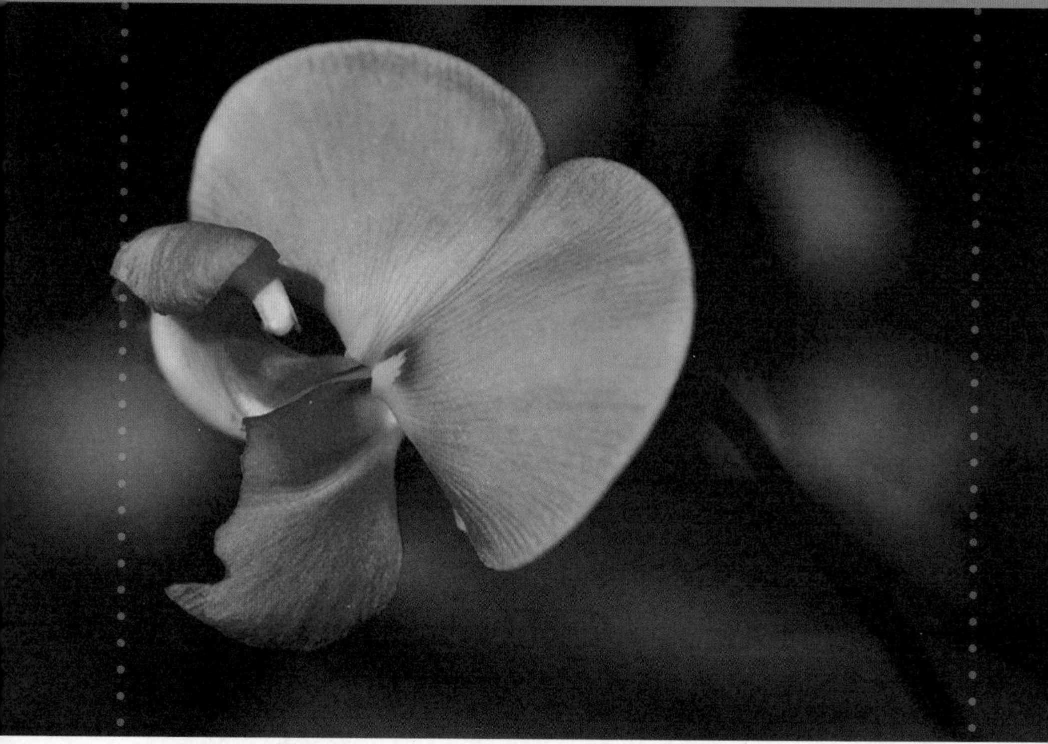

Scientific Name *Vigna vexillata* (L.) A.Rich.

Common Names Native Cowpea, Wild Cowpea, Zombi Pea, Bush Carrot.

Aboriginal Names Irrilm, Aanyjoo (Bardi) (Kenneally et al., 1996), Wanarrji (Gija) (Purdie et al., 2018), Bungga (Jaru) (Wightman, 2003), Ngalangka ninya (Kwini) (Cheinmora et al., 2017).

Field Notes Native Cowpea is a small prostrate or climbing perennial plant rising annually from a perennial rootstock. Its stems can be up to 6 m long. It has trifoliate, narrow leaflets with elongated tips. Its purple, blue or yellow pea-shaped flowers appear between February and June. Its fruit are narrow, cylindrical pods that can be up to 140 mm long. Native Cowpea is found in loamy soils in the Kimberley region of Western Australia, the Northern Territory and the east coast of Queensland and New South Wales (ALA, 2022; Fern, 2021; Native Plants Queensland, 2022; WAH, 2022). Native Cowpea is pantropical and occurs in

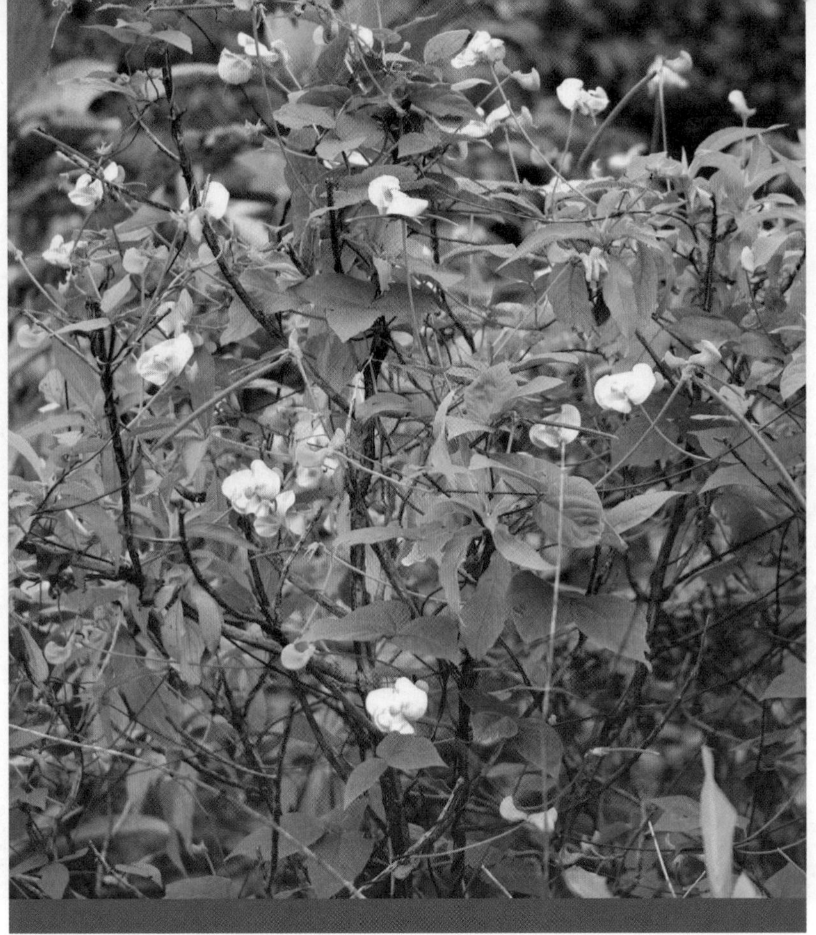

many Asian and South-east Asian countries, including India and Pakistan (Fern, 2021).

Medicinal Uses The roots of Native Cowpea were used as a mild laxative and were eaten to treat constipation (ANBG, 2000; Cock, 2011; Low, 1990).

Other Uses The tubers of the Native Cowpea are edible and were eaten raw or after they had been lightly roasted in hot ashes. The tubers, which are usually harvested in February and March, are reported to have a soft, creamy, tasty flesh and are particularly rich in protein (Cheinmora et al., 2017; Edwards, 2005; Fox & Garde, 2018; Kenneally et al., 1996; Purdie et al., 2018; Vigilante et al., 2013; Wightman, 2003). The young leaves and young pods are also edible and are eaten as a vegetable (Edwards, 2005). The seeds are edible also and are eaten as a pulse in India (Fox & Garde, 2018; Fern, 2021).

Native Fig

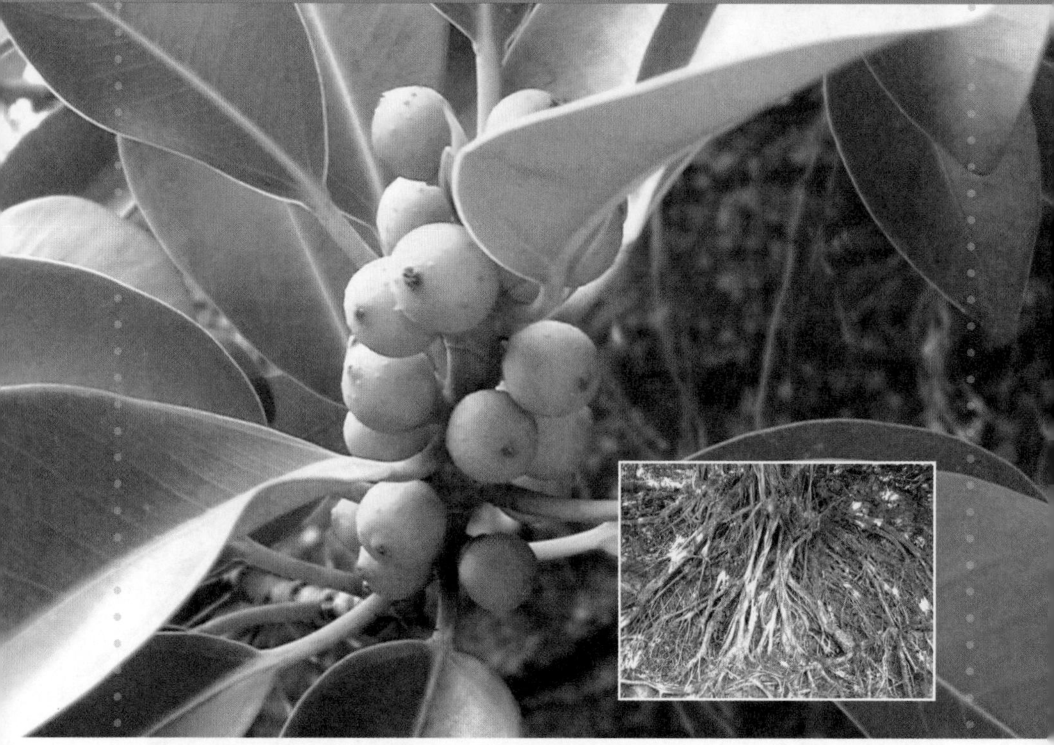

Scientific Name *Ficus platypoda* (Miq.) Miq., previously known as *Ficus leucotricha* (Miq.) Miq.

Common Names Native Fig, Desert Fig, Rock Fig.

Aboriginal Names Biyinyji (Bunuba) (Oscar et al., 2019), Guray, Gurir (Bardi) (Smith & Kalotas, 1985), Marrapanti, Ngilimirnti (Walmajarri) (Richards & Hudson, 2012), Binjili (Gaambera) (Karadada et al., 2011), Barramanbi (Wunambal) (Vigilante et al., 2013), Banggoornji, Banggoonji (Gija) (Purdie et al., 2018), Wijilgi, Wijirrgi (Jaru) (Deegan et al., 2010), Djamudet (Miwa) (Kimberley Specialists, 2020), Lakoorroo (Nyikina) (Young et al., 2012), Banggirndi (Gooniyandi) (Dilkes-Hall et al., 2019), Maraparnti, Wijirrki (Ngardi) (Cataldi, 2004), Mangaripinti, Witjirrki (Kukatja) (Valiquette, 1993), Binjili manya, Binjeli manya (Kwini) (Cheinmora et al., 2017; Crawford, 1982).

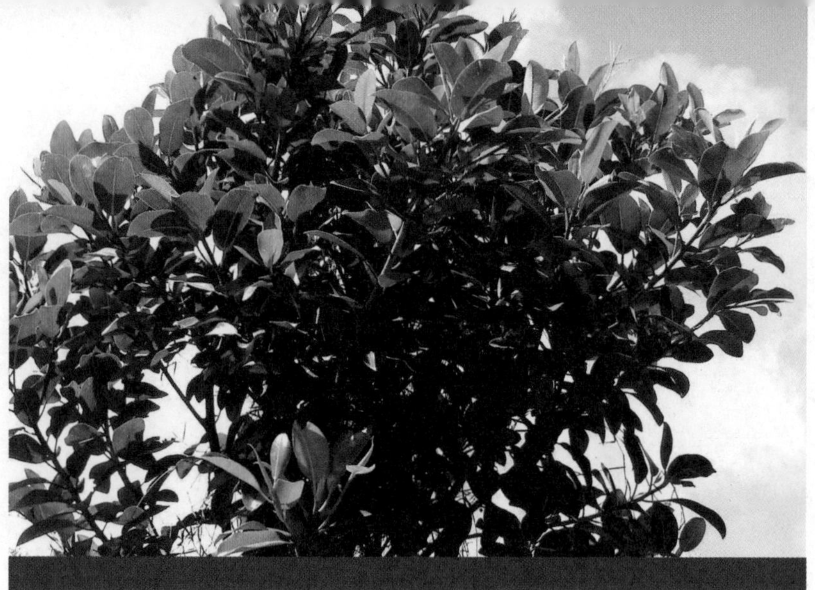

Field Notes Native Fig is a monoecious, lithophytic shrub or tree that grows up to 9 m in height. It has a finely textured grey bark and its branchlets are covered with fine hairs. Its leaves are alternate, elliptical to ovate and up to 160 mm long by 133 mm wide. Its male flowers appear between April and October and are dispersed among the fruitlets when the figs are ripe. Its tiny, hard globular fruit are about the size of marbles. Native fig occurs in sand, alluvium and loam over limestone, sandstone and granite on cliffs, hills, screes, uplands and granite rock pockets in the Pilbara and Kimberley regions of Western Australia, the Northern Territory, and Far North Queensland around the Gulf of Carpentaria (ALA, 2022; ATRP, 2020; WAH, 2022).

Medicinal Uses Old dry fruit were ground into a paste and mixed with water, which was eaten to treat indigestion, heartburn, stomach ache and diarrhoea (Smith, 1991). Kwini women used to put the sap on their breasts to stimulate lactation (Cheinmora et al., 2017).

Other Uses The fruit of the Native Fig are edible and were eaten raw when they were red and ripe between May and August. Old dry fruit that fell to the ground were collected and kept for a later date, either intact or ground to a paste and made into cakes (Cheinmora et al., 2017; Crawford, 1982; Kenneally et al., 1996; Low, 1991; Maiden, 1889; Oscar et al., 2019; Smith, 1991; Wightman, 2003).

Native Fuchsia

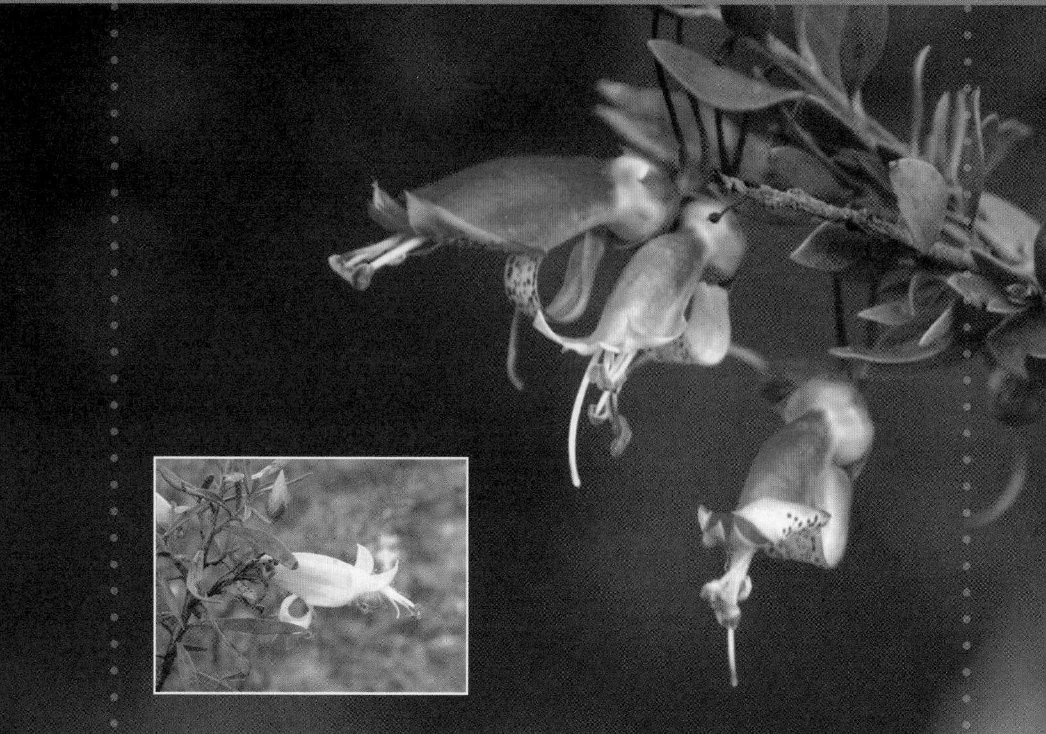

Scientific Name *Eremophila maculata* (Ker Gawl.) F.Muell.

Common Names Native Fuchsia, Spotted Emu Bush, Spotted Fuchsia Bush.

Aboriginal Names Wagila (Jaru) (Wightman, 2003), Mutarntilpa, Ngularnpa (Kukatja) (Valiquette, 1993), Wakila (Ngardi) (Cataldi, 2004).

Field Notes Native Fuchsia is a shrub that rarely grows over 3 m in height. Its glabrous, almost thread-like to almost circular leaves are up to 45 mm long and 18 mm wide. Its spotted, tubular flowers range in colour from red-pink to orange-yellow. Flowering is from May to November. Its fruit consist of four chambers, each containing one or more seeds. Native Fuchsia occurs in red sand, clay or sandy loam, on salt flats, claypans, floodplains, along watercourses and drainage lines, and in seasonally wet depressions. It is endemic to the southern reaches of the Kimberley

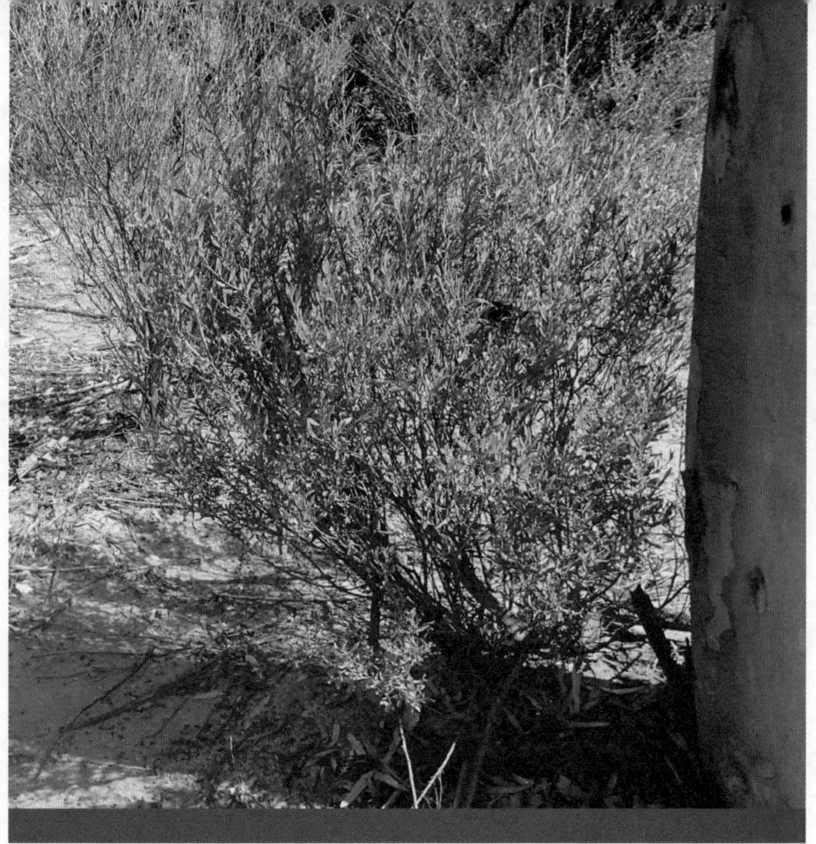

and most of mainland Australia except the far south-west, the far north-west and the Cape York Peninsula (ALA, 2022; ANPSA, 2022; WAH, 2022).

Medicinal Uses The Gija (or Kija) place leaves and twigs of Native Fuchsia over hot coals in a hole in the ground. A person with diarrhoea then puts their stomach over the steaming leaves and twigs, and the steam from them relieves their symptoms and the pain (Deegan et al., 2010; Wightman, 2003). Decoctions of the leaves and stems were used externally as a wash to bathe skin conditions, wounds and sores (Local Land Services Western Region, 2016). The vapours from crushed leaves were inhaled to clear the nasal passages (Australian Native Edible & Medicinal Seed Service, n.d.). The Ngardi used the leaves and stems for 'smoke medicine' to ease the symptoms of colds and influenza (Cataldi, 2004).

Other Uses The Gija often place leaves and twigs from Native Fuchsia in a campfire overnight to keep mosquitoes at bay (Wightman, 2003).

Native Hibiscus

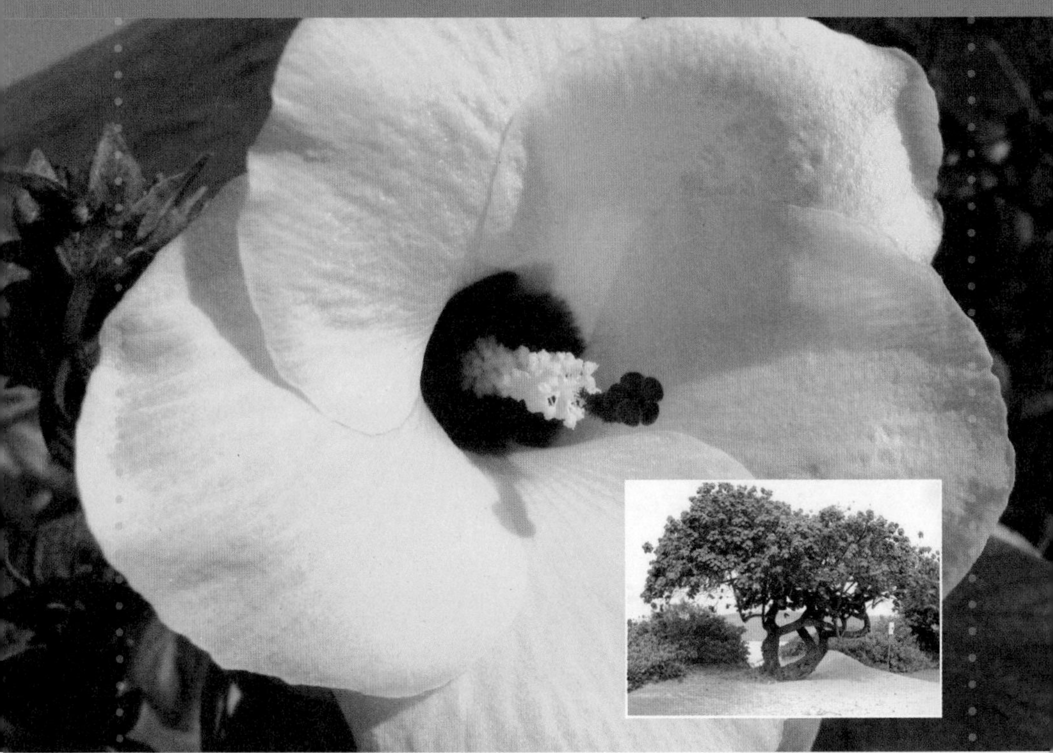

Scientific Name *Hibiscus tiliaceus* L.

Common Names Native Hibiscus, Beach Hibiscus, Coast Hibiscus, Coastal Cottonwood, Cotton Tree, Majagua, Coast Cottonwood, Cottonwood Hibiscus, Gatapa, Green Cottonwood, Sea Hibiscus, Native Rosella.

Aboriginal Names Laba (Wunambal, Gaambera) (Karadada et al., 2011), Yirulumal minya, Yurrurrumarl minya (Kwini) (Cheinmora et al., 2017).

Field Notes Native Hibiscus is a spreading tree that grows up to 5 m in height. It has large, heart-shaped leaves that are downy underneath, and bright yellow, round Hibiscus-type flowers with maroon centres that only last for one day before they fall. Flowering is in August in Western Australia. Its fruit are globose capsules about 25 mm long, with kidney-shaped seeds. Native Hibiscus occurs in swamps, in margins of saline coastal plains and pindan plains around the top coast of Australia, from the far north of the Kimberley region of Western Australia, the Northern Territory, the Torres Strait Islands, the Cape York Peninsula and down the east coast as far as Botany Bay (ALA, 2022; Medicinal Plants in Singapore, 2019; WAH, 2022). The plant is widespread throughout the tropics and subtropics of the world (ATRP, 2020).

Medicinal Uses In Australia, the slimy sap from the mucilaginous bark of Native Hibiscus was used as an antiseptic on cuts and other wounds to aid healing (Cock, 2011; Devanesen, 2000; Hiddins, 2001; MRCCC, 2020; Slockee, 2019). In Far North Queensland, decoctions of the leaves were used to bathe stingray stings (Edwards, 2005). Some Aboriginal groups applied a poultice of warmed leaves to leg ulcers and wounds to aid the healing process (Hiddins, 2001). Native Hibiscus is used in folk medicine in other countries. In the Philippines, infusions of the bark are taken internally to treat diarrhoea and dysentery. In other parts of the South Pacific, infusions of the leaves are used to aid in the delivery of a child. Infusions of the leaves are taken internally to treat postpartum discharges, coughs and sore throats. Leaves are ground into a paste, which is applied to sores, cuts, open wounds, boils and swellings to aid healing. Infusions of the leaves, roots and bark are taken internally for fever (Fern, 2021).

Other Uses The flowers and young leaves are edible raw or cooked as a vegetable (Hiddins, 2001). Maiden (1889) recounts that, 'The late M. Thozet says the aborigines (sic) of Central Queensland prize the root of this tree very much for food, and, in times of scarcity, eat the tops, which taste like sorrel'. The Kwini use the inner bark of Native Hibiscus to make cordage and use the straight branches to make fire sticks. They also use the long, straight branches to make fishing spear shafts (Cheinmora et al., 2017).

Native Lasiandra

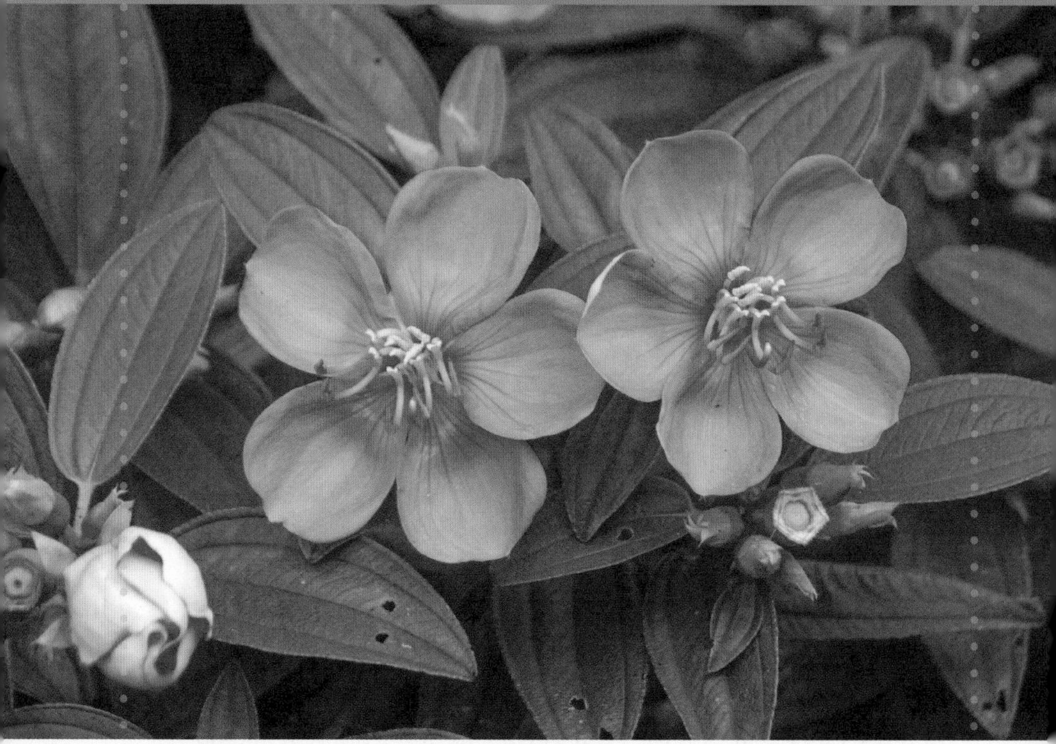

Scientific Name *Melastoma affine* D.Don., previously known as *Melastoma polyanthum* Blume.

Common Names Native Lasiandra, Blue Tongue.

Field Notes Native Lasiandra is an evergreen shrub growing up to 3 m in height. Its ovate leaves are covered in fine hairs, have longitudinal veins, and are up to 120 mm long and 40 mm wide. Its flowers occur on the ends of branchlets and are purple with five petals and sepals. In Australia, flowering is between May and November or January. Its fruit are small, black berries that appear straight after flowering. Native Lasiandra occurs in damp loam and rocky soils along creek beds, in wet-sclerophyll and rainforest habitats in the Kimberley region of Western Australia, the Northern Territory and down the east coast of Queensland and into New South Wales. It also occurs in India, Indonesia and Malaysia (ALA, 2022; Low, 1991; WAH, 2022).

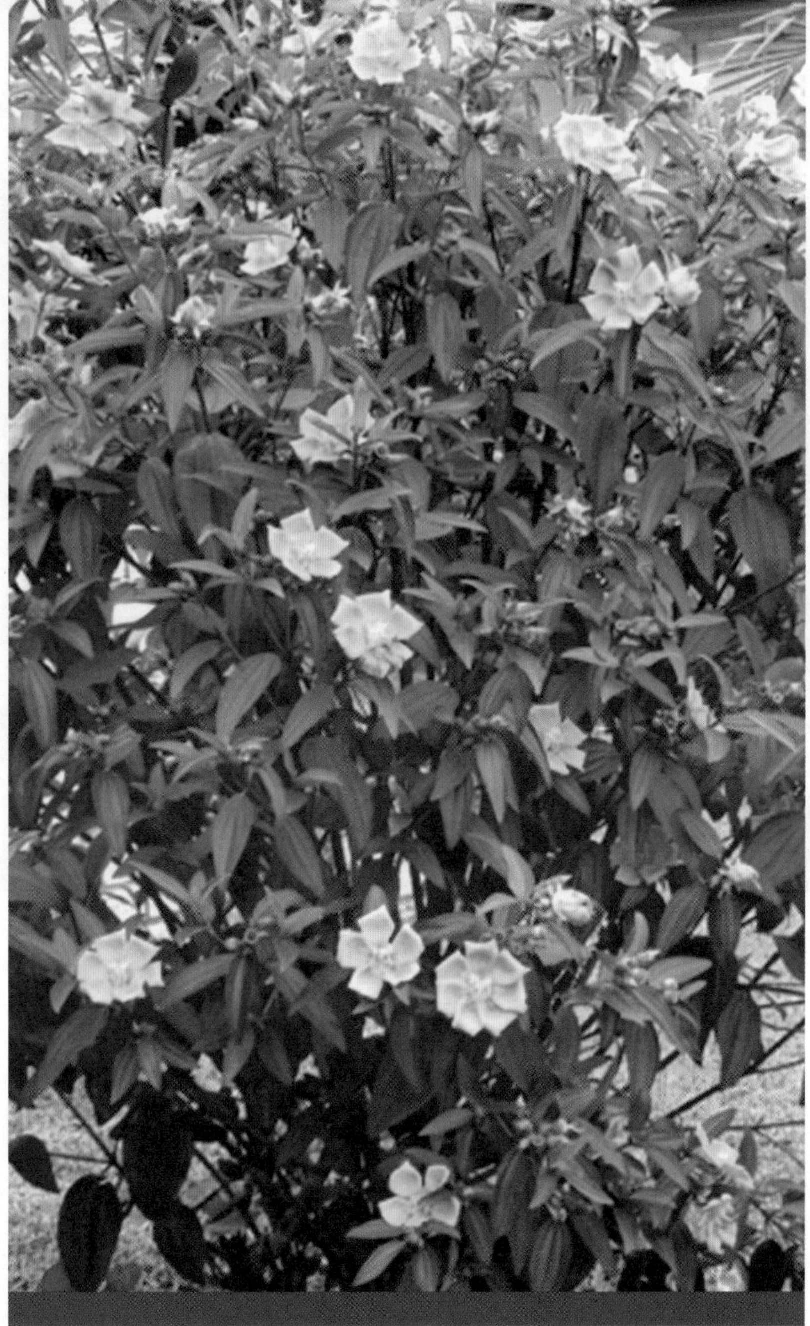

Medicinal Uses Decoctions of the leaves of Native Lasiandra were taken internally to treat diarrhoea and dysentery (Bailey, 1881).

Other Uses The berries of Native Lasiandra are edible but they stain the mouth, hence the common name 'Blue Tongue'. They are best eaten fresh straight off the tree (Australian Plants Society SA Region, 2022; Fox & Garde, 2018; Low, 1991; RFCA, 1993).

Native Myrtle

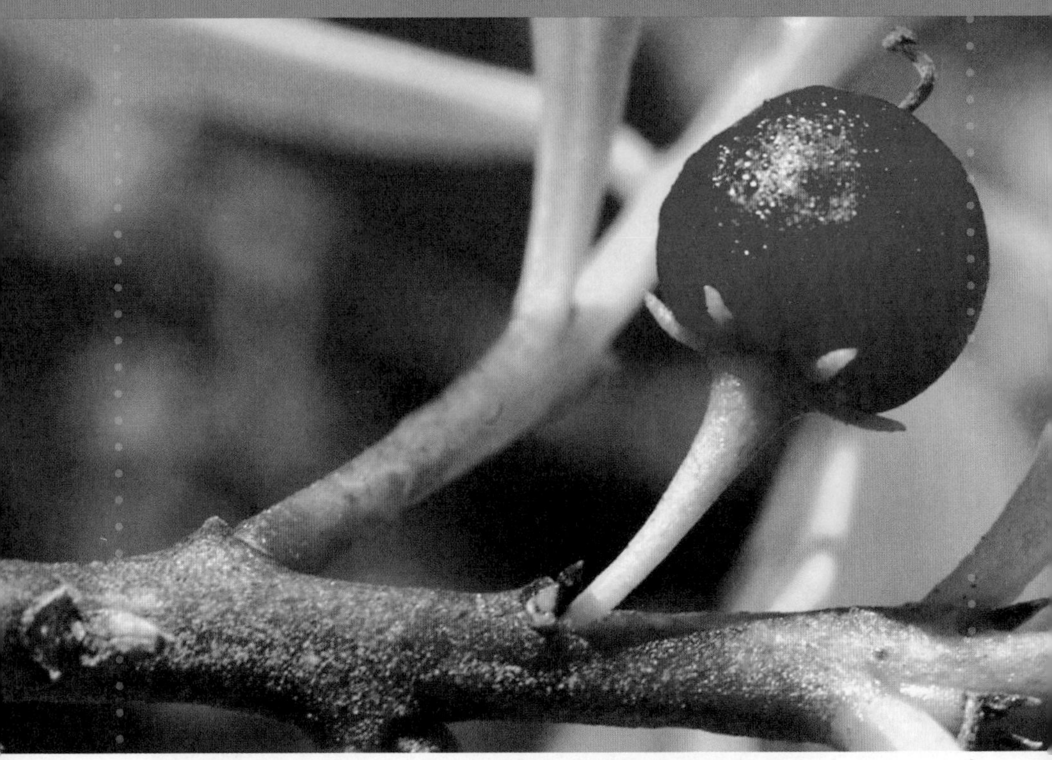

Scientific Name *Myoporum montanum* R.Br.

Common Names Native Myrtle, Water Bush, Boomeralla, Native Daphne, Western Boobialla.

Aboriginal Names Arninji (Wunambal, Gaambera) (Karadada et al., 2011), Madarrgoony (Gija) (Purdie et al., 2018).

Field Notes Native Myrtle grows as a spreading, much-branched shrub or tree up to 4 m in height. It has thin, green, lanceolate leaves and white, bell-shaped flowers with purple spots near the centre that appear from May to December. The fruit of the Native Myrtle are ovoid berries that are purple when ripe and up to 7 mm in diameter. Native Myrtle is found over most of mainland Australia except for the extremely arid areas (ALA, 2022; WAH, 2022).

Medicinal Uses Tuckerbush (2020) reports with reference to Native Myrtle, 'In Aboriginal culture the berries were eaten, the gum used for glue, and other parts of the plant used medicinally as a tonic,

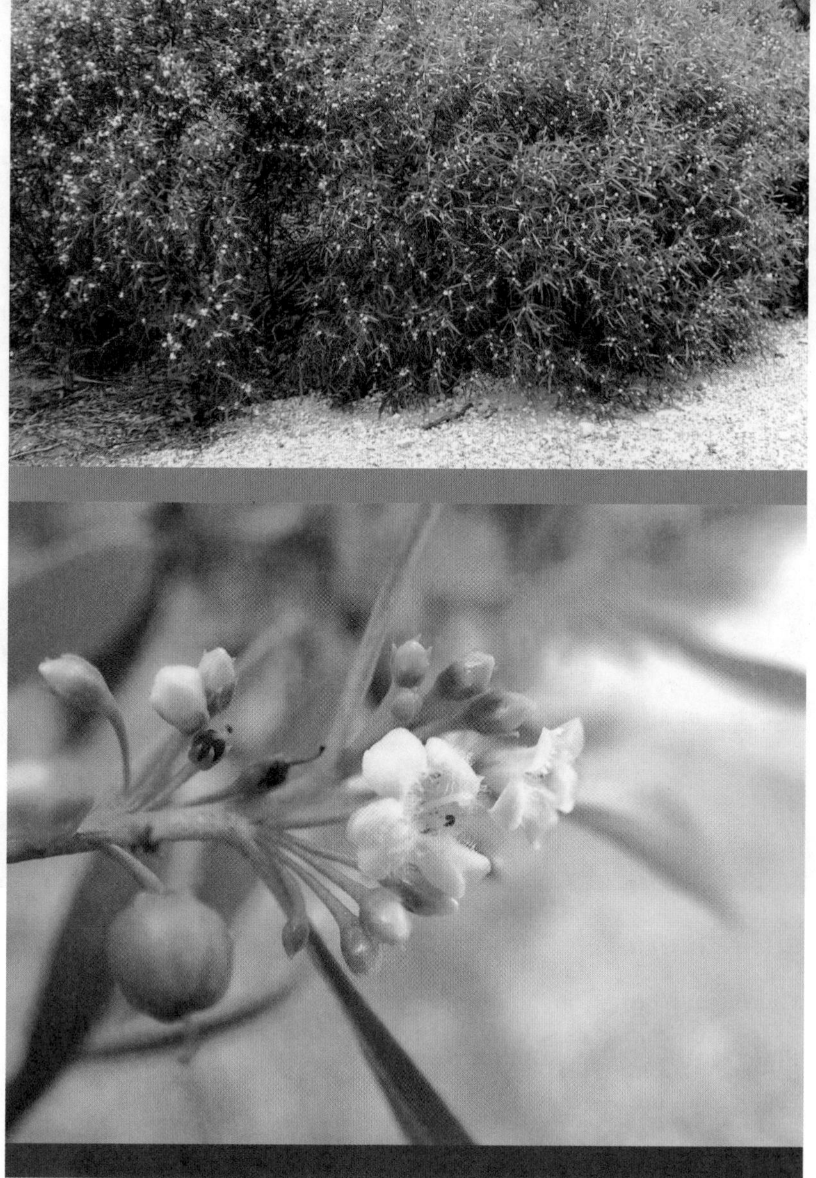

laxative, headache remedy and rheumatism treatment', but does not elaborate on which parts of the plant were used medicinally or the method of preparation. Coppin (2008) believes that the leaves are the part of the plant with medicinal properties.

Other Uses The small, purple fruit of Native Myrtle were a good snack food for Aboriginal people when ripe, but, although sweet, are reported to have a salty, bitter edge to them (Coppin, 2008; Cribb & Cribb, 1987; Low, 1991). The Wunambal Gaambera people did not eat the fruit (Karadada et al., 2011).

Native Plumbago

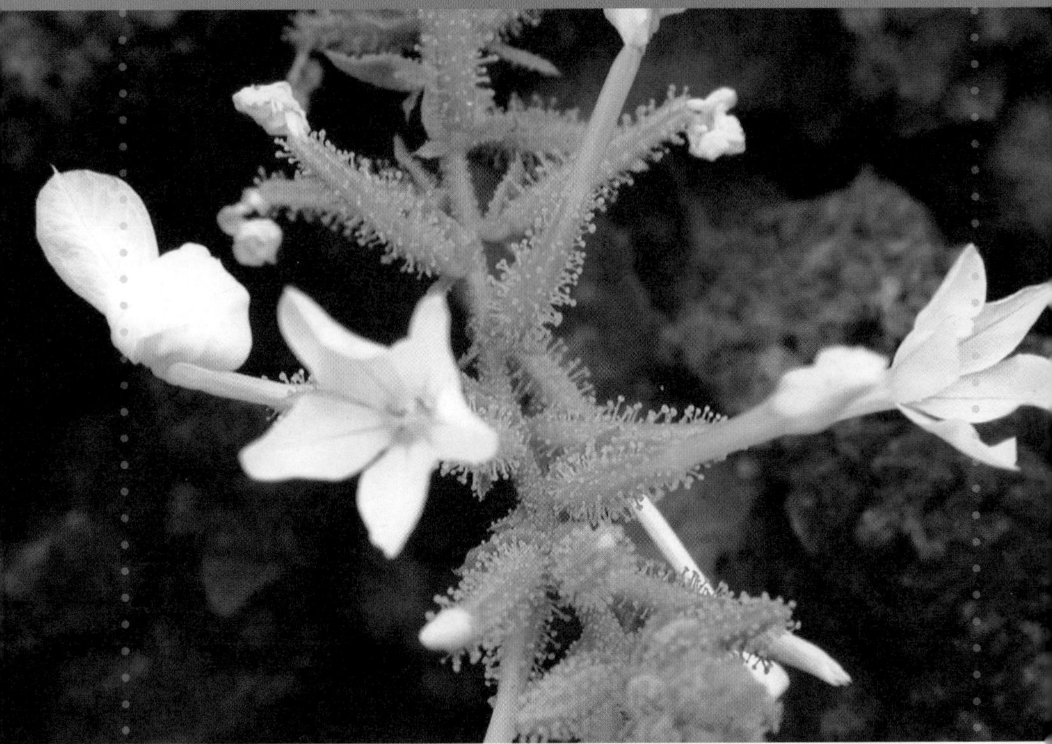

Scientific Name *Plumbago zeylanica* L.

Common Names Native Plumbago, Wild Plumbago, Leadwort.

Field Notes Native Plumbago is an erect or sprawling shrub that only grows up to 1.2 m in height. Its leaves are ovate, lance-elliptic or spatulate to oblanceolate and up to 90 mm long by 40 mm wide. Its white or white-blue flowers have five ovate petals and appear on 150 mm long, lanceolate bracts that have glandular, viscid rachises. Flowering in Western Australia is between January and August. Native Plumbago occurs in a variety of habitats in the Pilbara and Kimberley regions of Western Australia, the Northern Territory and Queensland, and many other tropical areas of the world, including Africa and South-east Asia (ALA, 2022; ATFP, 2022; WAH, 2022).

Medicinal Uses Native Plumbago is used in folk medicine across the tropics. Decoctions of the roots were used internally as an abortifacient in the early stages of pregnancy. Decoctions of the

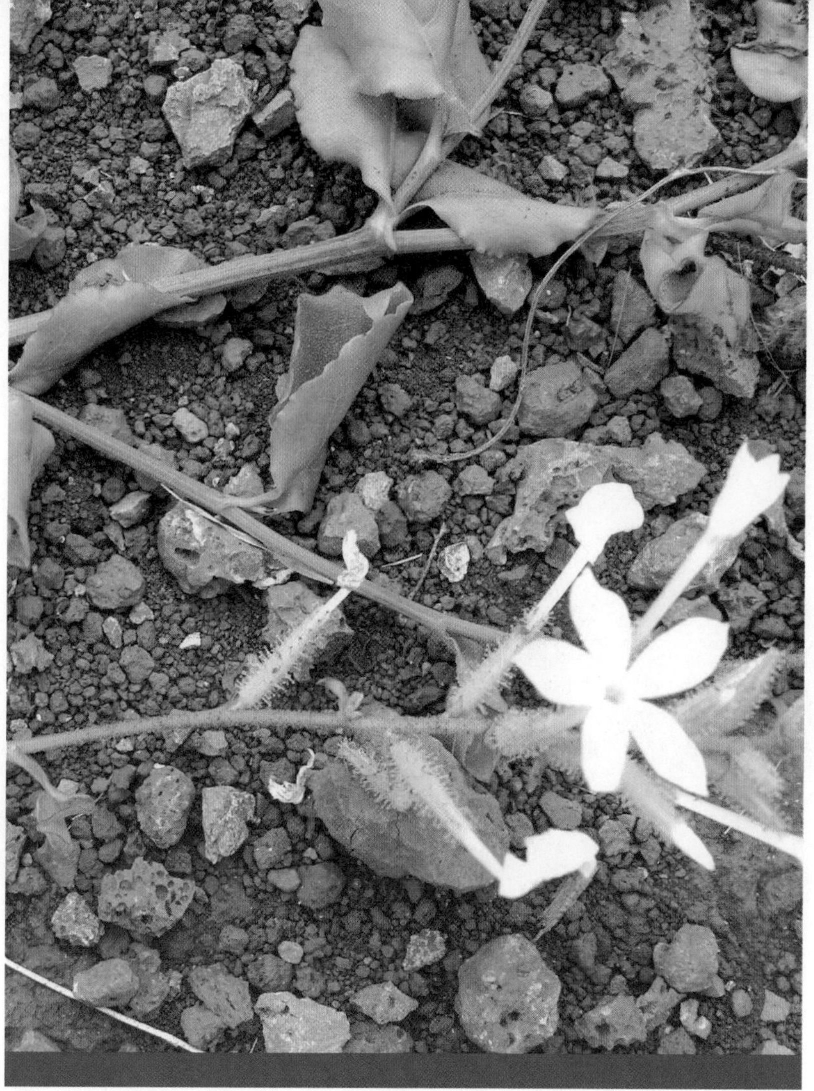

roots were also used externally as a remedy for skin conditions, including leprosy, scabies infestations, ringworm, dermatitis and acne, as well as for sores, leg ulcers, haemorrhoids and hookworm (Fern, 2021).

Native Poplar

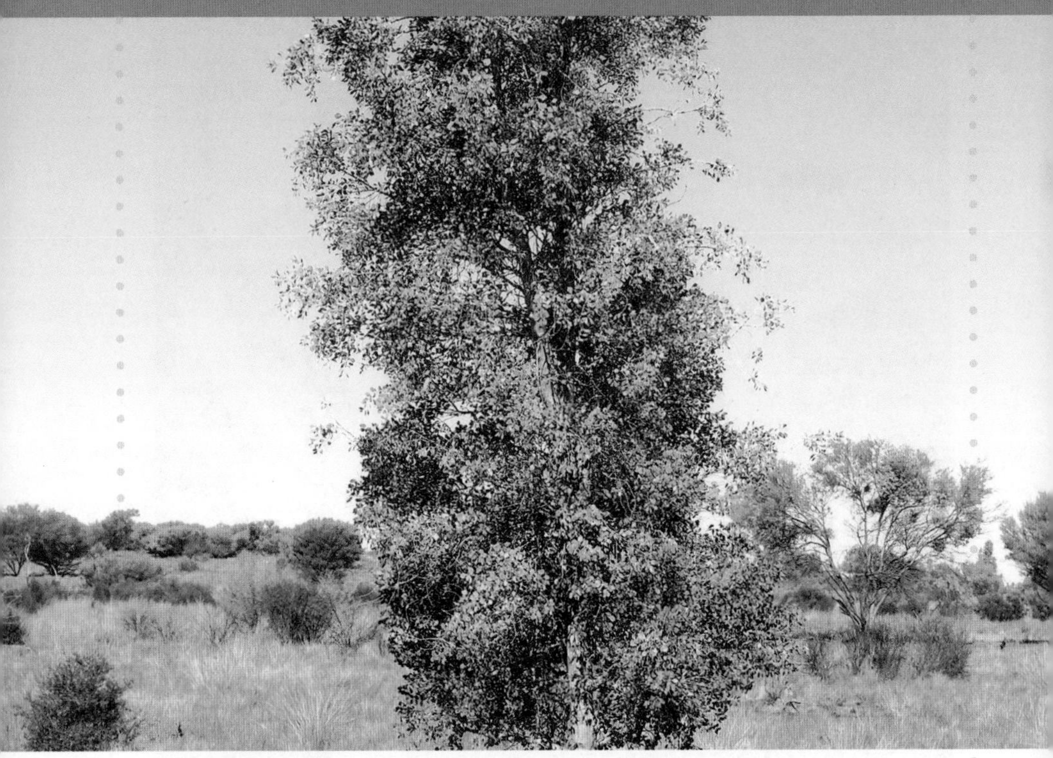

Scientific Name *Codonocarpus cotinifolius* (Desf.) F.Muell.

Common Names Native Poplar, Desert Poplar, Fire Tree, Bell Fruit Tree, Horseradish Tree, Quinine Tree, Medicine Tree, Firebush, Western Poplar, Toothache Tree.

Aboriginal Names Kantumi, Kalurti, Karturangu, Tjinatu, Yantuntu (Kukatja) (Valiquette, 1993), Karntuwangu (Ngardi) (Cataldi, 2004), Karntuwangu, Parntikari (Walmajarri) (Richards & Hudson, 2012), Garnduwangu (Yindjibarndi and Ngarluma), Gandilangu (Wajarri), Jimpirriny (Karajarri) (Willing, 2014).

Field Notes Native Poplar is a tall shrub or small tree that grows to around 10 m in height. The bark has dark red, yellow and green wavy patches. Its pale green, narrowly lanceolate, obovate, elliptic, more or less circular leaves are tapered at the ends but broader near the tips. Small, yellow-green male and female flowers appear in axillary racemes from April to October. Its bell-shaped fruit are

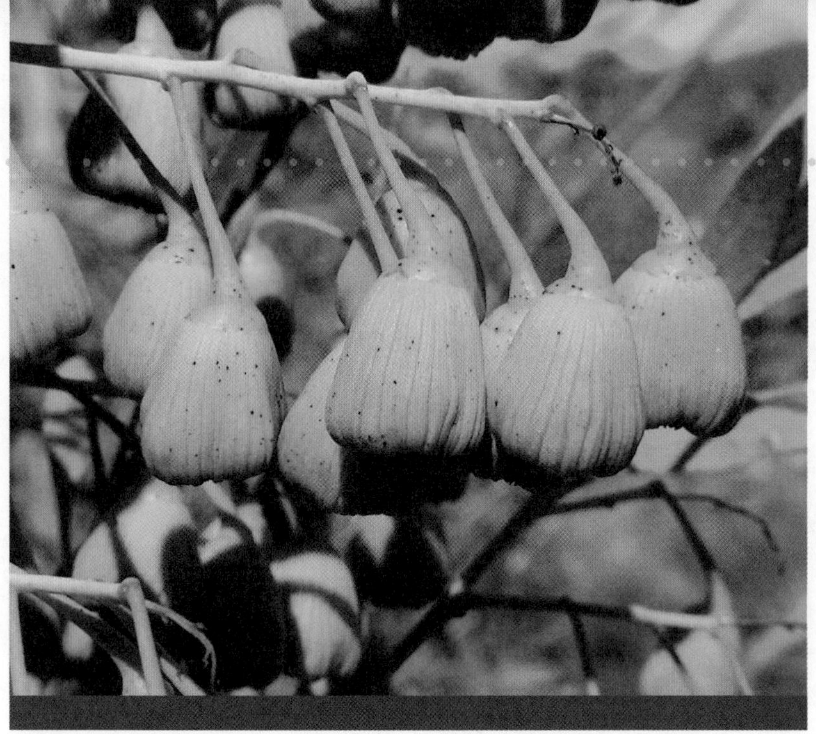

green and 7–12 mm long. Native Poplar occurs in red sand, loam and gravel in drier regions of mainland Australia, including those of the south-west, central and northern parts of Western Australia, as well as along the coast from Karratha to Broome in the Kimberley region (Lassak & McCarthy, 2001; WAH, 2022).

Medicinal Uses The roots, leaves and shoots of Native Poplar were chewed and used as a narcotic to ease toothache and general pain. Decoctions of the bark, roots and stems were used externally as an antiseptic wash for skin problems, such as eczema and sores; as a liniment to relieve rheumatic pain; and as a wash for colds, influenza and fever. The leaves were crushed and rubbed over the body to treat internal pain, the symptoms of colds and influenza, and to help heal sores and cuts. An infusion of a combination of Native Poplar and Maroon Bush (*Scaveola spinescens*; p. 328) was thought to be a good treatment for cancer of various types (Cock, 2011; Lassak & McCarthy, 2008; Smith, 1991). The Walmajarri chewed root bark to treat the symptoms of colds and influenza (Richards & Hudson, 2012).

Native Rosella

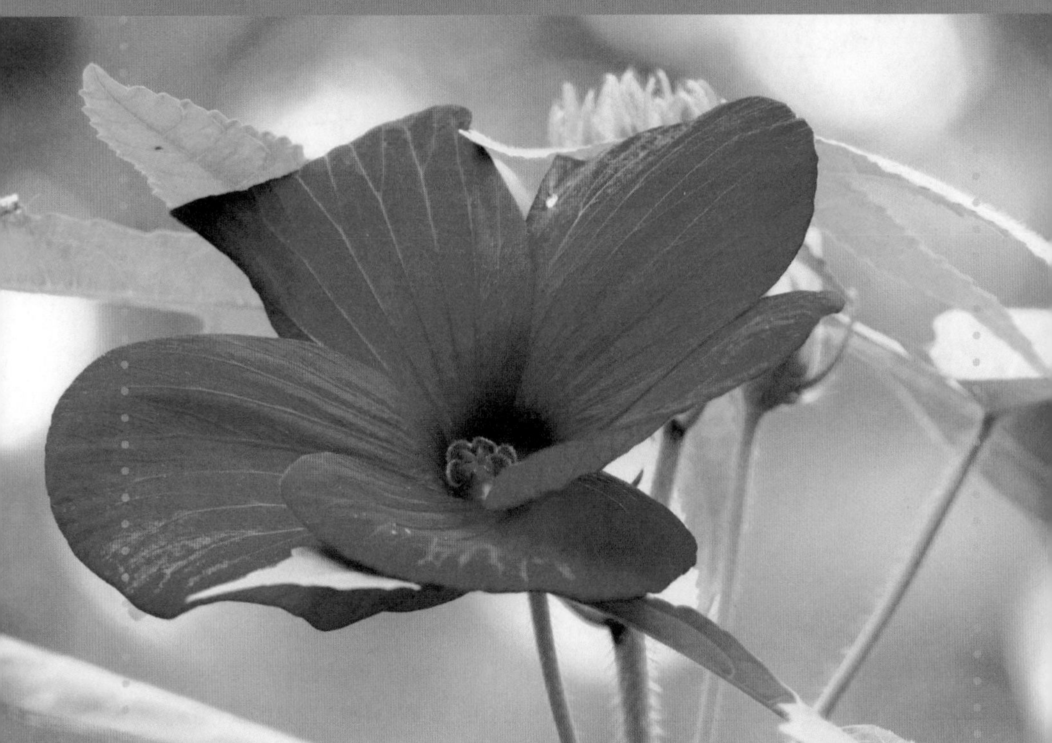

Scientific Name *Abelmoschus moschatus* subsp. *tuberosus* (Span.) Borss.Waalk., previously known as *Hibiscus rhodopetalus* (F. Muell) Benth.

Common Names Native Rosella, Musk Okra, Musk Mallow, Bush Carrot.

Aboriginal Name Nugu (Kwini) (Crawford, 1982).

Field Notes Native Rosella is a perennial herbaceous, trailing plant with soft hairy stems that spreads to around 2 m in diameter. It has an underground tuber, which it dies back to in the dry season. Its hairy, heart-shaped leaves have three to five lobes with serrated margins. Its flowers are round and Hibiscus-like, usually watermelon pink, sometimes white or cream, but always with a dark centre. Flowering is between October and April but the flowers only last for one day. Its fruit are tough papery capsules with black seeds. In Australia, Native Rosella occurs in open woodlands or grasslands,

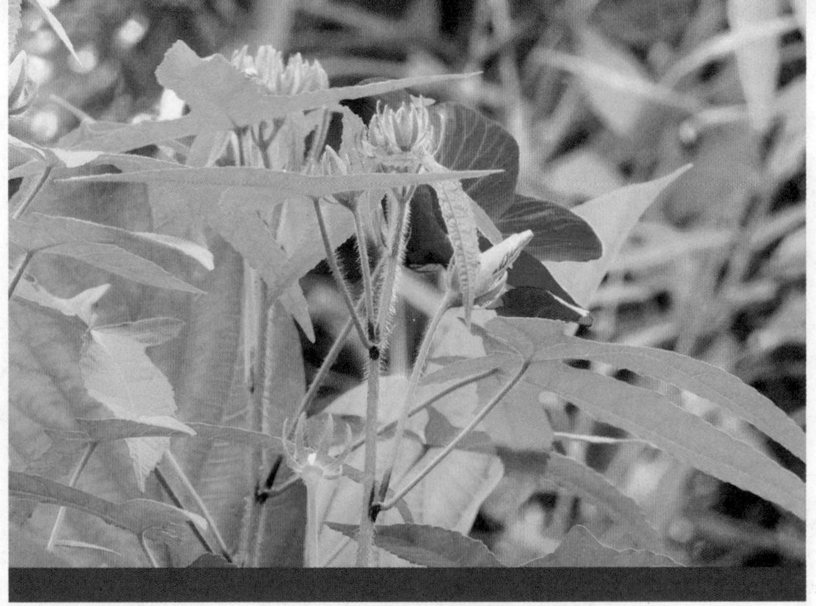

on rocky hillsides or on flat lands across the top end from the northern Kimberley region of Western Australia, through the Northern Territory and into north and eastern parts of Queensland (ANPSA, 2022; SMIP, 2022).

Medicinal Uses The essential oil made from Native Rosella is used in aromatherapy for the treatment of depression and anxiety, and can also be applied externally to treat cramps, poor circulation and arthritic pain (PFAF, 2022).

Other Uses The edible roots of Native Rosella look and are reported to taste like parsnip. The roots are cooked in hot ashes before they are eaten. They are harvested from May to November (ANPSA, 2022; Crawford, 1982; Hiddins, 2001; Isaacs, 1987). The leaves and shoots are also edible and may be eaten raw or cooked. The young seedpods are edible and are usually cooked and eaten as a vegetable, much like okra (ANPSA, 2022; SMIP, 2022).

Native Walnut

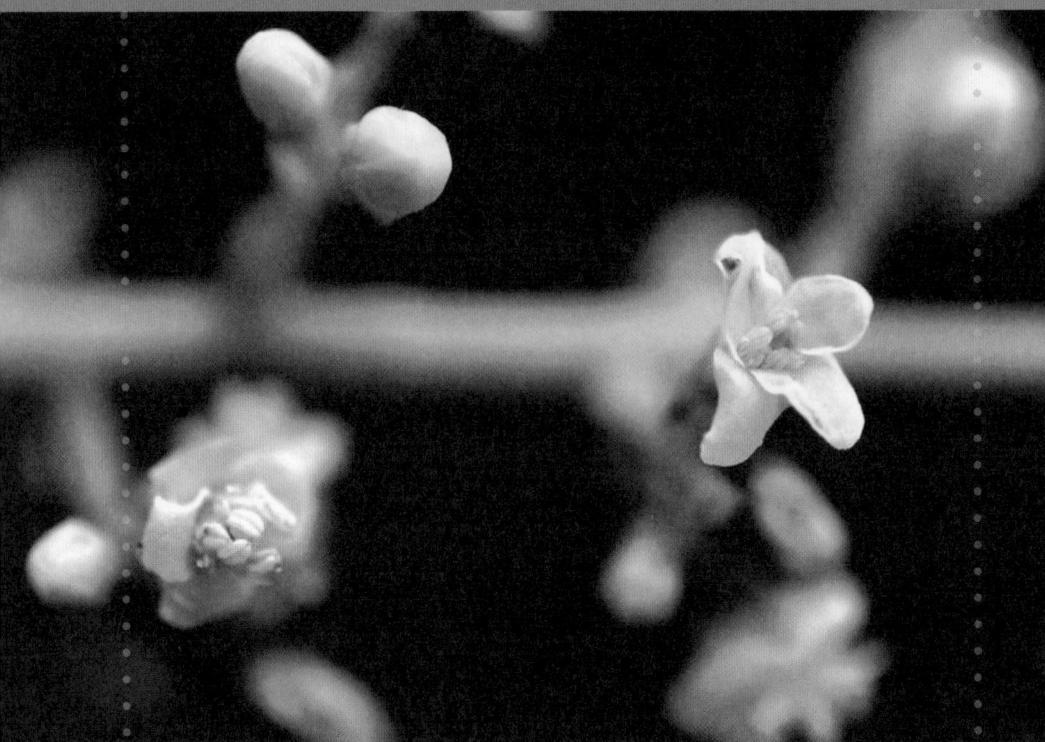

Scientific Name *Owenia reticulata* F.Muell.

Common Names Native Walnut, Desert Walnut.

Aboriginal Names Bandal (Nyangumarda), Lambilum, Lambilamb (Bardi) (Smith & Kalotas, 1985; Paddy et al., 1993), Limbalim (Nyul Nyul) (DAWE, n.d.), Karraparra, Makaly, Ngarlka, Tarripungu, Turtujarti (Walmajarri) (Richards & Hudson, 2012), Parntal (Karajarri) (Willing, 2014), Girla, Jurlurru, Yirlanggi (Jaru) (Wightman, 2003), Lawuwa (Kukatja) (Valiquette, 1993), Marrawaji (Walpiri) (Northern Tanami IPA, 2015).

Field Notes Native Walnut grows as a tree to 14 m in height. Its bark often appears black and corky. Its large green, ovate leaves have a prominent cream central vein and are up to 200 mm long. Its small white, star-shaped flowers appear any time from May to November. Its fruit are spherical and green with brown blotches, with a hard, woody shell inside. Native Walnut is found on stony

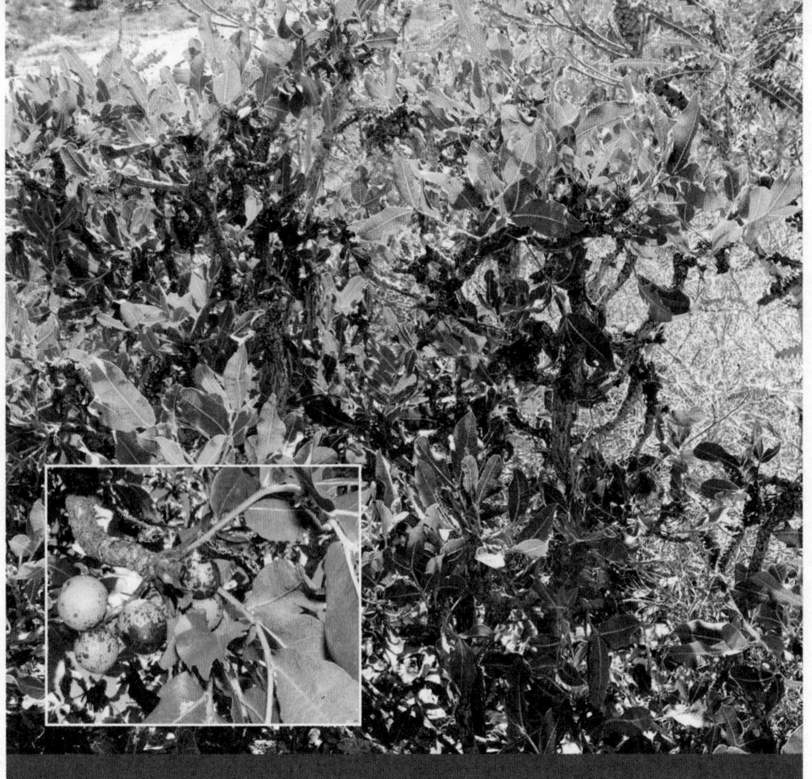

ridges, red sand dunes and plains across the top half of Australia, from the Pilbara and Kimberley regions in Western Australia to north-west Queensland (ALA, 2022; Lassak & McCarthy, 2001; WAH, 2022).

Medicinal Uses Crushed leaves and stems of Native Walnut, or decoctions of the leaves and young stems soaked in rags, were used as a poultice on sores and wounds. The kernels were roasted and crushed then rubbed on sores to aid the healing process (ExploreOz, 2019; Kenneally et al., 1996; Lassak & McCarthy, 2001; Native Tastes of Australia, 2022; Reid, 1986; Western Australia Now and Then, 2022). The leaves, bark and fruit were warmed on a fire and then applied as a poultice to areas of rheumatic pain (Paddy et al., 1993).

Other Uses The kernel of the fruit of Native Walnut is edible. The nut was roasted before it was cracked open and the kernel eaten. The shell is apparently extremely hard and is difficult to crack without shattering the kernel (Fern, 2021; Wightman, 2003). The sap or gum that oozes from wounds in the tree is also edible during the 'hot weather time' (December to March) (Wightman, 2003).

Needle-leaf Wattle

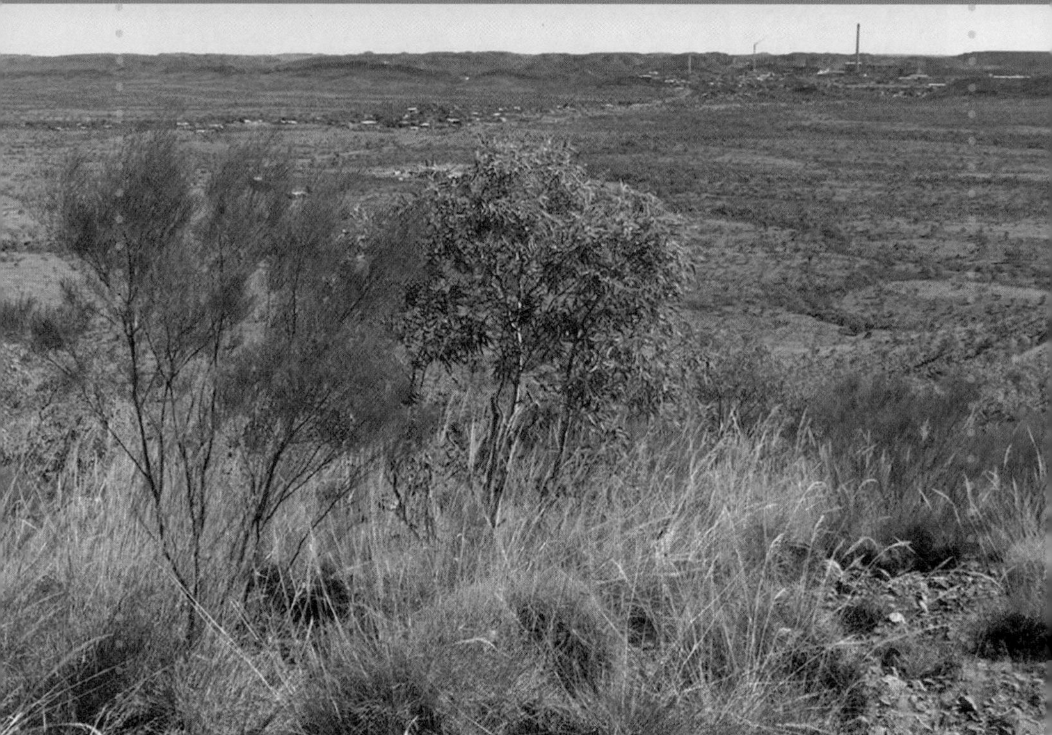

Scientific Name *Acacia orthocarpa* F.Muell.

Common Name Needle-leaf Wattle.

Aboriginal Names Binyinyi (W), Birrbirn (N) (Jaru) (Deegan et al., 2010).

Field Notes Needle-leaf Wattle is an erect, spreading or spindly shrub that grows to around 4 m in height. Its needle-like phyllodes can be up to 150 mm long. The yellow, cylindrical flower spikes have a length of up to 32 mm and can be present any time between March and October. Its fruit or seed pods are linear to oblanceolate in shape, taper towards the base and are up to 100 mm long. Needle-leaf Wattle occurs in sandy or stony soils, often over sandstone or ironstone, on rocky hills and rises, and on plains in the Pilbara and Kimberley regions of Western Australia, the Northern Territory and Queensland (ALA, 2022, WAH, 2022; World Wide Wattle, 2022).

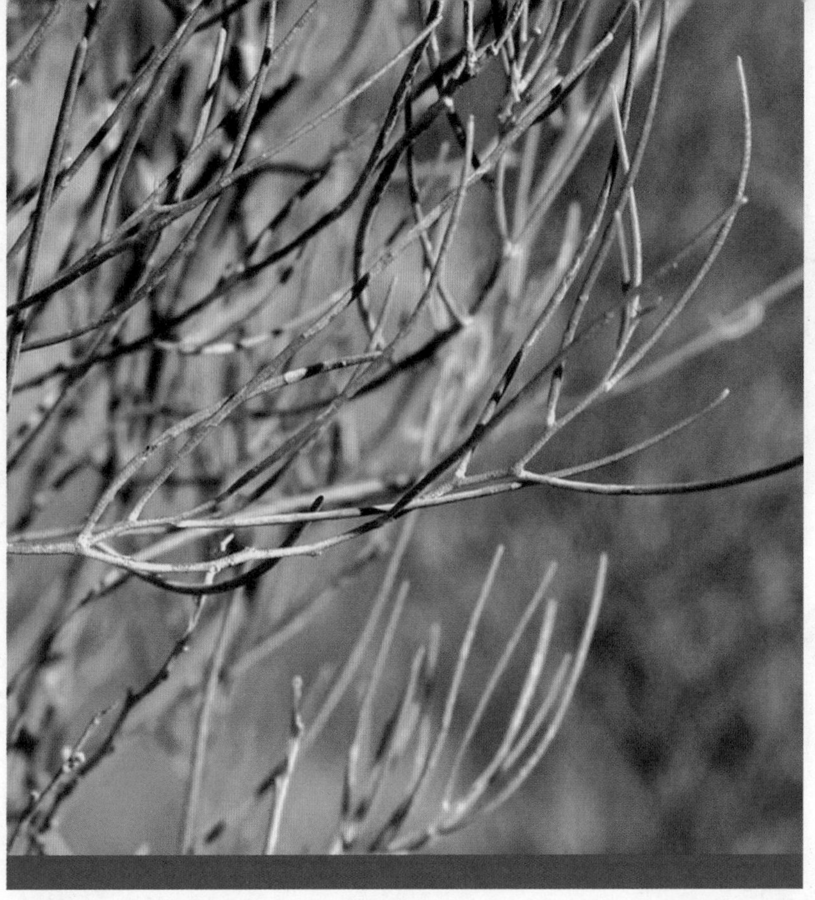

Medicinal Uses The branches from Needle-leaf Wattle are used by the Jaru for 'smoke medicine'. Branches are put on a dying fire and the smoke is used to treat the symptoms of colds, influenza and 'sore stomachs' (Deegan et al., 2010).

Ngurubi

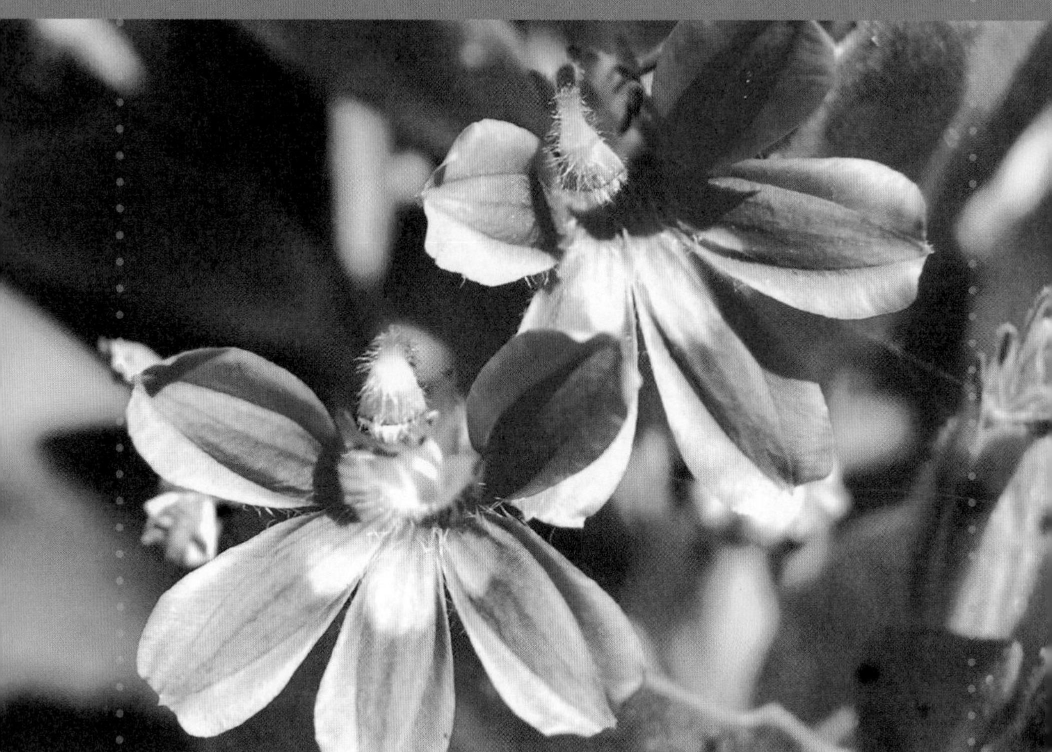

Scientific Name *Goodenia scaevolina* F.Muell.

Common Names Ngurubi, Blue Fan Flower.

Aboriginal Names Ngurubi, Ngurbi (Nyikina) (Smith & Smith, 2009).

Field Notes Ngurubi is an erect, much-branched, viscid plant that grows up to 1.5 m in height. It has ovate, green, serrated leaves and blue or white, fan-shaped flowers that appear between February and October. Ngurubi is found in shallow, stony soils on hill tops and slopes, and on sandstone outcrops in the Pilbara and Kimberley regions of Western Australia and in the western part of the Northern Territory (ALA, 2022; Lassak & McCarthy, 2001; WAH, 2022).

Medicinal Uses The roots of the Ngurubi plant growing nearer the sea were chewed and the juice swallowed as a cough suppressant (Lassak & McCarthy, 2001; Reid, 1986; Webb, 1959; Williams, 2013).

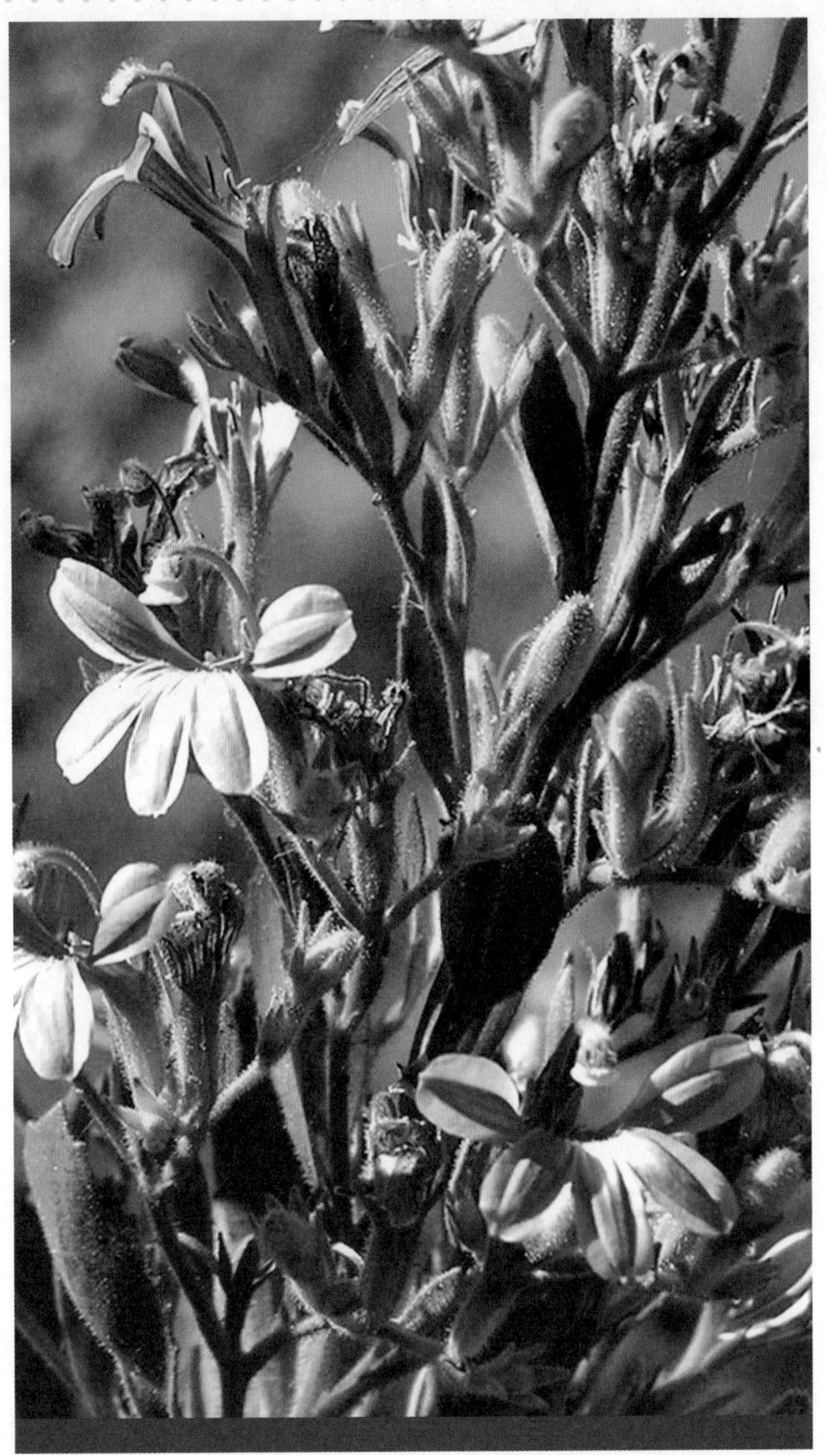

Nine-leaved Indigo

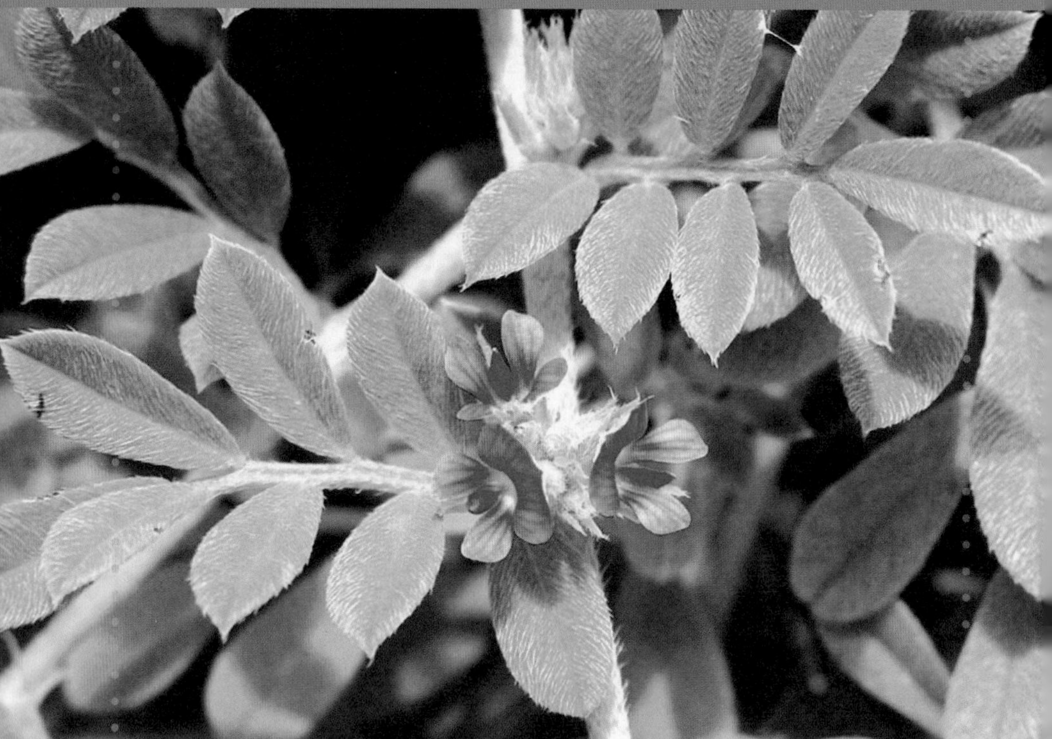

Scientific Name *Indigofera linnaei* Ali.

Common Names Nine-leaved Indigo, Birdsville Indigo.

Field Notes Nine-leaved Indigo is a prostrate to ascending, woody, hairy perennial herb with a tap root. It grows to around 500 mm in height with a spread of 1.5 m. Its compound leaves are up to 30 mm long with seven or nine obovate, alternate leaflets that are 15 mm long and 5 mm wide. Its bright red flowers are vermillion inside and appear from January to May. Nine-leaved Indigo occurs in sandy soils, along sandstone and limestone ridges, alongside rivers and creeks, and on rocky hillsides in the Pilbara and Kimberley regions of Western Australia, the Northern Territory, Queensland and the northern parts of South Australia and New South Wales (ALA, 2022; ATRP, 2020; Lassak & McCarthy, 2001; WAH, 2022). It also occurs in India, Indonesia, Laos, Myanmar, New Guinea, southern China, Thailand and Vietnam (Fern, 2021).

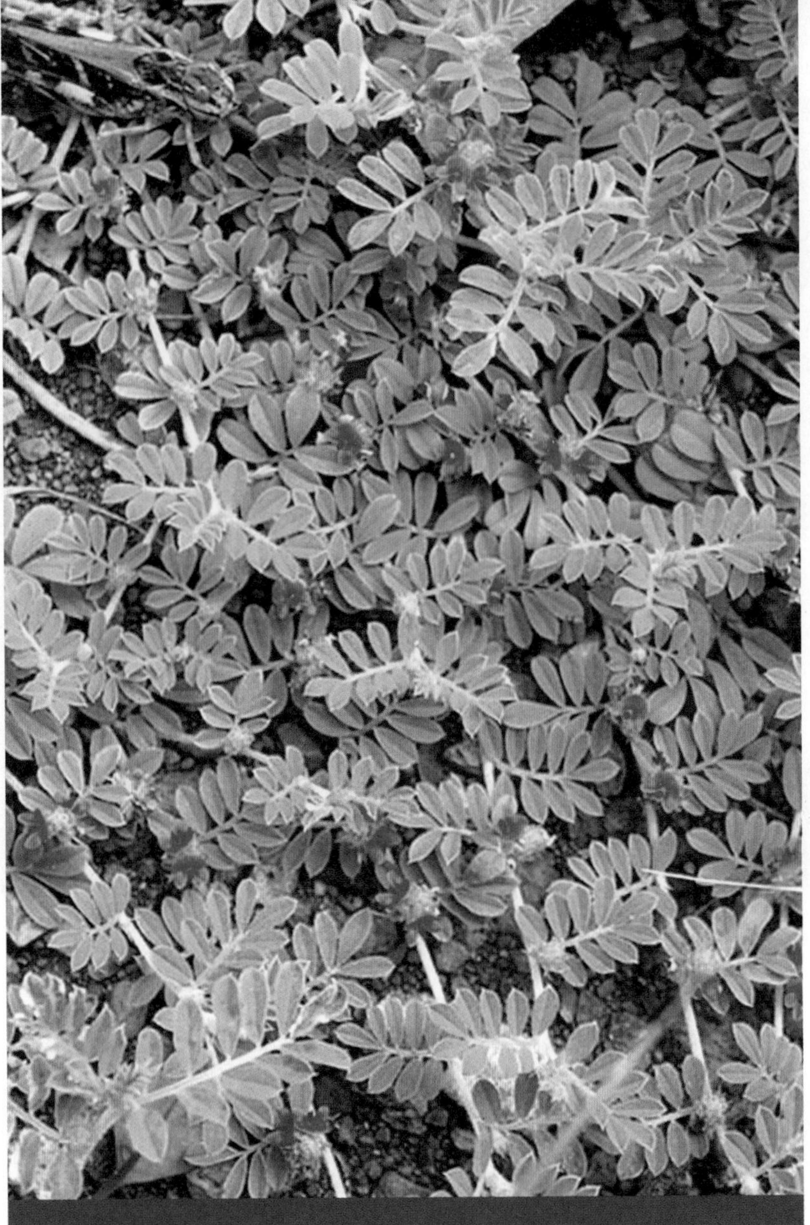

Medicinal Uses Infusions or decoctions of the whole plant were taken internally for coughs or for its diuretic properties (Lassak & McCarthy, 2001). The juice of the plant contains some ascorbic acid (vitamin C) (Fern, 2021).

Other Uses The seeds of Nine-leaved Indigo are edible and were usually only eaten when food was scarce in the areas where it grows. The seeds were usually ground into a powder (Fern, 2021).

Nodding Swamp Orchid

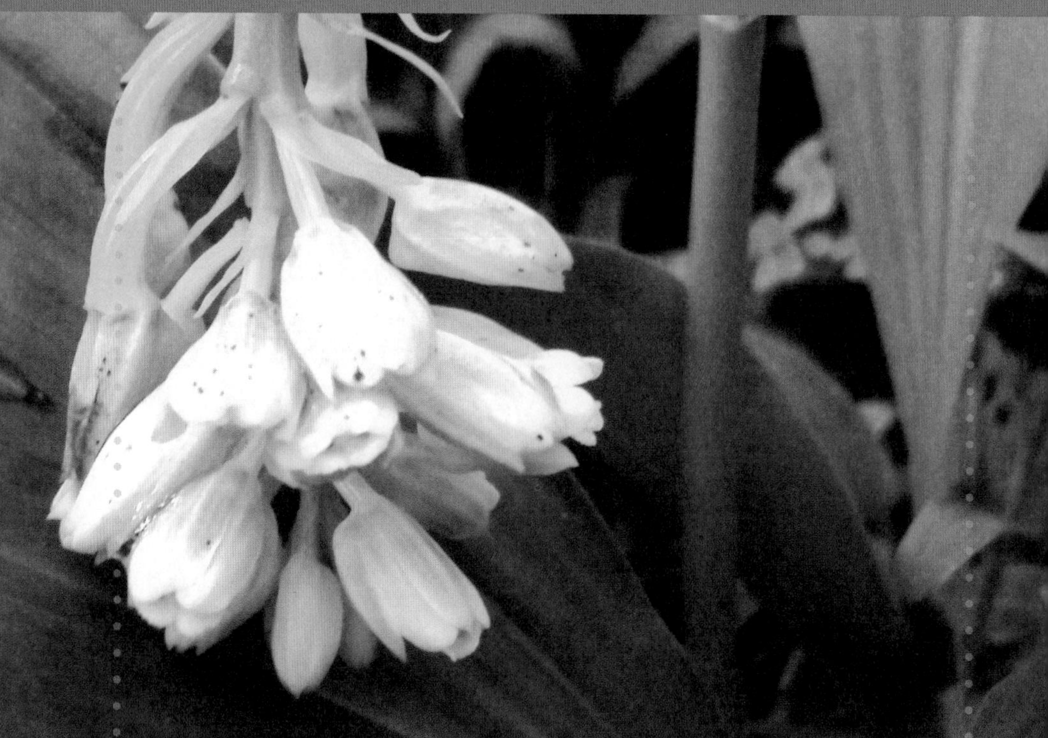

Scientific Name *Geodorum densiflorum* (Lam.) Schltr.

Common Names Nodding Swamp Orchid, Nodding Orchid, Shepherd's Crook Orchid, Pink Nodding Orchid.

Field Notes Nodding Swamp Orchid is a terrestrial, perennial orchid with shoots up to 300 mm long. Its edible pseudobulbs are up to 26 mm in diameter. Its long, ovate leaves are pleated along their length and up to 350 mm long. Each nodding flowering stalk is up to 400 mm long and produces up to 10 pink, orchid-type flowers that do not open fully, with sepals and petals up to 12 mm long. In Australia, flowering is between December and February. Nodding Swamp Orchid occurs in the Kimberley region of Western Australia, the Northern Territory and down the Queensland east coast as far as the border with New South Wales. It also occurs in tropical Asia and on some Pacific islands, including Fiji (ALA, 2022; PFAF, 2022).

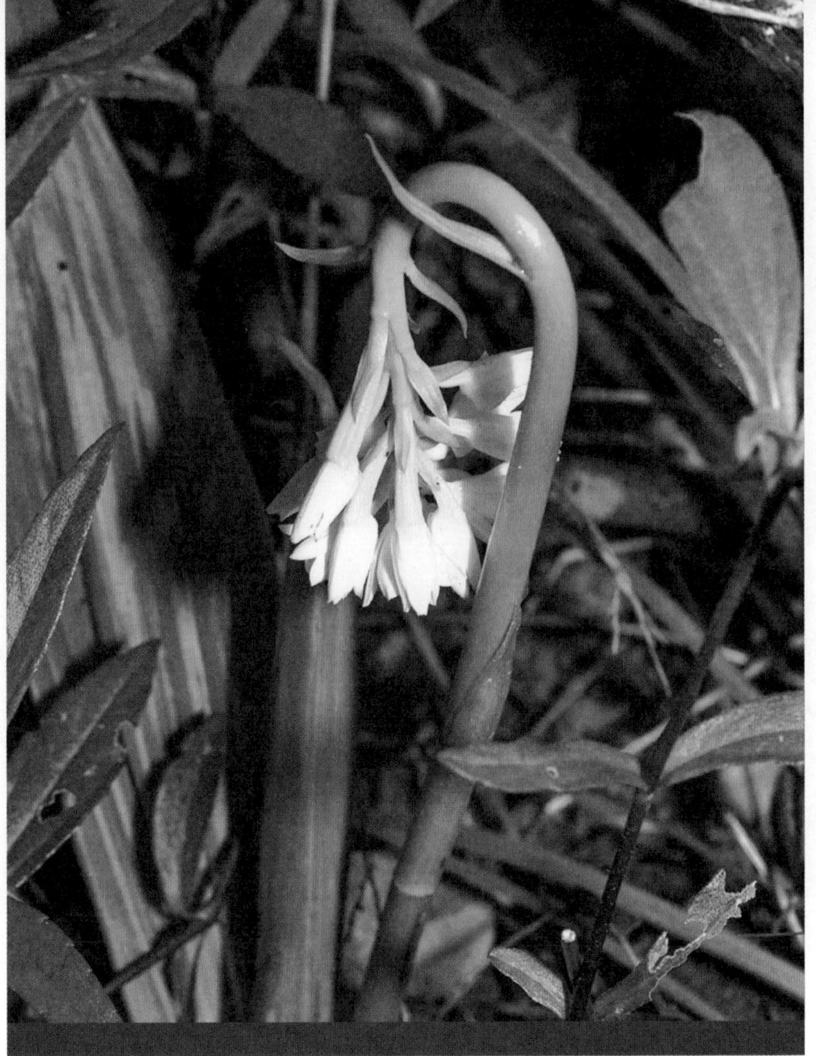

Medicinal Uses Poultices made from the crushed pseudobulbs of Nodding Swamp Orchid were applied to boils, carbuncles and abscesses to 'ripen them' or draw them out. The poultices were also applied externally to areas of rheumatic pain (Williams, 2010).

Other Uses The bulbs of Nodding Swamp Orchid are edible and were eaten raw as a snack by Aboriginal groups right across the top end of Australia (Williams, 2010).

Nonda

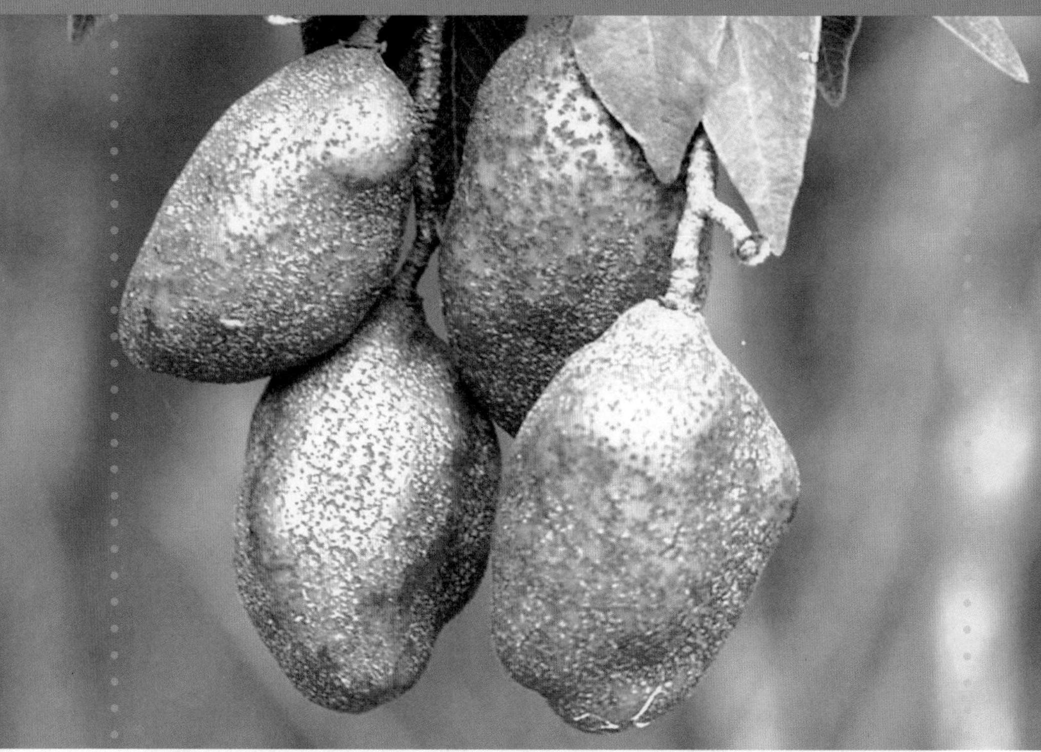

Scientific Name *Parinari nonda* Benth.

Common Names Nonda, Nonda Plum, Nonda Tree, Nunda Plum, Parinari.

Field Notes Nonda grows as a shrub or tree to around 6 m in height. The leaf blades are ovate and up to 80 mm long by 50 mm wide. In Australia, its small star-shaped, green-brown-yellow or white flowers are present between August and October. Its orange-brown fruit are ovoid-globular and roughly 40 mm long and 35 mm in diameter. Australian Tropical Rainforest Plants (2020) advise that the name 'Nonda' was given to this tree by Ludwig Leichhardt, a German explorer who explored parts of Queensland and the Northern Territory, but it is a 'misapplication of an Aboriginal name for a tree with some similarities in the Moreton Bay area'. Nonda occurs in sandy soils on sandy rises, in sandstone gorges and on creek banks across in the Kimberley region of Western Australia,

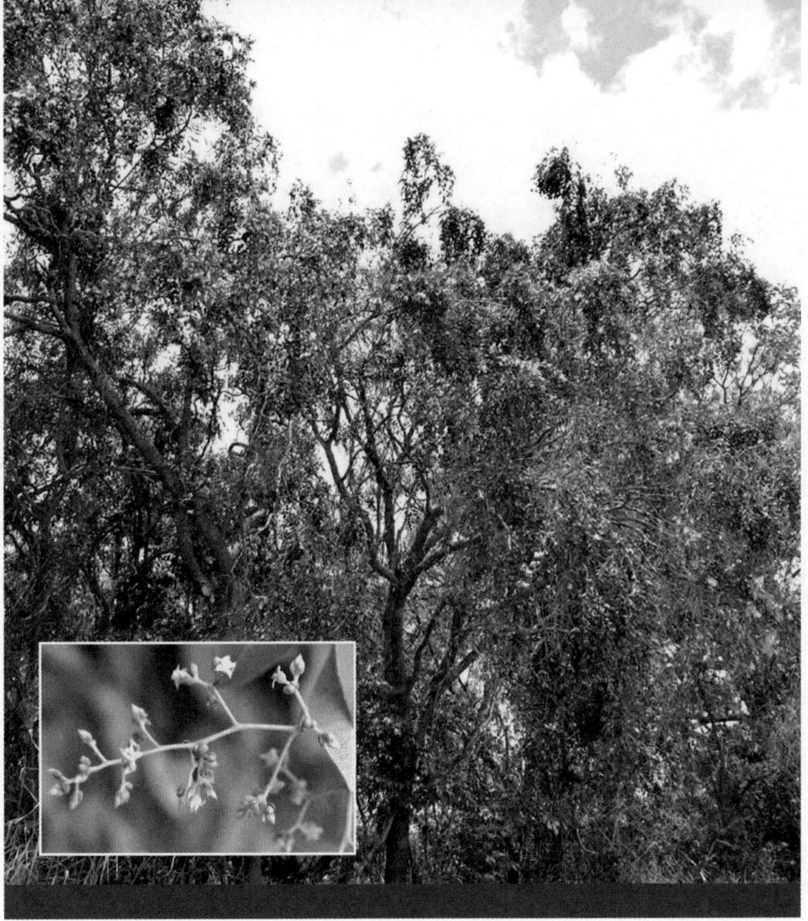

the Northern Territory and Far North Queensland. It also occurs in New Guinea (ALA, 2022; ATRP, 2020; WAH, 2022).

Medicinal Uses Aboriginal groups in Far North Queensland chewed the bark of the Nonda tree to ease the symptoms of colds and influenza. They also ate the fruit to settle an 'upset stomach'. A drink made from crushed old, dried fruit was sipped as a cough suppressant (Edwards, 2005).

Other Uses The flesh of the Nonda fruit is edible when ripe, which is usually in the dry season, but is reported to taste a bit like 'a mealy potato', and is slightly astringent (Cribb & Cribb, 1981; Fern, 2021; Hiddins, 2001; Maiden, 1889). Unripe fruit was often buried for a few days to ripen it. The mealy pulp was often ground to a dough-like substance, which was baked as Johnny cakes in hot ashes (Hiddins, 2001).

North Coast Wattle

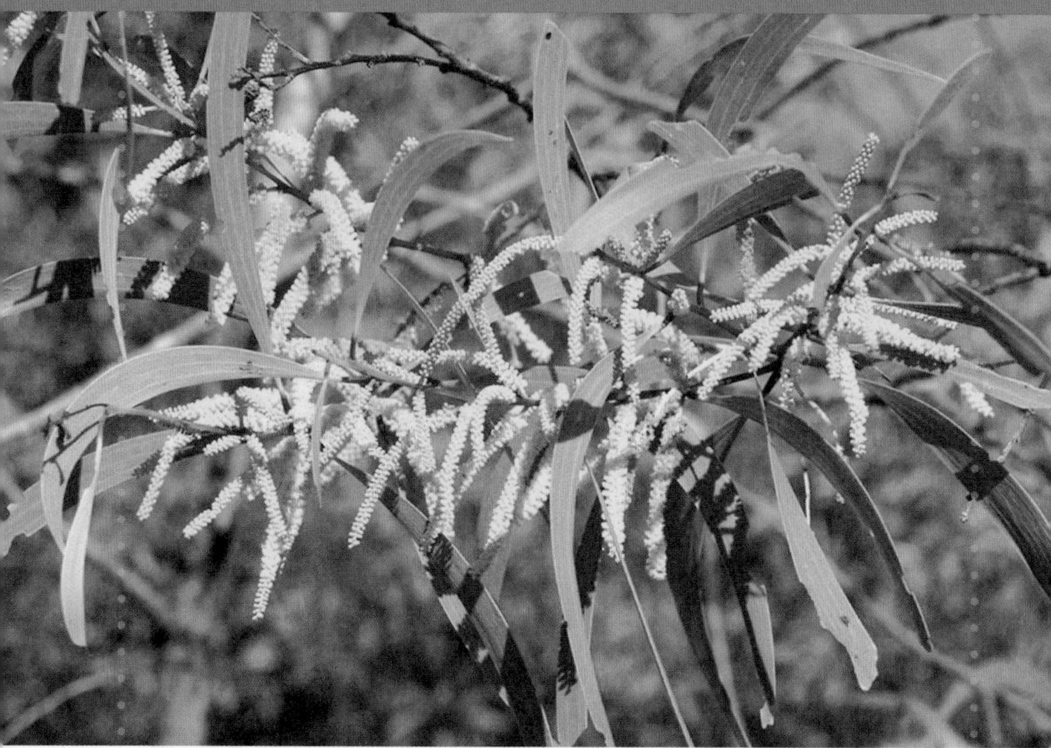

Scientific Name *Acacia leptocarpa* Benth.

Common Names North Coast Wattle, Hickory Wattle, Mangarr Mangal.

Aboriginal Name Mangarr manya (Kwini) (Cheinmora et al., 2017; Crawford, 1982).

Field Notes North Coast Wattle grows as a shrub or tree up to 10 m in height depending on conditions. It has dark grey to almost black bark. Its narrowly elliptic phyllodes are up to 210 mm long and 25 mm wide. Bright yellow flowers, present from autumn to spring, are borne on cylindrical spikes that are up to 70 mm long. Its fruit or seed pods are linear, curved or twisted, and up to 120 mm long and only 3 mm wide. North Coast Wattle occurs in open forest, in monsoon forest and rainforest margins in the northern Kimberley region of Western Australia, the top end of the Northern Territory, the Cape York Peninsula and southern Central Queensland

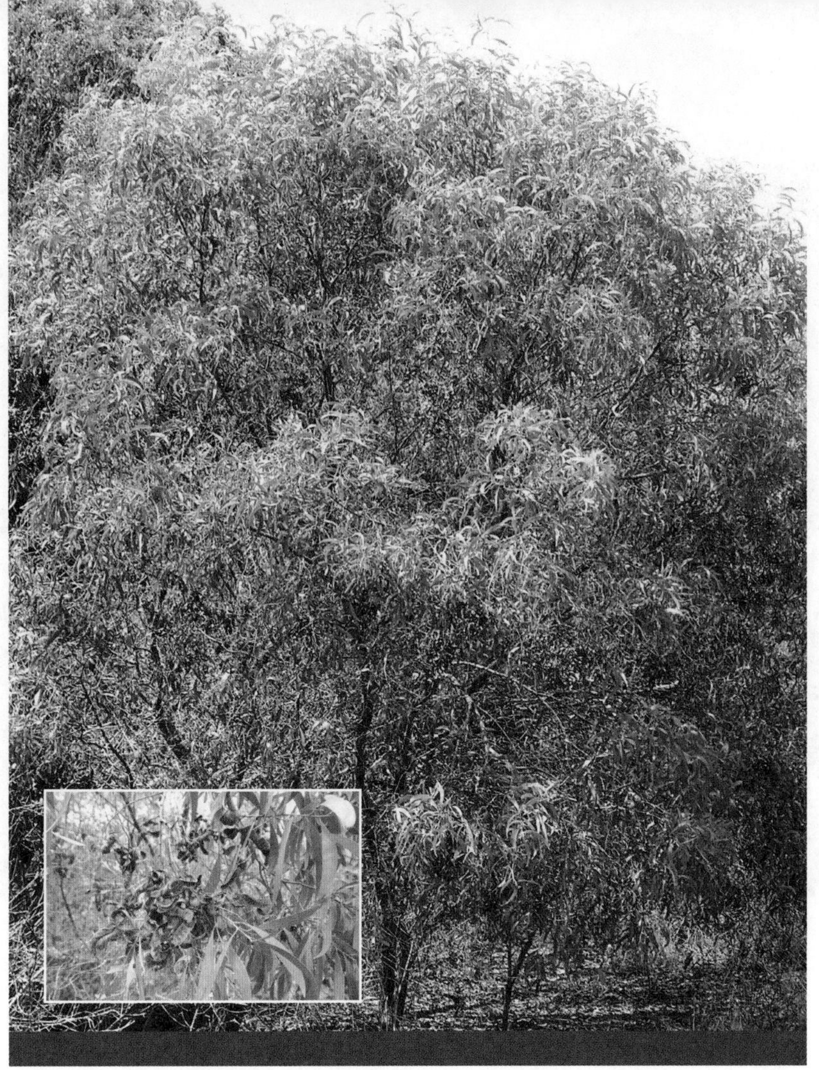

(ALA, 2022; World Wide Wattle, 2022).

Medicinal Uses Infusions of the crushed leaves were used to bathe sore eyes due to conjunctivitis (Cheinmora et al., 2017; Crawford, 1982; Native Tastes of Australia, 2022; Williams, 2011).

Other Uses The gum that oozes from wounds in the trunk of North Coast Wattle is edible (Queensland Bushfoods Association, 2022). The leaves and pods of North Coast Wattle contain saponin and can be rubbed with water to produce a soapy lather for washing. Crushed leaves, branches, bark, pods and seeds were used as 'fish poison' in some parts of the top end (Searle, 2020).

Northern Cane Grass

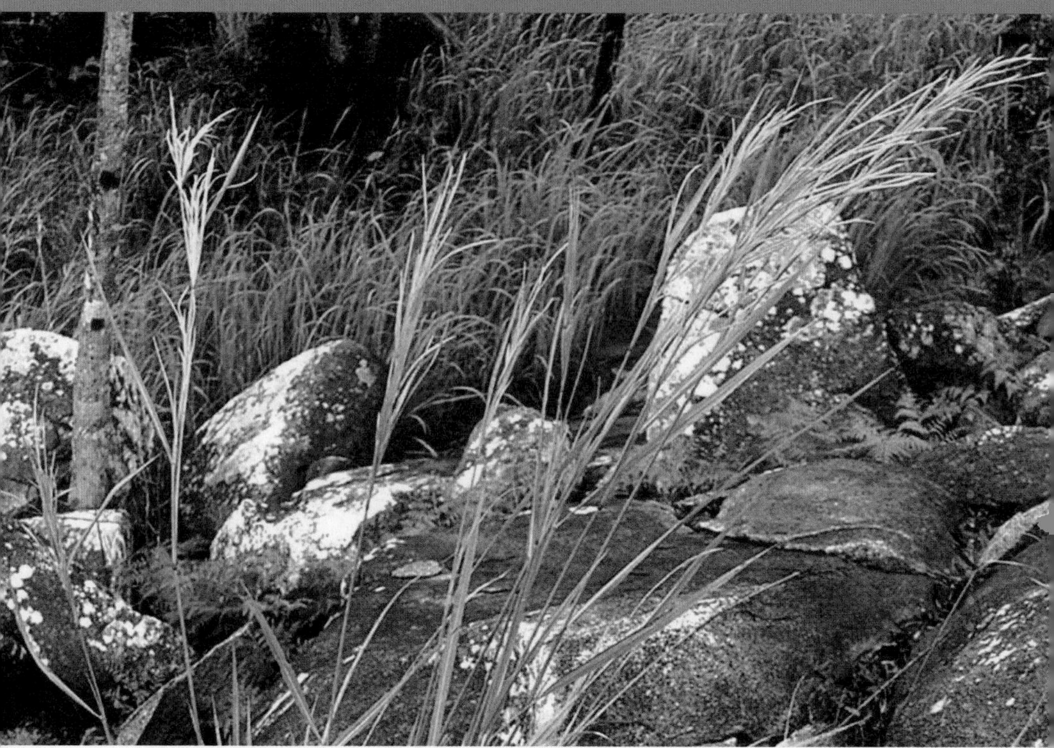

Scientific Name *Mnesithea rottboellioides* (R.Br.) de Koning & Sosef., also known as *Coelorachis rottboellioides* (R.Br.) A.Camus.

Common Name Northern Cane Grass.

Aboriginal Names Kilamperrji (Gija) (Wightman, 2003), Jawarl, Pantjin (Karajarri) (Willing, 2014).

Field Notes Northern Cane Grass is a rhizomatous, tufted perennial grass that grows to around 3.5 m in height. It has stout culms (stems) and green to olive-green leaf-blades that are up to 500 mm long and 20 mm wide. It has small green flowers that are present from March to August. Its seed heads are several finger-like branches crowded at the end of the stems. Northern Cane Grass occurs in grey-yellow sand or alluvium over sandstone, near creeks, swamps and around sandstone boulders all over the tropical north of Australia as well as tropical Asia (ALA, 2022; AusGrass2, 2022; SMIP, 2022; WAH, 2022).

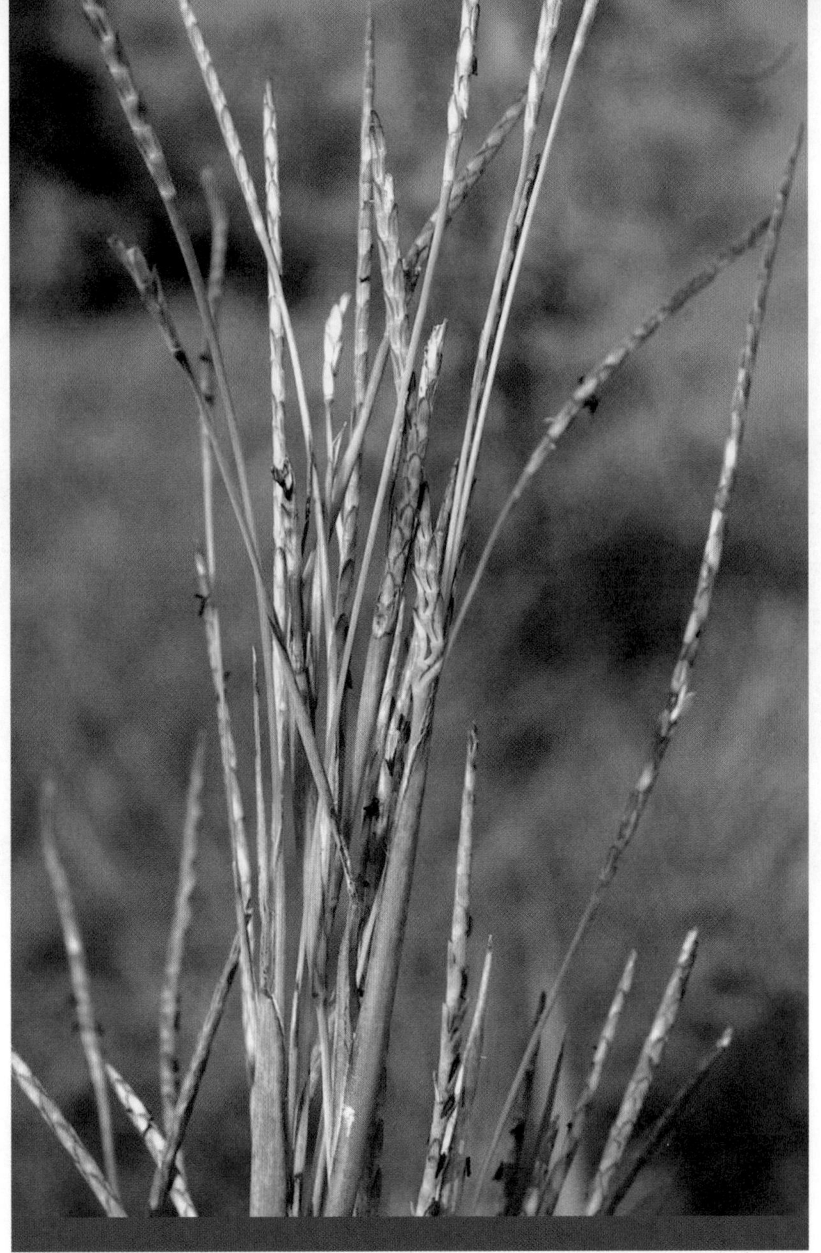

Medicinal Uses Decoctions of the leaves and culms were used externally as an antiseptic wash to bathe sores and wounds to aid the healing process (Smith, 1991).

Other Uses The rhizomes of Northern Cane Grass are edible and were roasted on hot coals before eating. The culms were carried on long walks in the dry season and sucked to provide the traveller with the sweet sap and a source of water (Smith, 1991).

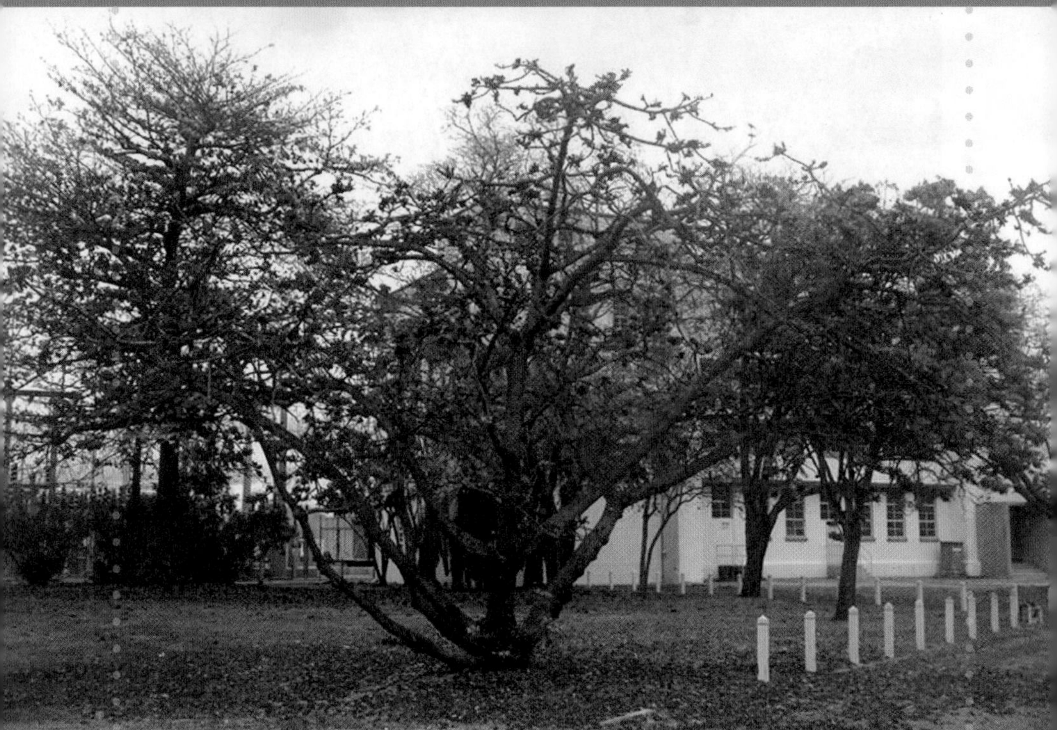

Scientific Names *Bombax ceiba* L., and *Bombax ceiba* var. *leiocarpum* A.Robyns.

Common Names Northern Cottonwood, Kapok, Kapok Tree, Red Kapok, Red Silk-cotton Tree, Red Flowered Kapok, Bombax, Semul, Silk Cotton Tree.

Aboriginal Names Wurndala (Wunambal, Gaambera) (Karadada et al., 2011), Wundala minya (Kwini) (Cheinmora et al., 2017).

Field Notes Northern Cottonwood is a deciduous tree that grows up to 20 m in height, often with buttress roots. Its trunk and branches are armed with short, stout thorns. Its elliptical leaves are up to 180 mm long and 55 mm across. Large, red, glossy flowers appear when the tree is leafless from August to September. Its fruit is a capsule roughly 100 mm long that is packed with cream fibrous material, which resembles kapok, that surrounds the seed. Northern Cottonwood occurs in sandstone or basalt soils in the Kimberley region of Western Australia, the top end of the Northern Territory, Cape York Peninsula and north-east Queensland. It also occurs in India and parts of South-east Asia (ALA, 2022; ATRP, 2020; WAH, 2022).

Medicinal Uses Various parts of the Northern Cottonwood tree are used in folk medicine in parts of Asia. The flowers are astringent and refrigerant and are used to treat skin problems. The young roots are diuretic and tonic and are used in the treatment of cholera, tubercular fistula, coughs, urinary tract infections, dysentery and impotency. Decoctions of the shoots were used to treat ulcers of the palate, syphilis, leprosy and spider or snakebites (Fern, 2021).

Other Uses The young roots of the Northern Cottonwood are edible after roasting (Barker, 1991; Fox & Garde, 2018; Hiddins, 2001; Kapitany, 2020; Vigilante et al., 2013). The flowers and leaves are also edible (Barker, 1991; PFAF, 2022). Some Aboriginal groups favoured the trunks of this tree for making dugout canoes. The inner bark was used for making cordage (Hiddins, 2001). The wood was used to make shields. The cotton-like kapok was used for ceremonial body decoration (Karadada et al., 2011).

Northern Kurrajong

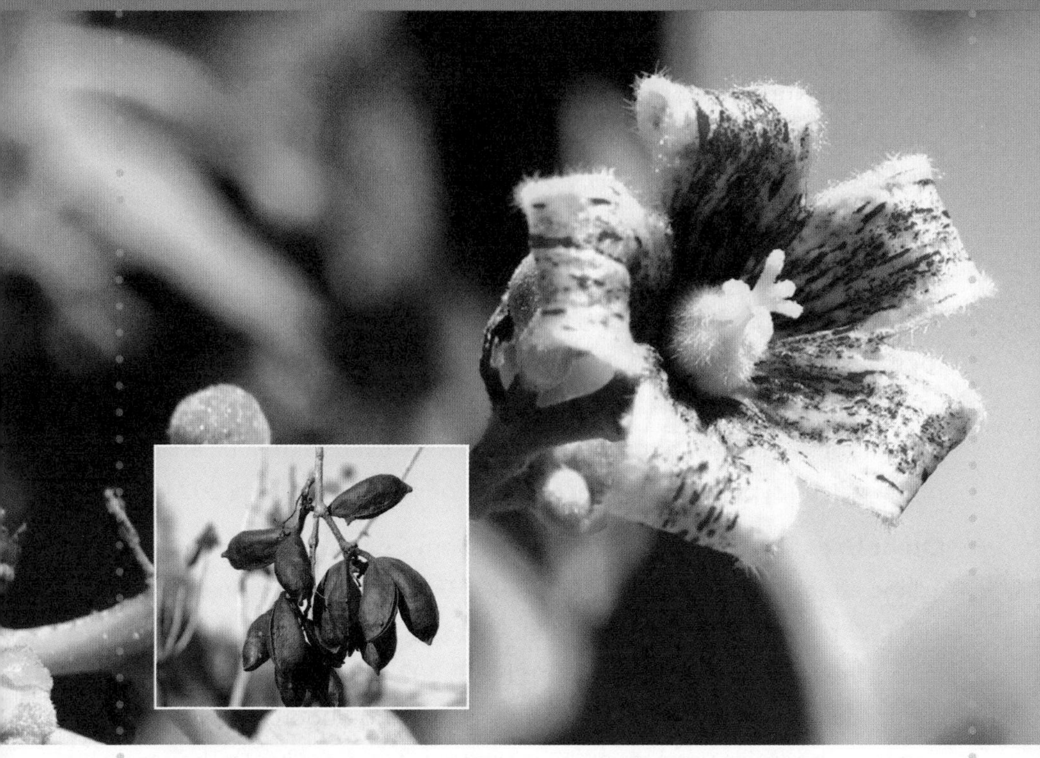

Scientific Name *Brachychiton diversifolius* R.Br.

Common Names Northern Kurrajong, Tropical Kurrajong, Kurrajong.

Aboriginal Names Jalarri (Bunuba) (Oscar et al., 2019), Jarlanba (Wunambal, Gaambera) (Karadada et al., 2011), Korr-korr, or Goor-goor (Bardi) (Young et al., 2012), Djalad (Kwini) (Crawford, 1982), Darlab (Yawuru), Kawoorrkawoorr (Nyul Nyul), Tarlap (Karajarri) (Kenneally et al., 1996), Werlalji, Therranggelji, Therrangkelji (Gija) (Purdie et al., 2018; Wightman, 2003), Wirlal (Jaru) (Wightman, 2003), Jalarr manya (Kwini) (Cheinmora et al., 2017), Kaworrkaworr (Nyikina) (Smith & Smith, 2009).

Field Notes Northern Kurrajong is a tree that has been sighted up to 25 m in height. Its leaves vary in shape, but most are heart-shaped. Its large, boat-shaped fruit or seed pods are pointy on both ends and open to reveal yellow seeds inside. Its attractive, yellow-green flowers with red centres appear from May to December in its native range but, in temperate climate areas, flowering occurs mainly in the summer months. In Western Australia, Northern Kurrajong occurs in red sandy soils over basalt and limestone, on stony hills and alongside rivers in the Kimberley region. It is also found in the top end of the Northern Territory and northern Queensland (ALA, 2022; ATRP, 2020; WAH, 2022).

Medicinal Uses Infusions of the leaves, bark and gum of Northern Kurrajong were used to treat skin sores, wounds and fever. Infusions of the inner bark were used as an eyewash to treat conjunctivitis (Herbalistics, n.d.; Williams, 2020). The gum was used as an antibacterial ointment to treat wounds, sores and leg ulcers (Williams, 2020).

Other Uses The seeds of Northern Kurrajong are edible and were eaten raw or roasted. The fine hairs have to be rubbed off the seeds before eating, as these can irritate the throat. The seed pods are available between September and late December. The flesh of the fruit is not eaten. The roots of young plants were also eaten raw or roasted after the skin was peeled off (Barker, 1991; Cheinmora et al., 2017; Crawford, 1982; Karadada et al., 2011; Kenneally et al., 1996; Oscar et al., 2019; RFCA, 1993; Wightman, 2003). The gum that oozes from wounds in the tree is also edible. The gum was usually cooked in hot ashes until it was brown, then ground to a powder, which was then mixed with water to make a sweet drink (Barker, 1991; Karadada et al., 2011; Kenneally et al., 1996; Vigilante et al., 2013). Fire sticks and spears were made from the wood of Northern Kurrajong, and cordage from the bark (Cheinmora et al., 2017; Crawford, 1982; SKIPA, 2022). Trunks from large, straight trees were used to make dugout canoes, which were used to hunt sea turtles (Cheinmora et al., 2017).

Northern Sandalwood

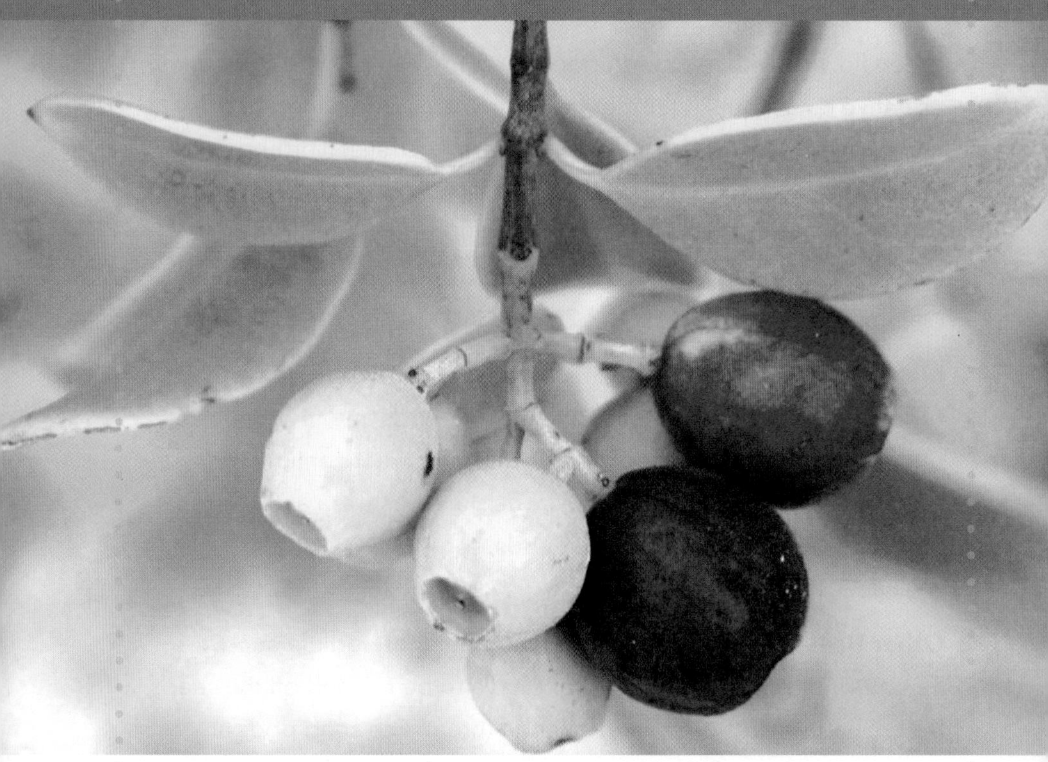

Scientific Name *Santalum lanceolatum* R.Br.

Common Names Northern Sandalwood, Plumbush, Plumwood, Bush Plum, Sandalwood, Tropical Sandalwood, Black Currant Tree.

Aboriginal Names Gooloomara (Miriwoong) (Leonard et al., 2013), Mulurri (Bunuba) (Oscar et al., 2019), Wuudaguuda (Wunambal, Gaambera) (Karadada et al., 2011), Mooloorr (Nyikina) (Young et al., 2012), Bolan, Tharragibberah, Gumamu (Nyikina), Mooloorr (Nyikina) (Smith & Smith, 2009), Bilalur (Bardi) (Smith & Kalotas, 1985), Bilooloorr (Bardi), Birrmankal (Nyul Nyul), Gumamu (Yawuru) (Kenneally et al., 1996), Woorlngooroony, Wurlnguruny (Gija) (Purdie et al., 2018), Miyaga, Miyarn, Nguman (Jaru) (Deegan et al., 2010; Wightman, 2003), Kanturanu, Mililiri, Munyurnpa, Munyunypa, Nganungu, Ngurnari, Nyuwari, Patutjuka, Yangurli (Kukatja) (Valiquette, 1993), Ngankurli (Ngardi) (Cataldi, 2004), Kartinykartiny (Nyangumarta), Kumamu (Karajarri) (Lands, 1997), Marrkirdi (Walpiri) (Northern Tanami IPA, 2015).

Field Notes Northern Sandalwood grows as a shrub or small tree to 7 m in height. It is hemiparasitic on roots of surrounding grasses and bushes which it relies on for some of its nutrients. The narrow fleshy, lanceolate leaves are bluish-green and around 80 mm long. Small, green-white-cream flowers with four small petals appear between January and October. The fruit are spherical berries that are almost black when ripe and up to 15 mm diameter. Northern Sandalwood occurs in red sand, sandy loam or clay along creeks and riverbeds, on red sand dunes over sandstone or on limestone ridges in a variety of habitats all over mainland Australia, except for Victoria and the south-west of Western Australia (ALA, 2022; Lassak & McCarthy, 2001; Native Plants Queensland, 2022; WAH, 2022).

Medicinal Uses The berries are thought to have slight narcotic properties. Decoctions of the scraped outer wood have been drunk for chest infections, such as bronchitis and pneumonia. Crushed leaves were used a poultice to aid in the healing of boils, skin sores and gonorrhoea. Infusions or decoctions of the mashed roots or leaves and bark were used as a liniment for rheumatic pain and as a skin wash to relieve itchy skin. They were also applied to the body to relieve general fatigue. The leaves were burnt as a smoking medicine to enable people to gather strength for long walks and to strengthen babies (Cock, 2011; Fern, 2021; Kenneally et al., 1996; Lassak & McCarthy, 2001; Reid, 1986; Smith, 1991; Webb, 1959; Williams, 2020). Decoctions of the leaves were used as a wash to treat colds and congestion. The leaves were also used as a 'steaming medicine' to treat colds and influenza (Purdie et al., 2018; Wightman, 2003; Williams, 2020) and warmed as a poultice to treat rheumatic pain (Kenneally et al., 1996; Paddy et al., 1993).

Other Uses The fruit of Northern Sandalwood are edible when black and ripe. The fruit are peeled and the white flesh (aril) inside is eaten. They contain good amounts of ascorbic acid (vitamin C). The fruit were often dried and kept for later consumption (Fern, 2021; Hiddins, 2001; Karadada et al., 2011; Lassak & McCarthy, 2001; Low, 1991; RFCA, 1993; Wightman, 2003; Young et al., 2012).

Northern Star Wattle

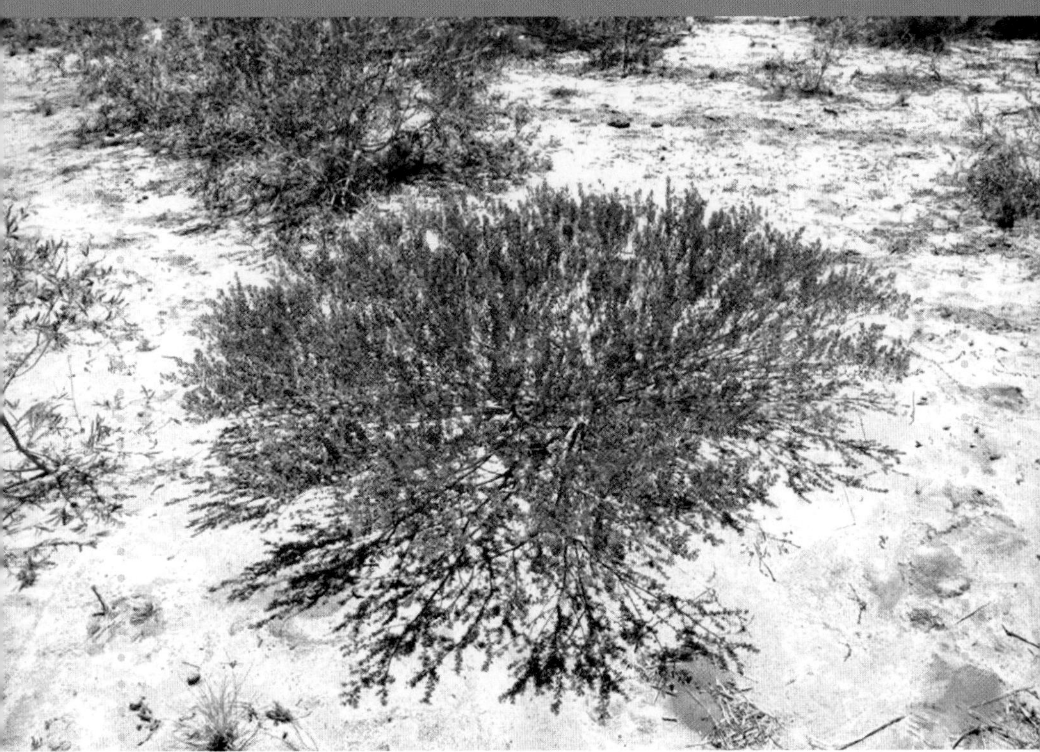

Scientific Name *Acacia stellaticeps* Kodela, Tindale & D.A.Keith.

Common Names Northern Star Wattle, Poverty Bush Glistening Wattle.

Aboriginal Name Parlmangu (Karajarri) (Willing, 2014).

Field Notes Northern Star Wattle is a low, dense shrub growing to 1.5 m in height and up to 3 m across. The bark is grey and smooth or finely fissured. The phyllodes are narrow elliptic-obovate, sometimes almost rounded, and up to 20 mm long and 12 mm wide. Its yellow, fluffy, globular flower heads are present from October to May. Its fruit or seed pods are flat, linear to narrowly oblanceolate or narrowly elliptic, up to 100 mm long and 10 mm wide, and explode when ripe to release the seeds. Northern Star Wattle occurs in red sand, stony sand and clay on flats, sand ridges and plains in the Kimberley, Pilbara and northern

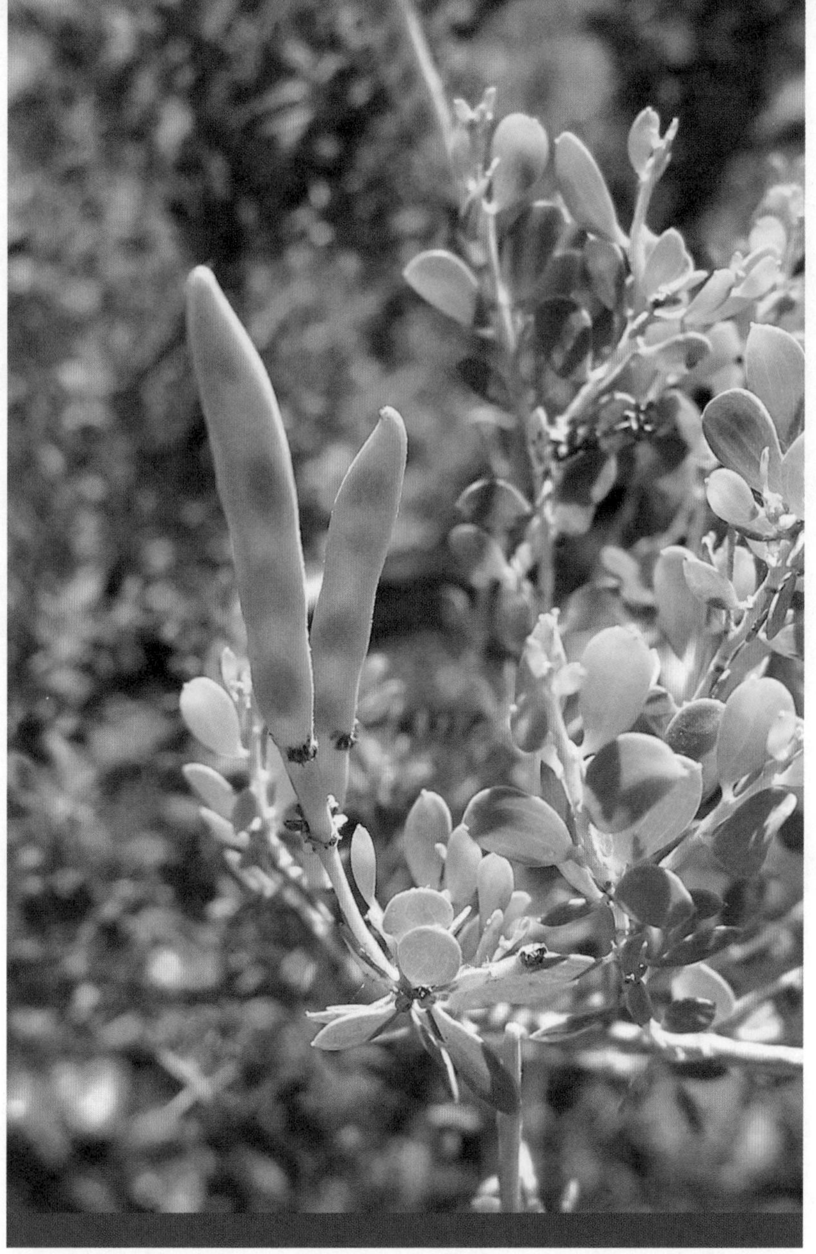

Goldfields regions of Western Australia (ALA, 2022; Maslin et al., 2010; WAH, 2022).

Medicinal Uses Decoctions of the phyllodes of Northern Star Wattle were used as an antiseptic wash to bathe sores and wounds, and to relieve itchy skin. The phyllodes are sometimes used for smoke medicine to relieve 'cold sick' or 'Kinkirrita', presumably the symptoms of colds and influenza (Willing, 2014).

Oakleaf Fern

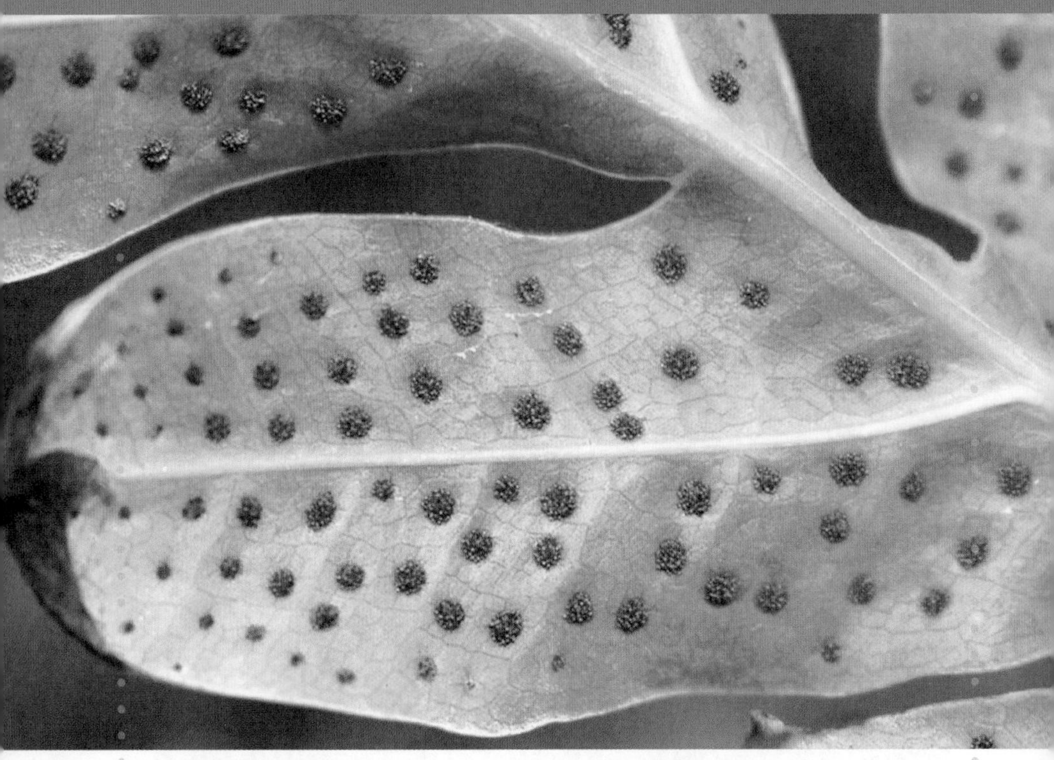

Scientific Name *Drynaria quercifolia* (L.) J.Sm.

Common Names Oakleaf Fern, Oakleaf Basket Fern.

Field Notes Oakleaf Fern is a rhizomatous, perennial fern that grows up to 1 m in height. It produces two leaf types: sterile 'nest' fronds near the base and longer deciduous fronds. The sterile fronds are brown, papery and up to 400 mm long and 300 mm wide. The fertile fronds are erect, smooth, light green, pinnate-lobed and 1 m long by 300 mm wide. They are divided into many strap-like lobes, each 330 mm long by 40 mm wide. Spores that look like reddish dots are produced on the underside of the fertile fronds. Oakleaf Fern occurs in peaty sand, in rock crevices, on rock shelves and in soil amongst boulders in the Kimberley region of Western Australia, the Northern Territory and Queensland. It also occurs in India and South-east Asia, including Malaysia, Indonesia, the Philippines, New Guinea and Fiji (Ferns of Western Australia, 2022; Fox & Garde, 2020; WAH, 2022).

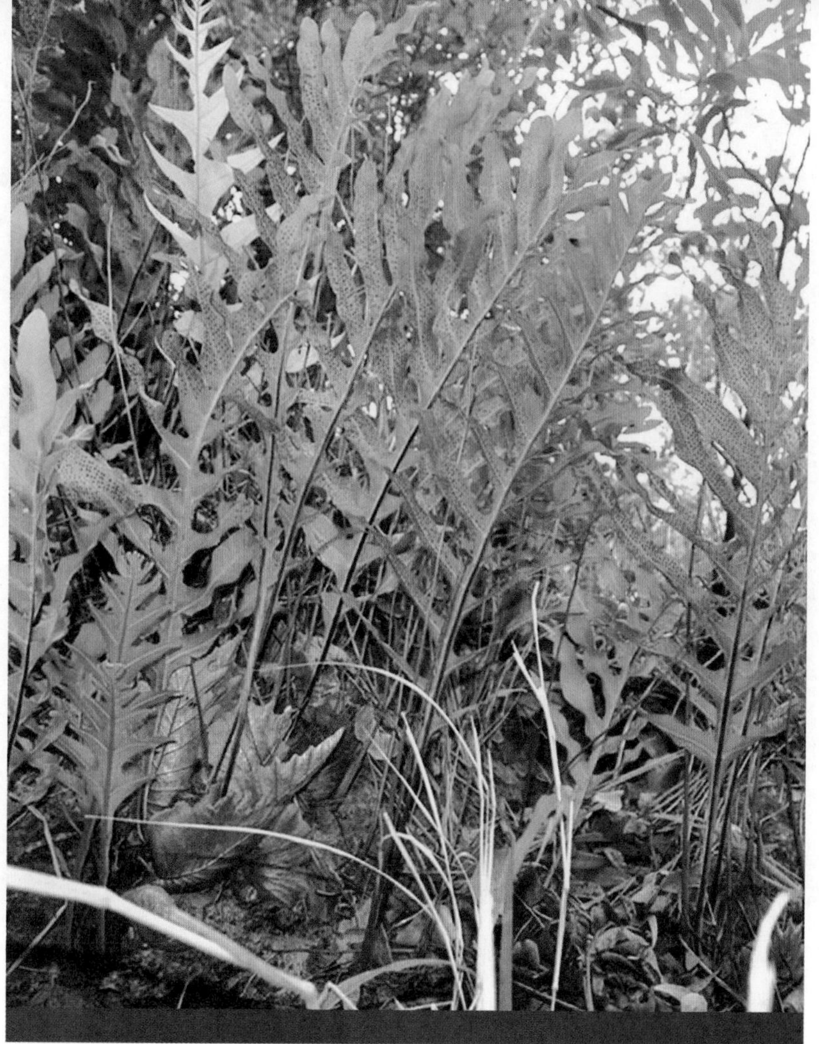

Medicinal Uses The leaves of Oakleaf Fern can be crushed and used as poultice to treat inflammation and swellings. The rhizomes are used in folk medicine in some Asian countries. The rhizome has astringent and bitter properties and is used as a tonic for the bowels. The rhizomes are also used in the treatment of typhoid fever, dyspepsia and coughs (Fern, 2021).

Other Uses The rhizomes of Oakleaf Fern were eaten by some Aboriginal groups across the far north of Australia when other food was scarce. The rhizomes were usually pounded with a stone, washed then baked in hot ashes (Fox & Garde, 2018).

Old World Forked Fern

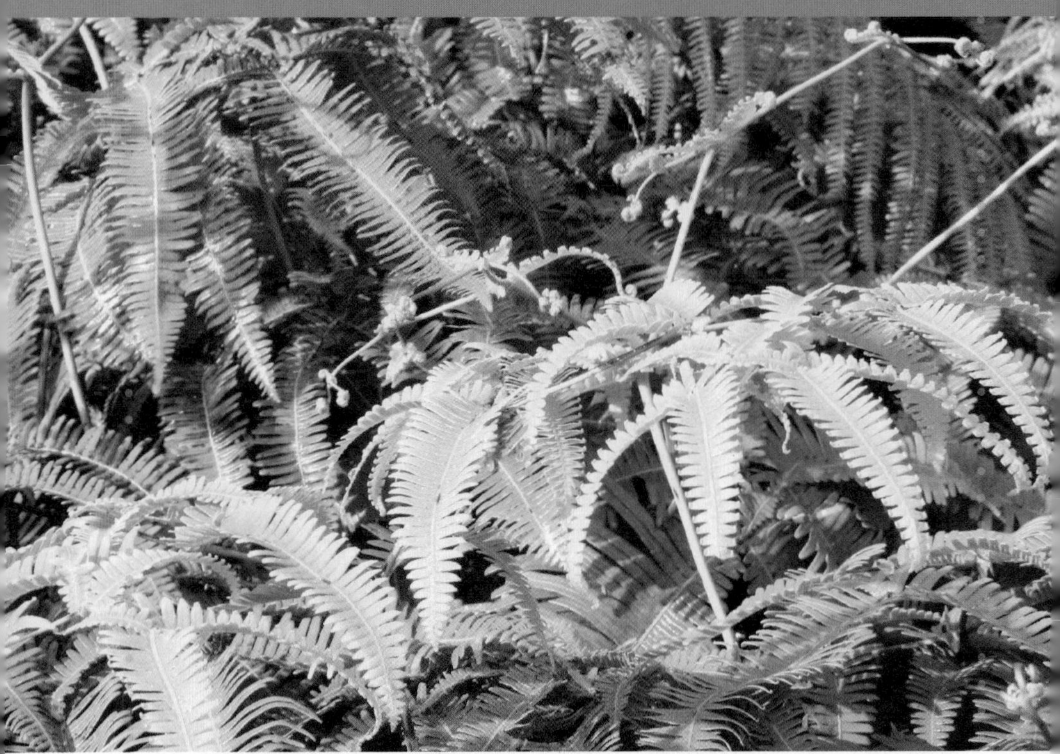

Scientific Name *Dicranopteris linearis* (Burm.f.) Underw., previously known as *Gleichenia dichotoma* (Thunb.) Hook.

Common Name Old World Forked Fern.

Field Notes Old World Forked Fern is a rhizomatous plant that spreads by cloning and is sometimes seen climbing on other plants. When climbing, the leafy branches can reach over 6 m long and they can climb to 10 m high when climbing trees. The leaves on the fronds are linear in shape and up to 70 mm long. The undersides of the leaves are hairy and sometimes waxy. In Australia, the fern is found forming thickets across the top end from the Kimberley region of Western Australia, through the Northern Territory and Far North Queensland, and down the east coast into northern New South Wales. It also occurs in tropical Africa, on the Indian subcontinent, in China, New Zealand, South-east Asia and on some Pacific islands (ALA, 2022; Fern, 2021; WAH, 2022).

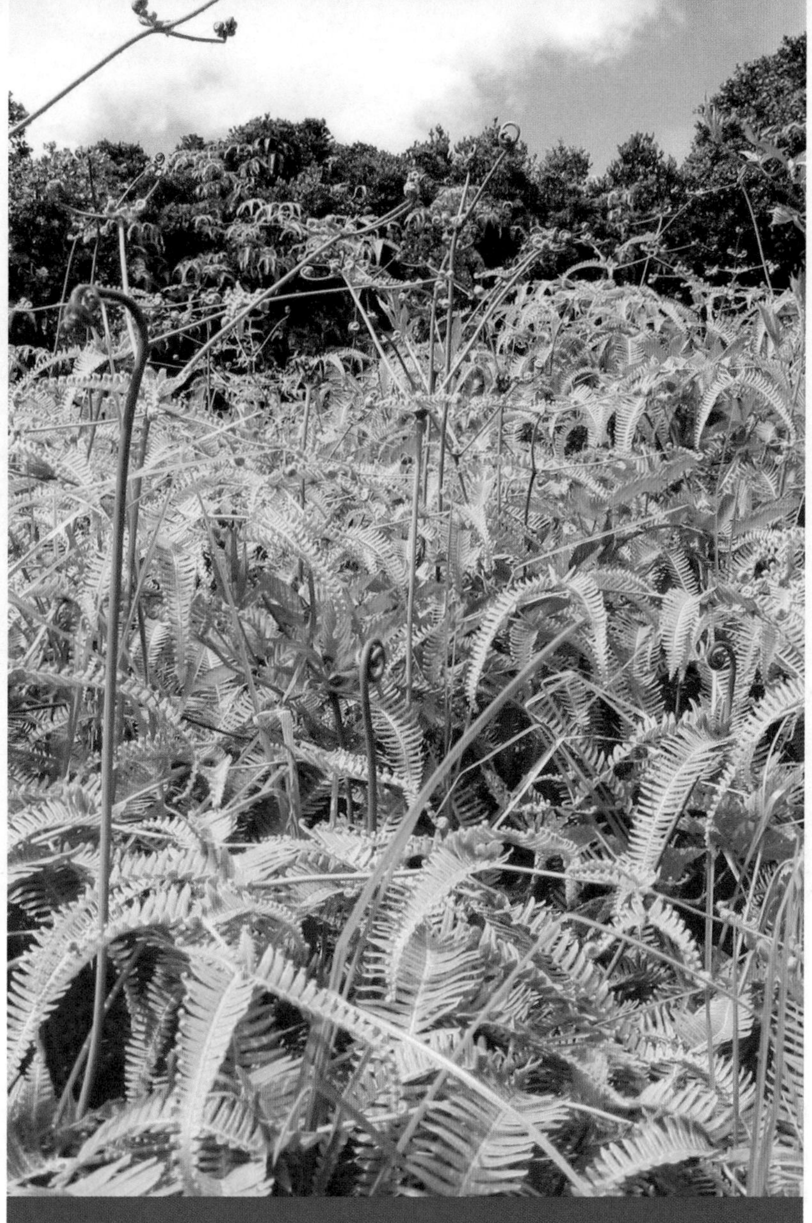

Medicinal Uses Old World Forked Fern is used in folk medicine in some countries. Crushed leaves were used as a poultice to treat wounds, cuts, boils, leg ulcers and sores. The rhizomes have been used internally to treat intestinal parasites (Fern, 2021).

Other Uses The rhizomes of this fern are a good source of starch and were used for food by some Aboriginal groups across Australia, as well as people of other tropical and sub-tropical countries (Fern, 2021; Maiden, 1889).

Onion Lily

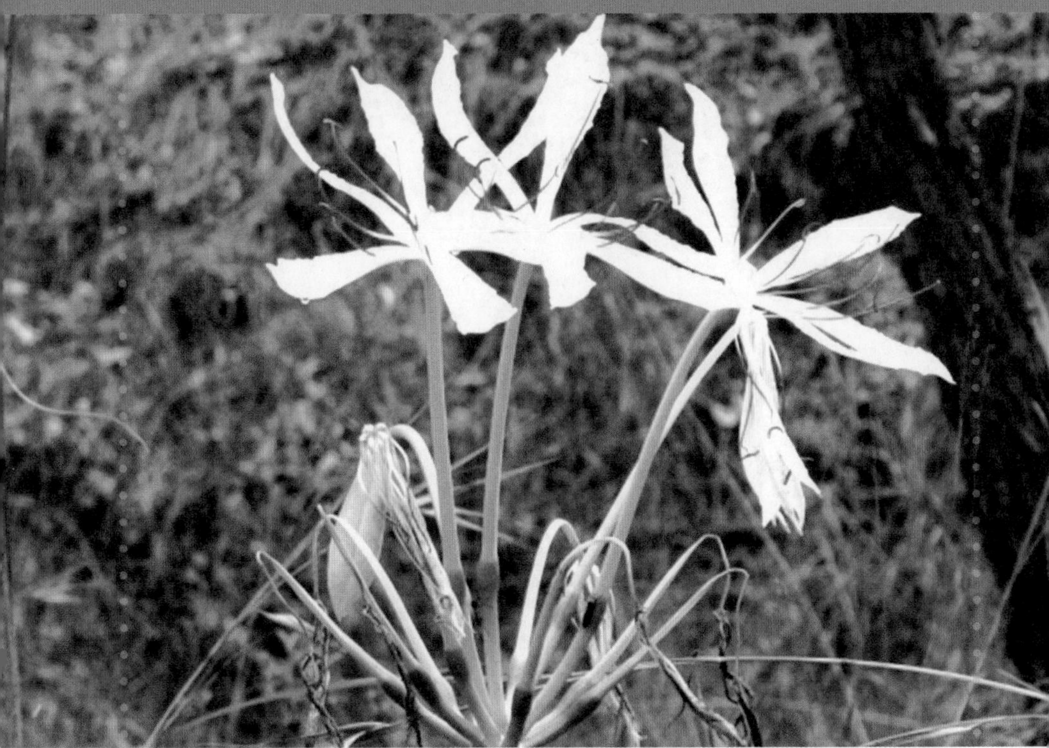

Scientific Name *Crinum arenarium* Herb., previously known as *Crinum angustifolium* R.Br.

Common Names Onion Lily, Bush Onion, Field Lily.

Aboriginal Names Dawadawarr (Bunuba) (Oscar et al., 2019), Alamarr (Wunambal, Gaambera) (Karadada et al., 2011), Barrjanggerrji, Baljanggarrji (Gija) (Purdie et al., 2018).

Field Notes Onion Lily is a herb that grows up to 1 m in height. Its linear leaves arise from the base. Its beautiful flowers are white with five long pointed petals and long pink to purple stamens. Onion Lily occurs on floodplains and in seasonally wet coastal and near-coastal areas of the Kimberley region and islands of northern Western Australia. It is also endemic to the Northern Territory and Queensland, where it is found as far south as Brisbane (ALA, 2022; Flora of Australia Online, 2022).

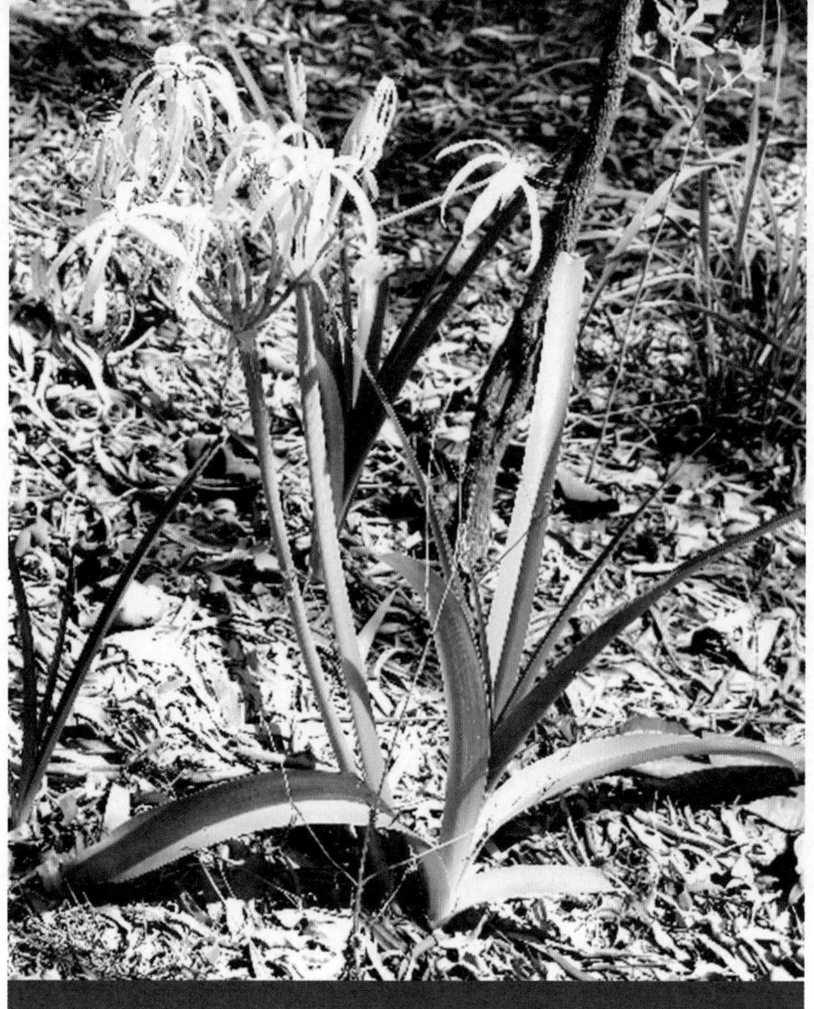

Medicinal Uses Infusions or decoctions of the crushed bulbs were used as an antiseptic wash on wounds and sores to promote healing, and as a treatment for leprosy (Low, 1990; Smith, 1991). Decoctions of the bulbs and leaves were used externally as a wash or liniment to relieve painful knees and hips due to arthritis (Smith, 1991).

Other Uses The root bulbs of the Onion Lily are edible but can be a bit bitter (Karadada et al., 2011; Vigilante et al., 2013). The Wunambal and Gaambera people smash the root bulbs up with a rock or stick until the pulp turns black. The remaining pulp is cooked for a long period. This method of preparation apparently makes the root bulbs taste better and less likely to make a person feel nauseous (Karadada et al., 2011).

Orange Jasmine

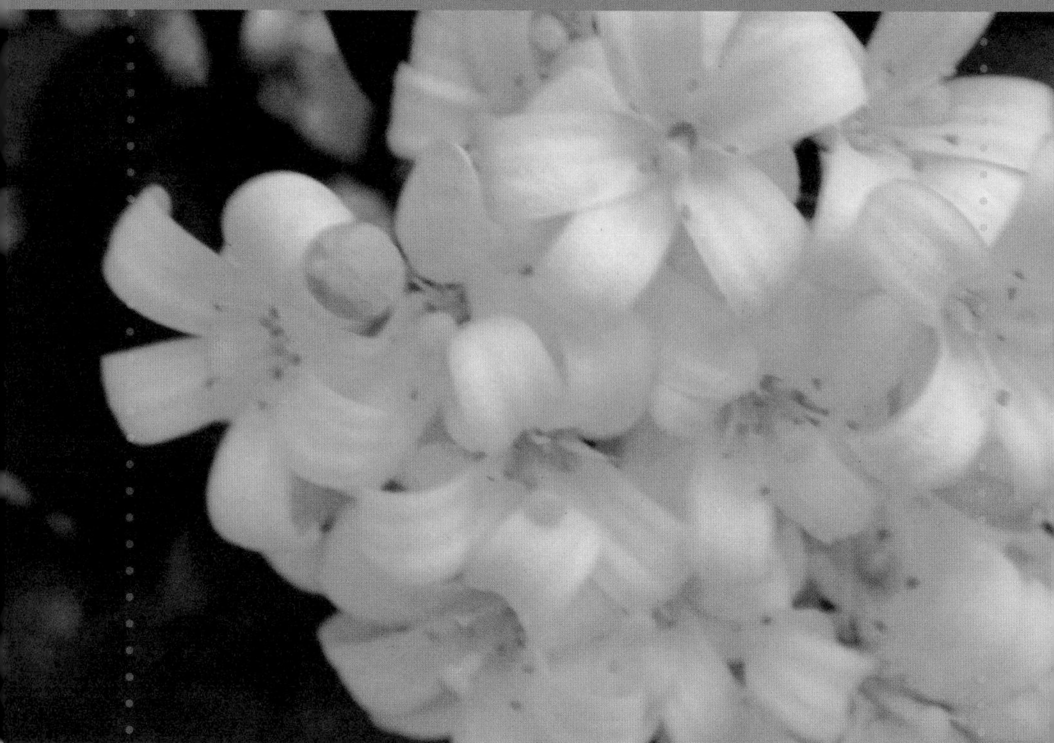

Scientific Name *Murraya paniculata* (L.) Jack. A similar plant, *Murraya paniculata* 'Exotica', is widely grown in the eastern states but is not native to Australia.

Common Names Orange Jasmine, Hawaiian Mock Orange, Chinese Box, Mock Orange, Burmese Boxwood, Chinese Boxwood, Cosmetic Bark Tree, Orange Jessamine, Satinwood, Chinese Myrtle, Jessamine, Lakeview Jasmine, Honey Bush, Murraya, Mock Lime.

Field Notes Orange Jasmine is a shrub or tree that grows up to 5 m in height. Its glossy, narrow-elliptic to ovate leaves are up to 70 mm long and 130 mm wide. Its fragrant white flowers have five petals that are up to 18 mm long and curved backwards. The fruit are ovoid berries up to 10 mm long and 14 mm in diameter. They turn from green to orange or bright red in colour as they mature. The fruit contain one or two teardrop-shaped seeds. Orange Jasmine occurs in sand, loam over sandstone or basalt in coastal areas,

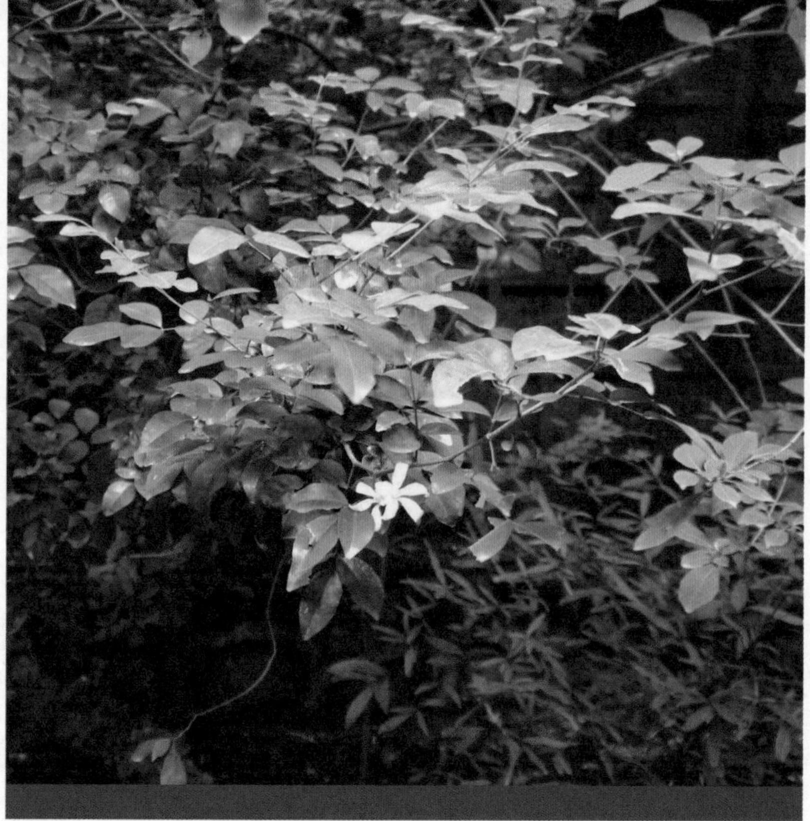

along creeklines and on scree slopes. It is native to the northern coast of the Kimberley region of Western Australia, the Northern Territory and Far North Qeensland. It also occurs in Cambodia, the Indian subcontinent, Indonesia, Laos, Malaysia, Myanmar, the Philippines, southern China, Sri Lanka, Taiwan, Thailand and Vietnam (ALA, 2022; WAH, 2022).

Medicinal Uses Decoctions of the leaves are used in folk medicine in Asia as an analgesic mouthwash for toothache, to treat diarrhoea and dysentery, and as a general analgesic. The decoctions can also be used externally as a liniment on painful joints and muscles due to arthritis. Powdered dry leaves are applied externally to fresh cuts to stem bleeding. Poultices of the fresh leaves are used to treat sprains and contusions (Fern, 2021; Health Benefits Times, 2020).

Other Uses The fruit of Orange Jasmine are edible though not very palatable. The flowers have been used in some countries to flavour tea and the leaves have been used to flavour curries (Fern, 2021).

Orange Spade Flower

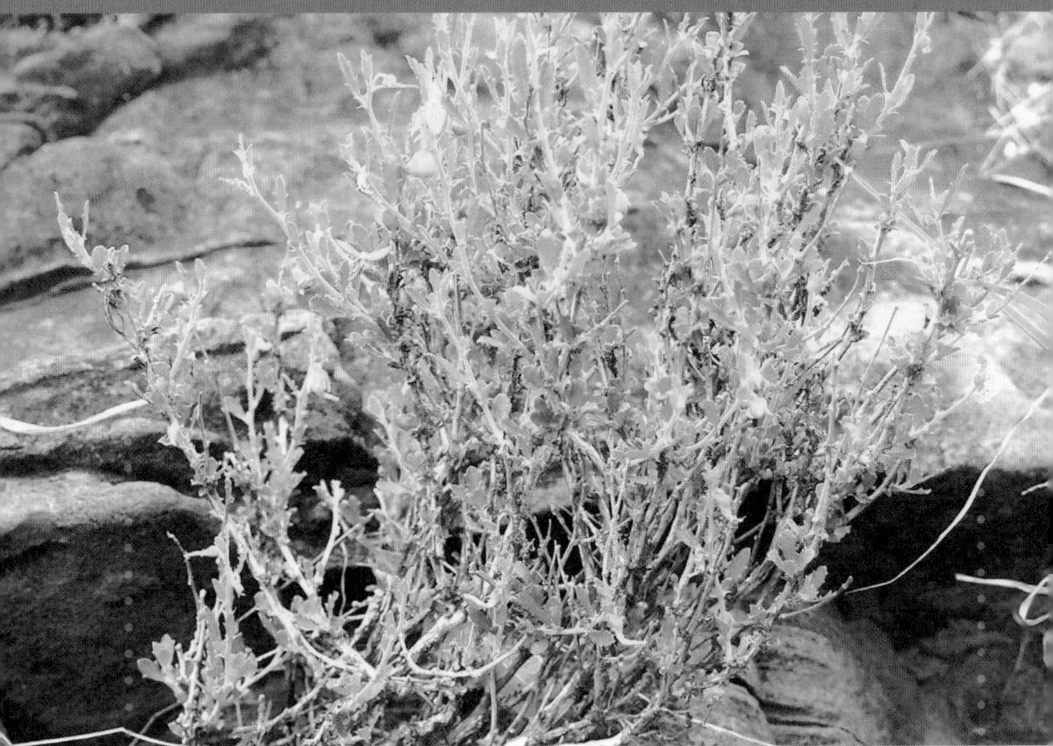

Scientific Name *Afrohybanthus aurantiacus* (Benth.) Flicker, previously known as *Hybanthus aurantiacus* (F.Muell. ex Benth.) F.Muell.

Common Name Orange Spade Flower.

Aboriginal Name Ngapurlu-ngapurlu (Kukatja) (Valiquette, 1993).

Field Notes Orange Spade Flower is a compact shrub that grows up to 600 mm in height. Its stems are scabrous or more or less glabrous. Its leaves are alternate or clustered, linear to lanceolate and up to 30 mm long. Its bright orange flowers have a large, spade-shaped lower petal hence the common name. Flowering can occur any time between May and October but usually occurs between June and July. Its fruit or seed pods are globose capsules that are up to 9 mm long. Orange Spade Flower occurs in the Pilbara and Kimberley regions of Western Australia, and the Northern Territory (ALA, 2022; eFlora.SA, 2022).

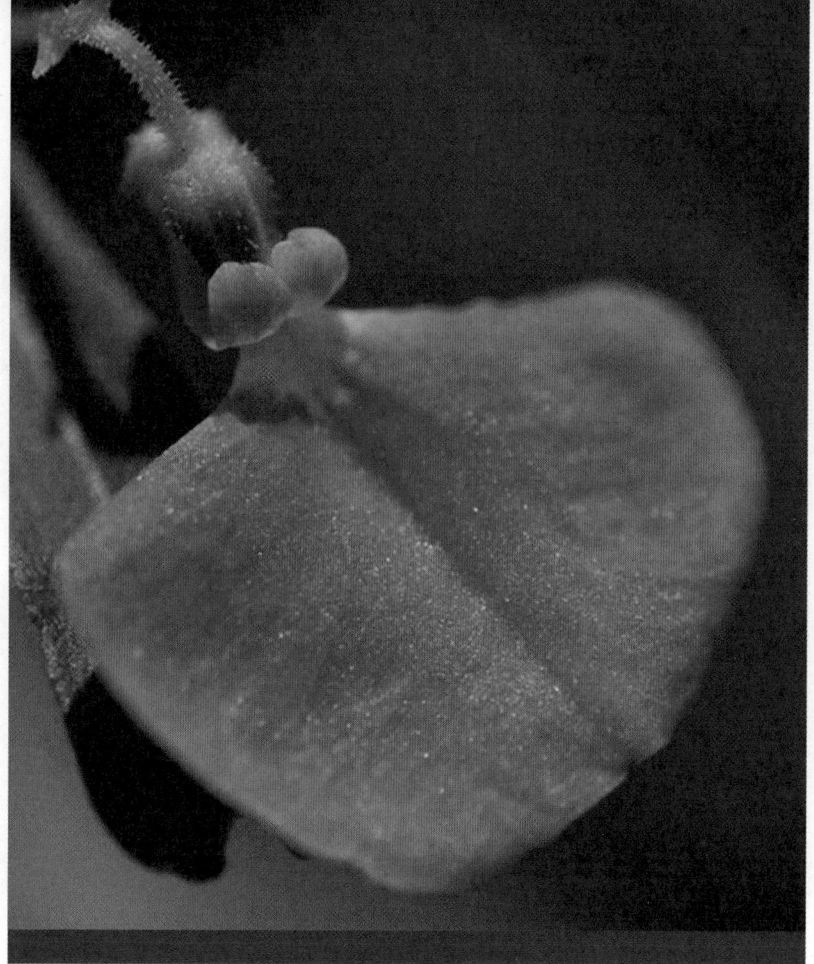

Medicinal Uses Sap from the Orange Spade Flower plant was applied to cuts and sores to aid healing. Vapours from the sap were inhaled to treat headaches and the symptoms of colds and influenza (Valiquette, 1993).

Pagurda

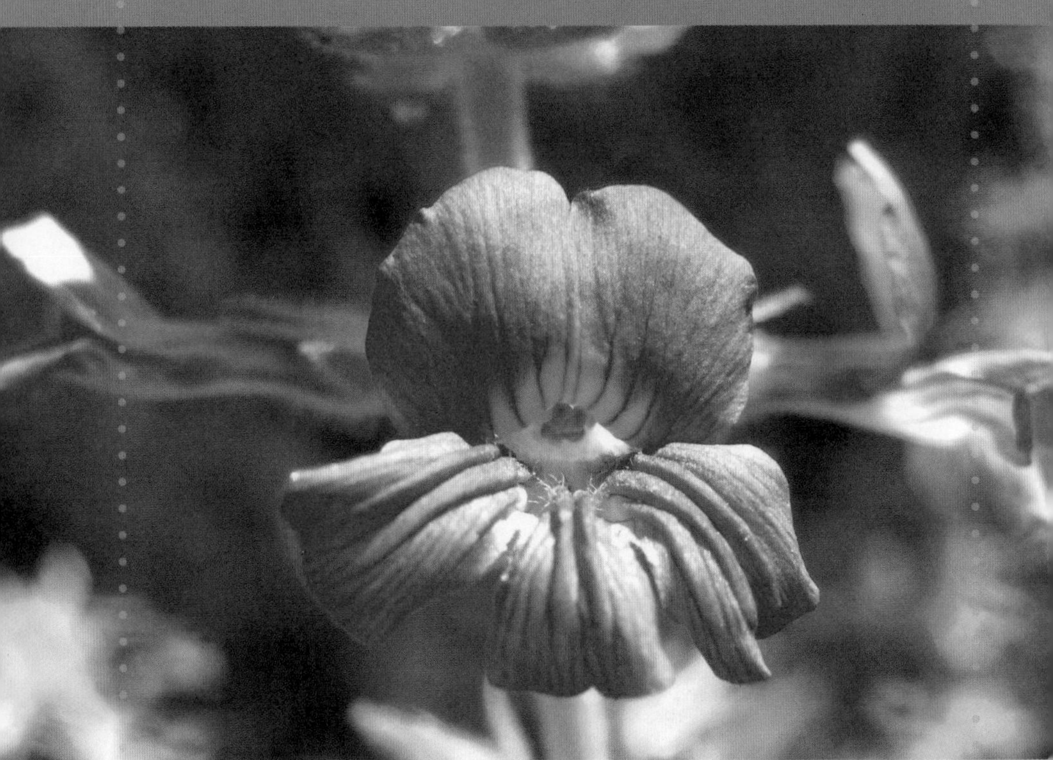

Scientific Name *Stemodia viscosa* Roxb.

Common Names Pagurda, Bluerod, Sticky Bluerod, Jirrpirinypa.

Aboriginal Names Ngunungunu (Bunuba) (Oscar et al., 2019), Minikuny-minyikunypa (Kukatja) (Valiquette, 1993).

Field Notes Pagurda grows as a sticky, strongly aromatic, decumbent to erect perennial herb or shrub up to 500 mm in height. Its leaves vary in shape and most are roughly elliptical and quite hairy. Its round, tubular blue-purple flowers appear between March and August. Pagurda occurs in sandy or clayey soils, often over sandstone, in creek and river beds, around waterholes and on floodplains in the Gascoyne, Pilbara and Kimberley regions of Western Australia, the Northern Territory and central Australia (ALA, 2022; Lassak & McCarthy, 2001; WAH, 2022).

Medicinal Uses Crushed leaves of Pagurda, probably held under the nose, were used to relieve the symptoms of colds and

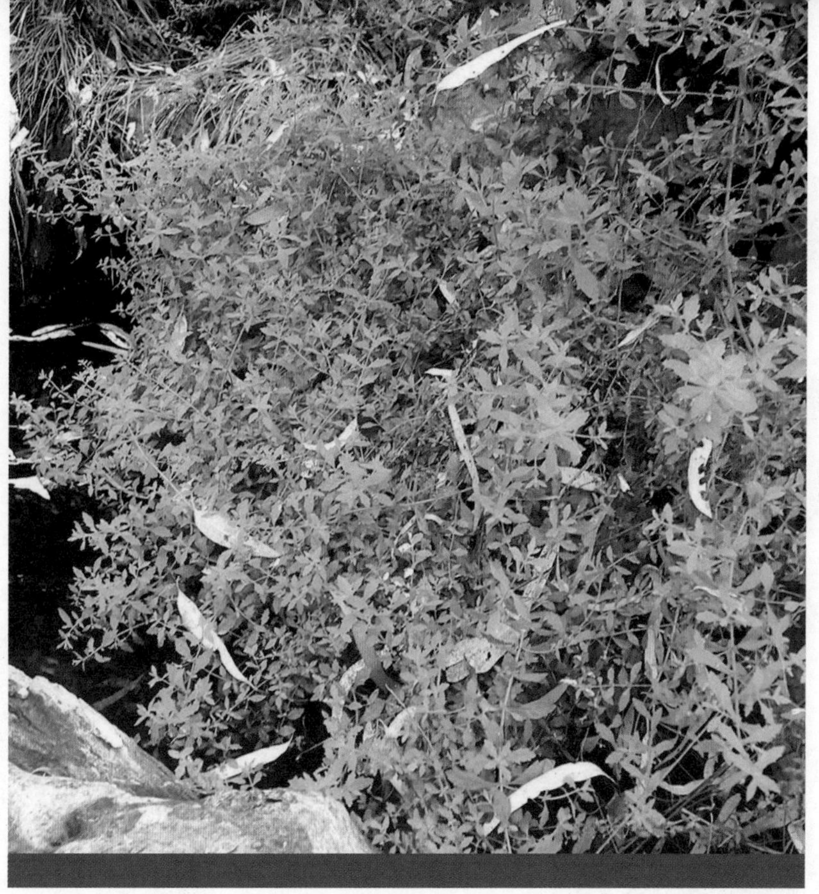

influenza. During times of contagious diseases, some Aboriginal groups made beds from the leaves covered with paperbark to keep babies healthy (Lassak & McCarthy, 2001; Low, 1990; Reid, 1986; Williams, 2013). Some Aboriginal groups ground the leaves and mixed the paste with fat to make a rubbing medicine, similar to Vicks, to treat the symptoms cold and influenza (Olive Pink Botanic Garden, 2010).

Papawitilpa

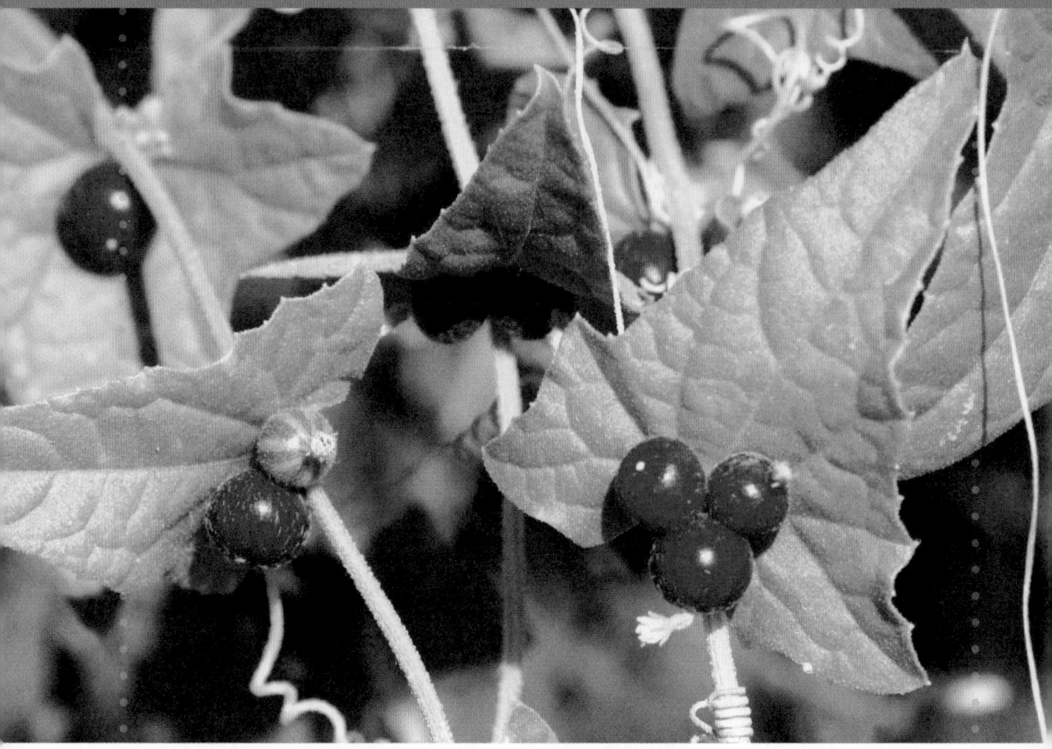

Scientific Name *Cucumis argenteus* (Domin) P.Sebastian & I.Telford.

Common Names Papawitilpa, Snake Vine.

Aboriginal Names Wantakapi-kapi, Waratji (Kukatja) (Valiquette, 1993).

Field Notes Papawitilpa is a trailing or climbing, monoecious, annual or perennial vine with arrowhead-shaped leaves. Its separate small, yellow male and female flowers on the same plant can be present all year round. Its globous fruit are initially green, red when ripe and only 8 mm in diameter. Papawitilpa occurs in a variety of habitats, including open shrublands, woodlands and hummock grasslands in the Pilbara and Kimberley regions of Western Australia, the Northern Territory, Queensland and South Australia (ALA, 2022; FloraNT, 2022).

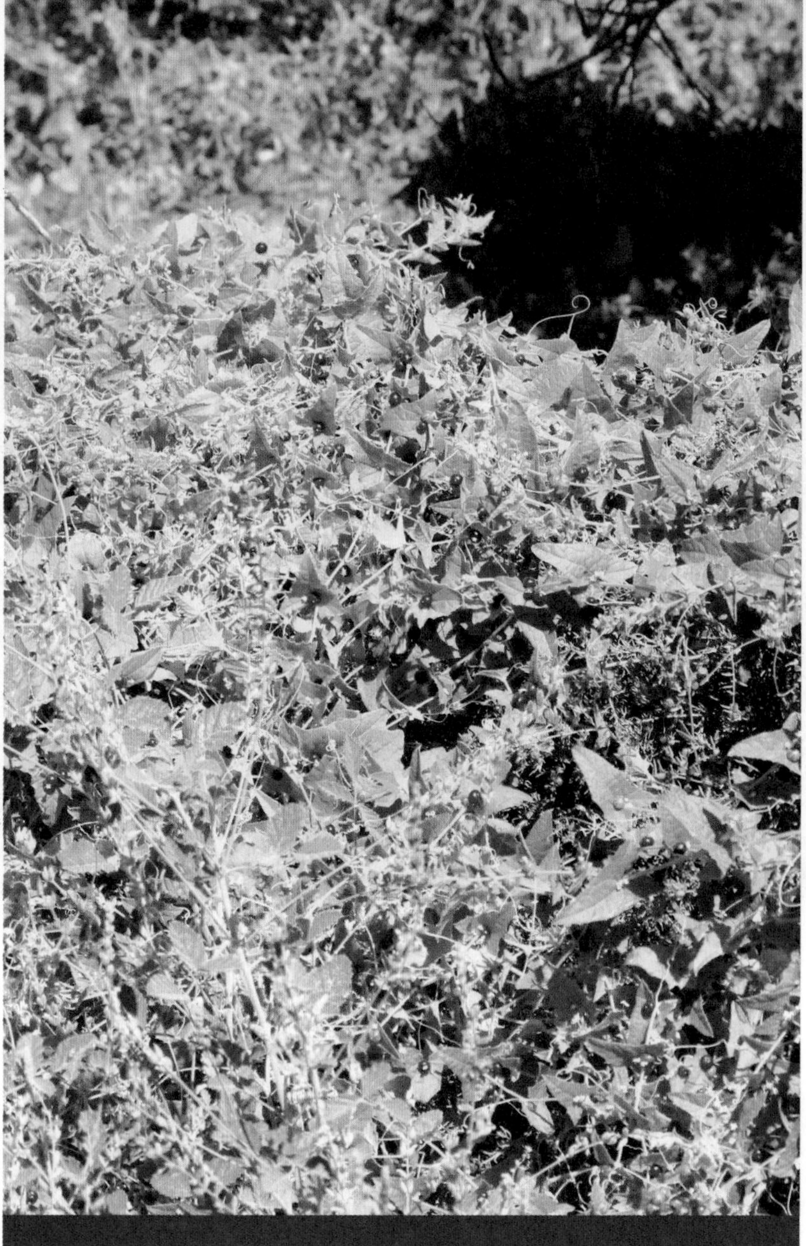

Medicinal Uses Compresses or poultices of the wetted and pulped leaves of the Papawitilpa vine were applied to the head to treat headaches and insomnia, (Morse, 2005). Pulp from the fruit is used as a liniment and rubbed on areas of rheumatic pain and sprains. The vine is sometimes wound around the head to treat headaches and insomnia (Valiquette, 1993).

Pemphis

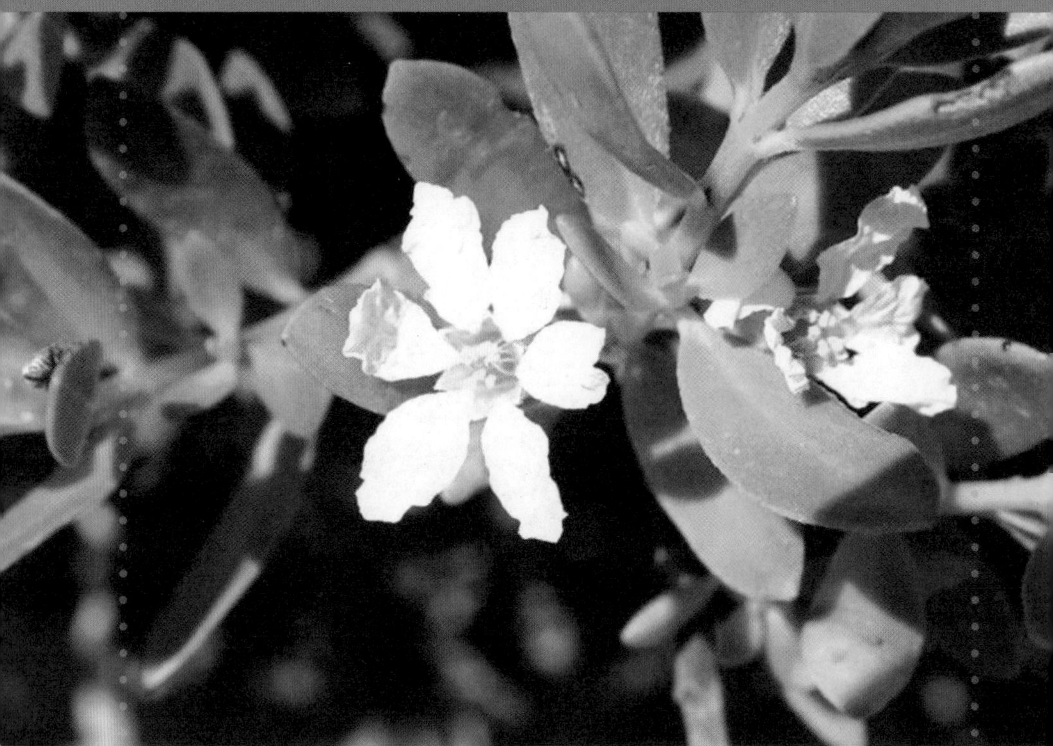

Scientific Name *Pemphis acidula* J.R.Forst. & G.Forst.

Common Names Pemphis, Digging Stick Tree, Kayu Burong.

Field Notes Pemphis is an evergreen mangrove growing as a shrub or densely branching small tree up to 8 m in height, but is occasionally found as a dwarf creeping shrub only 150 mm high. Its leaves are ovate and about 30 mm long and 9 mm wide. Its white to pink flowers have six small petals and six somewhat larger petals. They are present between March and July. The fruit are globose and about 6 mm long and 5 mm in diameter. Pemphis occurs in sand in coastal areas of the Kimberley region of Western Australia, the Northern Territory and the east coast of northern Queensland. It also occurs throughout most of the tropical Indo-Pacific region (ALA, 2022; ATRP, 2020; Fern, 2021; WAH, 2022).

Medicinal Uses The tip of a burnt Pemphis twig was applied to the site of a toothache to ease the pain (Low, 1990; Steptoe &

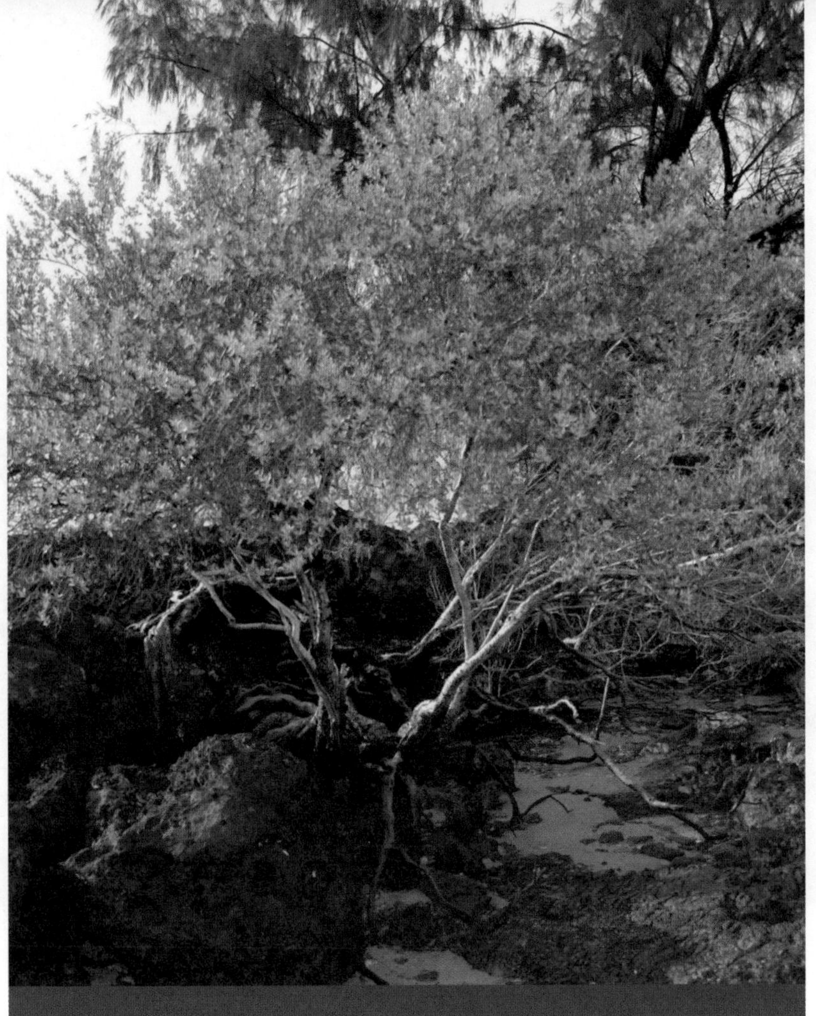

Passananti, 2012). Filtered infusions of the bark were used internally to induce uterine contractions to effect an abortion. Infusions of the bark were used to treat stomatitis (inflammation of the mouth and lips) (Fern, 2021).

Other Uses The thick, fleshy leaves of Pemphis are edible and are either used as a pot herb or eaten raw or boiled as a vegetable in parts of Africa and Asia. The fruit are also edible (Fern, 2021).

Pied Piper Bush

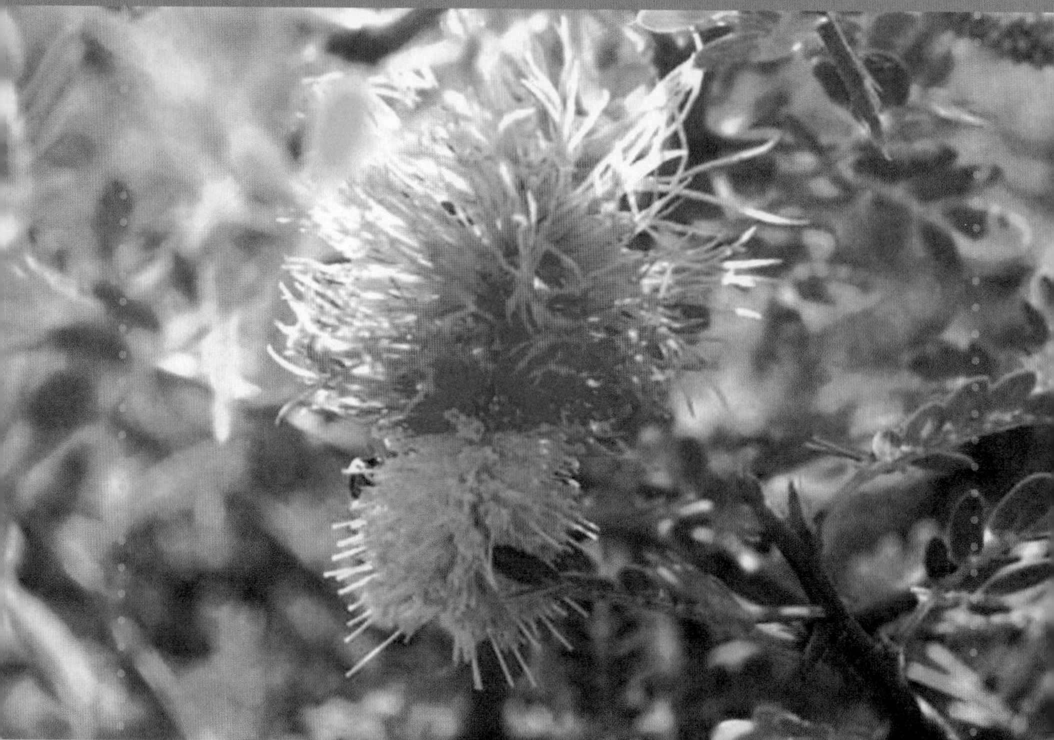

Scientific Name *Dichrostachys spicata* (F.Muell.) Domin.

Common Names Pied Piper Bush, Chinese Lantern, Thorn Bush.

Aboriginal Names Murrulumbu, Gulumarra (Jaru) (Wightman, 2003), Waka-waka (Kukatja) (Valiquette, 1993).

Field Notes Pied Piper Bush is a spreading or straggly, spiny shrub or tree that grows up to 6 m in height. Its leaves are bipinnate with five to seven ovate leaflets. Its fluffy flowers are a combination of yellow and pink-purple with 10 stamens. Flowering is between November and July. Its fruit or seed pods are linear, glabrous, flat, straight, curved or usually wavy and coiled and up to 65 mm long and 10 mm wide. Pied Piper Bush occurs in sand, sandy loam, loam, clay and stony clay soils along streams and on the border of swamps in the Pilbara and Kimberley regions of Western Australia, the Northern Territory, and the north-western part of Queensland (ALA, 2022; Flora of Australia Online, 2022; WAH, 2022).

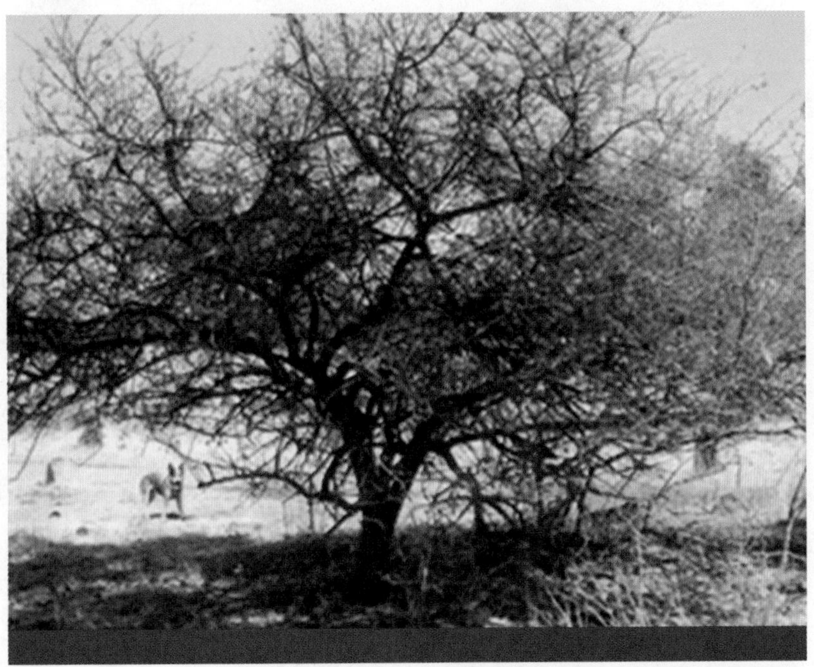

Medicinal Uses Decoctions of the bark of Pied Piper Bush are used as an antiseptic wash to treat skin sores and wounds. The washes are thought to dry the wounds and sores out and help them heal more quickly (Deegan et al., 2010; Wightman, 2003).

Pink River Apple

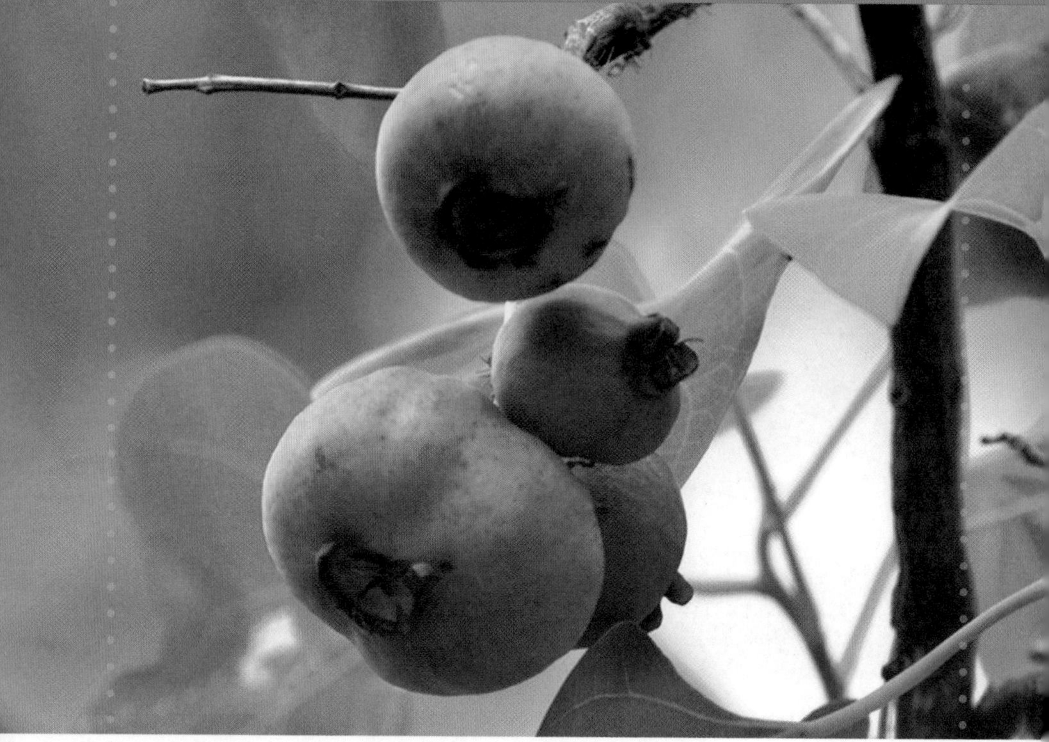

Scientific Name *Syzygium eucalyptoides* (F.Muell.) B.Hyland subsp. *eucalyptoides*.

Common Names Pink River Apple, Pink Bush Apple, White Bush Apple.

Aboriginal Names Gawoorriny, Roonggoony (Gija) (Purdie et al., 2018), Jinandarri (Jaru) (Wightman, 2003), Ngarûwarri minya, Ngarawarri minya (Kwini) (Cheinmora, et al., 2017).

Field Notes Pink River Apple grows as a shrub or tree up to 18 m in height. It has smooth whitish bark, and green, linear slender leaves. Its showy, cream-white flowers are usually present from May to November. Its white or pink globose fruit are small and fleshy. Fruiting occurs between November and February. Pink River Apple occurs in sand, sandstone or alluvium along watercourses and seasonally waterlogged depressions across the top end of Australia from the Kimberley region in Western Australia through the

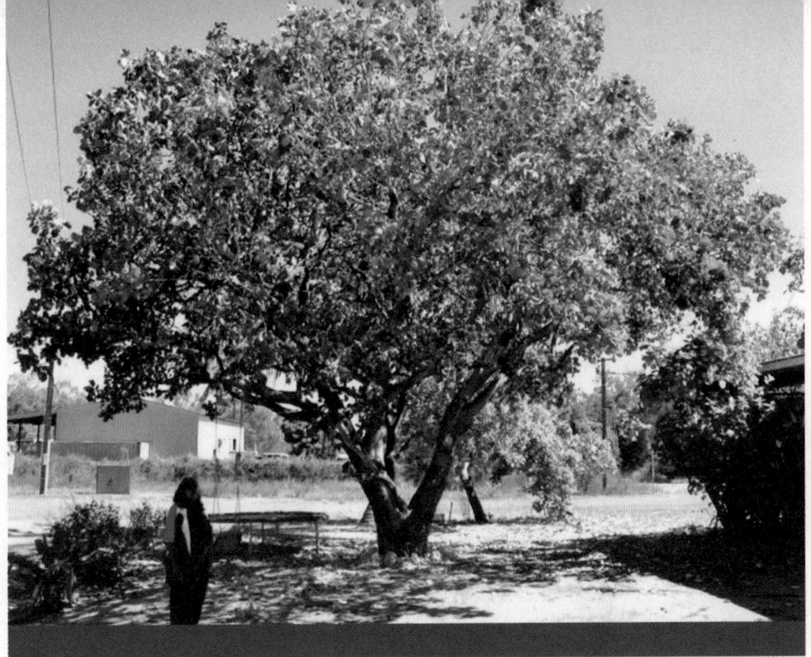

Northern Territory and into the Cape York Peninsula in Queensland (ALA, 2022; WAH, 2022).

Medicinal Uses Infusions of the crushed bark of Pink River Apple were used externally as a body wash to treat general malaise (Hiddins, 2001; SKIPA, 2022).

Other Uses The small fruit of the Pink River Apple are edible when pink and ripe. They are reported to be very tasty and much sought after. The fruit are available in the early wet season around December (Cheinmora et al., 2017; Edwards, 2005; Fox & Garde, 2018; Hiddins, 2001; Purdie et al., 2018; Wightman, 2003). The leaves can be chewed and are reported to 'have a pleasant taste and are favoured by children' (Cheinmora et al., 2017).

Pink Star Flower

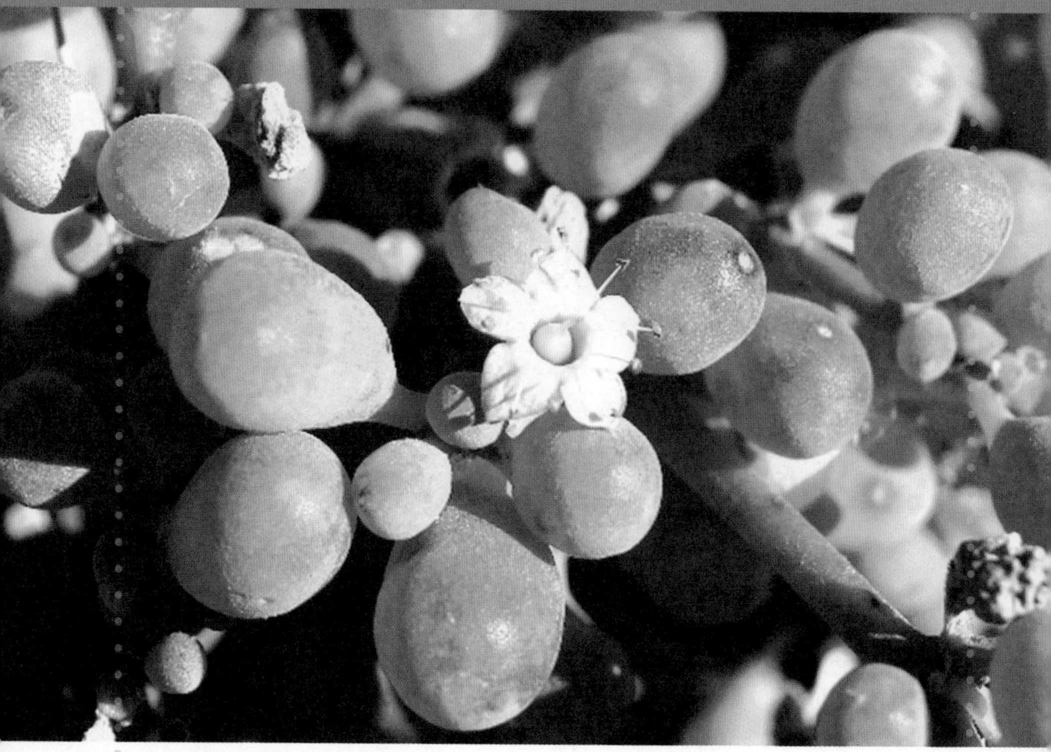

Scientific Name *Trianthema turgidifolium* F.Muell.

Common Name Pink Star Flower.

Field Notes Pink Star Flower is a decumbent, succulent, long-living herb that spreads over the ground. It has woody short stems. Its smooth, succulent, spatulate leaves are up to 20 mm long and 5 mm wide. A single small, pinkish-white, star-shaped flower grows from the base of the leaves. The Pink Star Flower is endemic to the Gascoyne, Pilbara and Kimberley regions of Western Australia as well as the south-western corner of the Northern Territory (ALA, 2022; WAH, 2022).

Medicinal Uses The antiseptic juice from the leaves of Pink Star Flower is applied directly to wounds and sores to aid healing, or into ears to treat earache due to an infection of the auditory canal (YMAC, 2016).

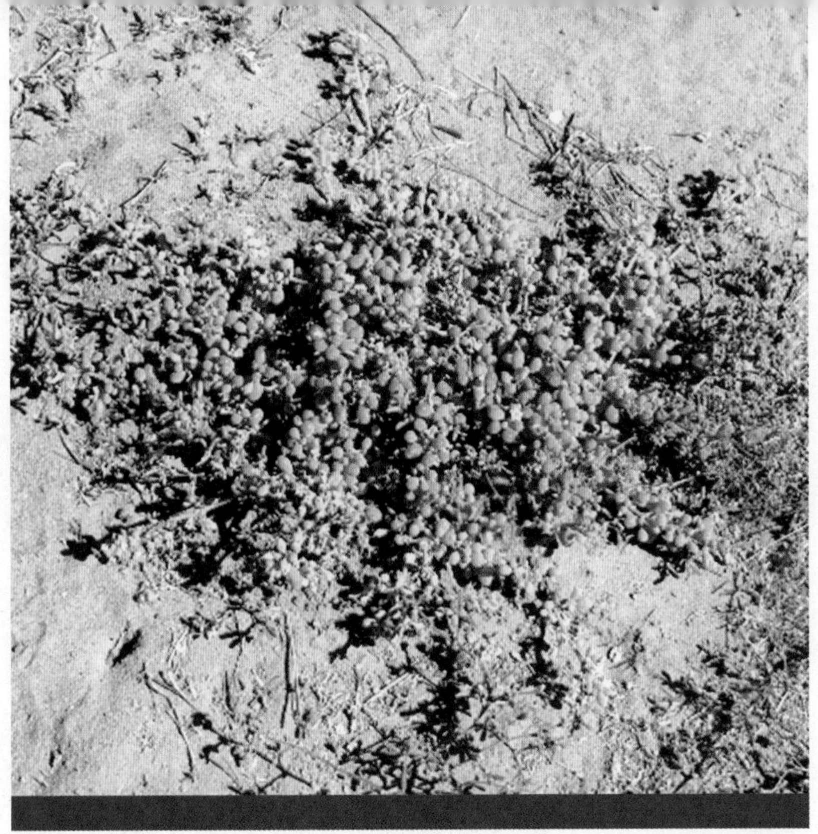

Other Uses The plant itself is not eaten, but an insect larva, which is longer than the regular Witchetty Grub, is found in this plant and is good to eat raw or lightly roasted (YMAC, 2016).

Pirrungu

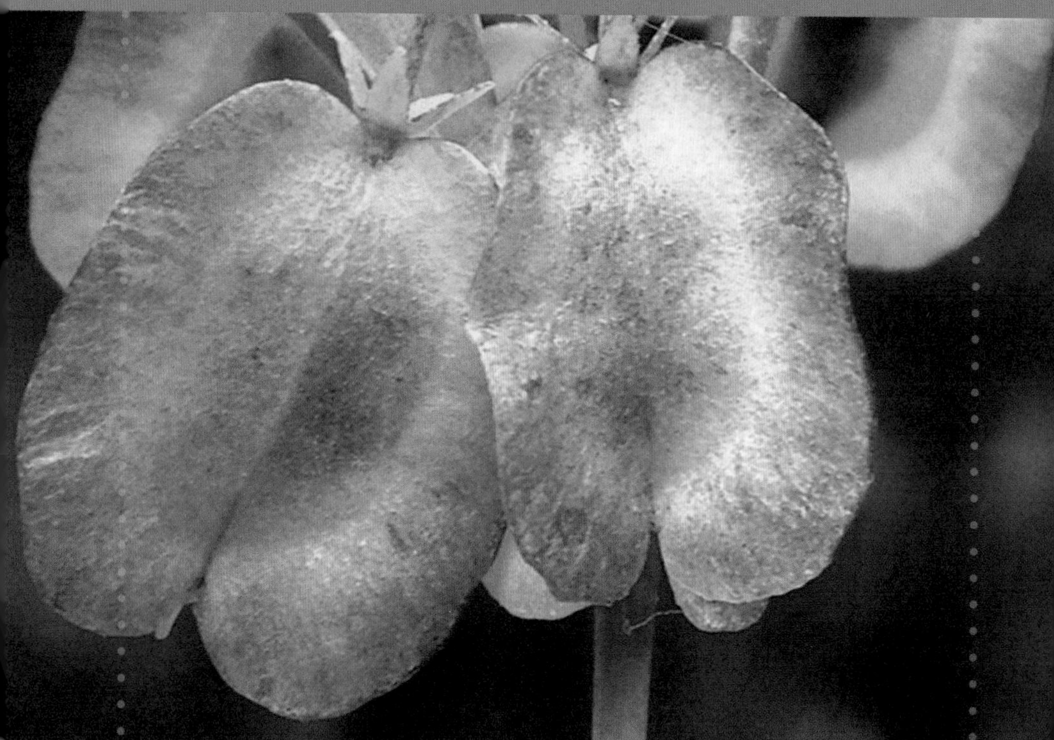

Scientific Name *Dodonaea lanceolata* F.Muell.

common Names Pirrungu, Hopbush.

Aboriginal Names Guradid (Bardi) (Smith & Kalotas, 1985).

Field Notes Pirrungu grows as a shrub up to 2 m in height. Its leaves are alternate, narrow, spear-shaped and up to 65 mm long and 15 mm wide. Its flowers appear from late autumn to spring and are petal-less. Its fruit are yellowish-green capsules with a winged appearance. Pirrungu is found in sand and loam over laterite, on rocky watercourses, stony ridges and hills in the Pilbara and Kimberley regions of Western Australia, as well as the Northern Territory and Queensland, with a couple of sightings in New South Wales near Nowendoc (ALA, 2022; Lassak & McCarthy, 2001; PlantNET, 2022; WAH, 2022).

Medicinal Uses The leaves of Pirrungu were bruised, cut up and boiled, then, after cooling, were applied as a liniment to various

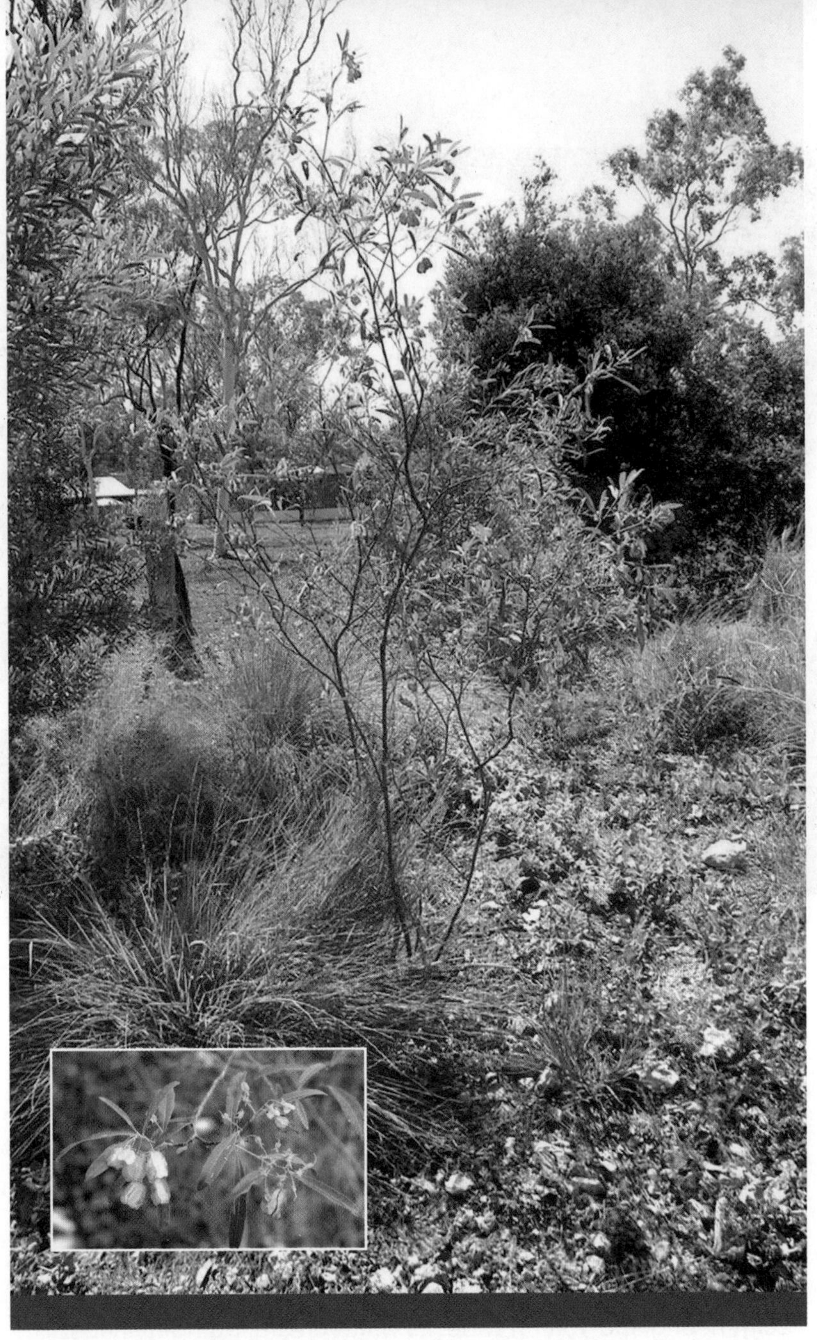

parts of the body for pain including arthritic and rheumatic pain and the pain of snakebite. Diluted decoctions of the leaves were taken internally for the same complaints, that is, as an analgesic (Lassak & McCarthy, 2001; Low, 1990; Reid, 1986; Webb, 1959; Williams, 2013).

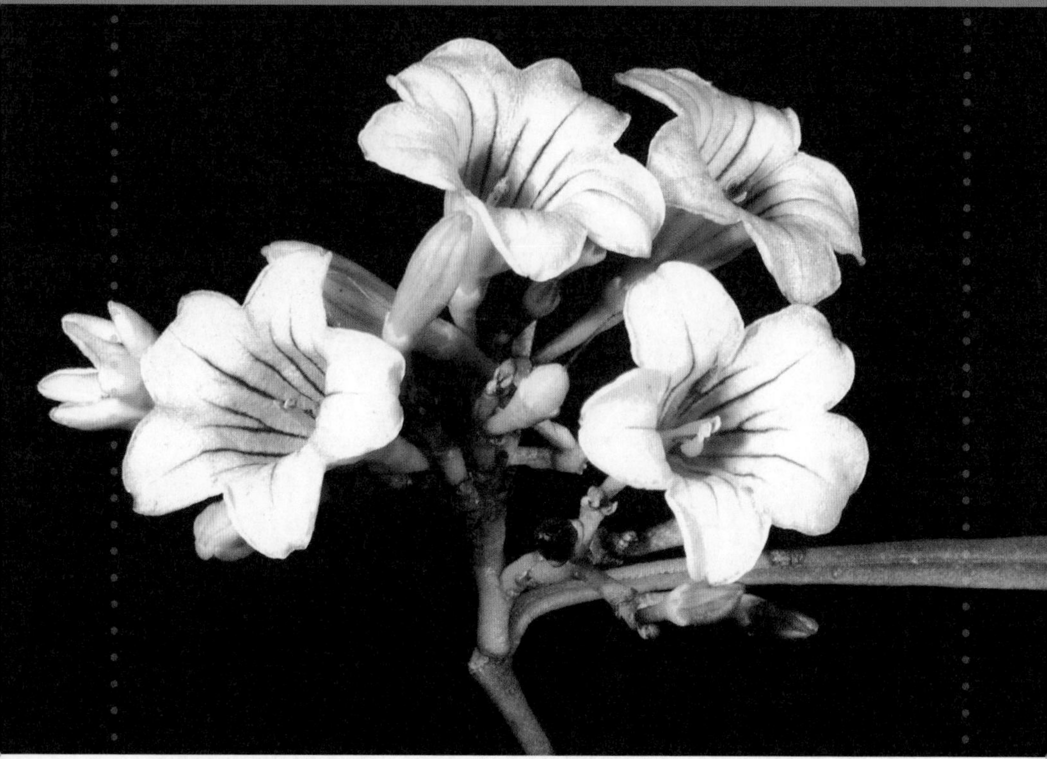

Scientific Name *Duboisia hopwoodii* (F.Muell.) F.Muell.

Common Names Pituri, Pitchuri Thornapple, Pitcheri, Pedgery, Bedjeri, Emu Bush, Emu Poison.

Aboriginal Names Nalwa, Walkaly (Ngardi), Janyungu (Ngardi, Warlpiri, Jaru, Walmajarri) (Cataldi, 2004), Tjanyungu, Walykalpa (Kukatja) (Cataldi, 2004; Valiquette, 1993).

Field Notes Pituri grows as a wispy shrub up to 4 m in height. Its leaves are narrowly elliptic or ovate-elliptic to linear, and up to 120 mm long and 13 mm wide. Its white-cream, trumpet-shaped flowers are present between June and November. Its fruit are globose or sub-globose, rarely ellipsoid, purple-black berries that are only 5 mm in diameter. Pituri occurs in yellow or red sand and sandy loam, on plains, low dunes and rises over most of Western Australia, including the southern reaches of the Kimberley. It also occurs in the southern part of the Northern Territory, most of South

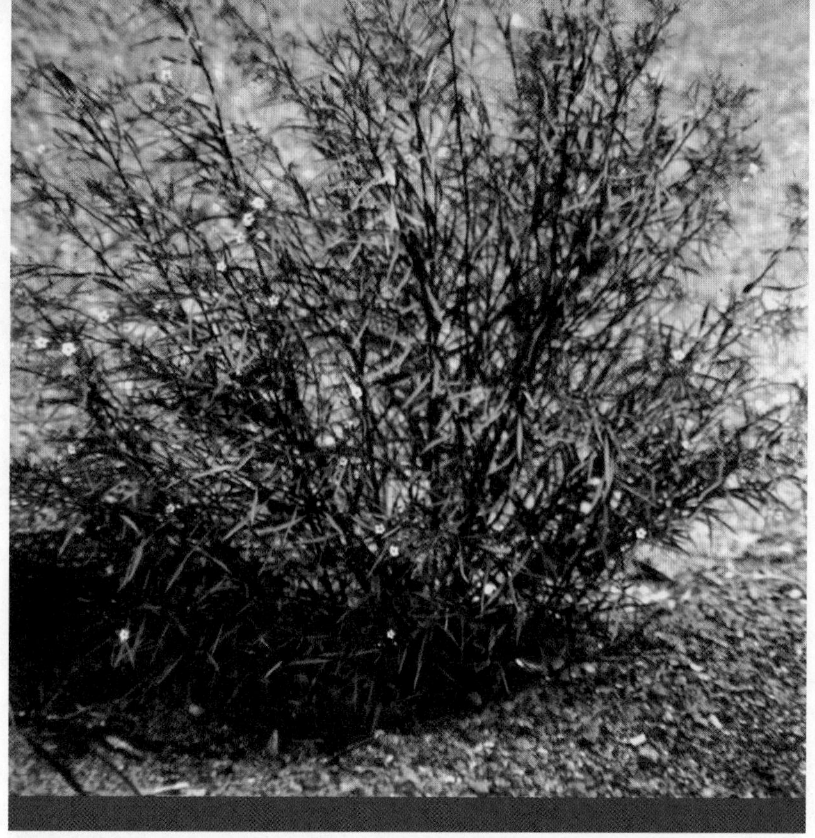

Australia, extending to central-western Queensland and western New South Wales (ALA, 2022; eFlora.SA, 2022; WAH, 2022).

Medicinal Uses Aboriginal Australians chewed the leaves of Pituri like tobacco for its nicotine and slight narcotic effect. The leaves contain the alkaloids nicotine, nor-nicotine, hyoscyamine and scopolamine, all in varying concentrations. The leaves are reported to curb hunger and thirst, and to invigorate people on long walks. Sometimes the leaves were mixed with the ash of other plants before they were chewed (eFlora.SA, 2022; Fern, 2021; Williams, 2013). Herbalistics (2022) reminds us that, 'Aboriginal tribes traded the dried leaves of this species over great distances before white settlement, being highly valued as a narcotic, stimulant'. The leaves also have analgesic properties (HerbResearch, 2022).

Other Uses The Ngardi put crushed Pituri leaves in waterholes to trap emus by making them groggy and easier to catch (Cataldi, 2004).

Pornupan

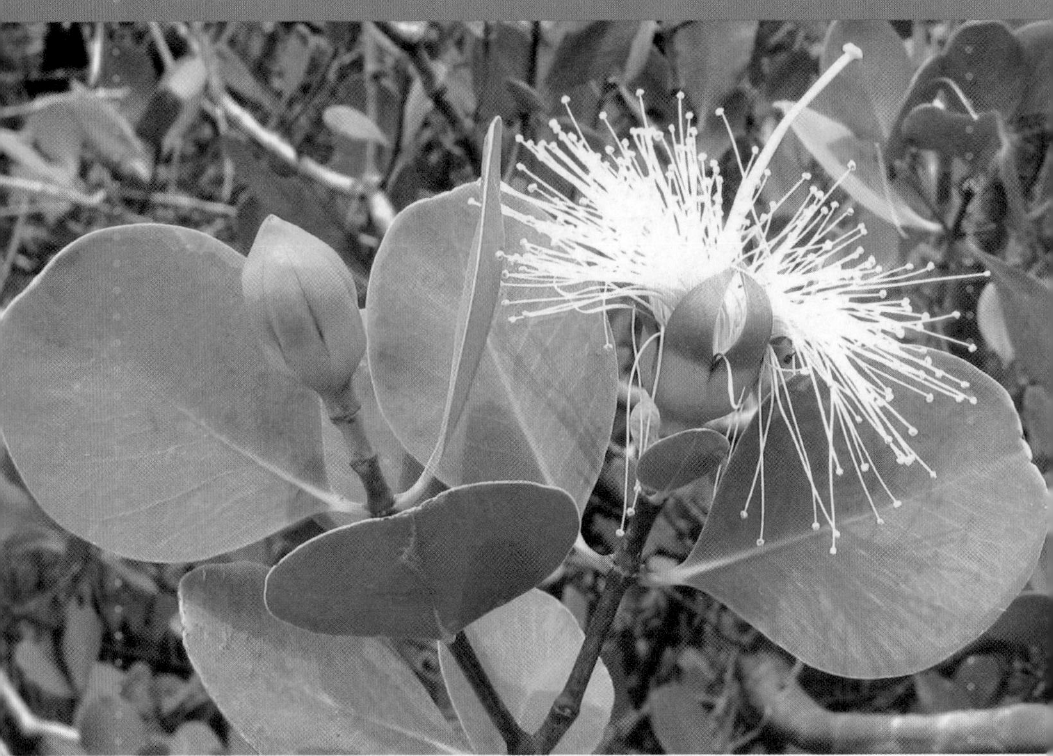

Scientific Name *Sonneratia alba* Sm.

Common Names Pornupan, Mangrove Apple, Pornupan Mangrove.

Aboriginal Names Jarrgarla (Wunambal, Gaambera) (Karadada et al., 2001), Djolor (Bardi) (Smith & Kalotas, 1985), Jolorr (Bardi) (Kenneally et al., 1996), Kulii (Kwini) (Cheinmora et al., 2017).

Field Notes Pornupan is a mangrove tree that grows up to 12 m in height. Its cracked to fissured bark is brownish, turning grey below the tidal mark. Its spiky flowers are white with a pink base and have up to eight linear sepals and eight petals. Flowering in the Kimberley is in February or from April to August. Its dark green fruit are globular, depressed berries up to 50 mm in diameter. Pornupan usually occurs on the seaward side of mangroves around the Kimberley and Northern Territory coasts and the east coast of Far North Queensland as far south as Cairns (ALA, 2022; WAH, 2022). It also occurs in eastern Africa, through the Indian Ocean and tropical

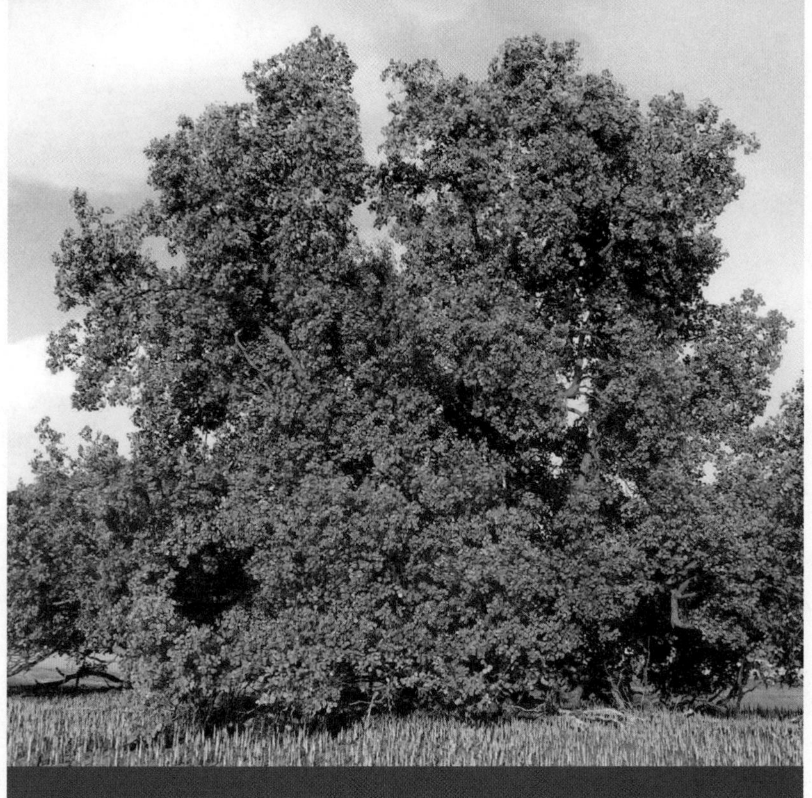

Asia, to the Philippines, Vanuatu and the Solomon Islands (Fern, 2021).

Medicinal Uses Decoctions of the bark were used to treat skin disorders and wounds (Thompson, 2020). The fruit was used to treat intestinal parasites and coughs (Fern, 2021).

Other Uses The fruit of Pornupan [mentioned on p420] are edible and can be eaten raw or cooked. The ripe fruit are reported to taste like cheese. The leaves are eaten as a vegetable in some countries (Fern, 2021). Nectar was sucked directly from the flowers (Kenneally et al., 1996; Smith & Kalotas, 1985). The wood often contains edible worms that are chopped out and eaten (Cheinmora et al., 2017). The wood from Pornupan was used by the Bardi to make shields (marga) (Kenneally et al., 1996; Smith & Kalotas, 1985).

Poverty Bush

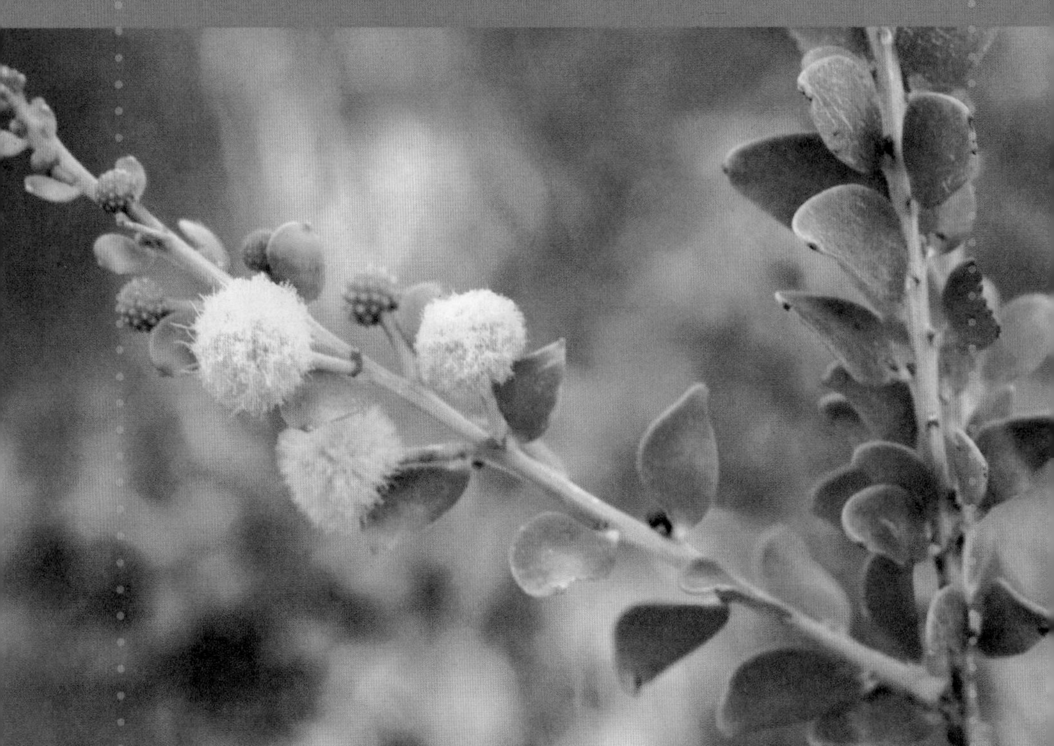

Scientific Name *Acacia translucens* Hook.

Common Name Poverty Bush.

Aboriginal Names Julurr (Wunambal, Gaambera) (Karadada et al., 2011), Balalagoord (Bardi) (Kenneally et al., 1996), Nyirrjarti, Purntalji (Walmajarri) (Richards & Hudson, 2012), Mantjangu, Ngarankura, Ngarawara, Parturtu (Kukatja) (Valiquette, 1993).

Field Notes Poverty Bush grows as a low or sometimes spreading, multi-branched or sometimes erect and slender shrub up to 3 m in height. Its phyllodes are elliptic to narrowly elliptic and approximately 20 mm long. Its yellow, spherical flower heads appear from March to November. Its fruit or seed pods are brittle, thinly woody, brown to black, narrowly oblanceolate to oblanceolate and up to 55 mm long and 10 mm wide. Poverty Bush is found in red sand and shallow soils over sandstone in the Pilbara and Kimberley regions of Western Australia and the western side of

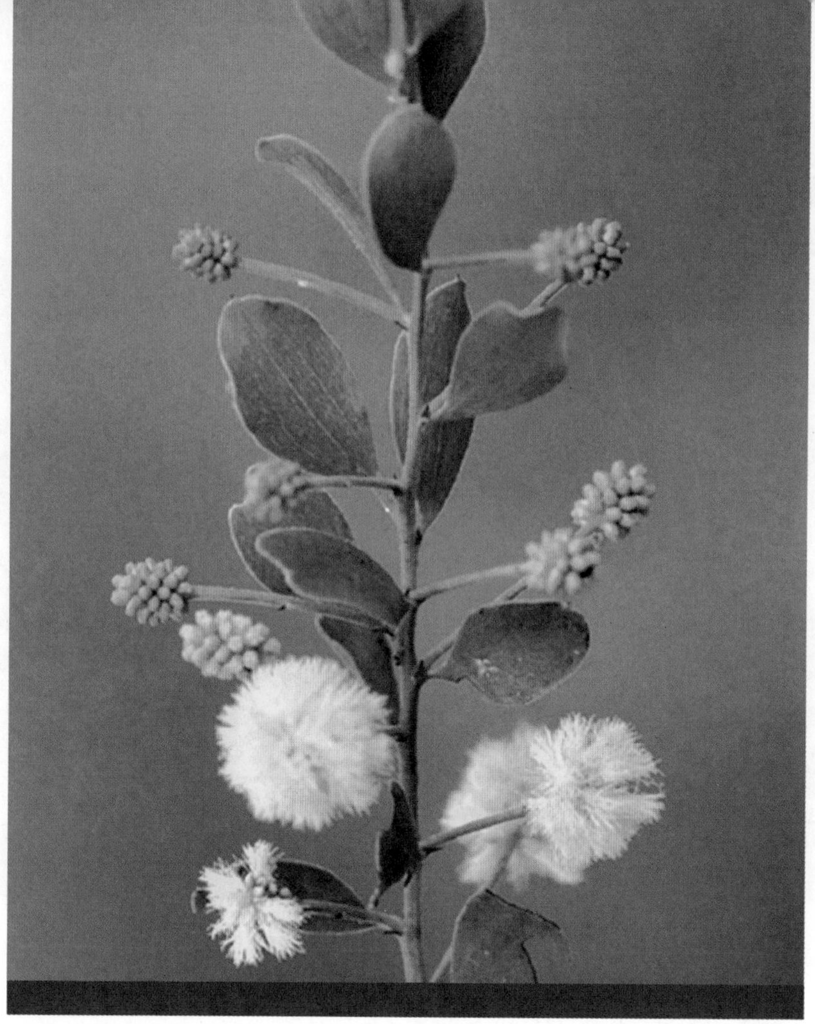

the Northern Territory (ALA, 2022; Lassak & McCarthy, 2001; WAH, 2022; World Wide Wattle, 2022).

Medicinal Uses Infusions or decoctions of mashed leaves and twigs of Poverty Bush were used externally as an antiseptic wash to bathe wounds and skin sores, and the head to relieve headaches (Lassak & McCarthy, 2001; Williams, 2011).

Other Uses Witchetty Grubs are often found in the roots of Poverty Bush. They are usually roasted briefly in hot ashes before they are eaten (Richards & Hudson, 2012).

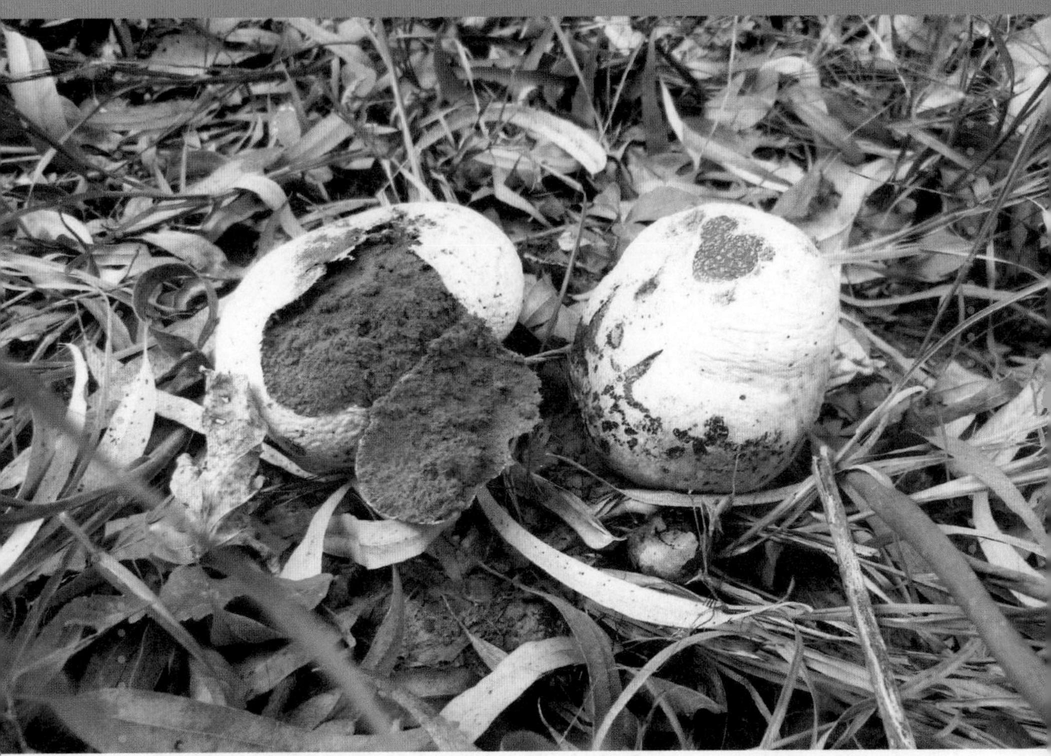

Scientific Names *Pisolithus tinctorius* (Micheli : Fr.) Coker & Couch, also known as *Pisolithus arhizus* (Scop.: Pers) Rauschert, and *Scleroderma tinctorium* Pers.

Common Names Puffballs, Horse Dung Fungus, Dead Man's Foot, Earth Balls.

Aboriginal Names Janbirra (Jaru) (Deegan et al., 2010), Jurntijarti (Walmajarri) (Richards & Hudson, 2012), Matjaputi, Matjarti, Puti-puti, Tupunganya, Turturtu (Kukatja) (Valiquette, 1993).

Field Notes Puffballs and other fungi of this species appear as common brown puffballs, pale to dark mottled brown in colour. They can grow up to 200 mm in diameter and 200 mm in height. As they age, the puffballs break down into a mass of powdery spores (Bougher, 2009). Puffballs are very common in disturbed leaf litter, especially around eucalypts. They are found throughout Australia and are indigenous to Western Australia. They are also found worldwide (Readford, 2011).

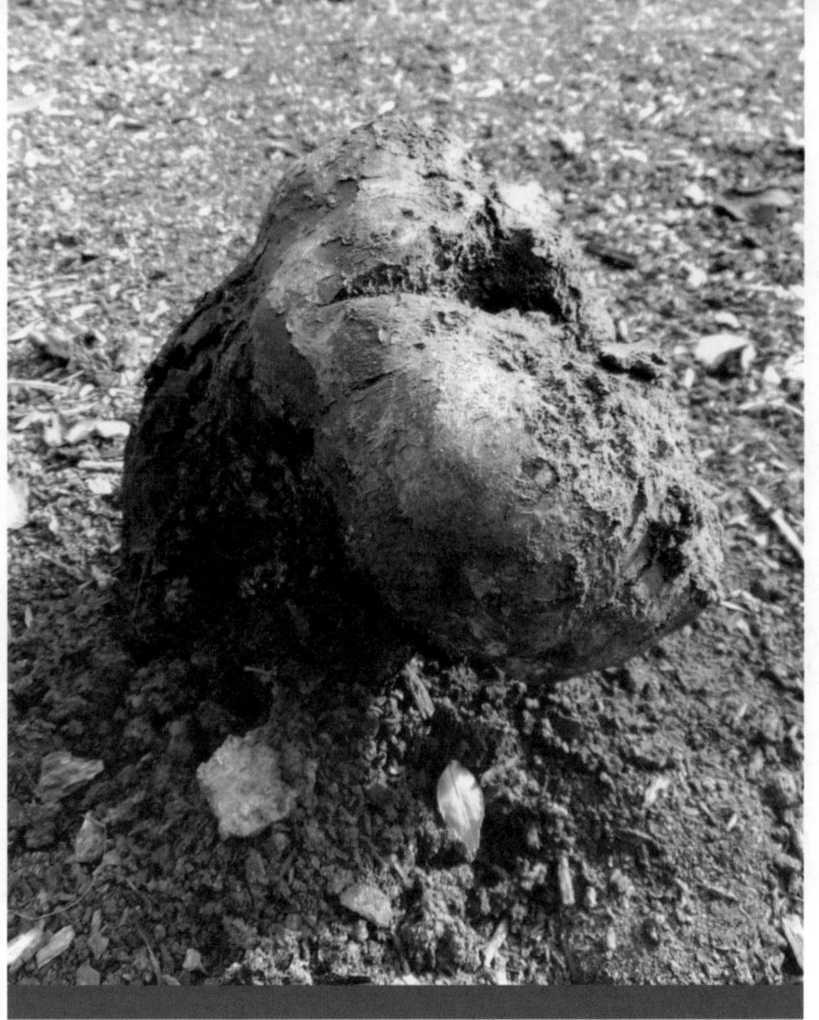

Medicinal Uses Puffballs have medicinal properties and were used by some Aboriginal groups. The fruit were broken open and the antiseptic spores were rubbed into wounds and sores to prevent infection and promote healing (Hansen & Horsfall, 2016; Lepp, 2012).

Other Uses The young fruiting bodies of Puffballs are edible (Deegan et al., 2010; Lepp, 2012; Richards & Hudson, 2012). The Jaru to the south of their country ate them; the northern Jaru did not (Deegan et al., 2010).

CAUTION: Care must be taken when identifying edible fungi as there are poisonous lookalikes.

Puncture Vine

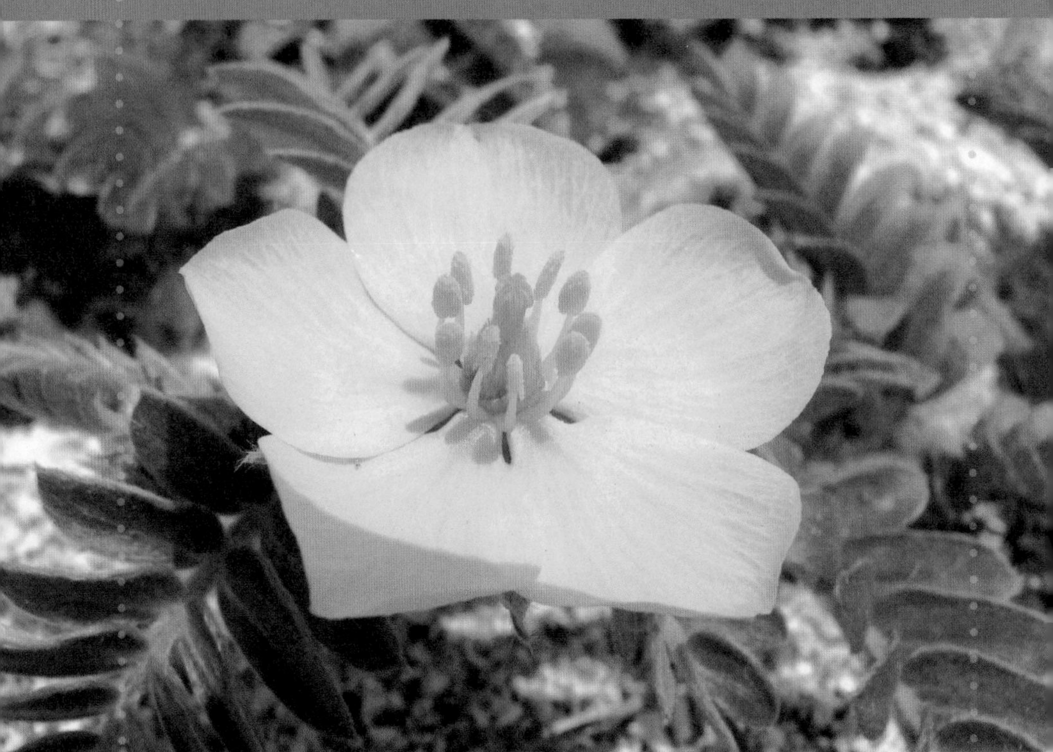

Scientific Name *Tribulus cistoides* L.

Common Names Puncture Vine, Caltrop, Bindi-eye, Goat's Head Burr, Jamaican Feverplant.

Field Notes Puncture Vine grows as a prostrate perennial herb with densely hairy branches up to 300 mm in height. It has small, ovate, opposite leaflets, and yellow buttercup-like flowers with five petals up to 18 mm long. The flowers are present at any time of the year. The fruit are spherical and around 16 mm in diameter with strong straight thorns and a median pair of spines. Puncture Vine occurs in sand or sandy loam, on dunes, rocky coasts and plains all over the top half of Australia but is more prevalent in coastal areas. It is pantropical and is found in the tropical regions of many other countries, especially near the coast (ALA, 2022; Fern, 2021; Lassak & McCarthy, 2001; WAH, 2022).

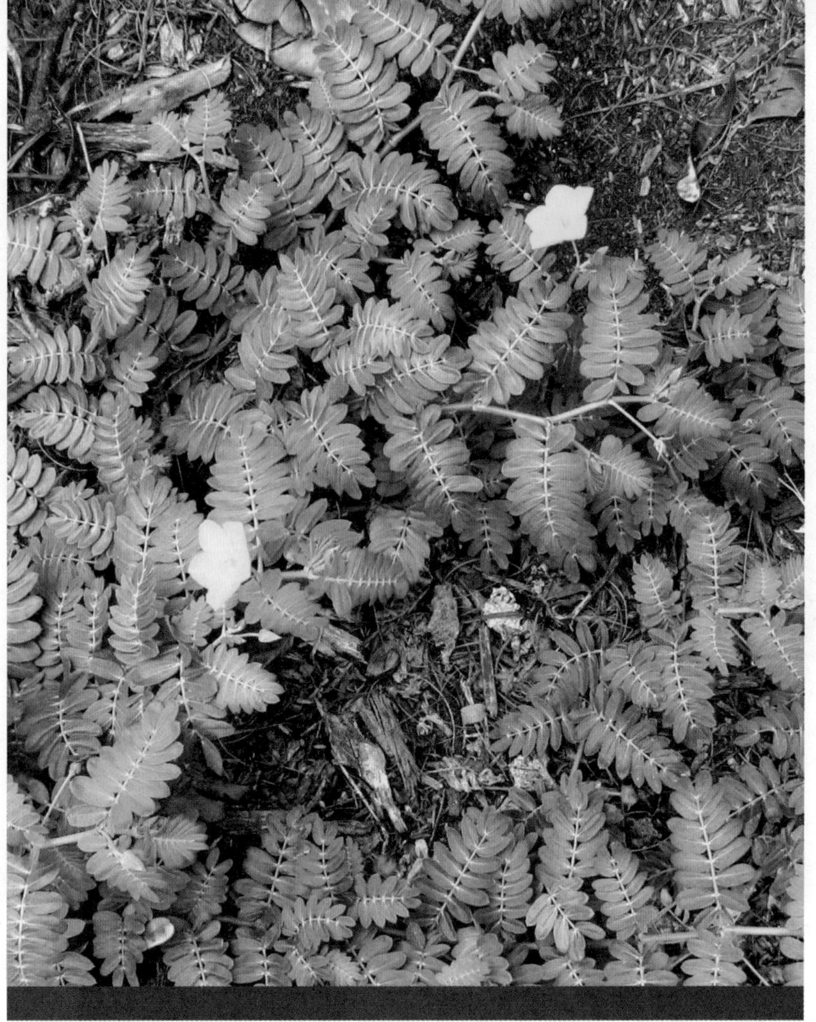

Medicinal Uses Puncture Vine is used in folk medicine in Australia, some Asian countries and Hawaii. Bruised leaves were held between the teeth and gums to relieve toothache (Lassak & McCarthy, 2001; Low, 1990). The plant is used to treat colds, malaria and urinary tract infections. Decoctions of the roots were given to children to relieve toothache. The leaves and roots were pounded and used as poultices that were applied to sores, leg ulcers and abscesses to hasten the healing process (Fern, 2021).

Other Uses The leaves can be cooked and eaten as a leafy vegetable (Fern, 2021).

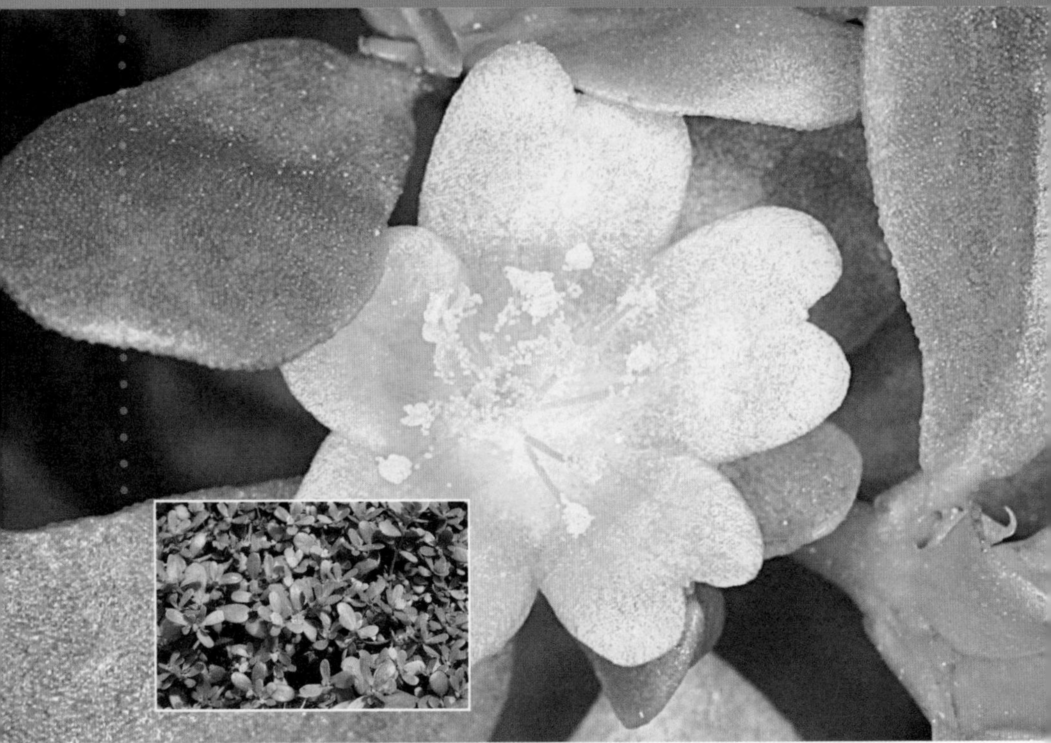

Scientific Name *Portulaca oleracea* L.

Common Names Purslane, Common Purslane, Pigweed.

Aboriginal Names Grassawassa (Nyul Nyul) (Kenneally et al., 1996), Wakati (Ngardi) (Cataldi, 2004).

Field Notes Purslane is a ground-hugging, annual plant with red stems, only growing up to 100 mm in height. Its small green, ovate, succulent leaves are about 25 mm long. Small yellow flowers, up to 10 mm in diameter, appear at the leaf base from April to May. The flowers contain small black seeds, which are dispersed after the flowers open. This plant is found all over Australia except for Tasmania (ALA, 2022; ANPSA, 2022; Kapitany, 2020; WAH, 2022). Two new forms of this plant have been discovered recently, Omega Gold and Omega Red, and are still being studied (Kapitany, 2020). Purslane has a 'cosmopolitan distribution' and is distributed widely in the tropical and sub-tropical areas of the world (Zhou et al., 2015).

Medicinal Uses Fern (2021) reports that, 'Purslane has been used in folk medicine since ancient times and is included in the World Health Organization's list of most widely used medicinal plants'. It is reported to have antibacterial, antiscorbutic, depurative, diuretic and febrifuge properties. The fresh juice of Purslane has been used in the treatment of strangury (blockage or irritation at the base of the bladder), coughs, sores, leg ulcers, wounds and numerous other ailments. Decoctions of the leaves were taken internally to treat stomach aches and headaches. Poultices made from crushed leaves were applied to burns to stave off infection. Both the leaves and the plant juice were used in the treatment of skin diseases and insect bites. Leaf juice was also used externally to treat earache. In China, the seeds of Purslane are used as a tonic and in the treatment of intestinal parasites, dyspepsia and opacities of the cornea (Fern, 2021; Williams, 2013; Zhou et al., 2015).

Other Uses The tiny black seeds of Purslane are ground to make flour for damper. Seeds are collected from May to June. The leaves and stems can be eaten raw, boiled or steamed as a green vegetable. The raw leaves are reported to taste like lettuce (Cataldi, 2004; Cribb & Cribb, 1981; Isaacs, 1987; Kapitany, 2020; Maiden, 1889). Purslane is reported to have the highest level of omega-3 fatty acids, essential for human nutrition, compared to any leafy green vegetable. Omega-3 fatty acids are thought to be important in preventing coronary artery disease, and for strengthening the immune system (Uddin et al., 2014). Some Aboriginal groups carried Purslane leaves with them on walks from one camp to another as a source of moisture when water was scarce (Dann, 2003).

Quinine Bush

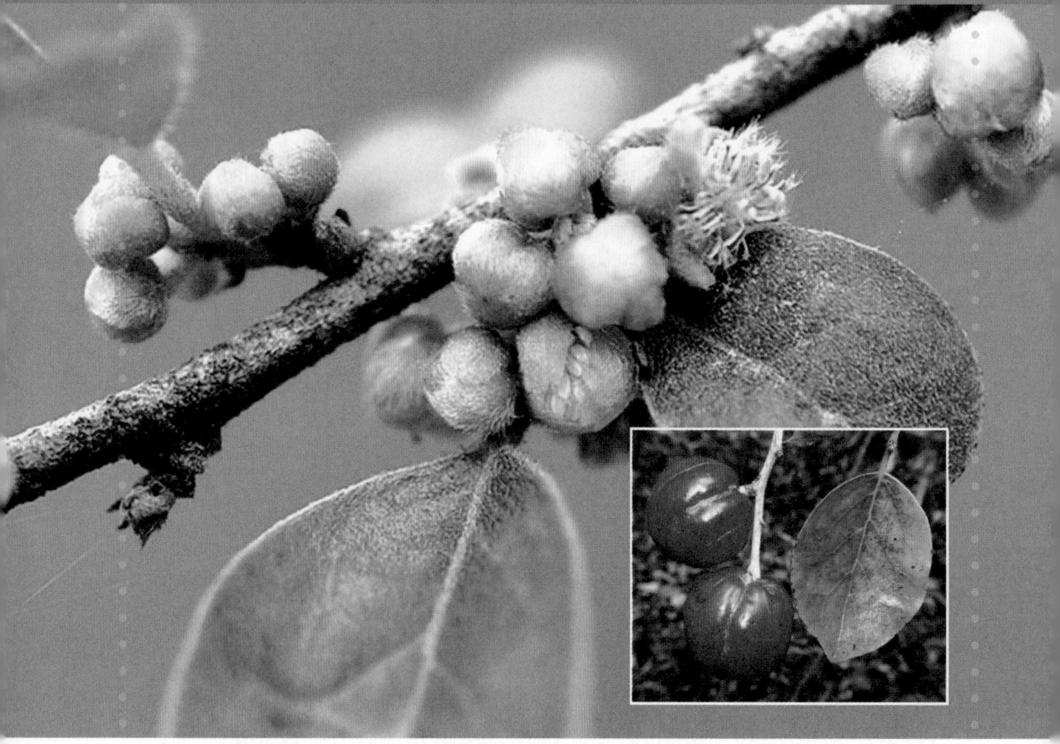

Scientific Name *Petalostigma pubescens* Domin.

Common Names Quinine Bush, Quinine Tree, Bitter Bark, Quinine Berry.

Aboriginal Names Wiljari (Wunambal, Gaambera) (Karadada et al., 2011), Dilngeri, Wildjari (the fruit) (Reid, 1986), Welrayiny (Gija) (Purdie et al., 2018), Mundurru (Jaru) (Wightman, 2003), Munturu (Kukatja) (Valiquette, 1993), Mardarrki, Dilngkûri winya, Wiljeri winya (the fruit) (Kwini) (Cheinmora et al., 2017).

Field Notes Quinine Bush grows as a shrub or tree to 7 m in height. It has green, broadly elliptical leaves up to 50 mm long that are densely covered in dull yellowish hairs and small white-yellow, insignificant flowers that are present any time between October and July. Its male flowers form in axillary clusters, whereas female flowers are solitary. Its fruit are yellow, globular, hairy and up to 20 mm in diameter, and split open to dispel the seeds when ripe.

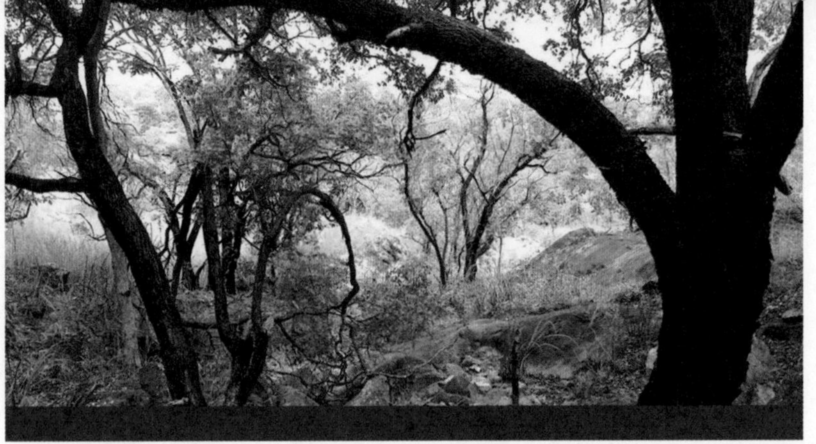

Quinine Bush occurs in sandy soils over sandstone, along creek lines, ridges, rocky slopes and on sandplains. This plant is endemic to the Kimberley region of Western Australia, the Northern Territory, Queensland, New South Wales and Papua New Guinea (ALA, 2022; Lassak & McCarthy, 2001; Noosa's Native Plants, 2022; WAH, 2022).

Medicinal Uses This plant was once thought to be the same as the Quinine Tree (*Petalostigma quadriloculare;* p. 432) but has recently been separated. It has the same medicinal properties. It was once thought the bark contained quinine, but studies have been inconclusive. Infusions of the bark or fresh fruit (one berry in a mug of water) have been used as an eyewash to treat conjunctivitis and as an antiseptic wash to treat wounds and sores. Fruit were held in the mouth to relieve toothache. The berries have been used in the past for the treatment of malaria (efficacy not recorded) (Cock, 2011; Crawford, 1982; Karadada et al., 2011; Lassak & McCarthy, 2001; Low, 1990; Reid, 1986; Webb, 1959). Infusions of the bark have been used as an antidote for opium overdose (SMIP, 2022).

Other Uses The fruit of the Quinine Bush are reported to be edible when ripe, but are quite bitter (City of Darwin, 2013). The wood of the Quinine Bush is very hard and was used to make woomeras or spear-throwers (Territory Native Plants, 2022).

Quinine Tree

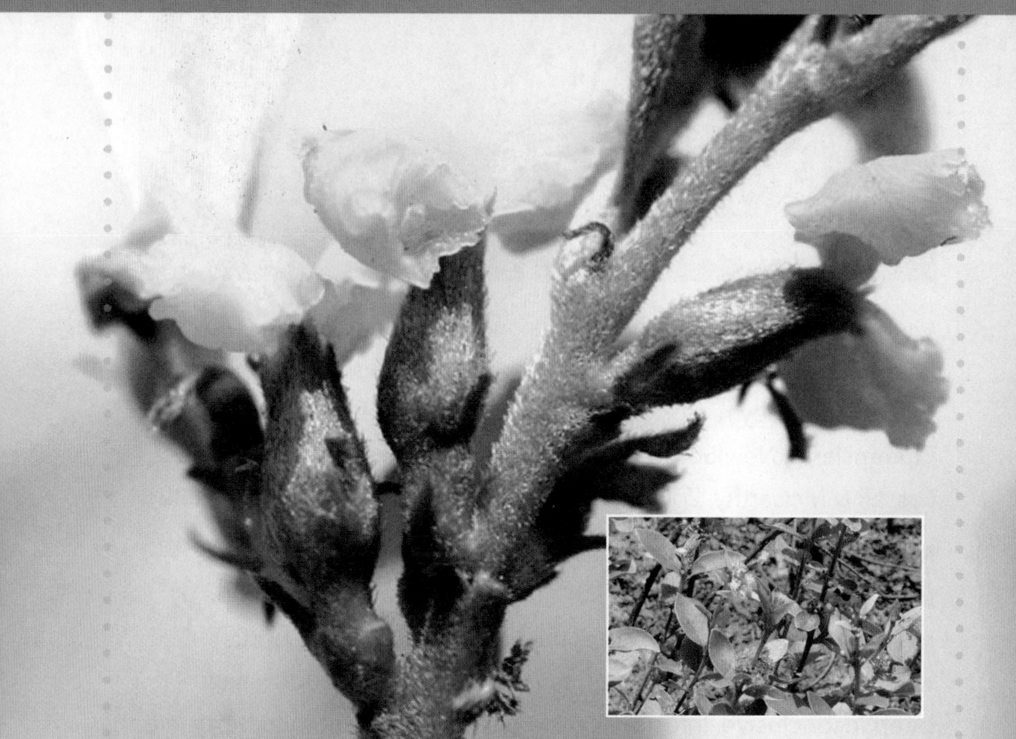

Scientific Name *Petalostigma quadriloculare* F.Muell.

Common Names Quinine Tree, Quinine Berry, Native Quince, Strychnine Bush, Bitter Crab.

Aboriginal Names Gooriwirring (Miriwoong) (Leonard et al., 2013), Dilngeri (plant), Wildjari (fruit) (Kwini) (Crawford, 1982; Reid, 1986).

Field Notes Quinine Tree grows as a diffuse shrub or small tree to 1.5 m in height. It has ovate leaves approximately 40 mm long, and small inconspicuous white-to-yellow flowers that appear between February and November. Its fruit are globular with three or four lobes and are orange to red as they age. The fruit are inedible and are considered poisonous. The Quinine Tree occurs in rocky loam over sandstone and on rocky hillsides in the Kimberley region of Western Australia and the Northern Territory, with a few sightings in northern Queensland (ALA, 2022; Lassak & McCarthy, 2001; WAH, 2022).

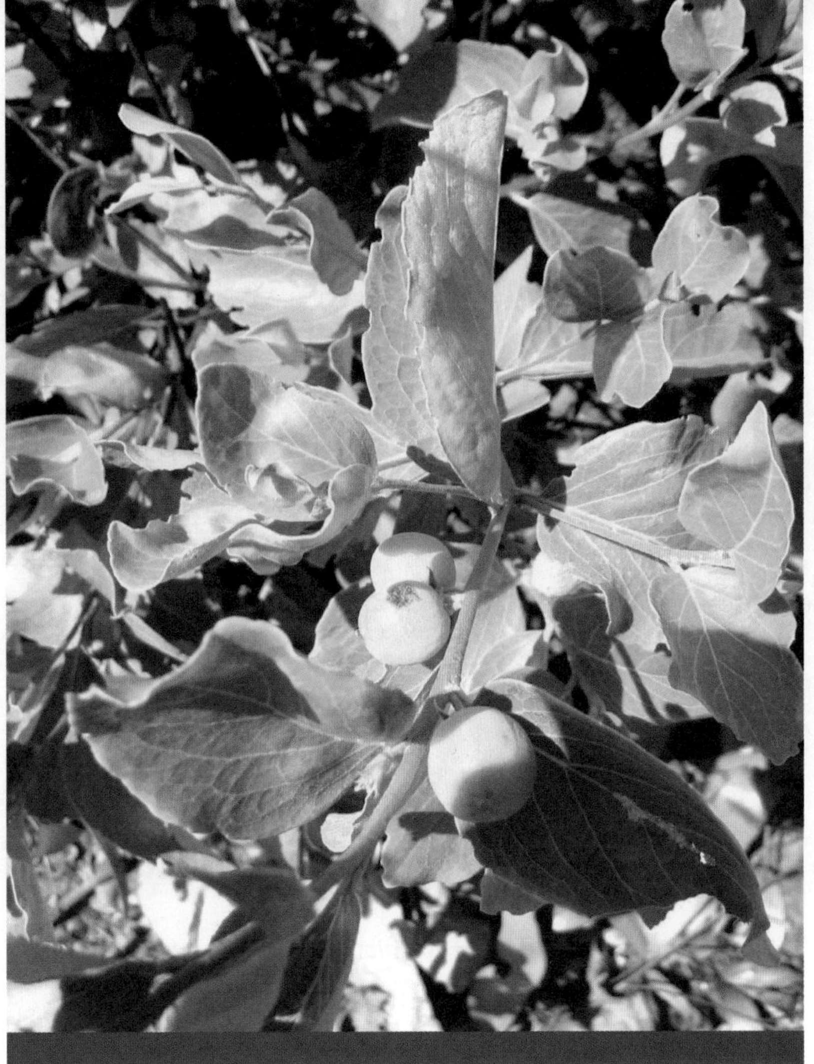

Medicinal Uses Infusions of the bark, leaves or fresh fruit (one berry in a mug of water) have been used as an eyewash to treat conjunctivitis and as an antiseptic wash for sores, cuts and skin ailments, such as scabies infestations and itchy skin. Fruit were held in the mouth to relieve toothache, but not swallowed. The berries have been used in the past for the treatment of malaria (efficacy not recorded) (Cock, 2011; Crawford, 1982; Isaacs, 1987; Lassak & McCarthy, 2001; Low, 1990; Reid, 1986; Smith, 1991).

Rag Weed

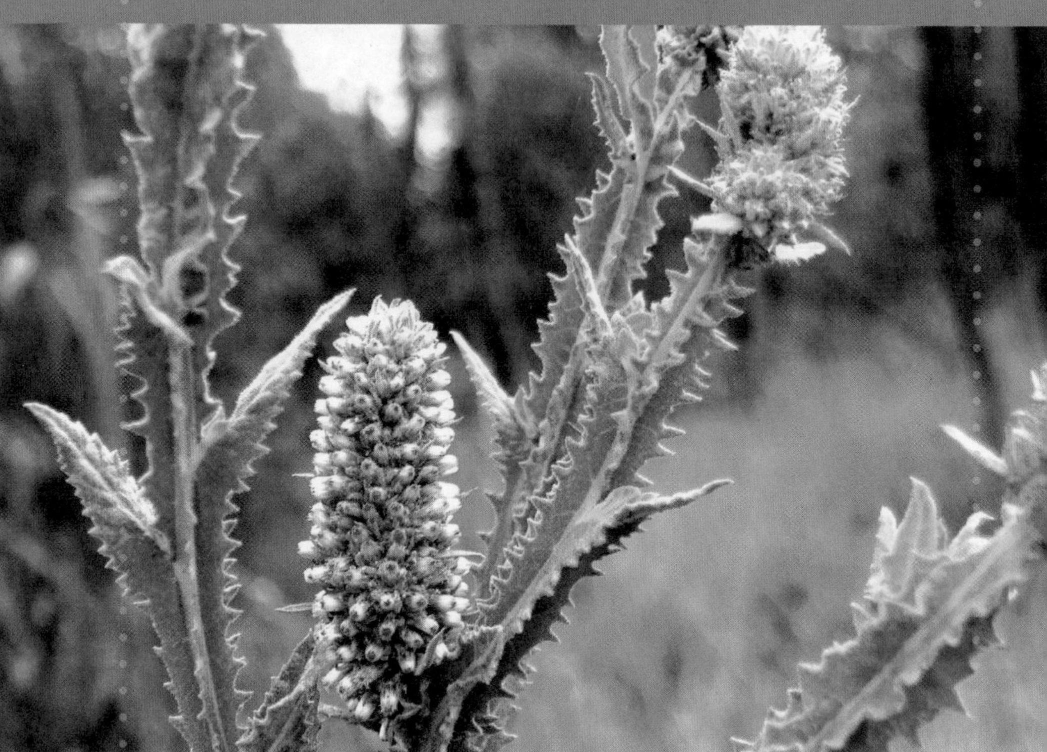

Scientific Name *Pterocaulon serrulatum* (Montrouz.) Guillaumin, previously known as *Pterocaulon glandulosum* F.Muell.

Common Names Rag Weed, Pterocaulon, Toothed Ragwort, Apple Bush.

Aboriginal Names Guriyimbiyimbi (Wunambal, Gaambera) (Karadada et al., 2011), Ngalili (Djawi) (Smith & Kalotas, 1985), Gooroongoony, Kurunguny (Gija) (Purdie et al., 2018), Manyani, Jujuminyiminyi (Ngardi) (Cataldi, 2004), Ngurnungurnu (Jaru) (Wightman, 2003).

Field Notes Rag Weed is a spreading or erect aromatic, perennial herb or shrub that grows to 1 m in height. It has broad leaves tapering at both ends, 20–50 mm long, with toothed margins and a wrinkled surface. The white, cream or pink flower heads occur at the end of stems and appear between May and October. Rag Weed often occurs in gravelly soils right across the top of tropical and

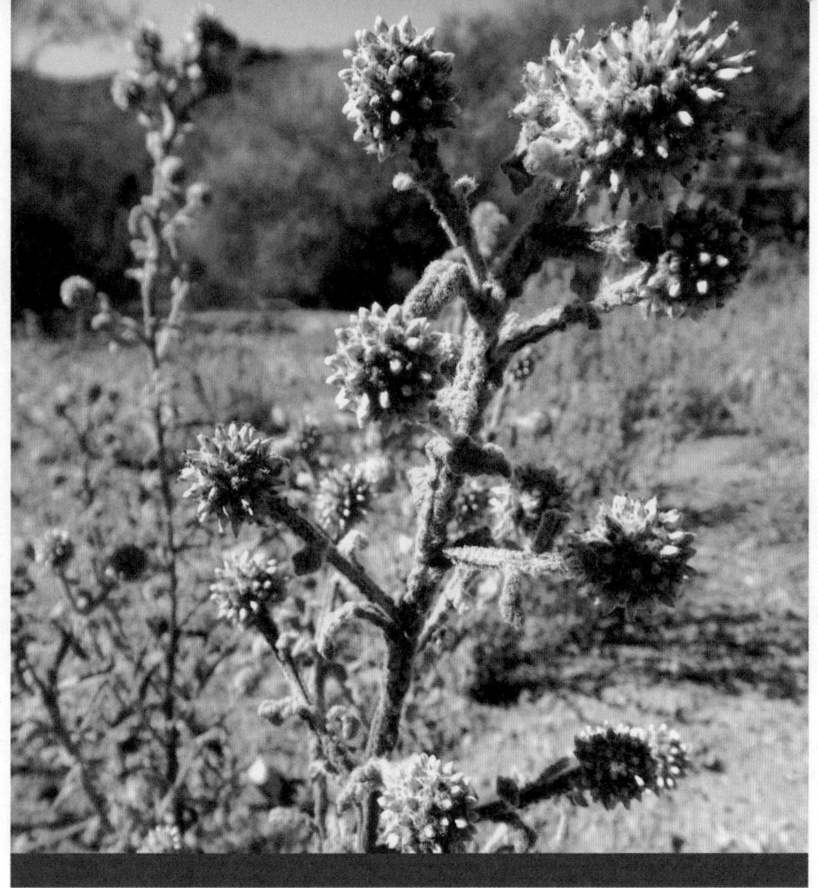

sub-tropical Australia, including the Pilbara and Kimberley regions of Western Australia (ALA, 2022; Lassak & McCarthy, 2001; SMIP, 2022; WAH, 2022).

Medicinal Uses The leaves of Rag Weed were chewed to relieve congestion of the lungs. The leaves were crushed and stuffed in the nose to relieve nasal congestion due to colds and influenza. Decoctions of the leaves were drunk for the same purpose. Crushed leaves were also applied as a poultice to wounds and sores to aid healing (Cock, 2011; Devanesen, 2000; Karadada et al., 2011; Lassak & McCarthy, 2001; Low, 1990; Smith, 1991; Webb, 1959; Wightman, 2003) and to painful joints and muscles to ease arthritic and rheumatic pain (Smith & Kalotas, 1985). In Central Australia, the Arrernte crushed the leaves and mixed them with animal fat from goannas or other animals and rubbed the salve on the chest, like Vicks, to relieve the symptoms of colds and influenza (SMIP, 2022).

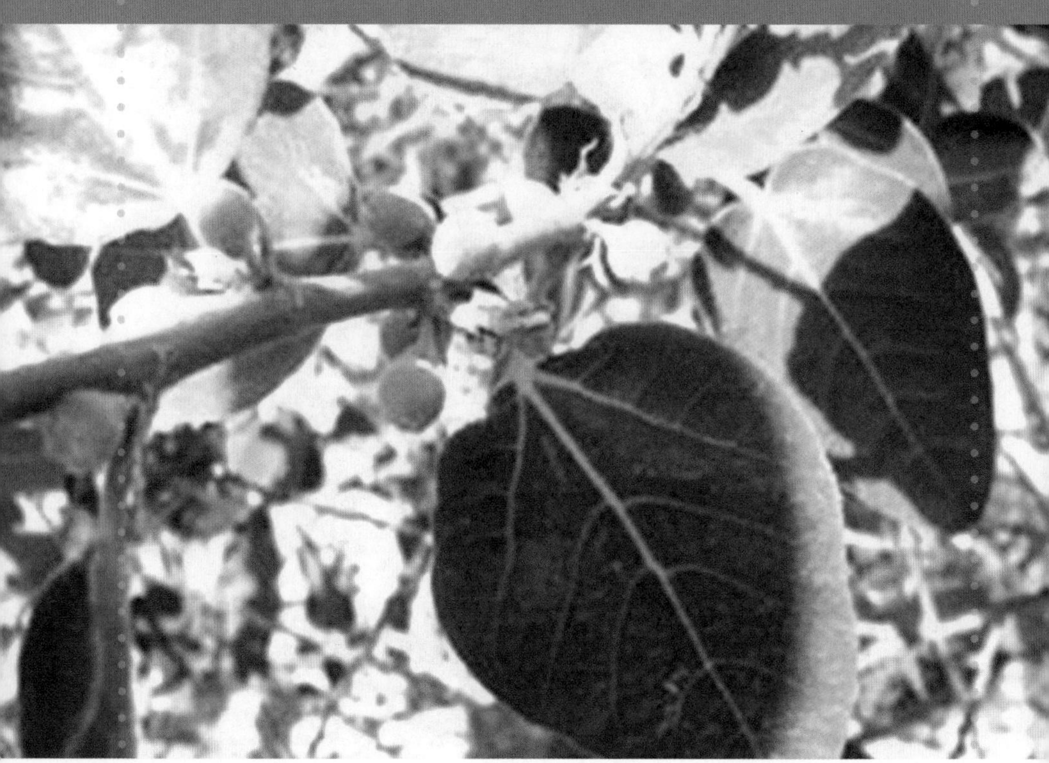

Scientific Names *Ficus aculeata* Miq., and *Ficus aculeata* var. *indecora* (Miq.) D.J.Dixon

Common Names Ranji, Sandpaper Fig.

Aboriginal Names Yinirri (Bunuba) (Oscar et al., 2019), Ngenji (Wunambal, Gaambera) (Karadada et al., 2011), Randji, Ranya (Bardi, Nyangumarta) (Smith & Kalotas, 1985), Ranyjamayi (Nyangumarta), Yingarrjiny, Yimarlji (Gija) (Purdie et al., 2018), Ranyja, Yinirr (Walmajarri) (Richards & Hudson, 2012), Yimarli (Gooniyandi) (Dilkes-Hall et al., 2019), Biijimbul, Minji manya (Kwini) (Cheinmora et al., 2017; Crawford, 1982). Ngamarnajina (Yawuru), Jirrib (Nyul Nyul) (Kenneally et al., 1996), Yimarl (Jaru) (Wightman, 2003), Jirrib (Nyul Nyul), Ranyja (Karajarri) (Moss et al., 2021).

Field Notes Ranji is a dioecious shrub or tree that grows to 15 m in height. Its bark is dark brown and fissured. Its ovate leaves, which are slightly pointed at the apex, are about 90 mm long by 60 mm

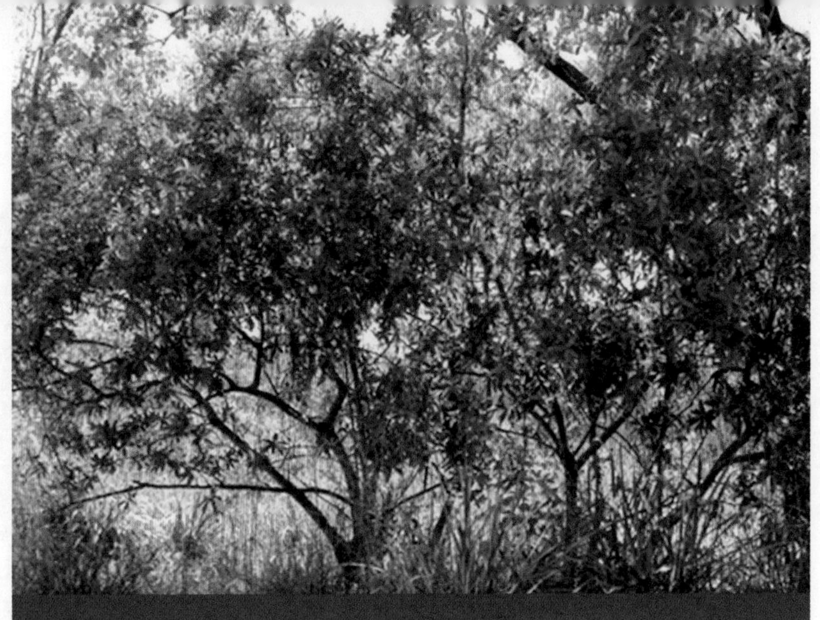

wide, and like sandpaper on both the upper and lower surfaces. Its figs are pedunculate, globular, form in clusters and are up to 10 mm in diameter. Ranji occurs in a variety of soils, on calcareous dunes, in vine thickets, on the edge of creeks, on floodplain margins, in gorges and at the base of cliffs. *Ficus aculeata* var. *indecora* only occurs in the Pilbara and Kimberley regions of Western Australia and the Northern Territory. *Ficus aculeata* also occurs in Queensland (ALA, 2022; ATRP, 2020; WAH, 2022).

Medicinal Uses The leaves of Ranji were warmed and applied as a poultice to bruises, sprains and areas of arthritic and rheumatic pain (Kenneally et al., 1996).

Other Uses The fruit of Ranji are edible when ripe and dark purple, between December and mid-March, and are usually warmed in hot ashes or sand before eating (Fox & Garde, 2018; Karadada et al., 2011; Kenneally et al., 1996; Smith & Kalotas, 1985; Vigilante et al., 2013; Wightman, 2003). The rough leaves of Ranji were often used as sandpaper, hence one of its common names, 'Sandpaper Fig' (Oscar et al., 2019; Smith & Kalotas, 1985; Wightman, 2003). The wood was used to make shields. Ash from burnt bark was mixed with Bush Tobacco (*Stemodia lythrifolia*) for chewing (Kenneally et al., 1996).

Ranji Bush

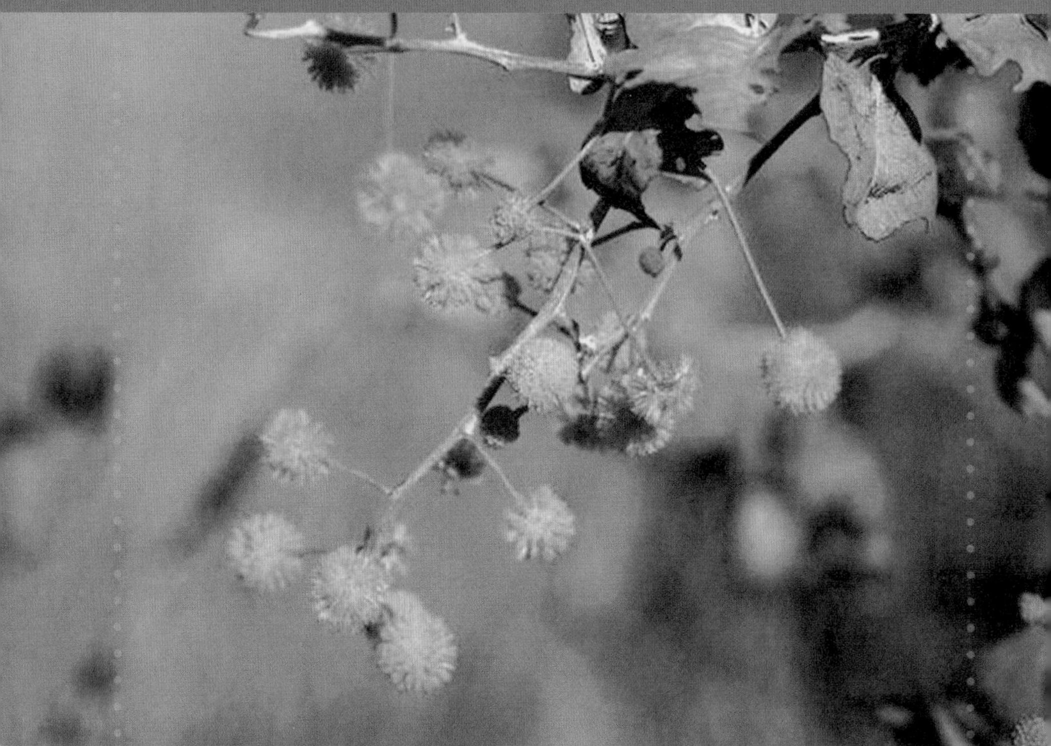

Scientific Name *Acacia pyrifolia* DC.

Common Names Ranji Bush, Kanji Bush.

Aboriginal Names Jiripali (Kurrama) (Young & Vitenbergs, 2007), Largarrbarra (Gija and Jaru) (Wightman, 2003).

Field Notes Ranji Bush is a wattle that grows as a shrub or tree up to 4.5 m in height. Its bark is smooth grey on main stems and yellow on the upper branches. Its blue-green, pear-shaped phyllodes are up to 75 mm long. The yellow flower heads are globular and occur in clusters between April and August. Ranji Bush is endemic to the Pilbara and Kimberley regions of Western Australia where it occurs in red-brown to yellow-brown sand, brown loamy clay, alluvial sand and skeletal soils on plains, along watercourses, lower slopes and on roadsides (ANPSA, 2022; WAH, 2022).

Medicinal Uses Decoctions of the inner red bark were used as an antiseptic wash to bathe sores, cuts and rashes, and were good for

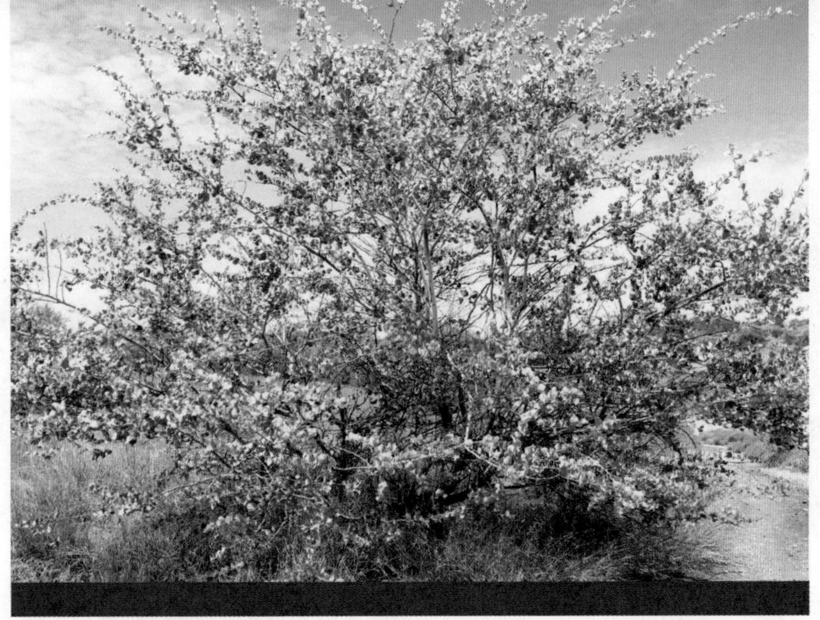

drying open wounds (Fern, 2021; Maslin et al., 2010; Webb, 1959; Young & Vitenbergs, 2007).

Other Uses The gum that oozes from wounds in the tree is edible and was eaten raw. The seeds are also edible and can be eaten raw or ground to flour to make Johnny cakes or damper (Bindon, 2014; Fern, 2021; Glasby, 2018).

Red Ash

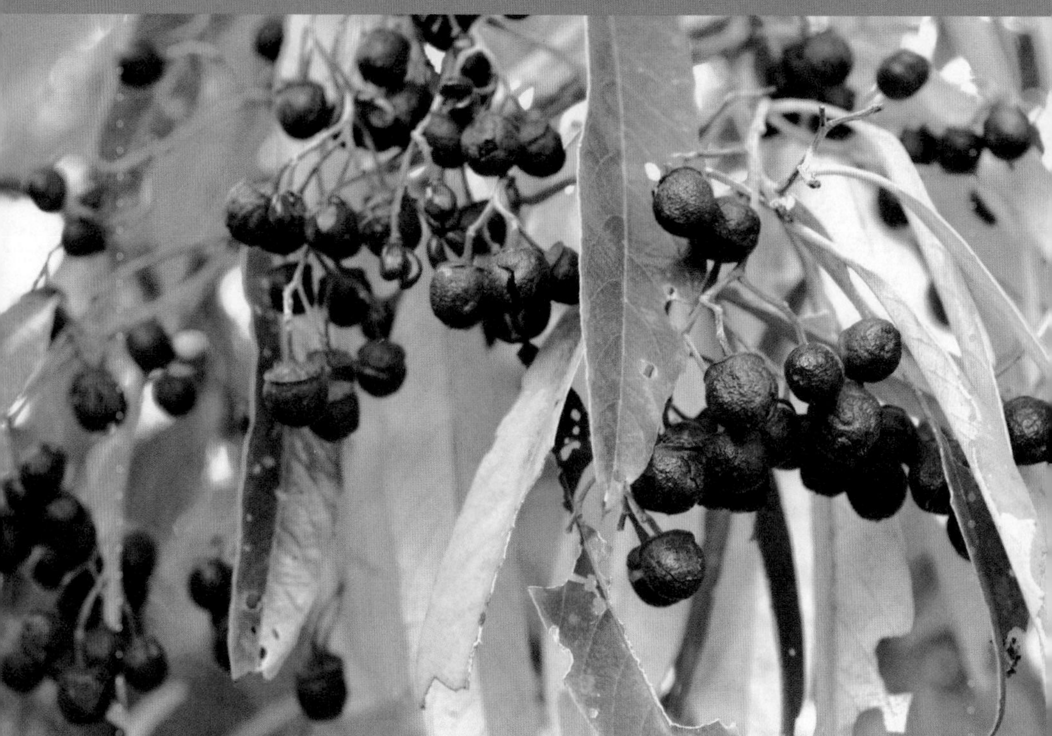

Scientific Name *Alphitonia excelsa* (Fenzl) Benth.

Common Names Red Ash, Leatherjacket, Coopers Wood, Soap Tree.

Field Notes Red Ash grows as a small or large tree to 21 m in warm moist conditions. It has grey bark on the trunk and rusty branches. Its leaves are ovate to lanceolate, blunt or pointy tipped, and up to 120 mm long. Its small, insignificant white flowers appear in clusters in late autumn and early winter. Its fruit are black, spherical to ovoid berries 5–9 mm in diameter. Red Ash occurs in or near rainforest areas in the Kimberley region of Western Australia, the Northern Territory, Queensland and down the east coast of New South Wales as far as the border with Victoria (ALA, 2022; ATRP, 2020; Lassak & McCarthy, 2001).

Medicinal Uses Infusions or decoctions of the crushed leaves of Red Ash were used to bathe the head to relieve headaches

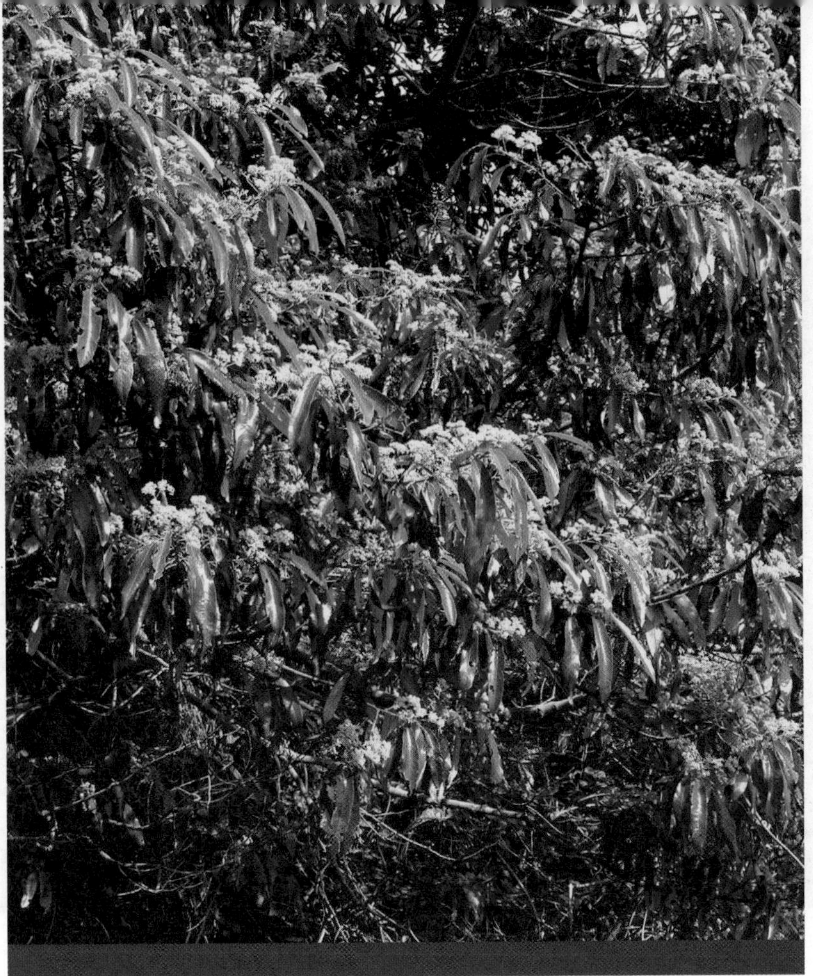

(Webb, 1959), the symptoms of colds and influenza, and as eardrops to treat earache due to inflammation of the auditory canal (Edwards, 2005). Warmed leaves were applied to sore eyes due to conjunctivitis. Decoctions of the bark, roots and wood were rubbed on the body as a liniment for rheumatic pain (Edwards, 2005; Webb, 1959). Decoctions of the bark and wood were gargled for toothache and were drunk as a tonic. Young leaf tips were chewed for an upset stomach (Cock, 2011; Lassak & McCarthy, 2001).

Other Uses The crushed leaves of Red Ash were used as bush soap, as the leaves are rich in saponin (Hiddins, 2001; Low, 1990). The berries and leaves were crushed and used as 'fish poison' to make it easier to catch fish (Hiddins, 2001).

Red Bush Apple

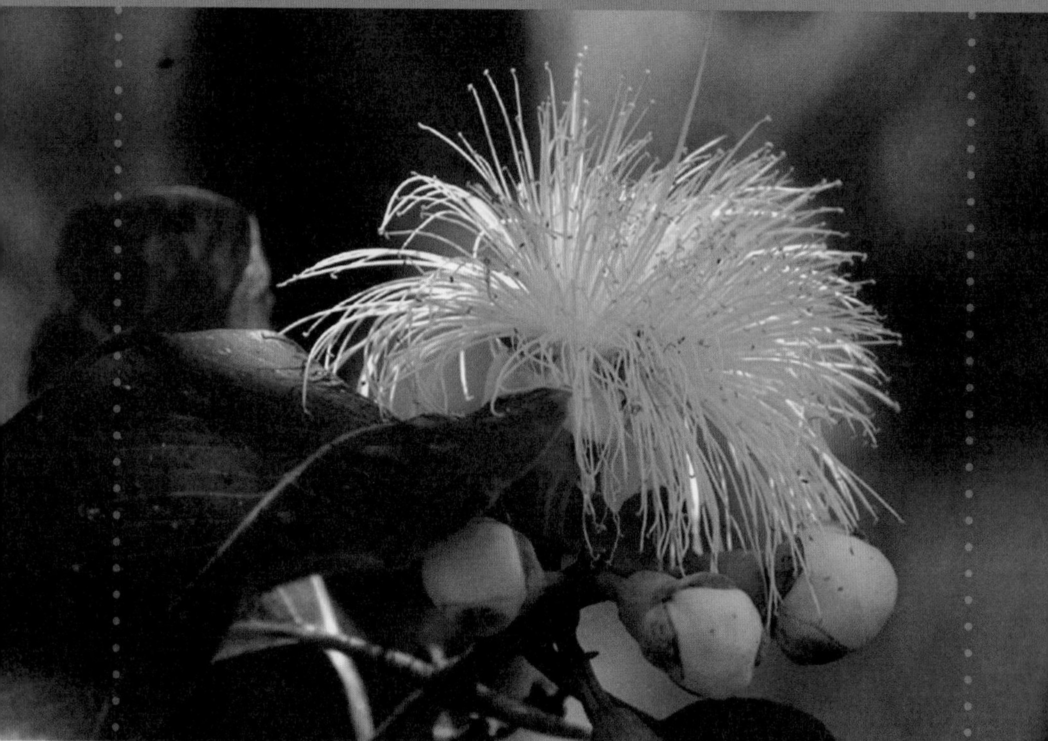

Scientific Name *Syzygium suborbiculare* (Benth.) T.G.Hartley & L.M.Perry.

Common Names Red Bush Apple, Wild Apple, Lady Apple, Red Wild Apple.

Aboriginal Names Ngalwarri (Wunambal, Gaambera) (Karadada et al., 2011), Illara (Bardi) (Smith & Kalotas, 1985), Ngarungurdukal minya, Ngarrungurdukal manya (Kwini) (Cheinmora et al., 2017).

Field Notes Red Bush Apple is a shrub or medium-sized tree that grows to 15 m high in good conditions. Its leaves are usually quite large, up to 190 mm by 130 mm, and come in various shapes. Its cream-white flowers have four lobes and appear between June and November. The fruit are deep red or pink, globular or ovoid, up to 70 mm long and 90 mm in diameter and strongly ribbed. The fruit are available during the wet season from October to March. Red Bush Apple occurs in sandy soils over sandstone, on

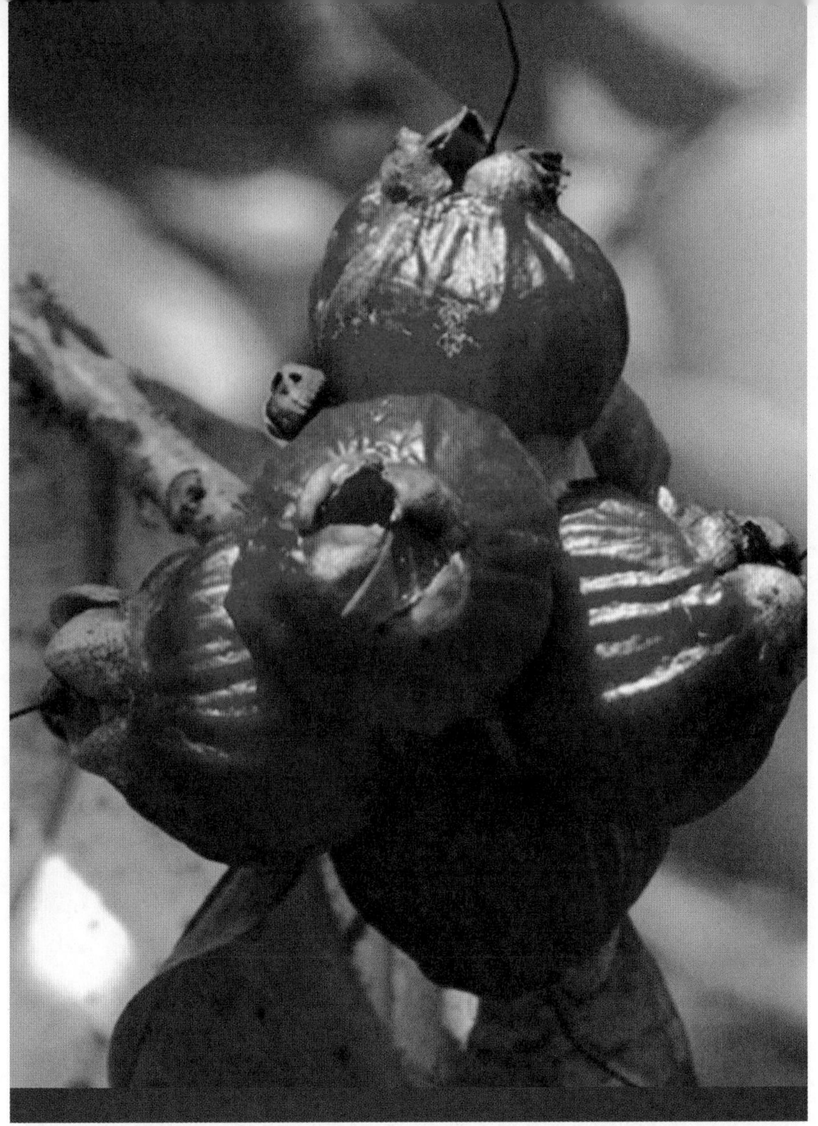

rocky sandstone hills and floodplains in the Kimberley region of Western Australia, the Northern Territory, the northernmost part of Queensland and New Guinea (ALA, 2022; ATRP, 2020; Fern, 2021; Lassak & McCarthy, 2001; WAH, 2022).

Medicinal Uses Infusions of the bark and roots of Red Bush Apple were taken internally for stomach pain. The fruit were boiled or baked in hot ashes, then the juice was drunk to ease chest congestion due to asthma and bronchitis (Cock, 2011; Fern, 2021; Lassak & McCarthy, 2001). Sometimes the leaves were heated and applied as a poultice to wounds and sores to aid healing and to stop bleeding. Pulp of the fruit was inserted into the ear to relieve earache (Hiddins, 2001; Low, 1990; Williams, 2020). Decoctions of the inner bark from the stems were used as an eyewash to treat conjunctivitis and to relieve tired, sore eyes. The decoctions were also used as an antiseptic wash to bathe sores and wounds. Small pieces of boiled inner bark were pushed into tooth cavities to ease the pain of toothache (Edwards, 2005; Smith, 1991). In Far North Queensland, the leaves were chewed, but not swallowed, to relieve the symptoms of colds and influenza (Edwards, 2005). Infusions of the leaves were taken internally to treat diarrhoea and stomach pain (Hiddins, 2001; Williams, 2020).

Other Uses The fragrant, spongy fruit of Red Bush Apple are edible; the flesh is crunchy with a sharp flavour. They were a good food source for Aboriginal groups where the fruit is found. They are a reasonable source of ascorbic acid (vitamin C) (Bindon, 2014; Cheinmora et al., 2017; Edwards, 2005; Fox & Garde, 2018; Hiddins, 2001; Karadada et al., 2011; Lassak & McCarthy, 2001; Low, 1991; Vigilante et al., 2013). The fruit are often smashed up and mixed with sugar and water before they are eaten (Karadada et al., 2011). Hard fruits were softened by putting them into hot sand next to a fire. Some Aboriginal groups in Queensland soaked the fruit for up to 24 hours to remove the saltiness before straining them and cooking them in a ground oven. The leaves were used to flavour meats that were cooked in a ground oven (Edwards, 2005).

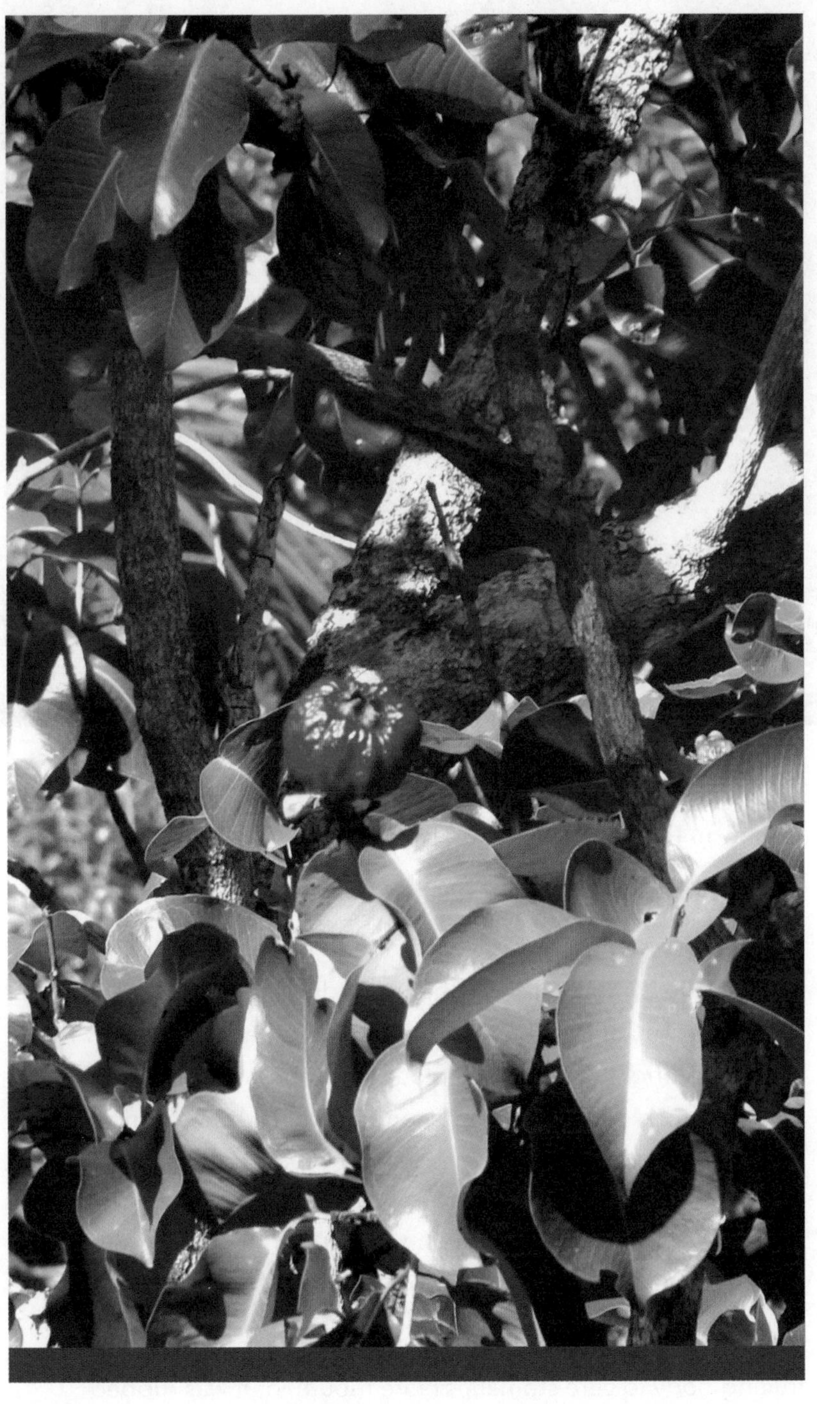

Red Fungus

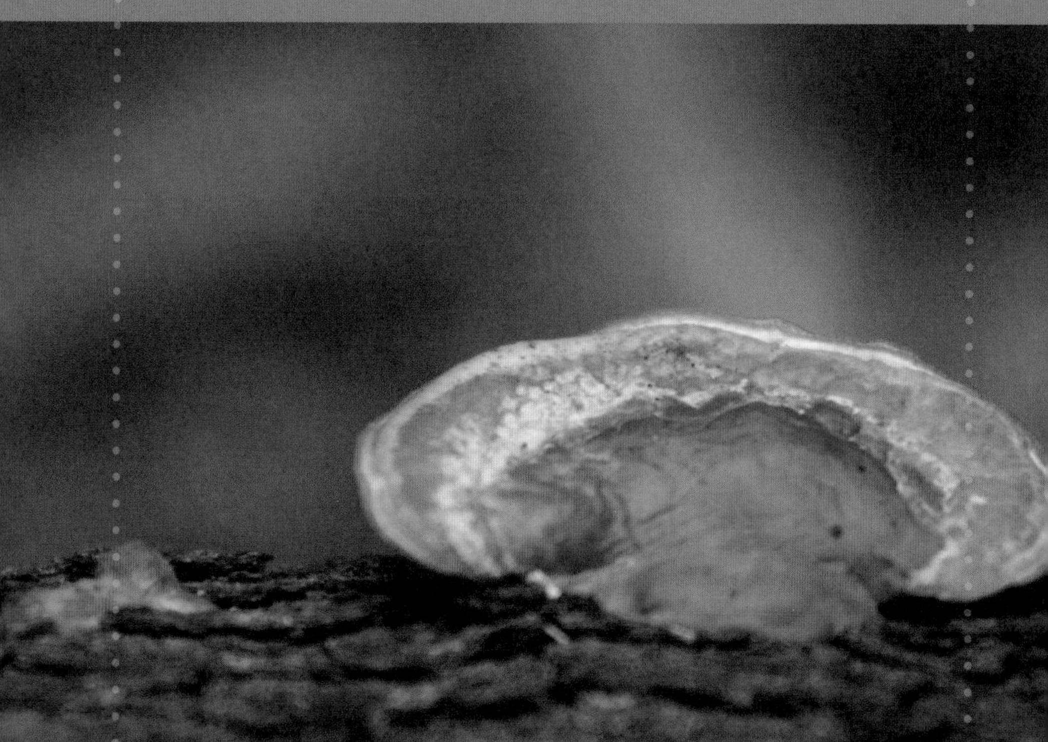

Scientific Name *Pycnoporus sanguineus* (L.) Murrill.

Common Names Red Fungus, Blood Red Bracket.

Aboriginal Name Tjawalirr-walirrpa (Kukatja) (Valiquette, 1993).

Field Notes Red Fungus is a bracket fungus that grows on dead or decaying wood. It grows either individually or in clusters. The fruiting bodies of Red Fungus contain both a cap and a stem. The caps are a bright red-orange colour and can vary in size but are found up to 140 mm in diameter and 5 mm thick. Red Fungus most typically occurs in tropical or sub-tropical regions of the world, including the Kimberley and south-west regions of Western Australia, the Northern Territory, Queensland and New South Wales (ALA, 2022; WAH, 2022).

Medicinal Uses Aboriginal people sucked on the bright orange fruiting body to cure stomatitis (sore mouth) or it was rubbed on cracked and sore lips. It was also given to babies as a natural

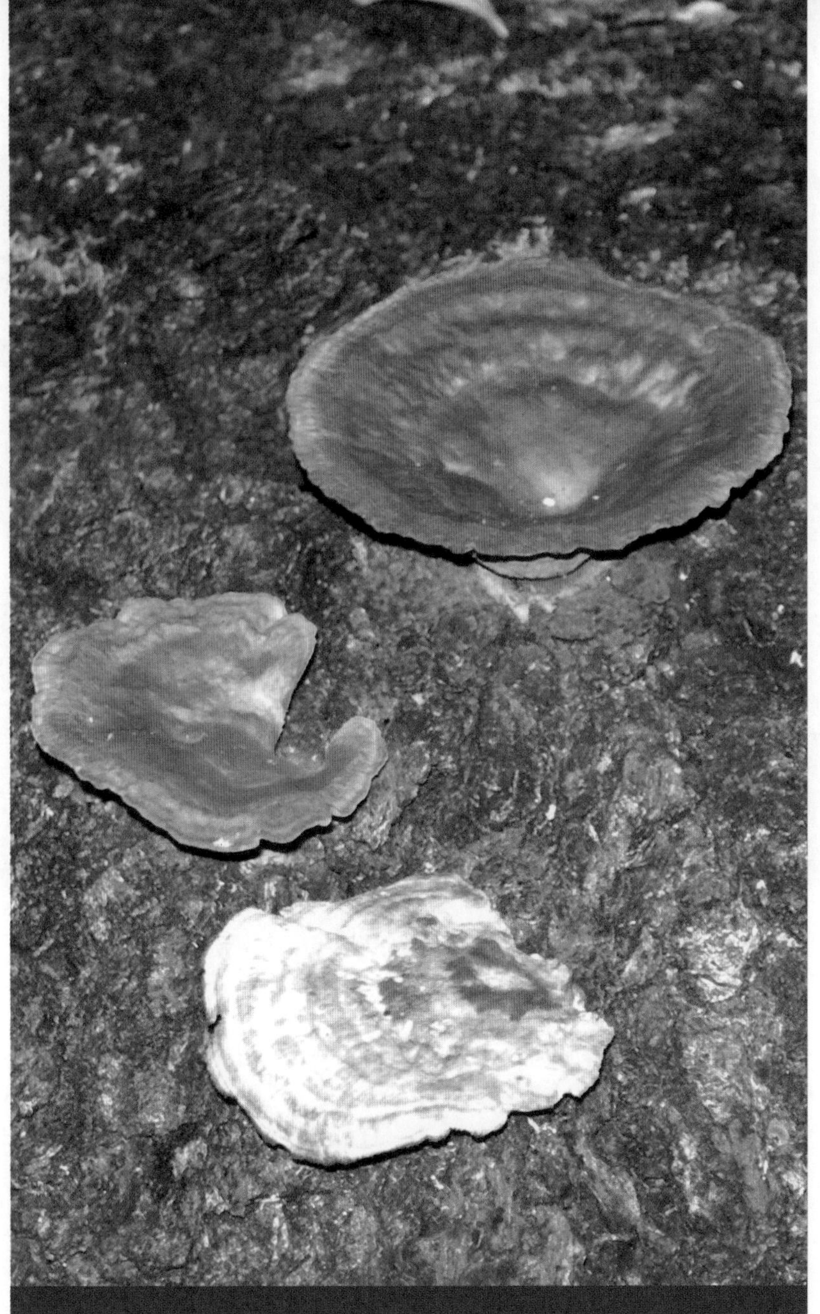

teething ring and to cure oral thrush (ANBG, 2022; Kamenev, 2011; Lepp, 2012; Smith, 1991).

Red Root

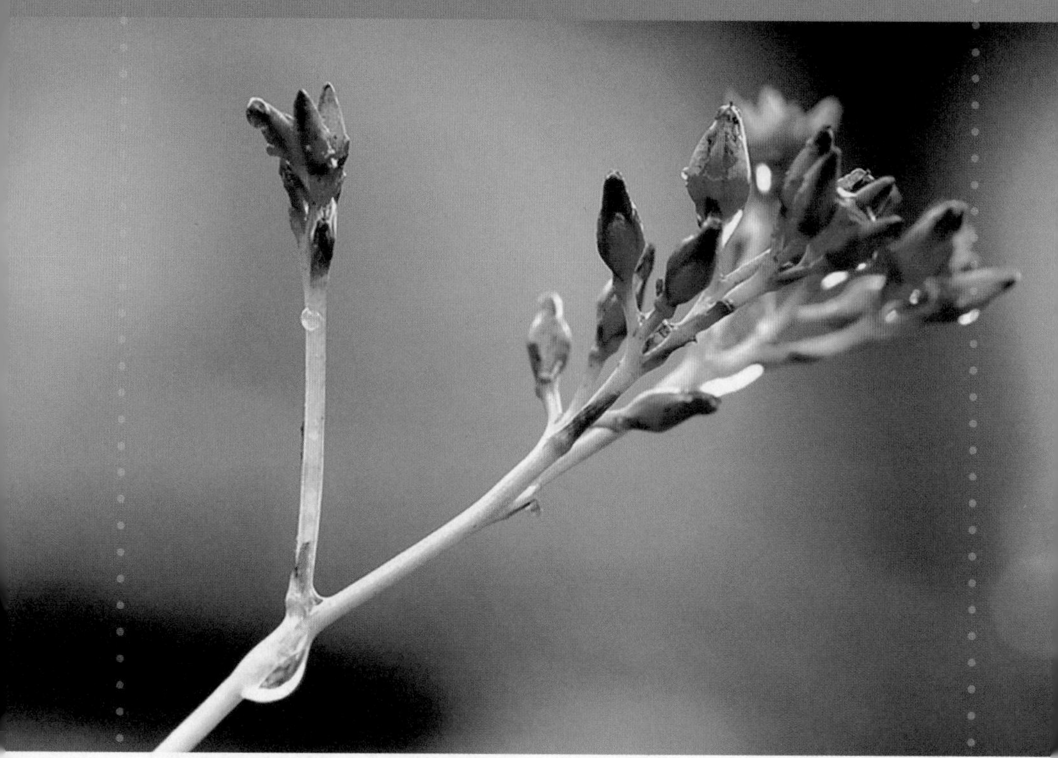

Scientific Name *Haemodorum ensifolium* F.Muell.

Common Names Red Root, Bloodroot.

Aboriginal Names Bilginje (Nyul Nyul), Kerrerlel, Minyngel, Minyngil (Gija) (Wightman, 2003).

Field Notes Red Root is a bulbaceous, perennial herb that grows up to 1.9 m in height. Its linear leaves are up to 10 mm wide and are basal with up to four arising from the base. Its small, red-brown flowers form in loose clusters of two to five along the divergent major branches, between March and June. Red Root occurs in sandy and rocky areas near creeks and low-lying places, and in sandy soil, in dry woodland and hummock grassland in the Kimberley region of Western Australia, and the adjacent areas of the Northern Territory as far east as Darwin (ALA, 2022; Flora of Australia Online, 2022; WAH, 2022).

Medicinal Uses The whole plant of Red Root was crushed and applied as a poultice on snakebites (efficacy not recorded) (Cock, 2011).

Other Uses The crushed, red-coloured tuber is added to fibre or cloth to dye it a red to brown colour (Wightman, 2003).

Redfruit Kurrajong

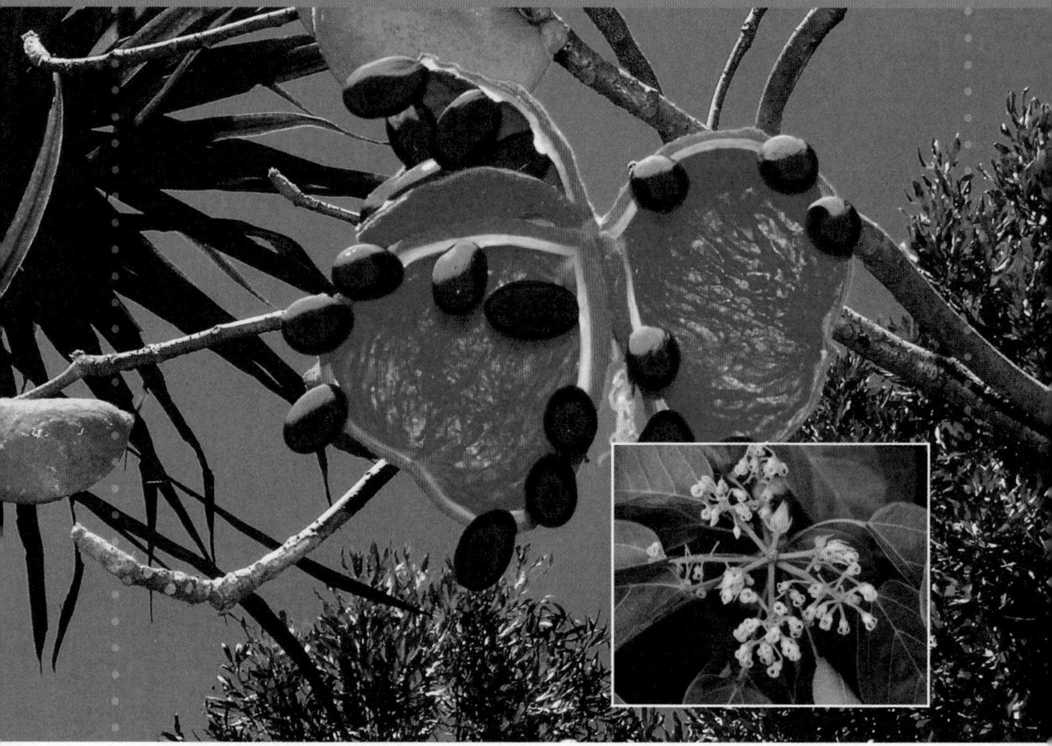

Scientific Name *Sterculia quadrifida* R.Br.

Common Names Redfruit Kurrajong, Orange Fruited Sterculia, Kuman, Orange Fruited Kurrajong, Smooth-seeded Kurrajong, Red Fruited Kurrajong, Peanut Tree, Scarlet-fruited Kurrajong, Small-flowered Kurrajong, White Crowsfoot, Native Peanut, Koralba.

Aboriginal Names Galala (Wunambal, Gaambera) (Karadada et al., 2011), Dalu manya (Kwini) (Cheinmora et al., 2017; Crawford, 1982).

Field Notes Redfruit Kurrajong grows as a deciduous shrub or tree to 20 m in height. It has elongated to heart-shaped leaves and green or yellow-green flowers that are clustered at the end of branchlets. Flowering is between February and June. Its fruit are bright red, woody capsules that occur in groups of five. Redfruit Kurrajong is found in sand over laterite, amongst sandstone boulders, on cliffs and ridge slopes in coastal areas of the Kimberley region of Western Australia, as well as the top end of the

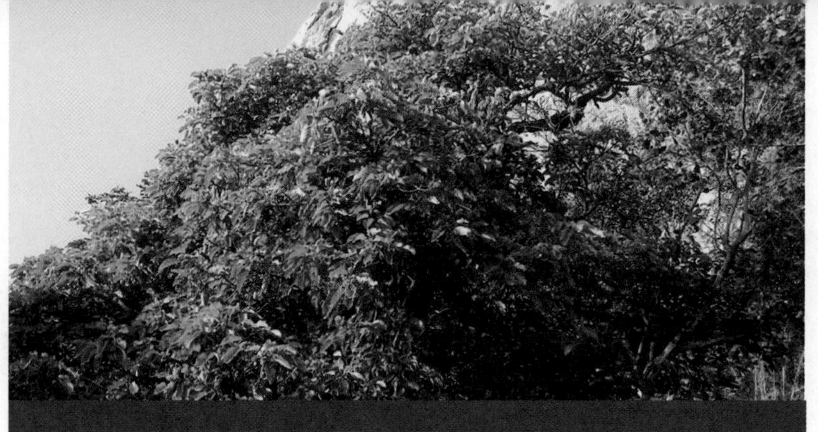

Northern Territory, Far North Queensland and down the east coast as far as the border with New South Wales (ALA, 2022; ATRP, 2020; Lassak & McCarthy, 2001; WAH, 2022).

Medicinal Uses Crushed leaves of the Redfruit Kurrajong were applied as a poultice to wounds and sores to aid healing. Infusions of the inner bark were used as an eyewash to relieve sore eyes due to conjunctivitis. Juice from the inner bark was dripped straight into the eyes for the same purpose or applied to cuts and wounds to aid healing (Fern, 2021; Hiddins, 2001; Lassak & McCarthy, 2001; Smith, 1991; Webb, 1959). Heated leaves were applied as a poultice to stings, including stingray and stonefish stings to relieve pain and itching (Low, 1990; Williams, 2020) and to wounds to aid healing (Cock, 2011; Fern, 2021; White & White, n.d.).

Other Uses The mucilaginous substance of the unripe fruit and seeds of the Redfruit Kurrajong are edible. The seeds were eaten either raw or roasted. The seeds are reported to taste something like peanuts. The tree bears fruit around October and November (Cheinmora et al., 2017; Crawford, 1982; Cribb & Cribb, 1981; Fox & Garde, 2018; Hiddins, 2001; Karadada et al., 2011; Low, 1991; Maiden, 1889; RFCA, 1993; White & White, n.d.). The leaves were sometimes cooked with meats as a sweetening agent (Low, 1991). The roots of young plants can be eaten raw or after they have been cooked in hot ashes or in a ground oven (Fern, 2021). The inner bark was used by some Aboriginal groups to make cordage (Hiddins, 2001).

Rhynchosia

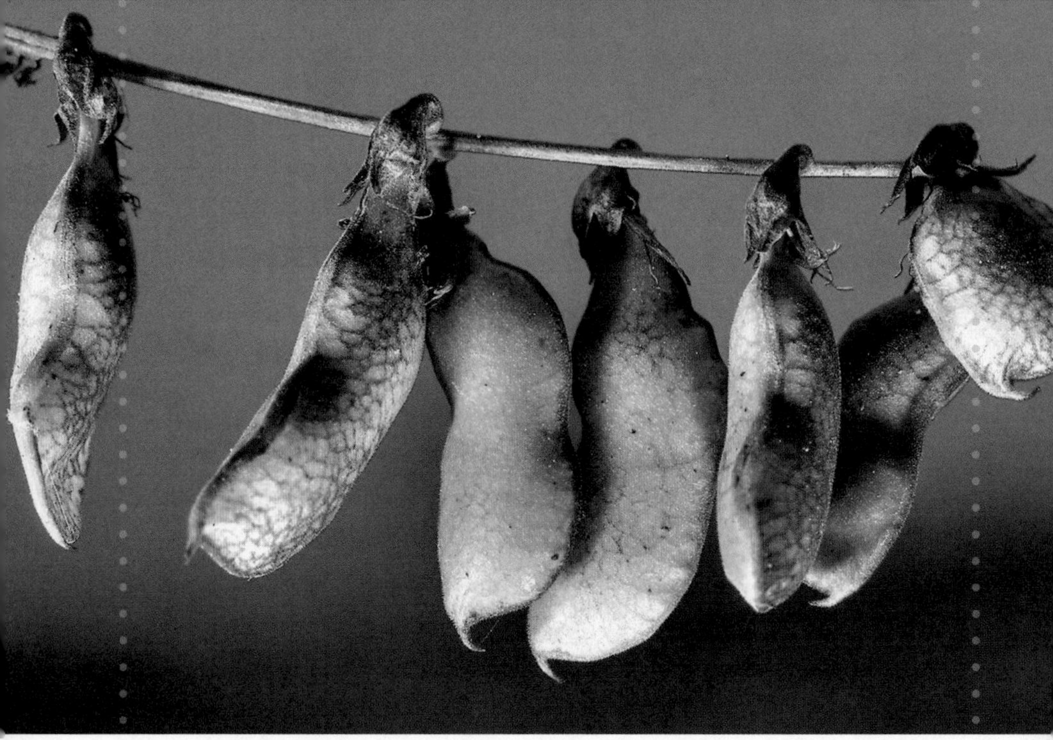

Scientific Name *Rhynchosia minima* (L.) DC.

Common Names Rhynchosia, Snout Bean, Burn Mouth Vine, Bush carrot, Jumby-Bean.

Aboriginal Name Yapili-pili (Kukatja) (Valiquette, 1993).

Field Notes Rhynchosia grows as a prostrate or twining perennial herb or climber that can climb to 3 m in height. Its leaves are ovate to rhomboid, up to 25 mm long and appear in clusters of three. The flowers are yellow with purple or brown veining and are up to 8 mm long, appearing in a raceme of up to 15 flowers. Flowering is any time between January and November. The fruit are seed pods, which are usually curved and up to 13 mm long and 4 mm wide. Rhynchosia is found in a variety of habitats in the Gascoyne, Pilbara and Kimberley regions of Western Australia, as well as the Northern Territory, Queensland, South Australia and as far south as central New South Wales in the east. It also occurs in Africa, the Americas,

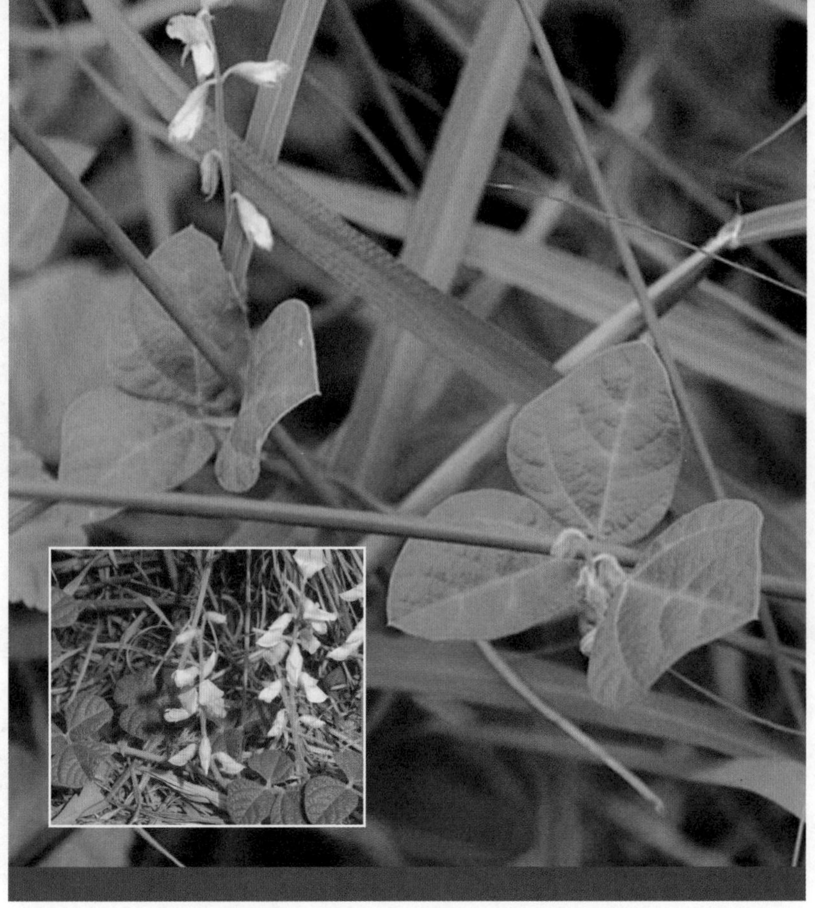

Asia, Indonesia and Malaysia (ALA, 2022; ATRP, 2020; Fern, 2021; Lassak & McCarthy, 2001; WAH, 2022).

Medicinal Uses Rhynchosia is used in folk medicine in many parts of the world where it grows. Decoctions of the root were taken internally to treat constipation and as an anthelmintic to expel intestinal parasites. They were also used to treat diarrhoea and dysentery. The leaves and roots were crushed and the resulting juice was applied externally to the anus to treat haemorrhoids. The leaves have abortifacient properties and have been used to induce abortions. The seeds have been used in the treatment of heart disease. The plant contains prodelphinidin, which is reported to have antibiotic properties (Fern, 2021).

Other Uses The carrot-like tubers of Rhynchosia are edible and were eaten raw or after they were roasted in hot ashes (Glasby, 2018).

River Fig

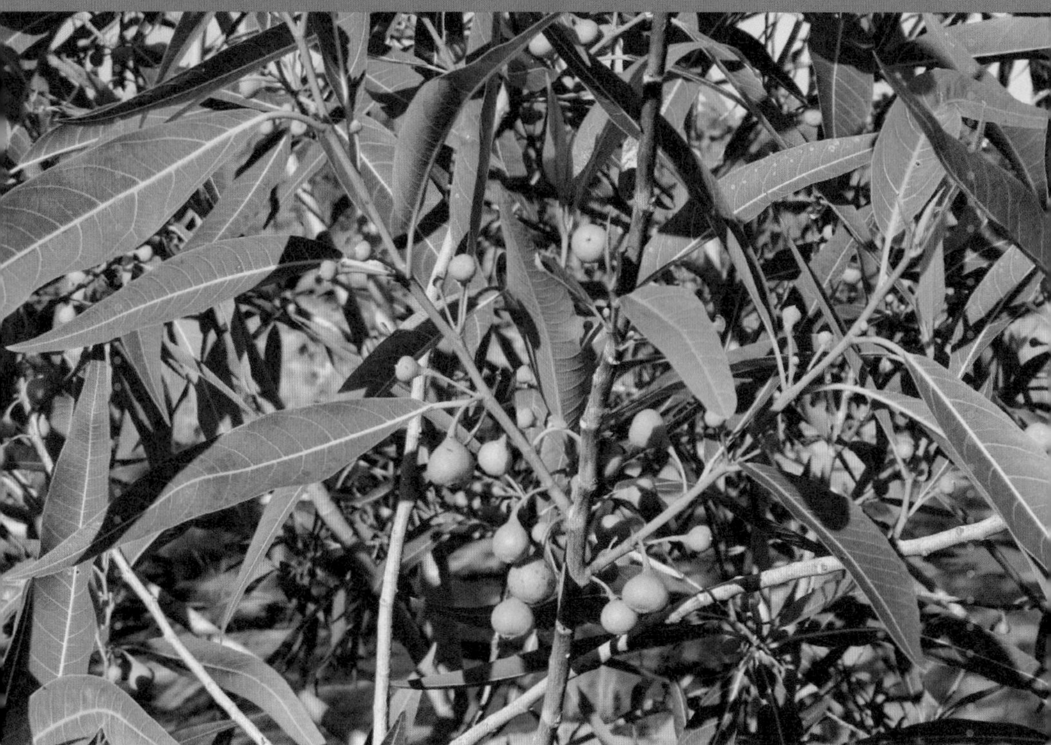

Scientific Name *Ficus coronulata* Miq.

Common Names River Fig, Peach-leaf Fig, Crown Fig.

Aboriginal Names Jamarndaj (Miriwoong) (Leonard et al., 2013), Julu (Bunuba) (Oscar et al., 2019), Jabayini, Ganambiny (Gija) (Purdie et al., 2018), Jabayi (W), Ngurlurr (N) (Jaru) (Wightman, 2003), Yalarra (Kwini) (Cheinmora et al., 2017).

Field Notes River Fig is a dioecious tree that grows to 15 m in height. Its branches are pendulous. Its leaves are alternate or occasionally opposite, narrowly elliptic, lanceolate or very rarely linear and up to 330 mm long. The leaf surfaces are slightly rough to the touch. Some leaves also have cystoliths, or hard stony structures, on their upper surface. Its male flowers appear on a peduncle any time of the year. Its globular fruit occur in the leaf axils and are up to 21 mm in diameter. River Fig is found in sandy soils, alongside rivers and creeks in the Kimberley region of

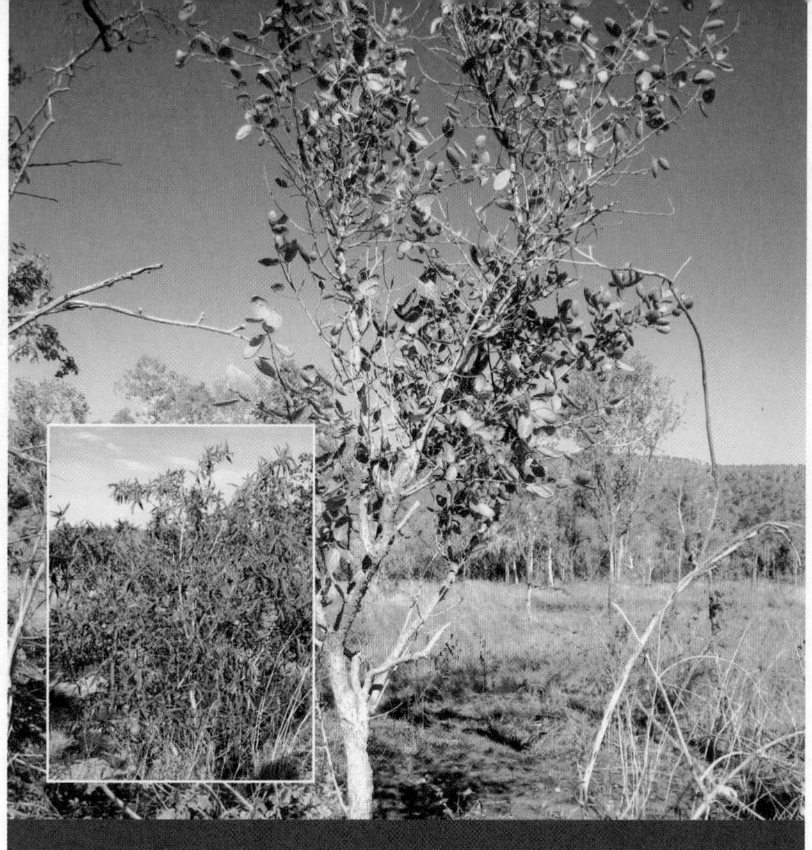

Western Australia and the northern half of the Northern Territory (ALA, 2022; ATRP, 2020; WAH, 2022).

Medicinal Uses The milky latex exuding from broken twigs or leaves of River Fig was dabbed directly onto wounds, sores and cuts to aid healing and to protect them from dirt. It was also applied directly onto boils and carbuncles to help draw them out. Decoctions of the fresh leaves and branches were applied as an antiseptic wash to sores and wounds to aid healing (Smith, 1991).

Other Uses River Fig fruit were eaten raw when ripe and soft in the late dry to early wet season (Smith, 1991; Wightman, 2003). The leaves and bark of River fig were used as 'fish poison' by the Gija. The stunned fish floated to the top of the water and were easy to collect (Purdie et al., 2018; Wightman, 2003). The fruit were used as fish bait when other baits were scarce (Wightman, 2003). The bark was used to make strong cordage (Oscar et al., 2019).

River Mangrove

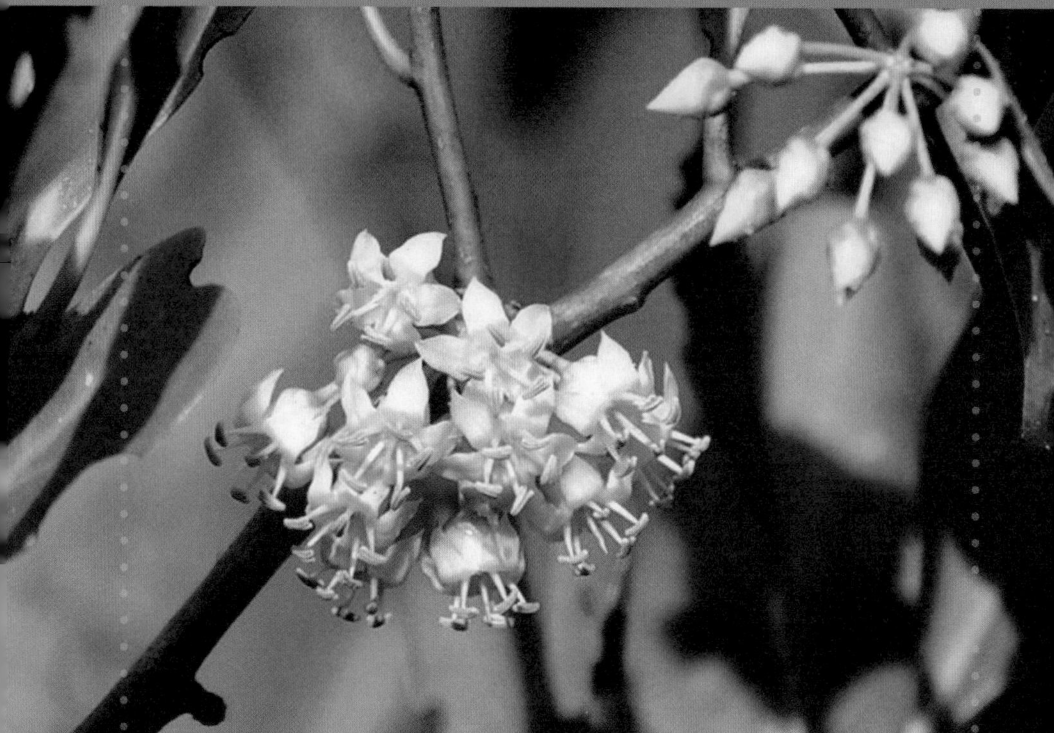

Scientific Name *Aegiceras corniculatum* (L.) Blanco.

Common Names River Mangrove, Black Mangrove.

Aboriginal Names Marlawarn (Miriwoong) (Leonard et al., 2013), Oorroolboorr (Bardi) (Kenneally et al., 1996), Urulbur (Bardi) (Smith & Kalotas, 1985), Limi (Wunambal, Gaambera) (Karadada et al., 2011), Kulii (Kwini) (Cheinmora et al., 2017).

Field Notes River Mangrove grows as a shrub or small tree up to 7 m in height. Its obovate leaves are up to 100 mm long and 50 mm wide and are leathery and minutely dotted. It has fragrant, small white flowers that appear in clusters of 10 to 30. Flowering in Australia is from April to October. Its fruit are light green to pink in colour, a curved horn-shape and up to 75 mm long. River Mangrove grows in mud in estuaries and tidal creeks, usually at the seaward edge of the mangrove zone. In Australia, it grows around the northern coastline from Exmouth in Western Australia to the south

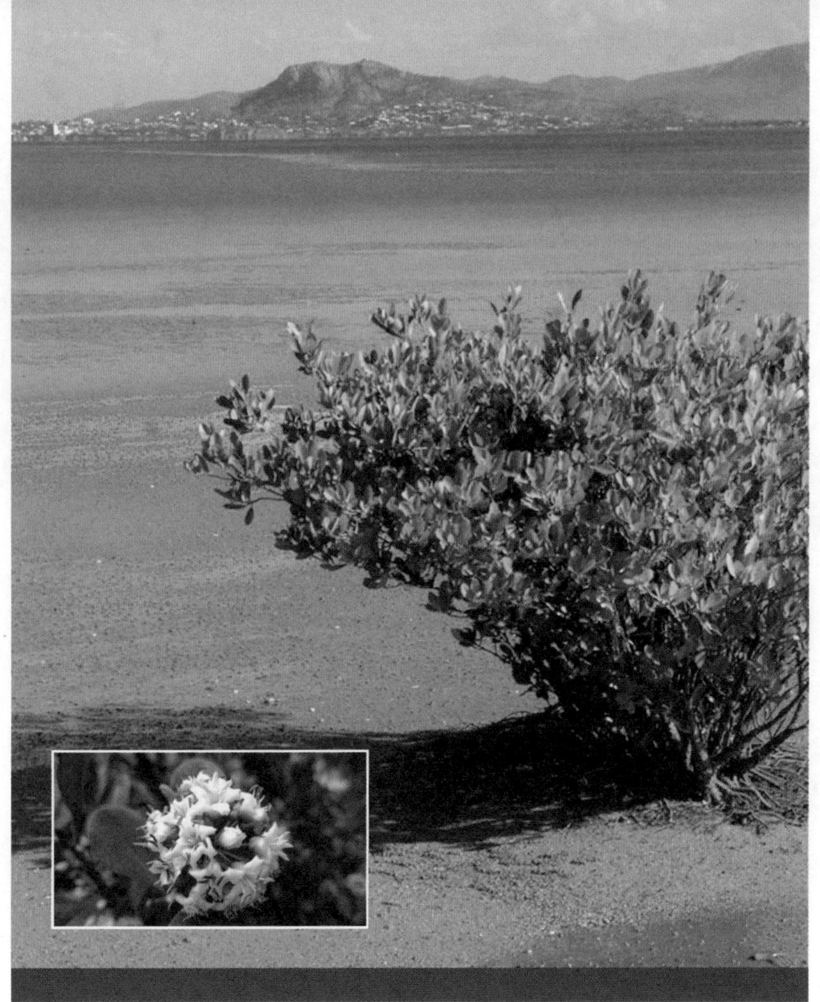

coast of New South Wales. It also occurs in India, through South-east Asia to southern China and in New Guinea (ALA, 2022; Lassak & McCarthy, 2001; WAH, 2022).

Medicinal Uses Decoctions of the leaves, or the juice extracted from squeezing the leaves, were used as eardrops for earache (a remedy for women only). Decoctions were taken internally to treat chest infections (Lassak & McCarthy, 2001; Low, 1990).

Other Uses The leaves, bark and wood were used as 'fish poison' to make the fish easier to catch (Kenneally et al., 1996; Smith & Kalotas, 1985).

River Teatree

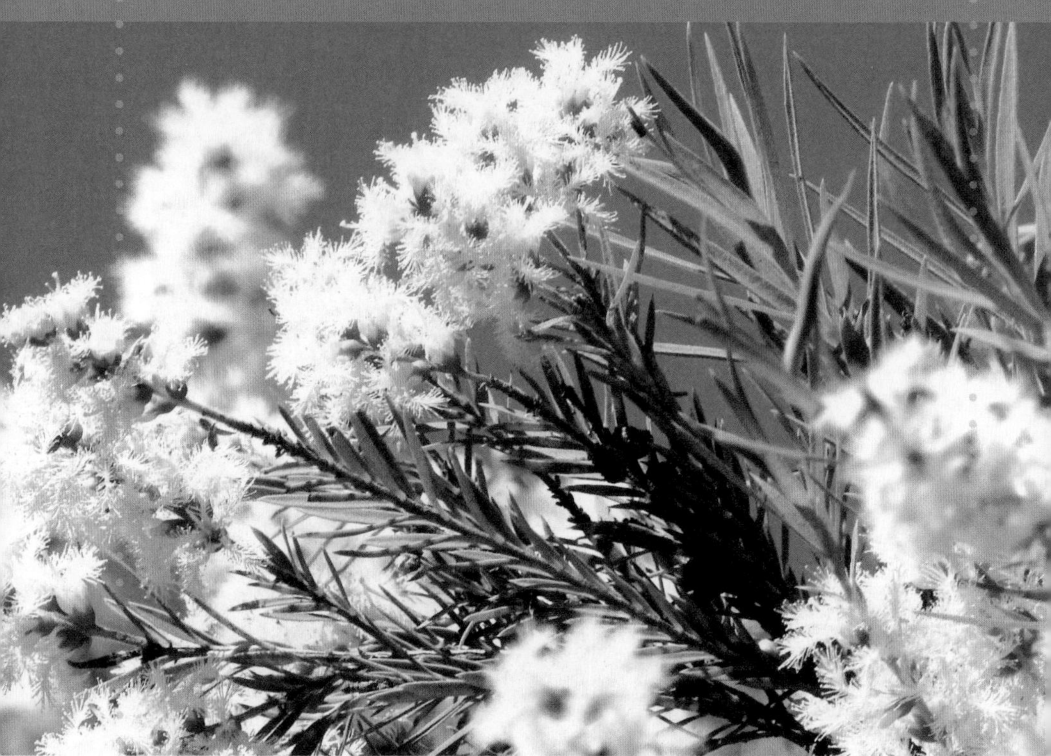

Scientific Name *Melaleuca bracteata* F.Muell.

Common Names River Teatree, Black Tea Tree, Honey Myrtle.

Aboriginal Names Woongenji or Wengenji (Gija) (Purdie et al., 2018), Wungun (Jaru) (Wightman, 2003).

Field Notes River Teatree is a shrub or small tree which grows to 15 m in height. It has a very dense canopy. The bark is smooth on young stems and on older stems can be hard and fissured. The leaves are twisted and grow to 20 mm long. The flowers are white or cream and grow in cylindrical spikes between May and January. River Teatree occurs in alluvial soils along small watercourses in the Pilbara and Kimberley regions of Western Australia, parts of the Northern Territory, central Australia and the east coast of Queensland and New South Wales (ALA, 2022; NSW Government Local Land Services, n.d.; WAH, 2022).

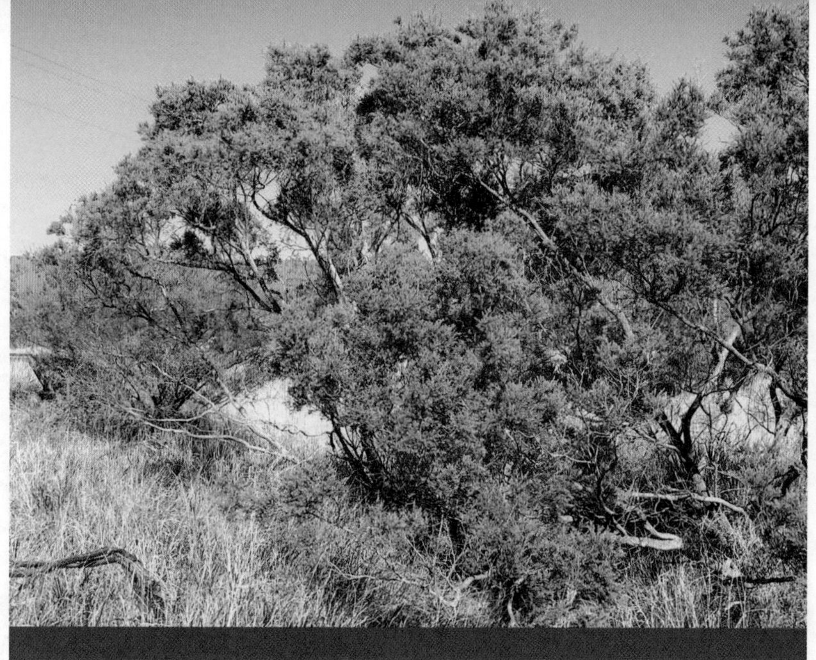

Medicinal Uses Teatree oil produced from the leaves, bark and flowers of melaleucas is well known as a treatment for minor cuts, burns, abrasions, pimples, bites, stings and fungal infections, such as dermatophytosis (ringworm, tinea or athlete's foot) and fungal nail infections. Traditionally, leaves were crushed and held under the nose for the relief of headaches, coughs and nasal congestion. Decoctions of the leaves were also rubbed on the forehead for headaches, and the steam inhaled for the symptomatic relief of colds and influenza. Infusions of the leaves were drunk in small quantities to relieve coughs and were rubbed over the body for generalised aches and pains (NSW Government Local Land Services, n.d.).

Other Uses In some parts of Australia the leaves of some teatrees were drunk as a type of tea. The nectar can be sucked from the flowers or added to water to produce a sweet drink (Cicada Woman Tours, 2013; NSW Government Local Land Services, n.d.). Like other teatrees (paperbarks), the flexible and absorbent bark was quite useful for shelters, bandages, blankets, coolamons and a type of food wrapping or container (Cicada Woman Tours, 2013; NSW Government Local Land Services, n.d.).

Rock Grevillea

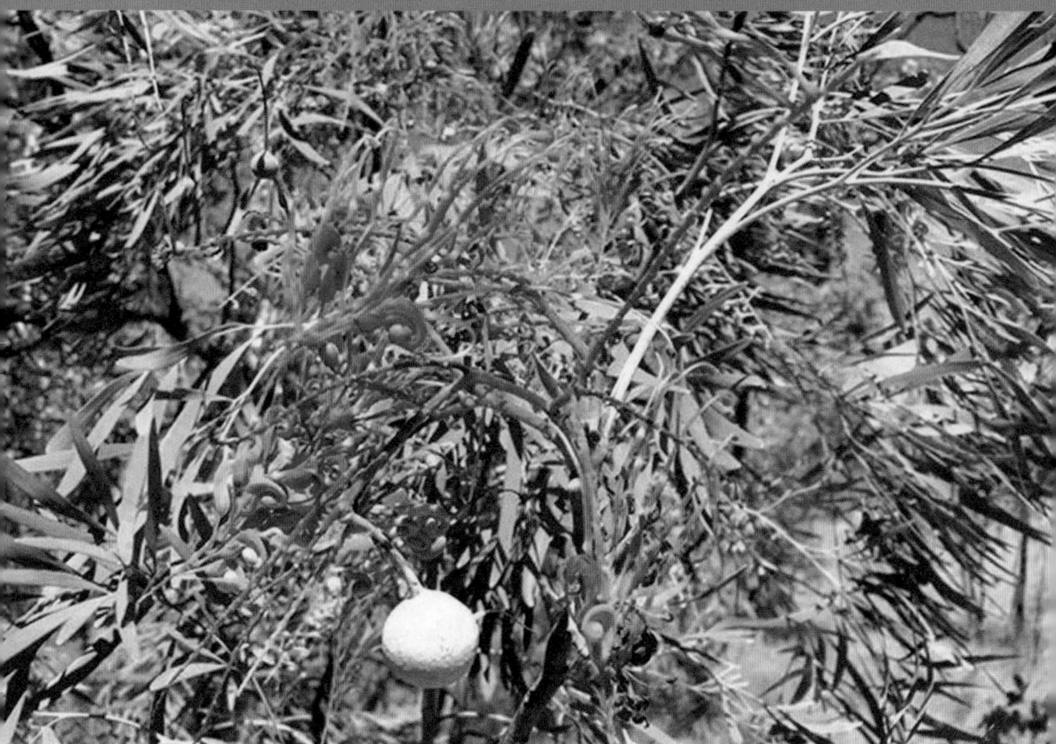

Scientific Name *Grevillea heliosperma* R.Br.

Common Names Rock Grevillea, Red Grevillea.

Aboriginal Names Miljirli (Walmajarri) (Richards & Hudson, 2012), Jamoordoo, Djamudu (Bardi) (Smith & Kalotas, 1985).

Field Notes Rock Grevillea is a small spreading, sparingly branched, sometimes lignotuberous shrub or tree that grows to around 8 m in height. It has thick, rough, brown bark. There are about 11 or 12 leaflet blades per compound leaf, with each leaflet measuring up to 130 mm long by 35 mm wide. The leaflets are longitudinally veined, with three to five veins slightly more prominent than the rest. The beautiful red or pink, spider-like flowers are present between May and September. Its fruit are green woody, round pods about 30 mm in diameter that turn brown as they age. Rock Grevillea occurs in sandy clay or red loam, commonly on sandstone or laterite, on rocky hillsides, plateaus or

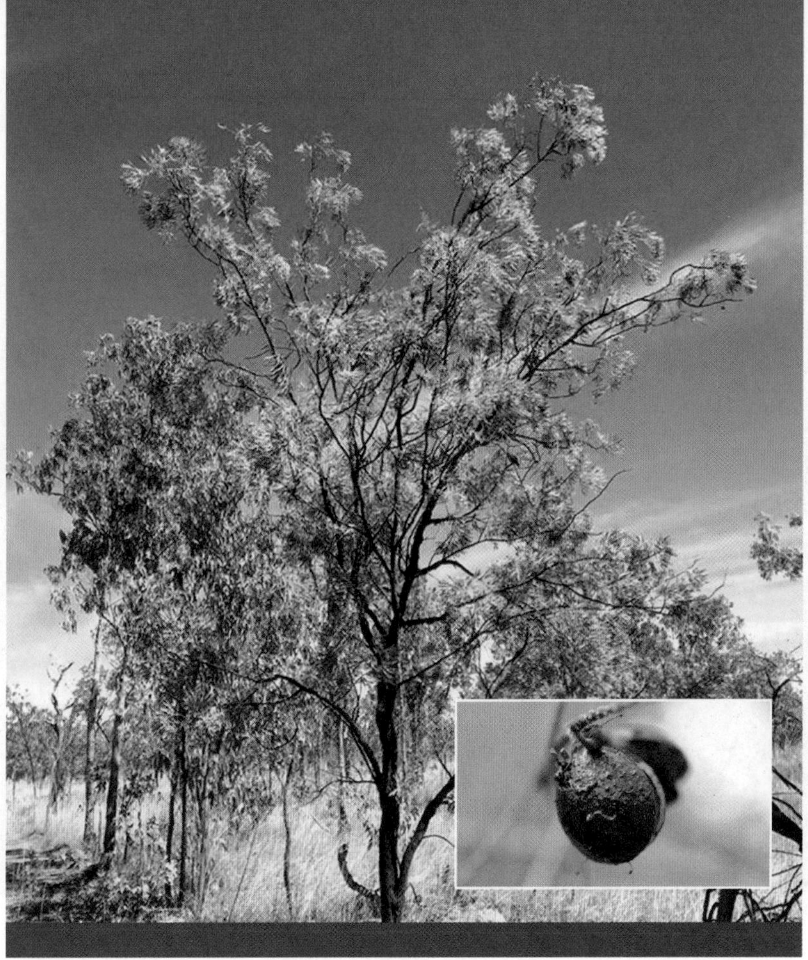

other rocky sites in the Kimberley region of Western Australia and the northern half of the Northern Territory, with rare sightings in Far North Queensland (ALA, 2022; ANPSA, 2022; WAH, 2022).

Medicinal Uses Decoctions or infusions of chopped-up bark and leaves were used as an antiseptic wash to treat skin conditions, such as infected sores, wounds and scabies infestations (Smith, 1991; Williams, 2011).

Other Uses The seeds of Rock Grevillea are edible and are usually eaten raw (Fox & Garde, 2018; Kenneally et al., 1996). The gum, called 'gudju' by the Bardi, that oozes from wounds in the tree is edible (Kenneally et al., 1996; Smith & Kalotas, 1985). Nectar was sucked straight from the flowers. Alternatively, the flowers were dipped in water to make a sweet drink (Kenneally et al., 1996).

Salt Wattle

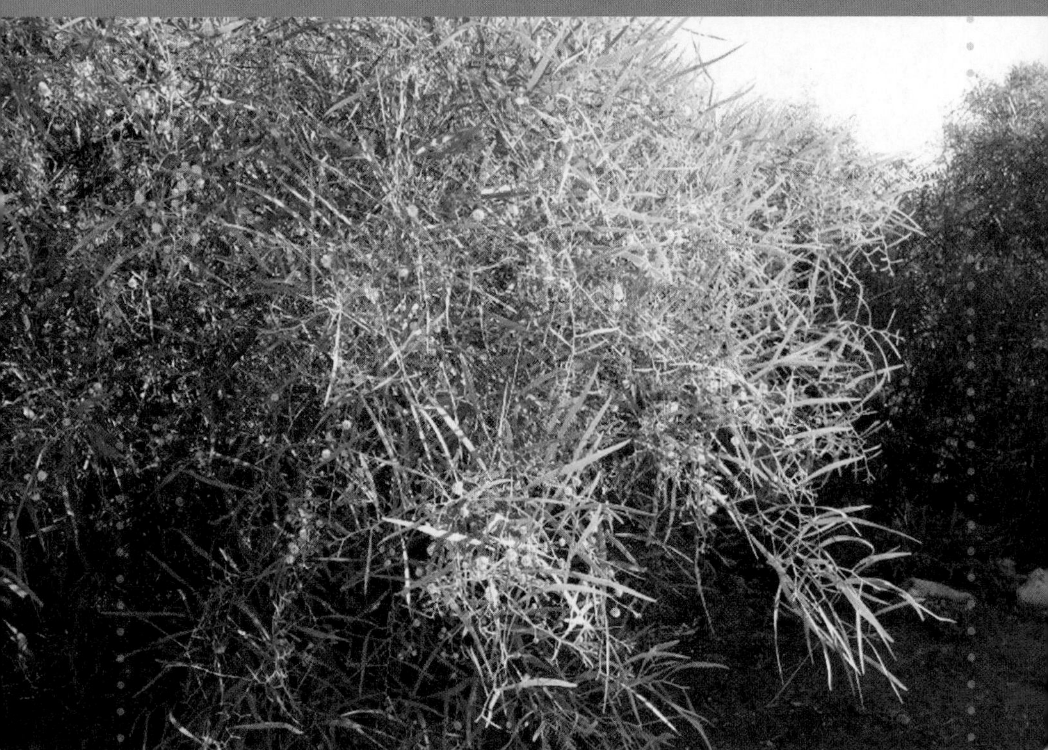

Scientific Name *Acacia ampliceps* Maslin.

Common Names Salt Wattle, River Wattle, Spring Wattle.

Aboriginal Names Merenyji, Mirinji (Gija) (Purdie et al., 2018), Mardiwa, Mardiya, Marduwa (Jaru) (Wightman, 2003).

Field Notes Salt Wattle grows as a bushy, glabrous shrub or tree to a height of around 8 m. Its phyllodes are lanceolate, drooping and up to 200 mm long. Its globular flower heads are clusters of pale-cream to light-yellow flowers. Flowering is between May and August. Its woody fruit or seed pods are long and narrow, up to 120 mm long and 6 mm wide and are present from late August to December. Its seeds are black with a dark red aril. Salt Wattle occurs in sand or sandy soils alongside creeks and rivers, on coastal sand dunes, floodplains and salt flats in the Pilbara and Kimberley regions of Western Australia, as well as the western half of the Northern Territory (ALA, 2022; Maslin et al., 2010; WAH, 2022).

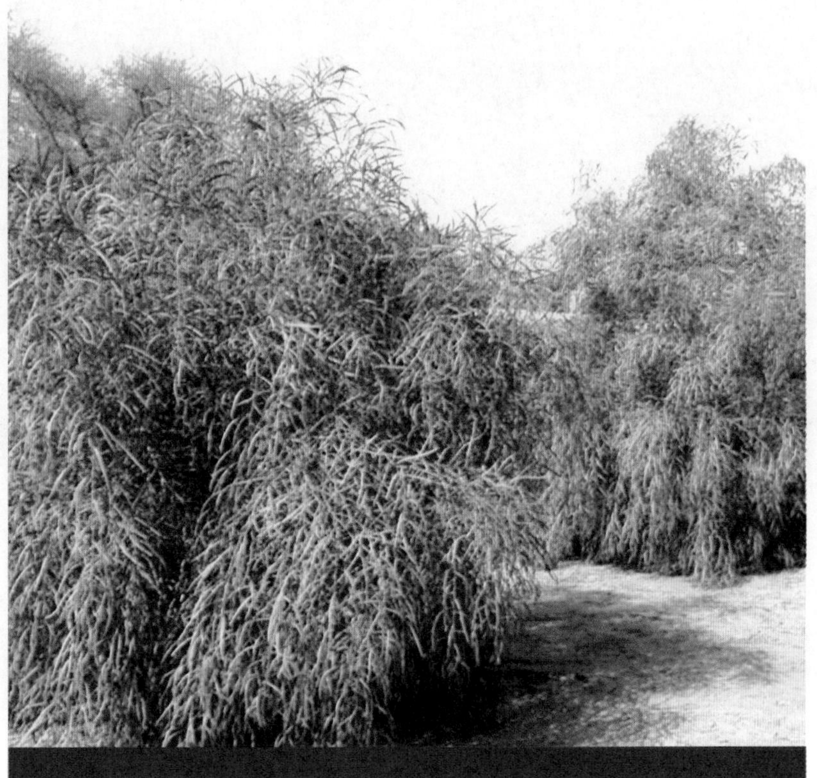

Medicinal Uses Decoctions of the bark were used externally by some Aboriginal groups as an antiseptic wash for wounds and skin sores, and to bathe sore eyes to treat conjunctivitis (Maslin et al., 2010).

Other Uses The gum that oozes from wounds in the Salt Wattle tree is edible and is eaten straight off the tree or mixed with water to make a sweet drink (Maslin et al., 2010; Wightman, 2003). The seeds are also edible and were generally ground to paste or eaten without preparation (Bindon, 2014; Fern, 2021; Kenneally et al., 1996). The Gija boiled the gum of Salt Wattle and mixed it with different coloured ochre to make bush paint (Wightman, 2003).

Saltwater Paperbark

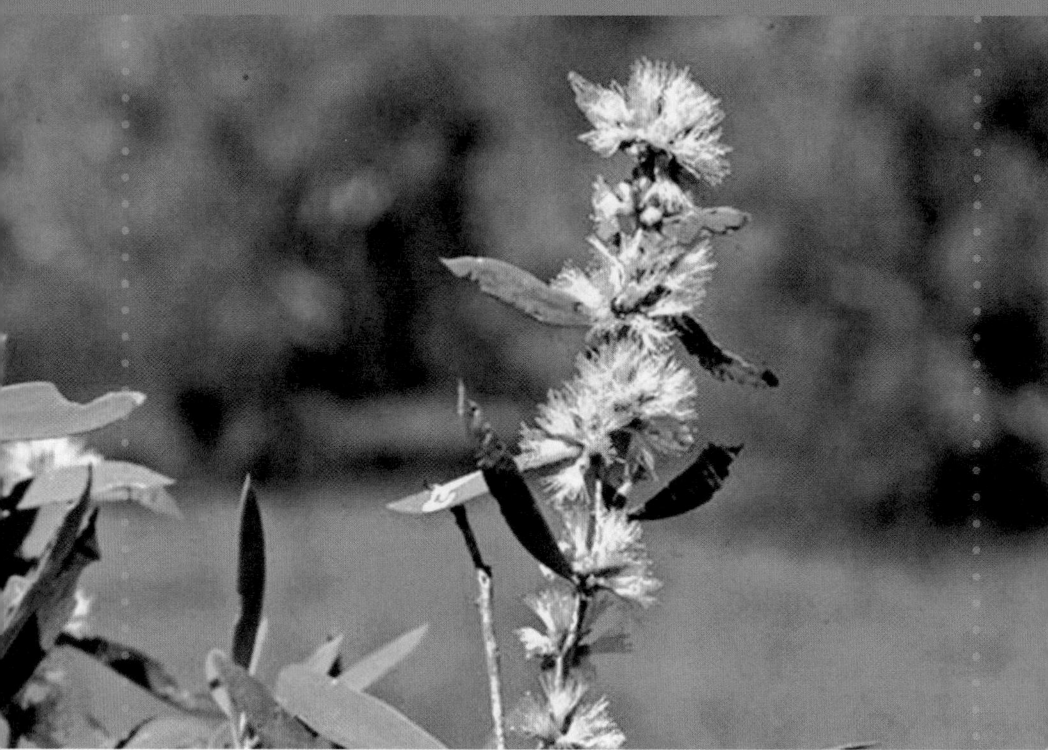

Scientific Name *Melaleuca alsophila* Benth., previously known as *Melaleuca acacioides* F.Muell. (misapplied).

Common Names Saltwater Paperbark, Flying-fox Paperbark.

Aboriginal Names Gooloongoorr (Nyul Nyul) (Dobbs et al., 2015), Loonyjoomard (Bardi) (Kenneally et al., 1996), Lundjamada (Bardi) (Smith & Kalotas, 1985), Jinjilji (Gija) (Purdie et al., 2018; Wightman, 2003), Wumulurru (Kwini) (Cheinmora et al., 2017), Jurnkurl (Karajarri) (Willing, 2014), Moorrka (Nyikina) (Smith & Smith, 2009).

Field Notes Saltwater Paperbark grows as a shrub or tree to 15 m in height. Its leaves are ovate to lanceolate and vary in length. Its white-cream bottlebrush-type flowers are present between March and October. Its fruit are cup or barrel-shaped woody capsules about 2 mm in diameter. Saltwater Paperbark is found in sandy soils that are often saline, along watercourses, in swamps, on floodplains, coastal flats and in saline habitats in coastal and near-coastal areas

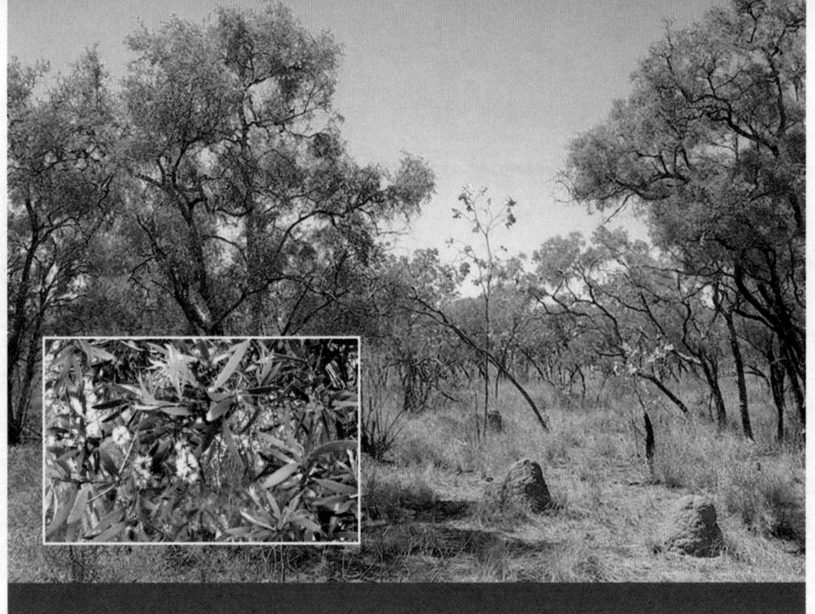

of the Pilbara and Kimberley regions of Western Australia, and the north-west corner of the Northern Territory (ALA, 2022; SKIPA, 2022; WAH, 2022).

Medicinal Uses Decoctions of the leaves of Saltwater Paperbark were taken internally after meals as a cough suppressant and to relieve the symptoms of colds and influenza. Crushed leaves were held under the nose and the vapours inhaled to clear blocked sinuses due to sinusitis and to relieve the symptoms of colds and influenza (Edwards, 2005; SKIPA, 2022; Smith, 1991; Williams, 2011). Aboriginal groups in Far North Queensland used decoctions of the leaves as a wash to treat general malaise. They also boiled the leaves and applied them as a poultice to treat catfish stings (Edwards, 2005).

Other Uses Aboriginal people in the Kimberley have used the trunk of the Saltwater Paperbark to build shelters. Native beehives are often found in the trunk and branches of this tree and are a good source of sugarbag or honey (Kenneally et al., 1996; SKIPA, 2022). The bark was burnt in campfires to repel mosquitoes (Kenneally et al., 1996; Smith & Kalotas, 1985). The swellings that appear on the tree can be a good source of a small amount of water (Cheinmora et al., 2017; Kenneally et al., 1996).

Sand Palm

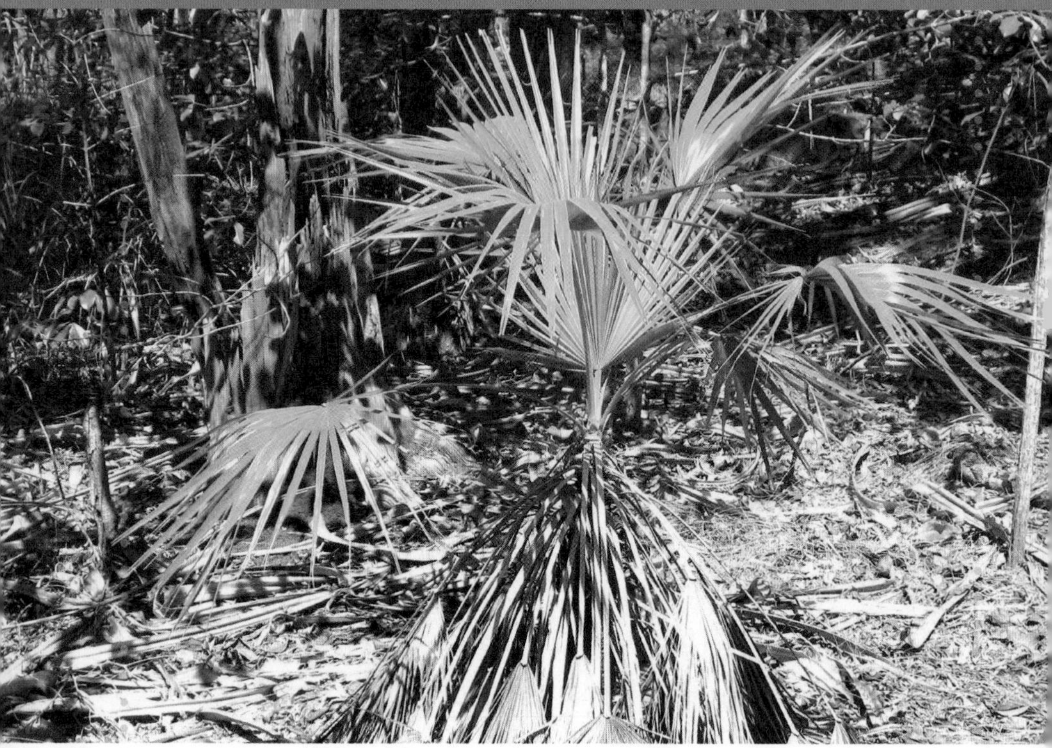

Scientific Name *Livistona leichhardtii* F.Muell., also known as *Livistona humilis* R.Br. and previously known as *Livistona lorophylla* Becc.

Common Names Sand Palm, Common Sand Palm, Fan Palm.

Aborigina Names Yalarra, Dangana (Wunambal, Gaambera) (Karadada et al., 2011), Yarranu manya, Dangana manya (Kwini) (Cheinmora et al., 2017).

Field Notes Sand Palm is a small, slender palm that grows up to 7 m in height. It has eight to fifteen fan-shaped leaves in a globose crown that are up to 500 mm long, with petioles up to 700 mm long. This palm is sexually dimorphic, that is, there are separate male and female plants. Its small flowers are yellow and up to 4 mm across. Its fruit are shiny, purple-black, ellipsoid, pyriform or obovoid, and up to 19 mm long and 10 mm in diameter. Sand Palm is found in open forest and woodland growing in deep sandy soils,

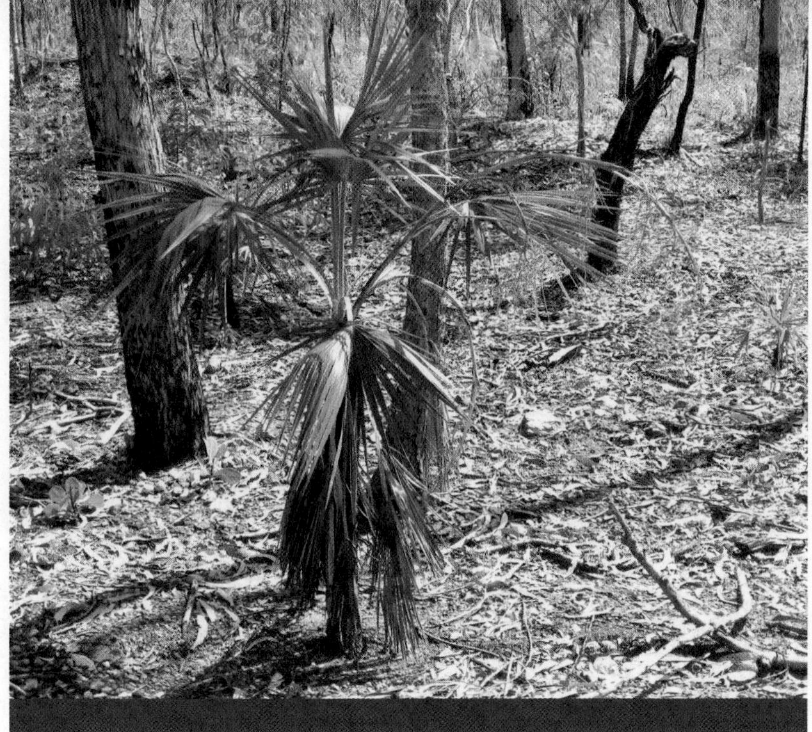

across the top half of the Kimberley region of Western Australia and the Northern Territory (ALA, 2022; Palm Pedia, 2015).

Medicinal Uses The core of the stem is pounded and made into a drink, which is used to treat coughs, colds, sore throats, chest infections, diarrhoea and tuberculosis. Poultices of the crushed stem core were applied to the lower back to relieve back pain (ALA, 2022; Devanesen, 2000).

Other Uses The fruit of the Sand Palm are edible. The heart (central growing tip) can also be eaten, either raw or roasted (Cheinmora et al., 2017; Fox & Garde, 2018; Karadada et al., 2011; Vigilante et al., 2013). The Kundjeyhmi people of the Kakadu National Park eat the pith of the smaller Sand Palms about 1 m high that they call 'An-marrabbi'. The trunk of the palm is put on the fire to slowly roast overnight and the pith is eaten the next day (Fox & Garde, 2018). The new leaves of Sand Palm were used to make baskets and dilly bags (Cheinmora et al., 2017; Karadada et al., 2011). The stems and leaves were used in the past to make wet season shelters (Karadada et al., 2011).

Sandhill Wattle

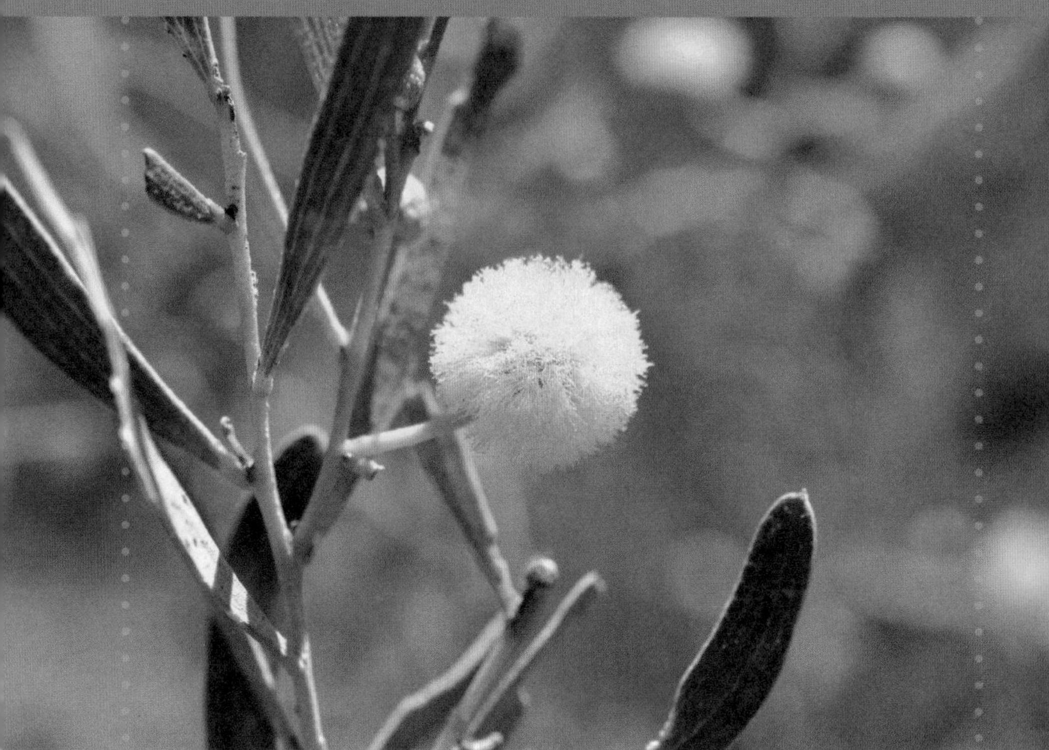

Scientific Name *Acacia dictyophleba* F.Muell.

Common Names Sandhill Wattle, Spear Wattle, Waxy Wattle, Feather-veined Wattle.

Aboriginal Names Langkur, Lungkun (Nyangumarta), Langkirr, Ngarturti, Mantalpa, Mulyarti, Ngakarrkalalya, Wartarti (Kukatja) (Valiquette, 1993), Marrja, Ngatarruku (Ngardi) (Cataldi, 2004).

Field Notes Sandhill Wattle is an erect, compact to spreading, or sometimes spindly and straggly, resinous shrub that grows to 4 m in height. Its blue-grey oblanceolate phyllodes are up to 85 mm long and 28 mm wide. Its yellow, ball-shaped flower heads are present between March and September. Its fruit are light brown, oblong, papery pods that are up to 90 mm long and 16 mm wide. Sandhill Wattle occurs in red sand, on sand dunes, sandplains and stony plains in the Pilbara and southern Kimberley regions of Western Australia, the Northern Territory and Queensland (ALA, 2022; Maslin et al., 2010; WAH, 2022).

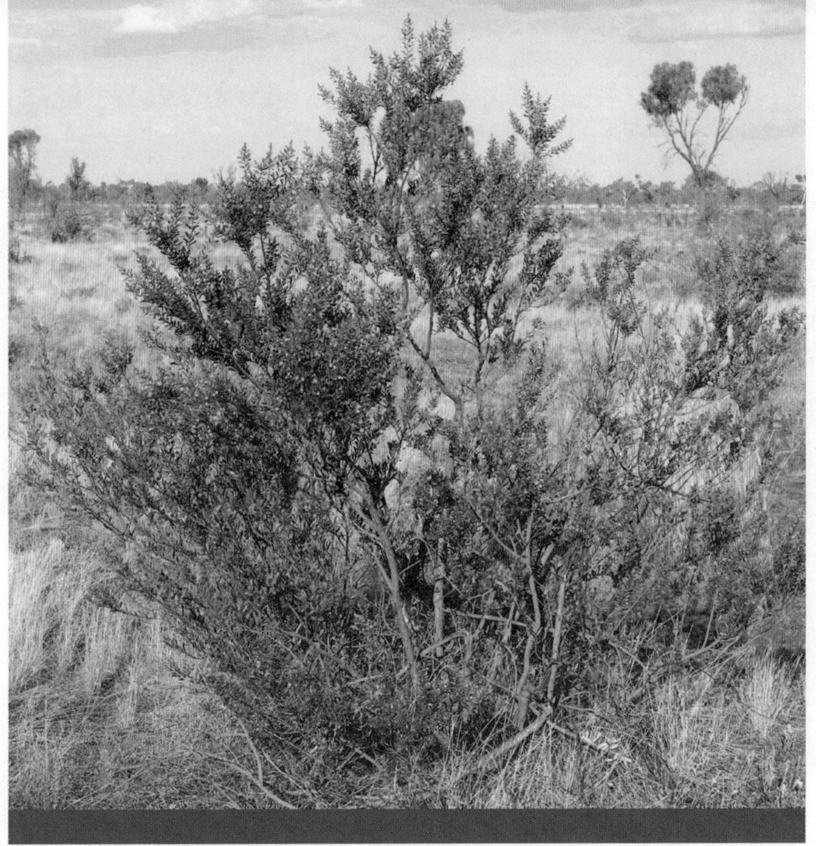

Medicinal Uses The leaves of Sandhill Wattle were used as 'smoke medicine' for mothers and newborn babies to strengthen them after birth. Young girls were also smoked with the leaves at the onset of menstruation (Cataldi, 2004; Williams, 2011).

Other Uses The seeds of Sandhill Wattle are edible and were ground to flour to make damper or Johnny cakes, which were baked in hot ashes or just eaten as a paste (Bindon, 2014).

Sandpaper Fig (*Ficus opposita*)

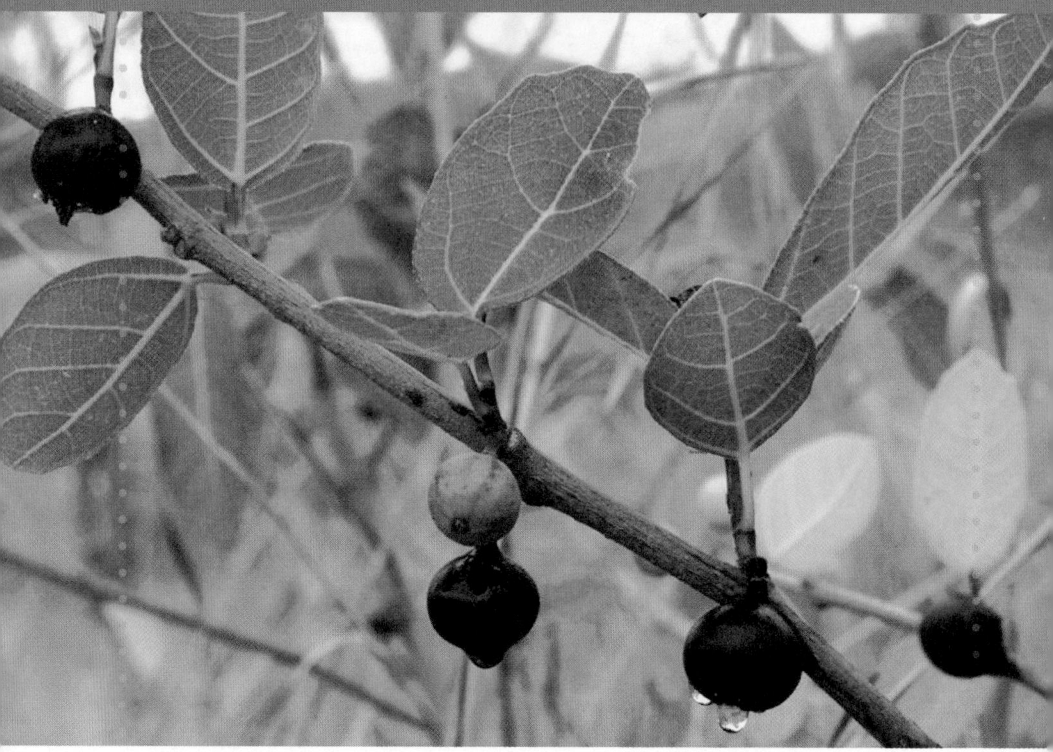

Scientific Name *Ficus opposita* Miq.

Common Names Sandpaper Fig, Figwood.

Aboriginal Names Ranyja, Yinirr (Walmajarri) (Richards & Hudson, 2012), Ngamarnajina (Yaruwu, Karajarri), Raanyja (Bardi), Jirrib (Nyul Nyul), Ranyja (Nyangumarta) (Lands, 1997), Jirribi (Nyikina) (Smith & Smith, 2009).

Field Notes This Sandpaper Fig grows as either a shrub or small tree to around 3 m in height. Its ovate leaf blades are up to 140 mm long and 60 mm wide and are usually rough (like sandpaper) on the upper surface. Its fruit are globular to depressed globular and up to 20 mm in diameter, with the outer surface pubescent (covered with short, soft and erect hairs) and usually black and shiny when ripe. This Sandpaper Fig occurs in open forest, monsoon forest and beach forest in the Kimberley region of Western Australia, the Northern Territory and Queensland. It also occurs in parts of South-east Asia (ALA, 2022; ATRP, 2020).

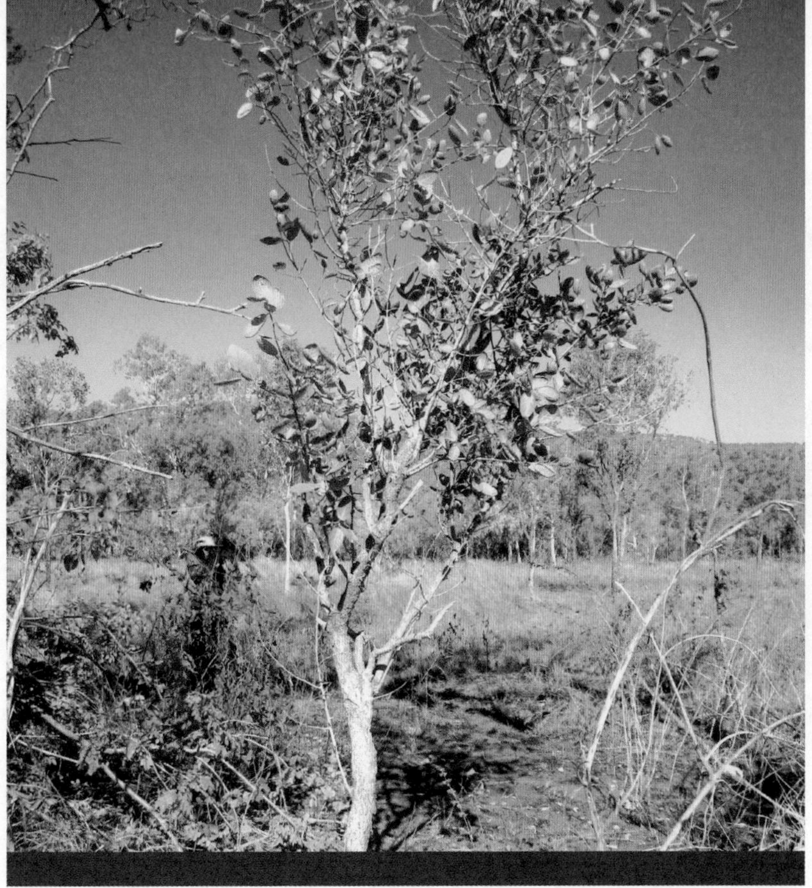

Medicinal Uses The leaves of this Sandpaper Fig were warmed over hot ashes and were used as a poultice and applied to bruises, swellings and areas of rheumatic pain. This was practised right across the top end of Australia by Aboriginal groups (Kane, 2022). The rough leaves and milky latex of the plant were used to treat ringworm: the ringworm area would be abraded with the leaves, then the milky latex would be applied to the area requiring treatment (Calvert, n.d.; Wet Tropics Management Authority, n.d.). Decoctions of scrapings of the inner bark from the stem and the roots were taken internally frequently in small doses to treat diarrhoea, and also used as an eyewash to treat conjunctivitis (Grier, n.d.).

Other Uses The fruit of this Sandpaper Fig are edible when black and ripe (Richards & Hudson, 2012) and have a high ascorbic acid (vitamin C) content (918 mg per 100 g) (Flavel, 2018). They are reported to be more palatable than some other native figs (ALA, 2022).

Sandpaper Fig (*Ficus scobina*)

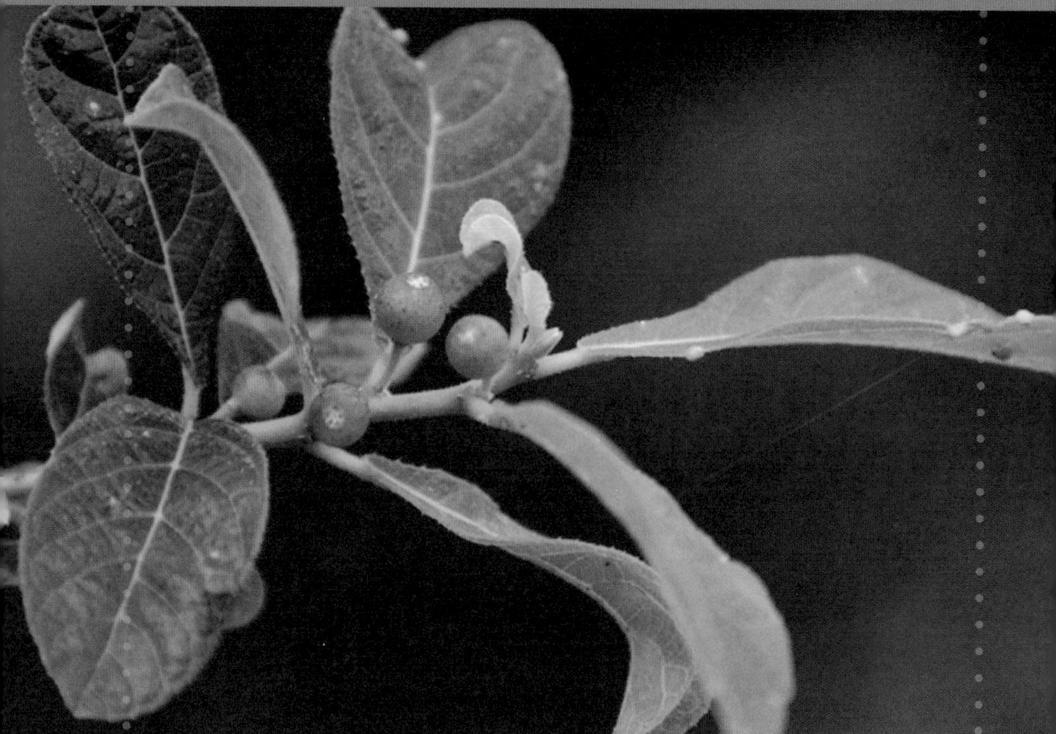

Scientific Name *Ficus scobina* Benth.

Common Name Sandpaper Fig.

Aboriginal Names Ranyja (Walmajarri) (Richards & Hudson, 2012), Yingarrjiny (Gija) (Wightman, 2003).

Field Notes Sandpaper Fig is a dioecious tree or shrub that grows up to 8 m in height. It has dark brown bark and rough, obovate leaves, opposite or alternate, that are up to 160 mm long and 80 mm wide. Its small fruit are globular and only around 10 mm in diameter. Sandpaper Fig occurs in alluvium, often alongside creeks, in the Kimberley region of Western Australia and the Northern Territory (ALA, 2022; ATRP, 2020; WAH, 2022).

Medicinal Uses Decoctions of the white, inner bark were sipped to treat diarrhoea (Wiynjorrotj et al., 2005).

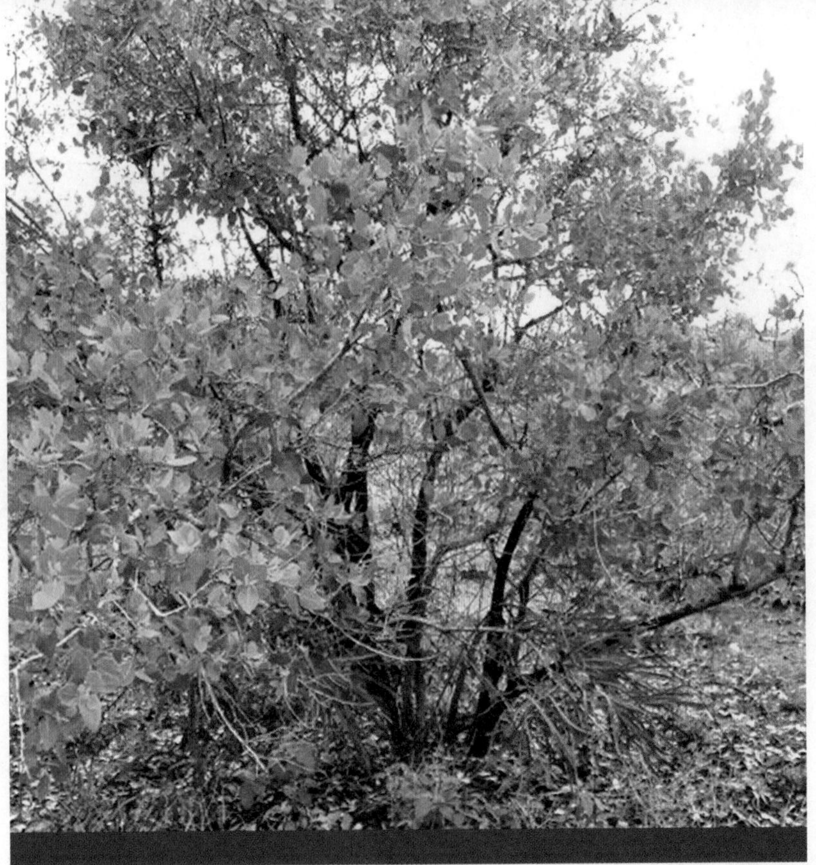

Other Uses The figs from this Sandpaper Fig tree are edible when purple or black, soft and ripe, appearing from March to April. They are sometimes warmed in hot ashes before eating (City of Darwin, 2013; Fox & Garde, 2018; Roebuck Bay Working Group, n.d.; SKIPA, 2022; Smith, 1991; Wightman, 2003). The rough leaves of Sandpaper Fig are used like sandpaper to smooth wooden objects, such as boomerangs and didgeridoos (Wiynjorrotj et al., 2005).

Saw-edged Spurge

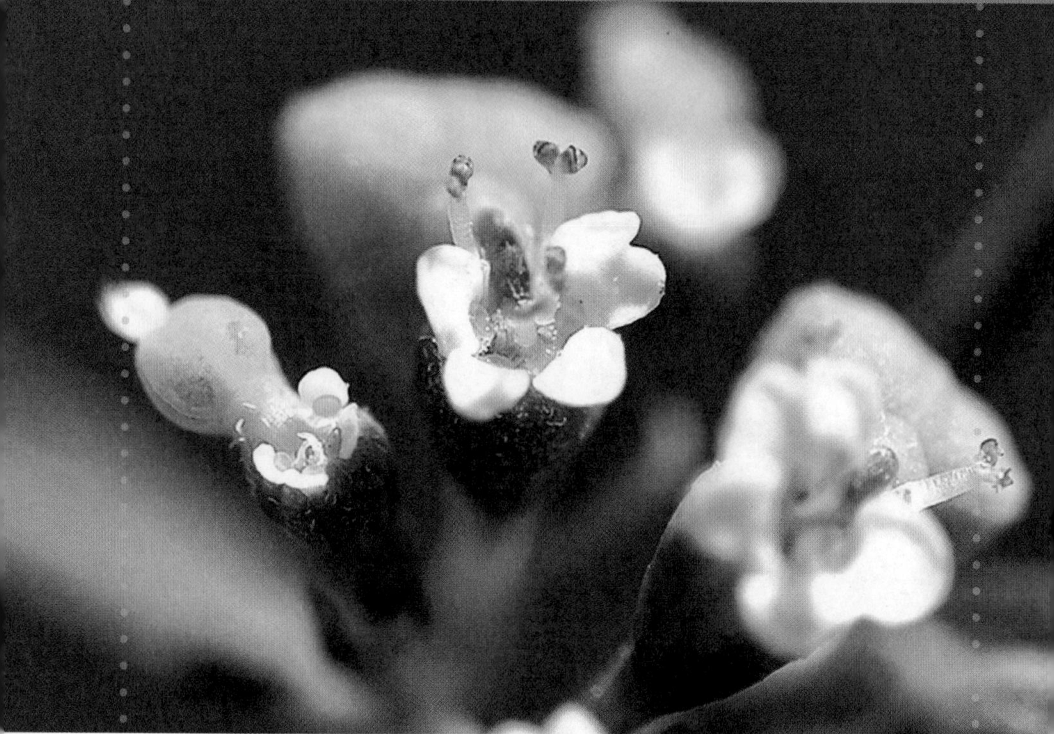

Scientific Name *Euphorbia bifida* Hook. & Arn., previously known as *Euphorbia vachellii* Hook. & Arn.

Common Name Saw-edged Spurge.

Field Notes Saw-edged Spurge is an erect, annual herb that only grows to around 800 mm in height. Its leaves are opposite, long elliptic to widely linear with toothed margins and up to 25 mm long by 5 mm wide. Its small, white flowers have four petals. Its small seed capsules containing three seeds are only 2 mm in diameter. Saw-edged Spurge occurs along the edge of creeks, across the top end of Australia from the Kimberley region of Western Australia, through the Northern Territory and Queensland, and down the east coast as far as northern New South Wales. It also occurs in southern China, India, Indonesia, Japan (Ryukyu Islands), Malaysia, Myanmar, the Philippines, Sri Lanka, Taiwan, Thailand, Vietnam and on some Pacific islands (ALA, 2022; PlantNET, 2022; WAH, 2022).

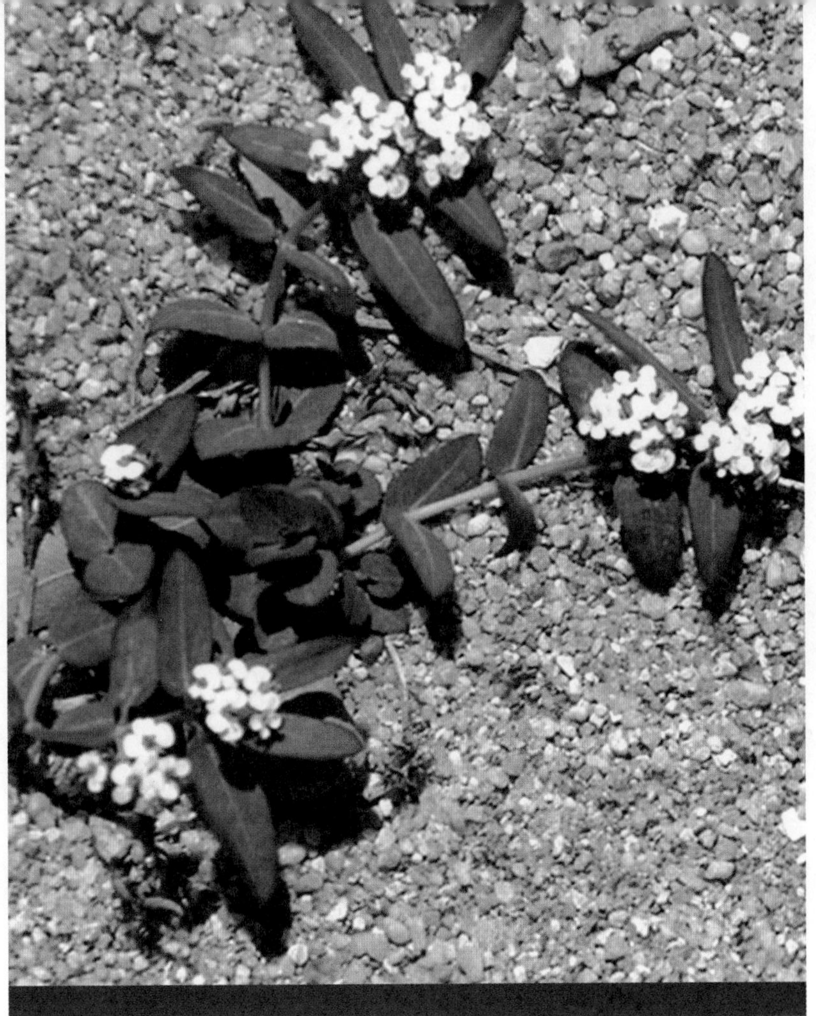

Medicinal Uses Aboriginal groups in Far North Queensland chewed the whole Saw-edged Spurge plant without swallowing it to treat 'upset stomachs'. Decoctions of the whole plant were applied topically as an antiseptic wash to treat skin sores and wounds (Edwards, 2005).

Scarlet Bloodroot

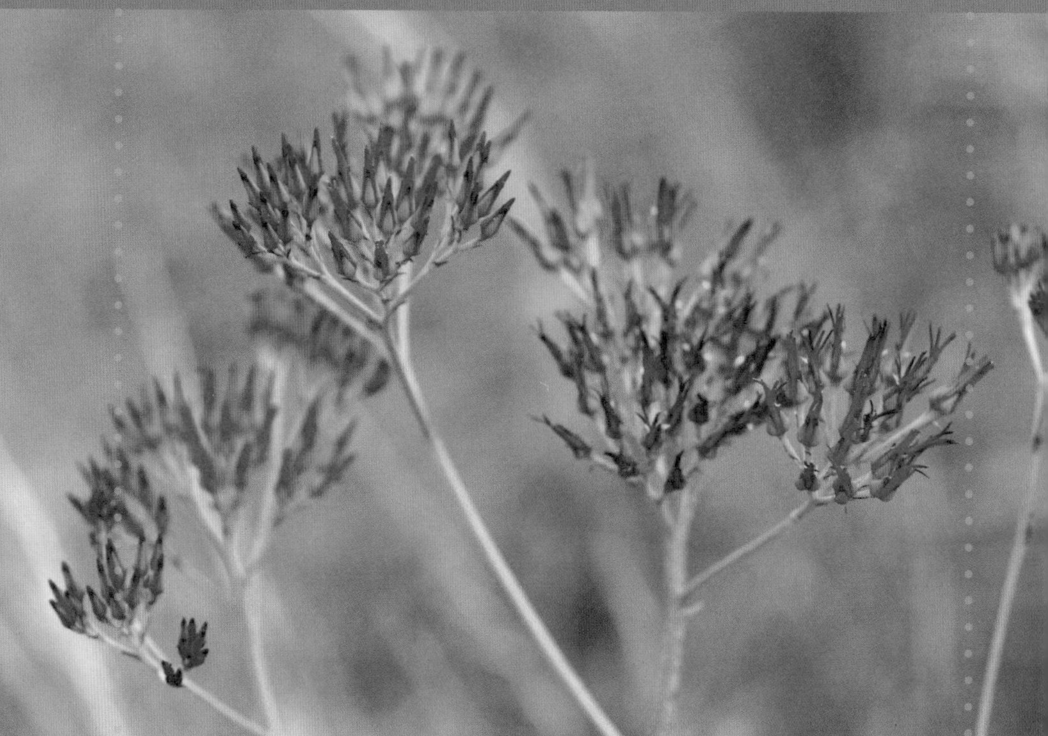

Scientific Name *Haemodorum coccineum* R.Br.

Common Names Scarlet Bloodroot, Bloodroot, Red Root.

Field Notes Scarlet Bloodroot is a perennial herb with flower stalks that can grow up to 1 m in height. It has basal, strap-like leaves arising from an underground rhizome that are up to 60 mm long and 10 mm wide. Its deep-red or orange-red flowers form in clusters on long, stiff stems. These plants usually die back to the rhizome in the winter or dry season and regrow in the summer or wet season. Scarlet Bloodroot occurs in open woodland habitats, on gravelly or shallow lateritic soils and sandstone in the east Kimberley region of Western Australia, the Northern Territory and Far North Queensland. It also occurs in New Guinea (ALA, 2022; ANPSA, 2022).

Medicinal Uses Decoctions of the crushed roots of Scarlet Bloodroot were used as an antiseptic wash that was applied

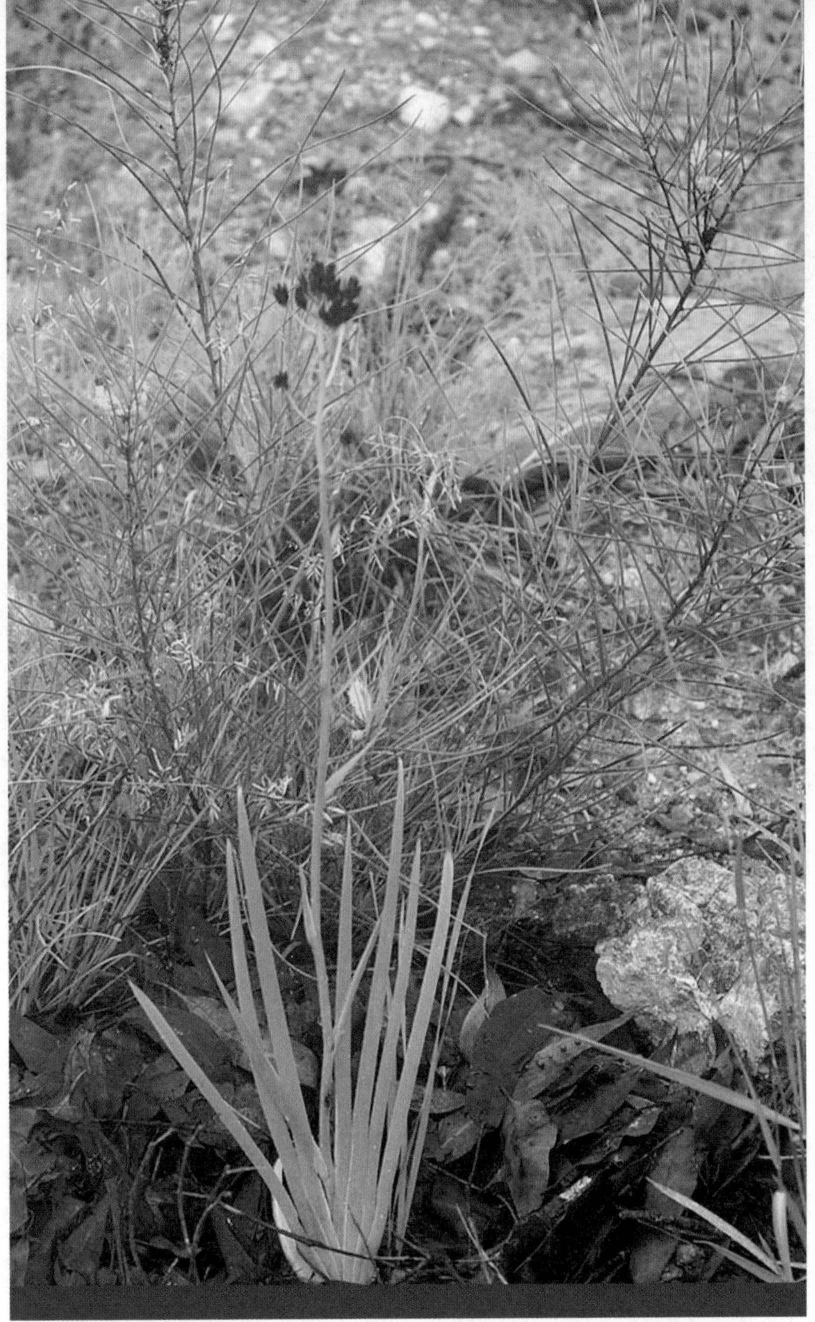

externally to skin sores and wounds to aid the healing process (Williams, 2012).

Other Uses The bulbous roots of Scarlet Bloodroot are reported to be edible (Lindsay, 2004).

Scentgrass

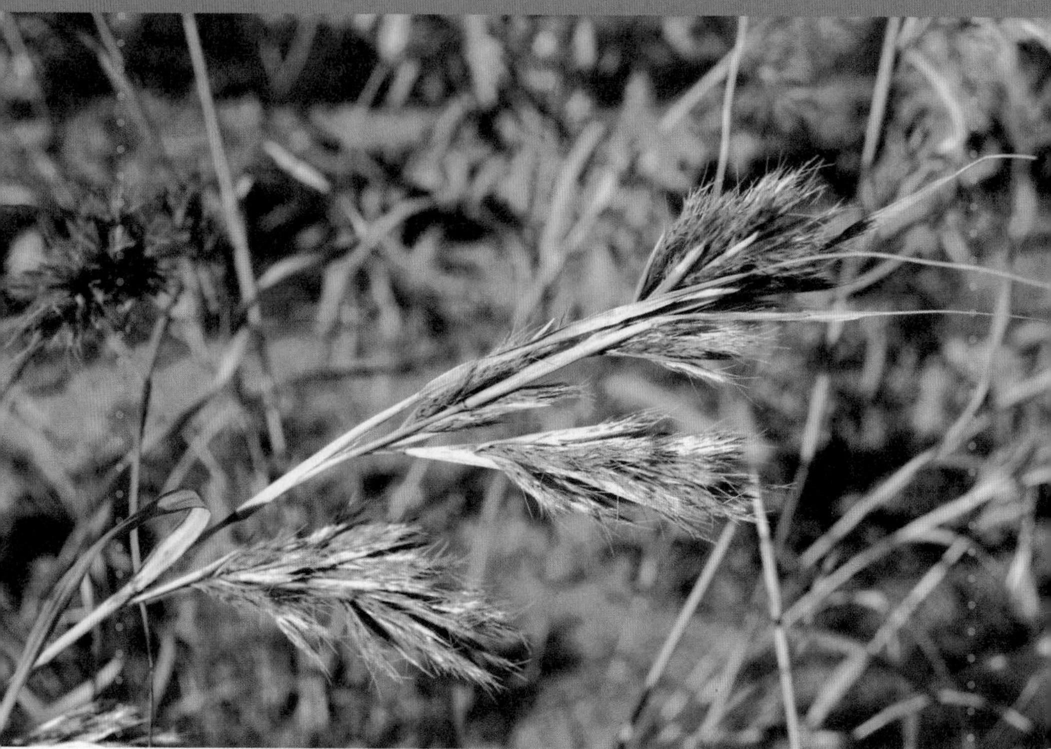

Scientific Name *Cymbopogon ambiguus* A.Camus.

Common Names Scentgrass, Lemon Grass, Native Lemon Grass, Australian Lemon Grass.

Aboriginal Names Karltu-karltu, Warakatji, Yawula (Kukatja) (Valiquette, 1993), Majal (Kwini) (Cheinmora et al., 2017).

Field Notes Scentgrass grows in tufty clumps to around 1.8 m in height. Its leaves are long and basal. The leaves and stems have a lemony scent when crushed. The green flowers that appear in clusters at the top of the stalks can be seen from November to December or from January to June. Scentgrass grows on rocky hills, exposed granite and on roadsides that have shallow loam or clay soils. It also grows beside creeks in stony uplands. Scentgrass occurs all over mainland Australia (ATRP, 2020; Bowman et al., 2000; WAH, 2022).

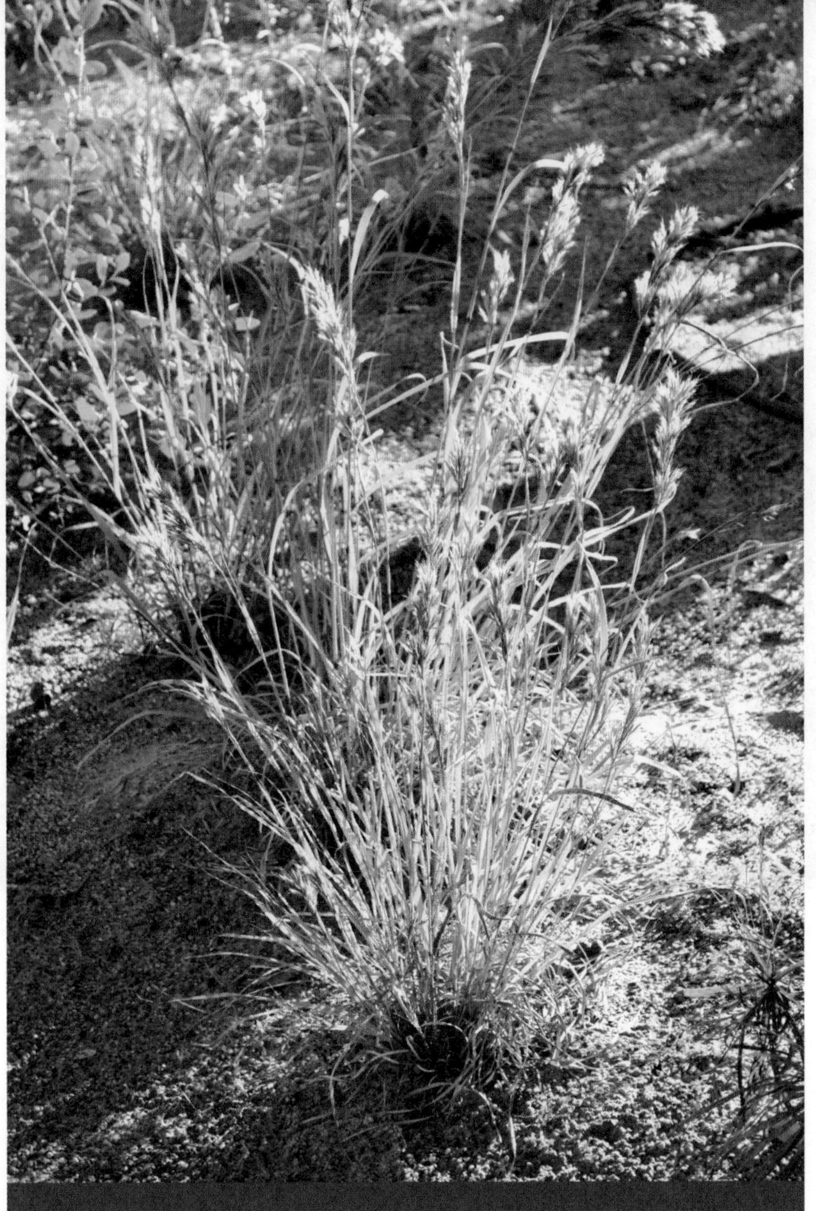

Medicinal Uses Decoctions of the leaves, stems and roots of Scentgrass were used for bathing the body to treat general malaise and as an antiseptic wash for sores, skin rashes, cramps, earache, scabies infestations and sore eyes due to conjunctivitis. Small amounts of the decoctions were drunk to relieve sore throats and diarrhoea (Devanesen, 2000). The leaves were crushed and the vapour inhaled for 'chest complaints' (Pearn, 2004).

Scraggy Wattle

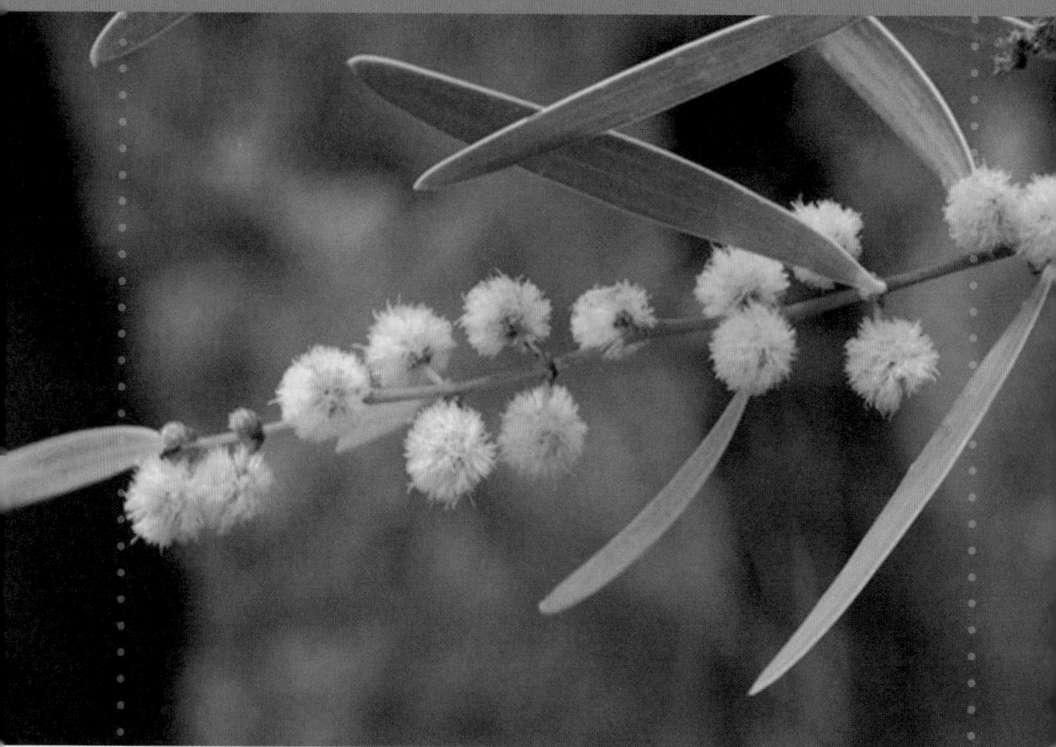

Scientific Name *Acacia multisiliqua* (Benth.) Maconochie.

Common Name Scraggy Wattle.

Field Notes Scraggy Wattle is a spindly shrub or tree that grows to 5 m in height. Its phyllodes are narrowly elliptic, usually slightly incurved and up to 65 mm long and 13 mm wide. Its yellow, ball-shaped flowers are present between February and August. Its seed pods are linear, raised over and constricted between seeds, and up to 65 mm long and 5 mm wide. Scraggy Wattle occurs in sandy soils over sandstone or alluvium on rocky slopes in the Kimberley region of Western Australia, the Northern Territory and Queensland (ALA, 2022; WAH, 2022; World Wide Wattle, 2022).

Medicinal Uses A handful of crushed fresh phyllodes of Scraggy Wattle was gently boiled in water and the steam inhaled to clear nasal congestion due to colds, influenza and sinusitis (Searle, 2020; Subhan, 2016; Williams, 2011). Alternatively, the phyllodes were

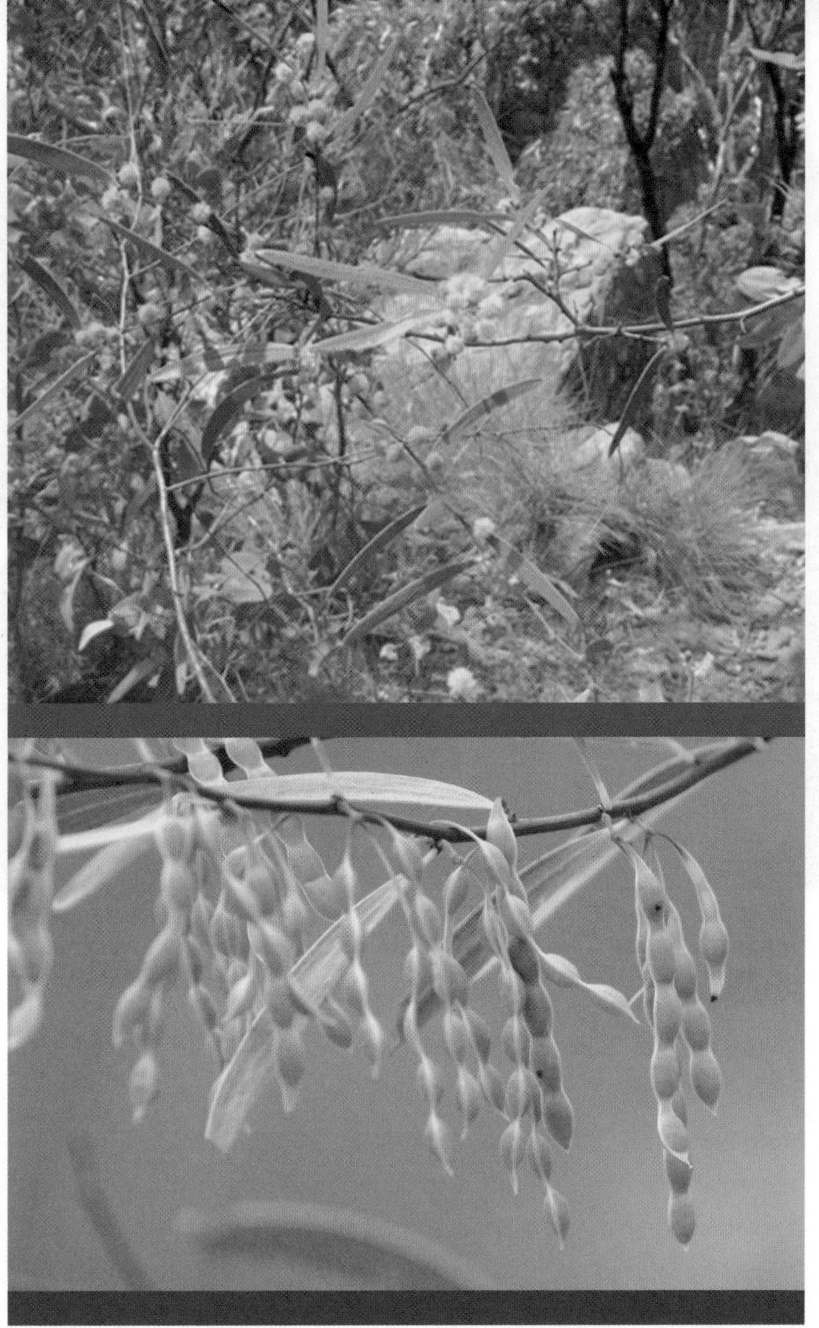

crushed in the hand and the vapours inhaled for the same purpose (Williams, 2011).

Scrambling Clerodendrum

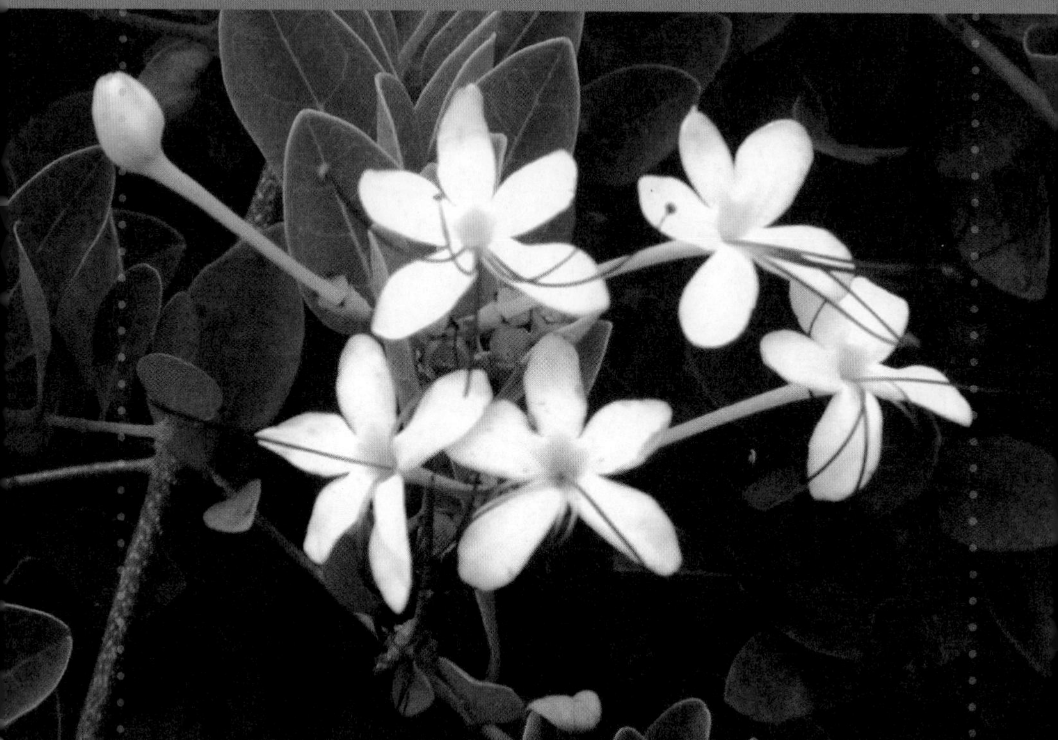

Scientific Name *Clerodendrum inerme* (L.) Gaertn.

Common Names Scrambling Clerodendrum, Harmless Clerodendron, Wild Jasmine, Sorcerers Bush, Seaside Clerodendrum.

Field Notes Scrambling Clerodendrum grows as an untidy vine or shrub up to 4 m in height, with stems to 30 mm in diameter. Its glabrous leaves are elliptic to narrowly elliptic or ovate to lanceolate, and up to 110 mm long and 55 mm wide. Its white, star-shaped flowers have five petals and long, red stamens. Its fruit are black drupes that are up to 20 mm long by 15 mm in diameter, have four segments and are borne on a calyx. Scrambling Clerodendrum occurs in proximity to the sea in the Kimberley region of Western Australia, the Northern Territory and down the Queensland coast as far south as north-eastern New South Wales. It also occurs in tropical and sub-tropical Asia and on some Pacific

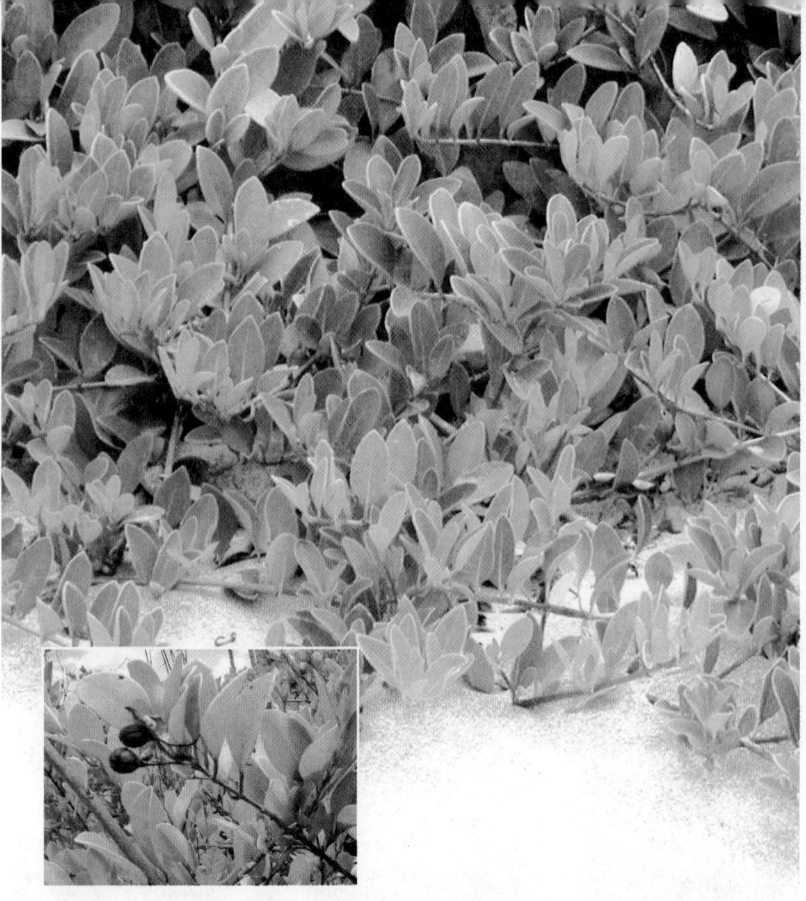

islands (ALA, 2022; ATRP, 2020; FloraNT, 2022; WAH, 2022).

Medicinal Uses Scrambling Clerodendrum is used in folk medicine throughout Asia. In Thailand and the Philippines, decoctions of the roots were taken internally to treat fever and as a general alterative (tonic). The leaves were crushed and used as a poultice to resolve swelling. In Indonesia, the seeds are used to treat an upset stomach and are reported to be good for treating seafood poisoning. In Thailand, a decoction of the leaves or poultices of ground leaves are used in the treatment of skin diseases and itchy skin. The root can be boiled in oil and used externally as a liniment for rheumatic pain (Fern, 2021).

Other uses The fruit of Scrambling Clerodendrum are edible, although a bit spongy. They were eaten by some Aboriginal groups across the top end of Australia (Cribb & Cribb, 1981).

Screwpine

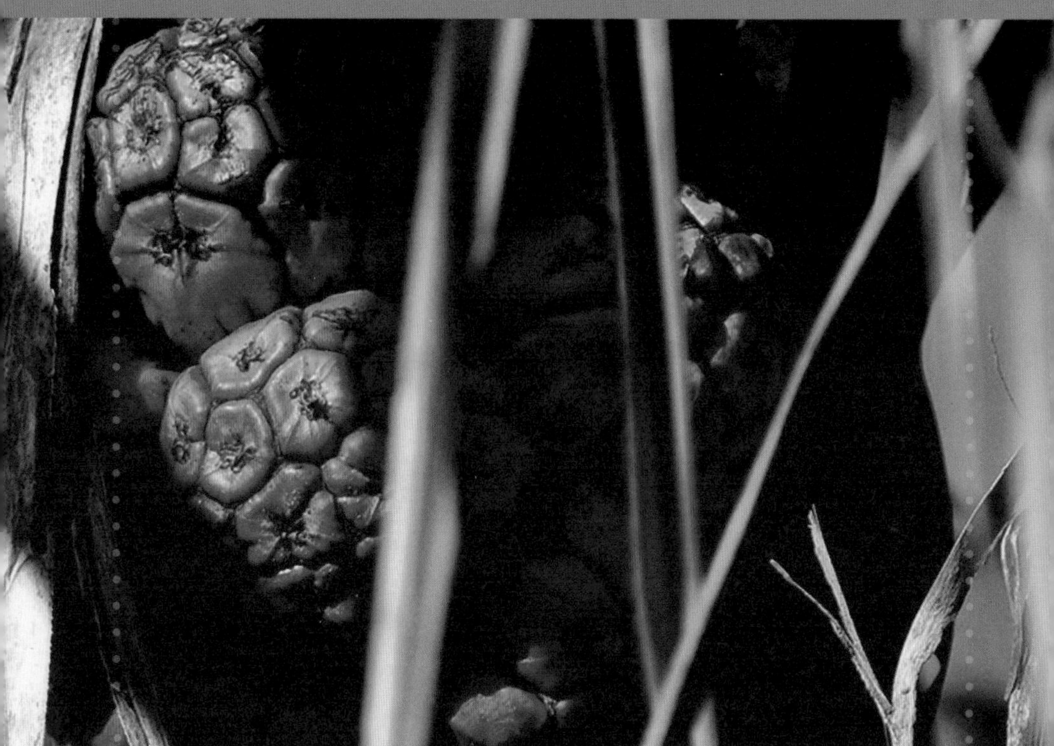

Scientific Name *Pandanus spiralis* R.Br.

Common Names Screwpine, Screw Palm, Spring Pandanus, Pandanus.

Aboriginal Names Jarrmirdany (Yawuru, Karajarri) (Lands, 1997), Wirnbeng (Miriwoong) (Leonard et al., 2013), Yarrari (Bunuba) (Oscar et al., 2019), Ganandurr, Yirawala (Wunambal, Gaambera) (Karadada et al., 2011), Iidool, Idul (Bardi), Manbang, Munbung (Nyul Nyul) (Smith & Kalotas, 1985), Wirniny (Gija) (Purdie et al., 2018), Wagwire (Yawuru) (Kenneally et al., 2018), Jangarra, Wirnbu (Jaru) (Wightman, 2003), Tjilkarr-tjilkarrpa, Tjulkarr-tjulkarrpa (Kukatja) (Valiquette, 1993), Jangkularru wunu (Worrorra) (Clendon et al., 2000), Jangarna manya, Kanandurr manya (Kwini) (Cheinmora et al., 2017). The Bardi call the nuts 'gamba' (Kenneally et al., 1996).

Field Notes Screwpine is a tree-like monocot (palm) that can reach up to 10 m in height. Its long, prickly leaves spiral upwards from its

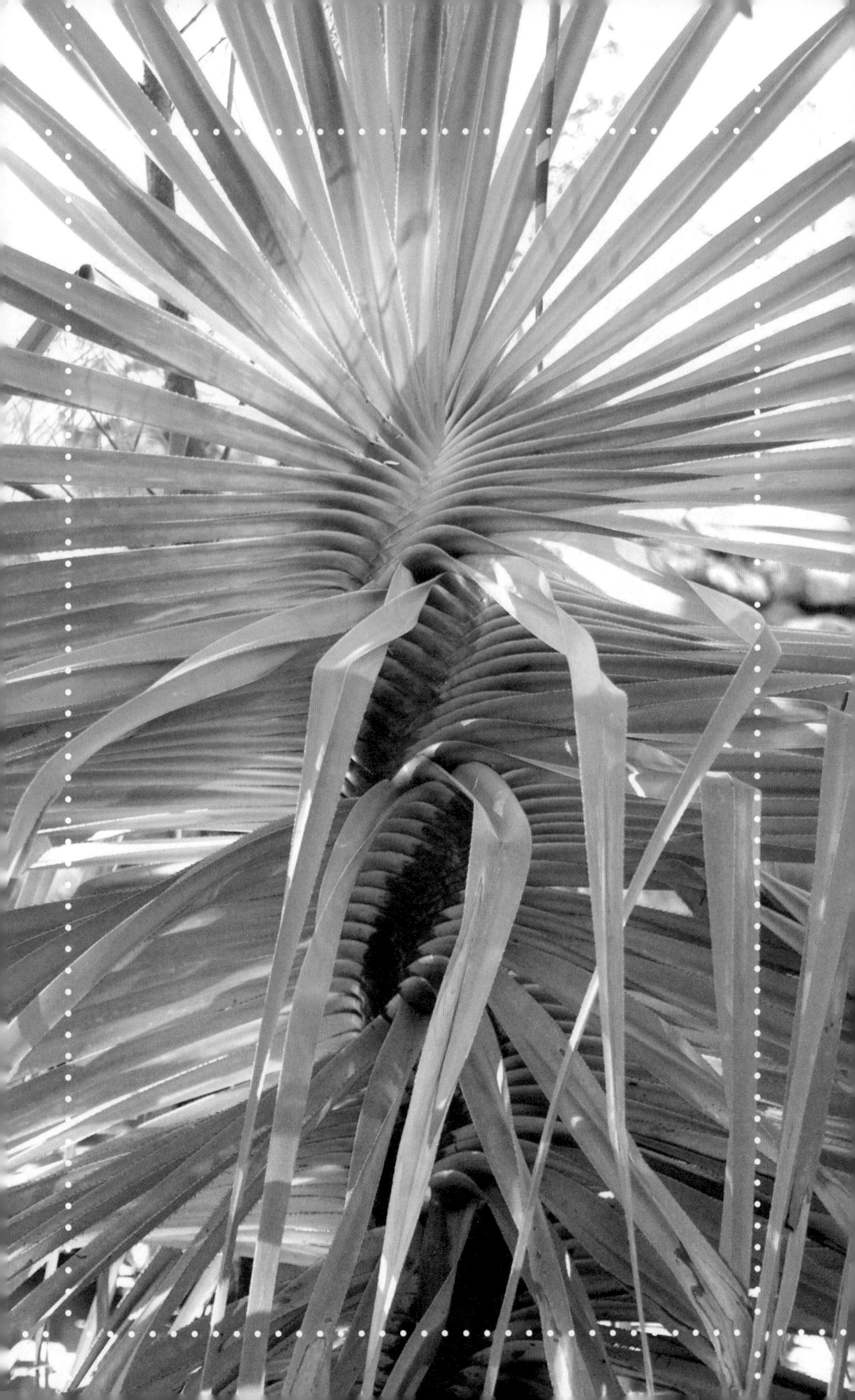

slender trunk. Its white flowers are small and form in dense clusters, with male and female flowers on different trees. Its fruit are orange to red syncarps made up of several individual drupes. The fruit are present from September to November. Screwpine occurs in sand, loam, clay and alluvium over sandstone, alongside creeks and rivers, in valleys, on swampy grasslands, on beaches and coastal dunes in the Kimberley region of Western Australia, the Northern Territory and northern Queensland (ALA, 2022; Lassak & McCarthy, 2001; WAH, 2022).

Medicinal Uses The inner core of young Screwpine was eaten for stomach cramps and to relieve diarrhoea (Lassak & McCarthy, 2001; Low, 1990; Smith, 1991). Infusions of the exposed roots were applied externally to the head to relieve the symptoms of colds, influenza and headaches (Cheinmora et al., 2017; Low, 1990; Reid, 1986). Decoctions of the roots were used externally as a medicinal wash to treat scabies infestations. The upper, young sections of the stem were cleaned of leaf bases, crushed, heated on hot coals, then applied as a poultice to painful areas of the body for pain relief. The soft white basal sections of the leaves were chewed to treat mouth ulcers and sore throats (Smith, 1991).

Other Uses The nuts or kernels of the seeds of Screwpine are eaten raw or roasted after the skin has been removed (Cheinmora et al., 2017; Edwards, 2005; Karadada et al., 2011; Low, 1991; Maiden, 1889; Purdie et al., 2018; Reid, 1986; Smith, 1991; Wightman, 2003). According to Low (1991), the seeds 'taste deliciously nutty raw or roasted' and were an important Aboriginal food because of their fat and protein content. Fern (2020) believes that the pulp of the fruit is edible if it is cooked 'in order to destroy a deleterious substance' that causes stomatitis (sore lips and a blistered tongue). The fruit are available in June (Kenneally et al., 1996). The inner base of young leaves is also edible and was eaten raw (Cheinmora et al., 2017; Maiden, 1889; Smith, 1991). The leaves of Screwpine are used by some Aboriginal groups to make baskets, mats

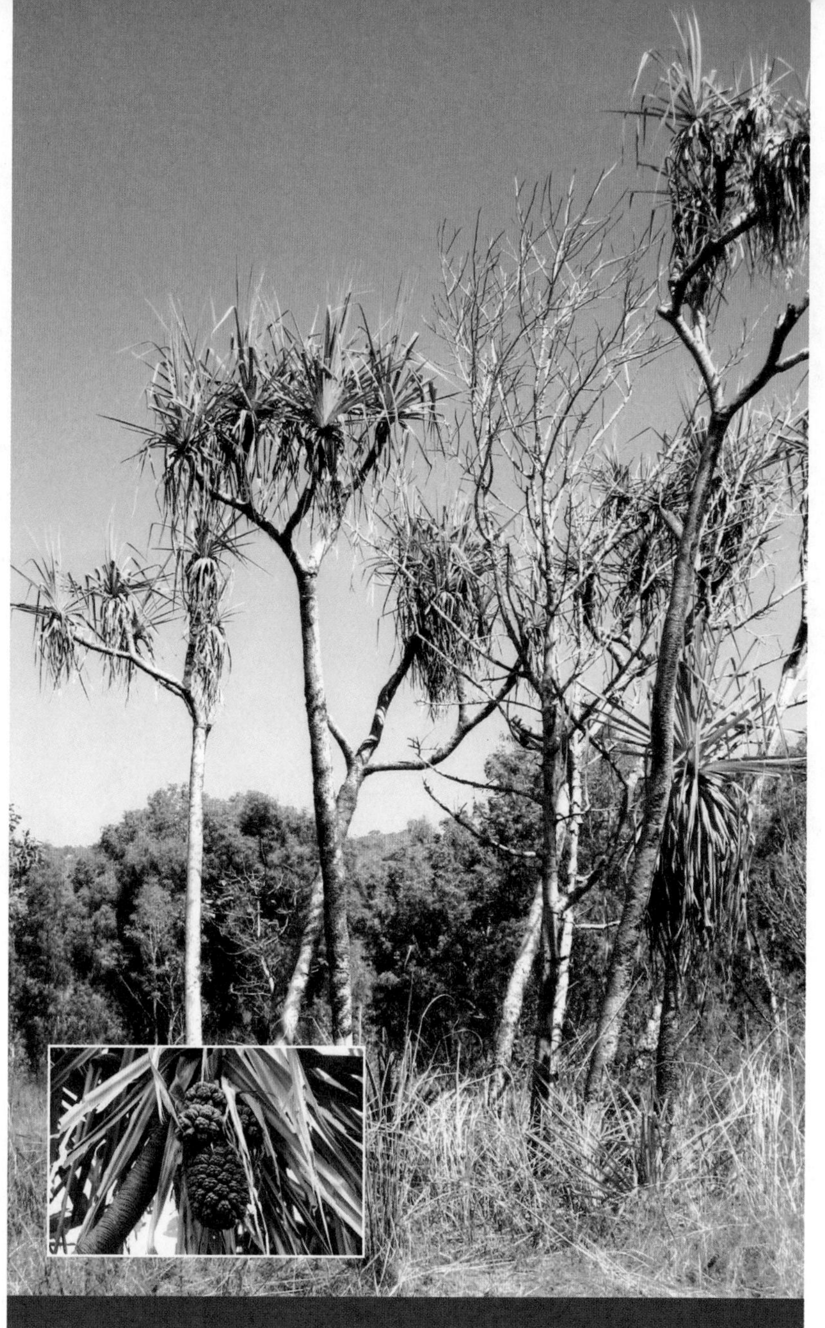

(Cheinmora et al., 2017; Purdie et al., 2018; Wightman, 2003) and footwear (Karadada et al., 2011; Kenneally et al., 2018).

Scurvy Grass

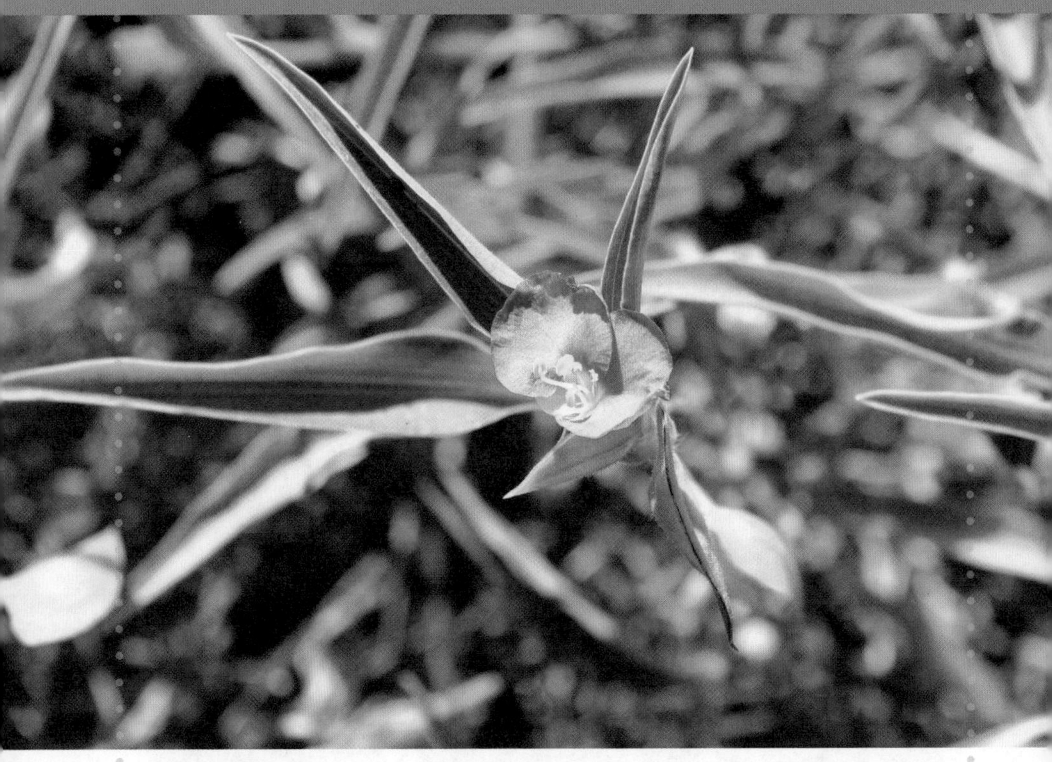

Scientific Name *Commelina ensifolia* R.Br.

Common Names Scurvy Grass, Wandering Jew, Scurvy Weed.

Aboriginal Name Buwerrku manya (Kwini) (Cheinmora et al., 2017).

Field Notes Scurvy Grass is a prostrate or semi-prostrate perennial or annual herb that grows up to 300 mm in height. Its leaves are lanceolate and up to 120 mm in length. Its blue flowers have two petals and are about 20 mm in diameter. They can be present at any time of the year. Scurvy Grass occurs in sandy clay, lateritic soils and clay over basalt and sandstone, on floodplains, seepage areas and rocky grounds in the Pilbara and Kimberley regions of Western Australia, the Northern Territory, Queensland and New South Wales. It is also endemic to India and Sri Lanka (ALA, 2022; ATRP, 2020; WAH, 2022).

Medicinal Uses The swollen lateral roots of Scurvy Grass are cooked for a short period then eaten as an analgesic (Cheinmora

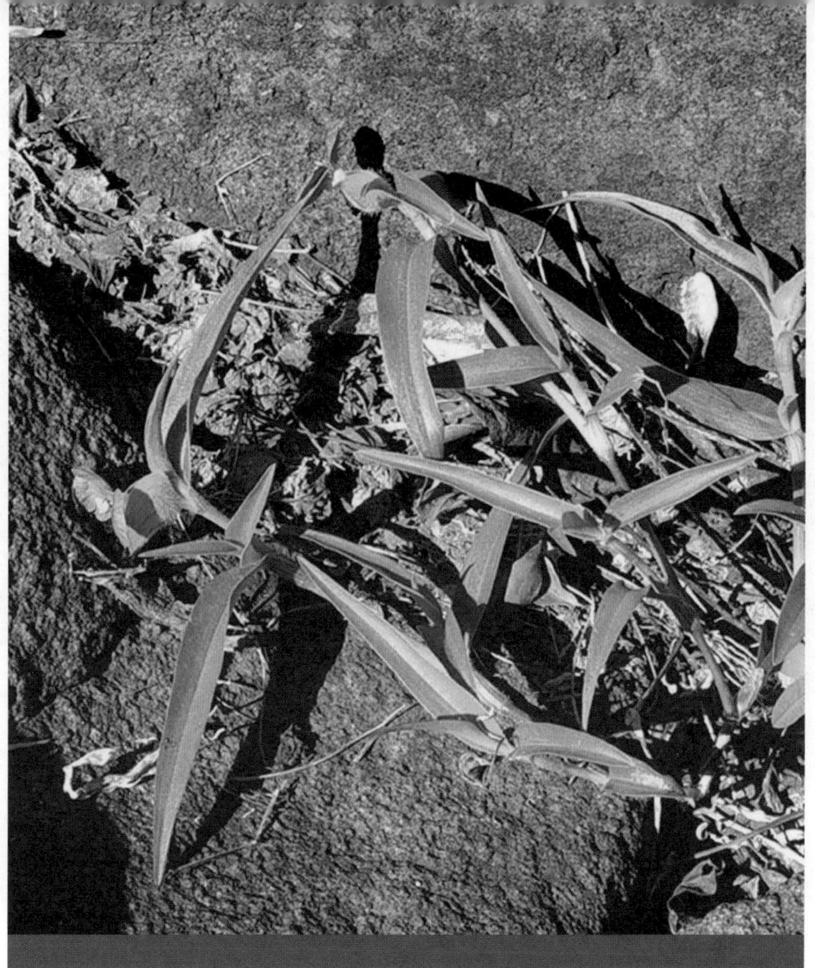

et al., 2017). It is also used in Ayurvedic medicine in India and Sri Lanka where decoctions of the whole plant are used as a diuretic and an anti-inflammatory. The juice of the root is taken internally for indigestion (Sindhuja et al., 2012).

Other Uses Some Aboriginal groups cooked and ate Scurvy Grass leaves as a vegetable, which probably prevented them from getting scurvy, as the leaves are high in ascorbic acid (vitamin C) (Low, 1990). The roots, which are harvested between May and November, are edible and are usually cooked in hot ashes or in ground ovens before eating (Cheinmora et al., 2017; Crawford, 1986; Fox & Garde, 2018; Vigilante et al., 2013).

Scurvy Weed

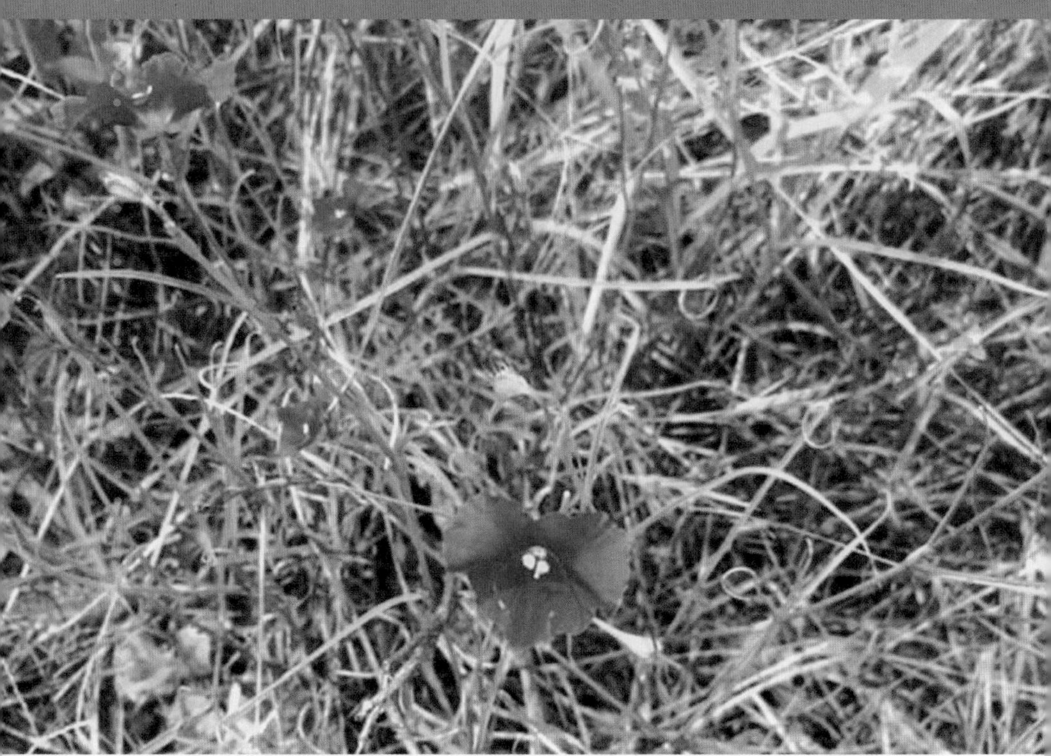

Scientific Name *Commelina ciliata* Stanley.

Common Names Scurvy Weed, Commelina.

Field Notes Scurvy Weed is a prostrate or semi-prostrate perennial or annual plant that grows to around 700 mm in height. It has thin leaves and round blue flowers that are present between March and August. Scurvy Weed occurs in clay and black soils, on floodplains and beside creeks in the Kimberley region of Western Australia, the Northern Territory and Queensland (ALA, 2022; WAH, 2022).

Medicinal Uses Scurvy Weed is reported to be a good source of ascorbic acid (vitamin C). The leaves of Scurvy Weed were eaten by some Aboriginal groups in the Kimberley to prevent scurvy (Woodall et al., 2010).

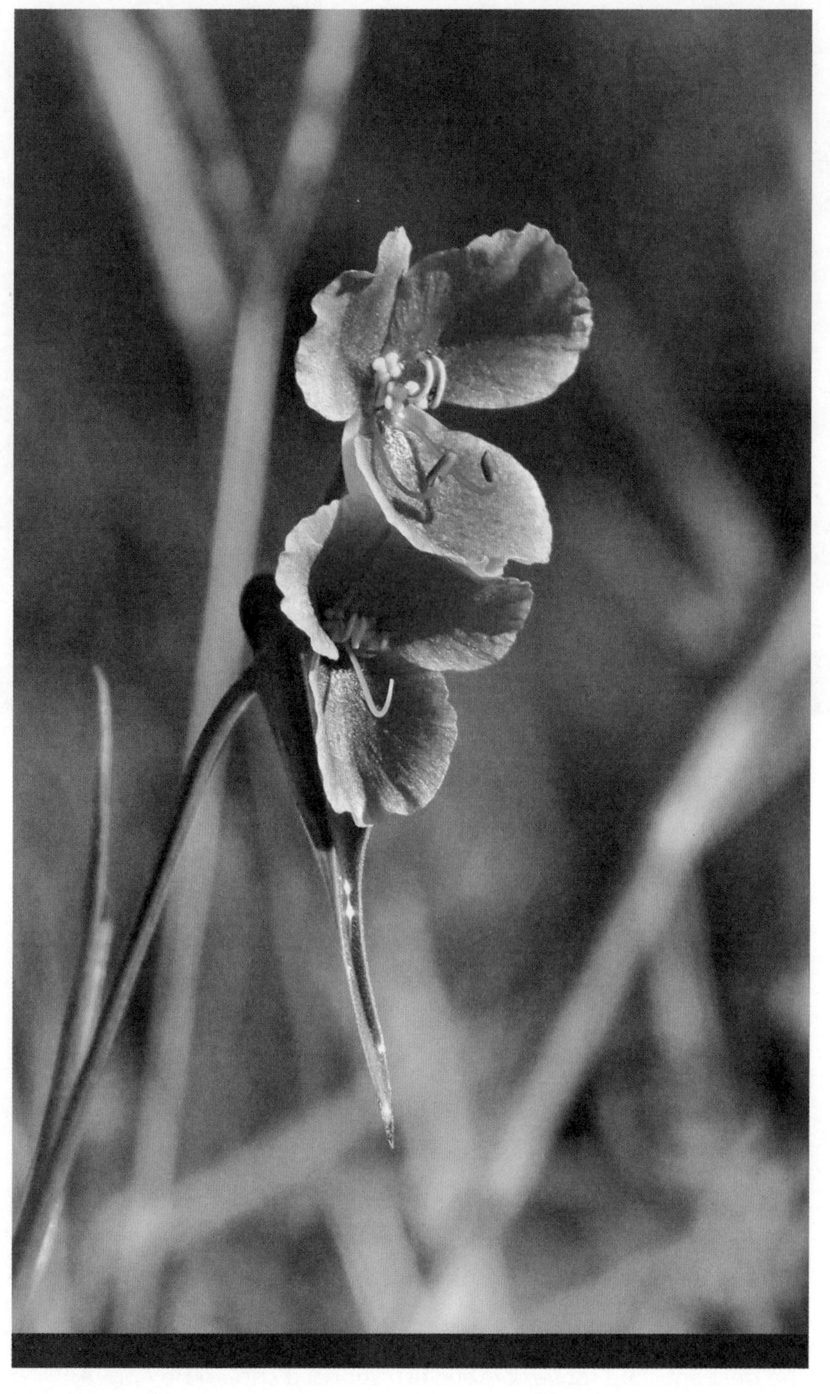

Sea Purslane

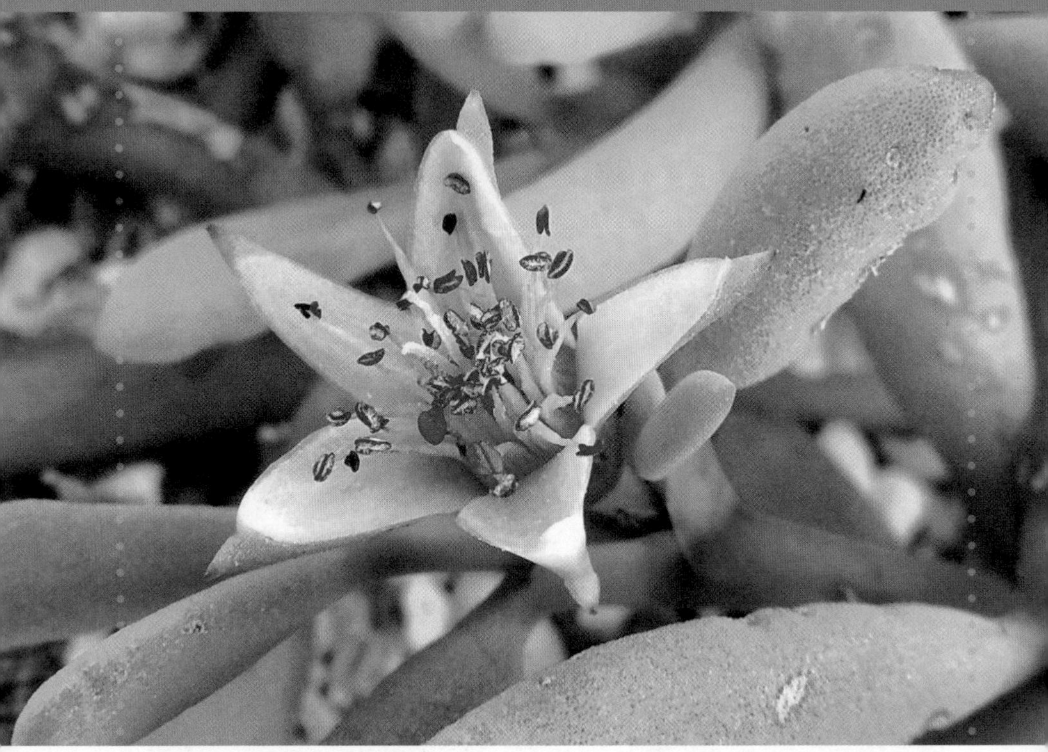

Scientific Name *Sesuvium portulacastrum* (L.) L.

Common Name Sea Purslane.

Aboriginal Name Kumardu (Kwini) (Cheinmora et al., 2017).

Field Notes Sea Purslane is a sub-erect to sprawling perennial plant. It has succulent, glossy green, linear or lanceolate leaves that are up to 70 mm long and 15 mm wide. Its pink-purple, star-shaped flowers are present between March and December. Sea Purslane occurs in sandy clay over coastal limestone and sandstone, on tidal flats and salt marshes around the northern coastline from the Pilbara and Kimberley regions in Western Australia to the northern beaches in New South Wales (ALA, 2022; WAH, 2022). It also occurs in other tropical and sub-tropical areas of the world (Fern, 2021).

Medicinal Uses Decoctions of Sea Purslane are reported to be the best antidote for venomous fish stings. It should be applied externally for an extended period (Fern, 2021). Sea Purslane leaves

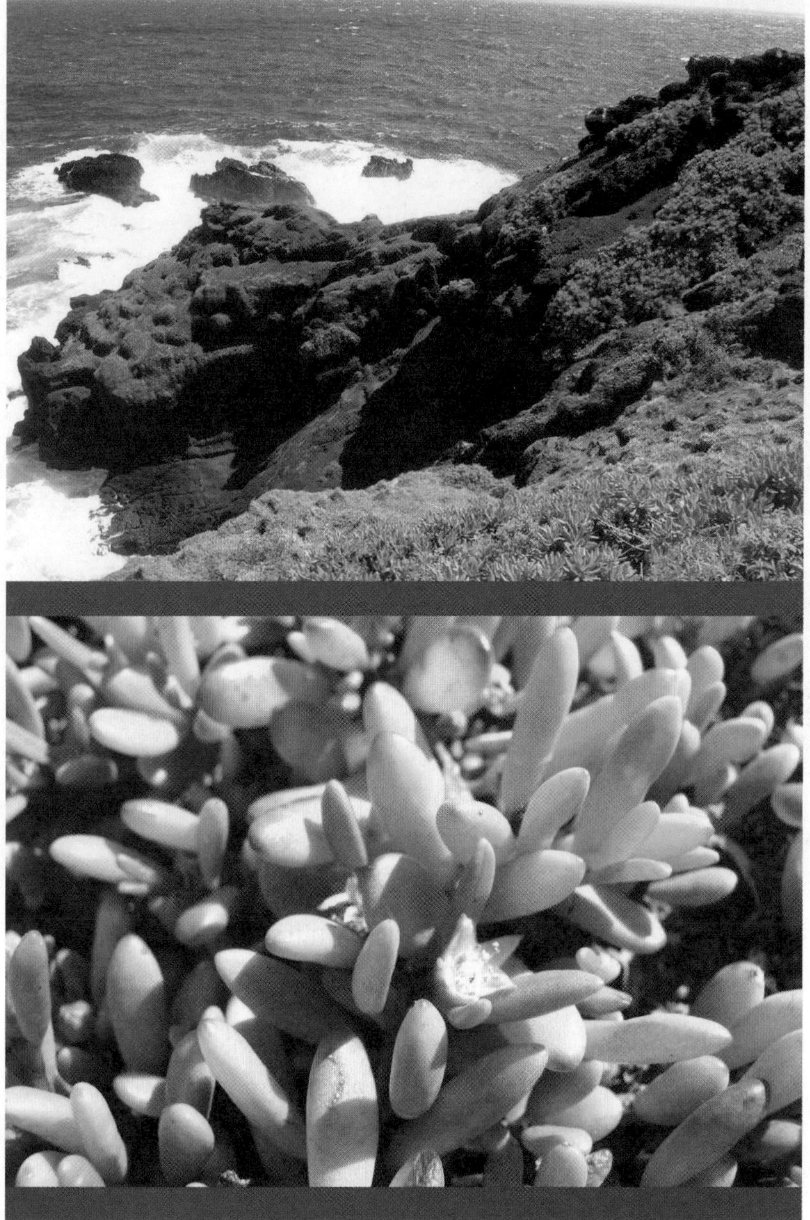

are reported to be a good source of ascorbic acid (vitamin C) (Tuckerbush, 2022). The plant has a long history of use in folk medicine to treat fever, scurvy and urinary tract infections (Kaur & Nitika, 2015). Studies of the leaf's essential oil has revealed antibacterial, antifungal and antiviral properties (Williams, 2020).

Other Uses Sea Purslane leaves can be eaten raw or cooked as a vegetable but have a slight salty flavour (Cheinmora et al., 2017; Fern, 2021; Kaur & Nitika, 2015; Low, 1991).

Signal Mistletoe

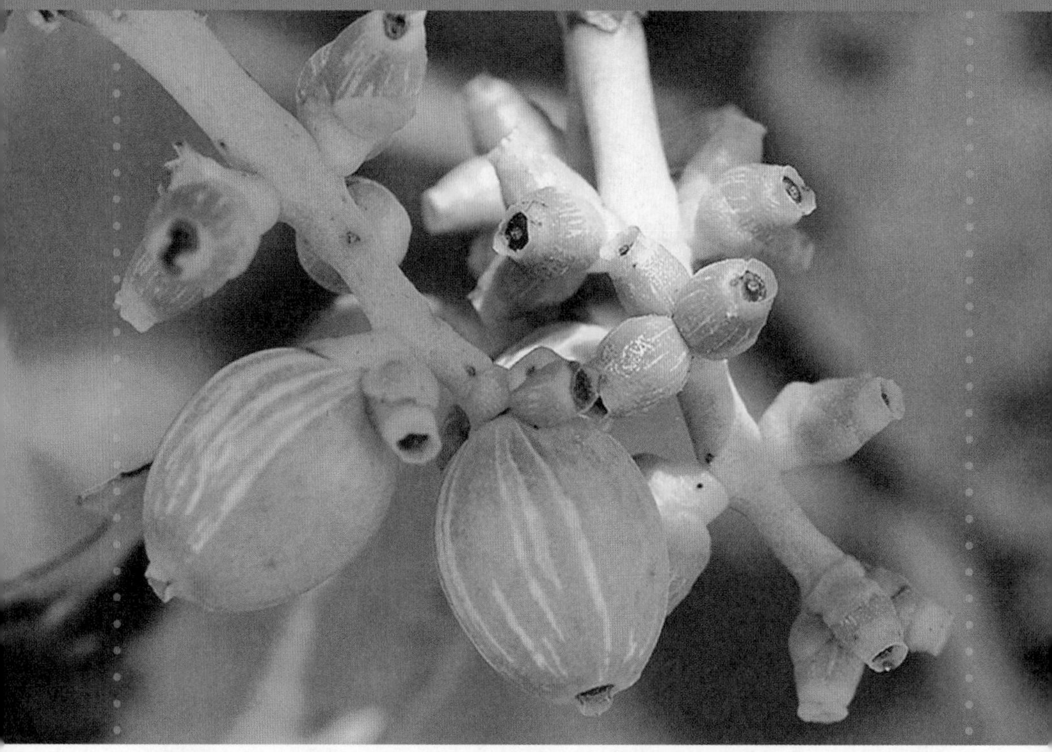

Scientific Name *Decaisnina signata* (Benth.) Tiegh.

Common Name Signal Mistletoe.

Field Notes Signal Mistletoe is an aerial shrub that is hemiparasitic on the branches of host trees. Its leaf blades are broadly lanceolate to orbicular, thick and leathery and up to 165 mm long. Its red, green and yellow tubular flowers are borne in triads and are present around August. Its fruit are ovoid drupes about 10 mm long. Signal Mistletoe occurs on Tropical Banksia (*Banksia dentata*), and on monsoon and other woodland forest species in the north of the Kimberley region of Western Australia, the Northern Territory and the Cape York Peninsula in Queensland (ALA, 2022; ATRP, 2020; WAH, 2022).

Medicinal Uses Decoctions of the leaves of Signal Mistletoe were taken internally, a small amount at a time, to relieve the symptoms

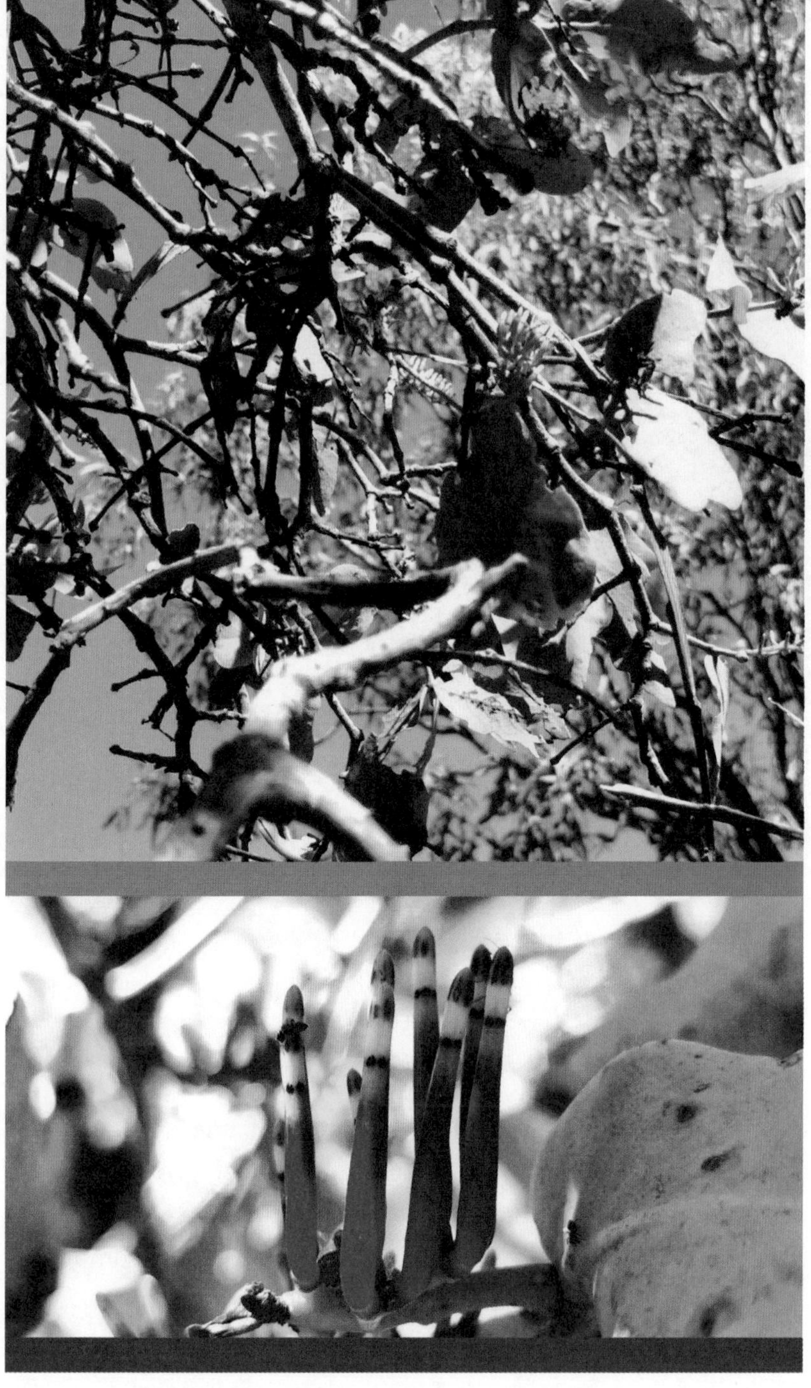

of colds and influenza, including coughs and chest congestion (Wiynjorrotj et al., 2005).

Other Uses The fruit of Signal Mistletoe are edible when ripe (Guse, 2005).

Silky Grevillea

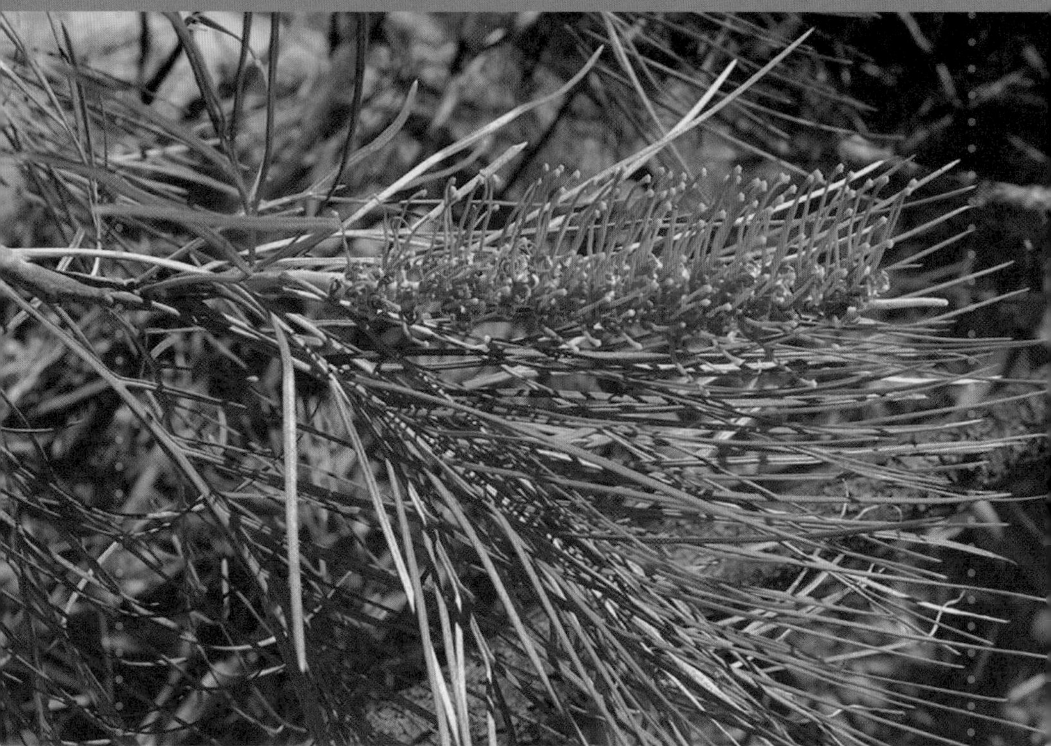

Scientific Name *Grevillea pteridifolia* Knight.

Common Names Silky Grevillea, Darwin Silky Oak, Ferny-leaved Silky Oak, Fern-leaved Grevillea, Golden Grevillea, Golden Tree, Golden Parrot Tree.

Aboriginal Names Gali-Galing (Miriwoong) (Mirima Dawang Woorlab-gerring 2017), Jarni (Jaru) (Deegan et al., 2010),Balmangan (Wunambal, Gaambera) (Karadada et al., 2011), Jawilyiny (Gija) (Purdie et al., 2018; Wightman, 2003), Marrimbulnu, Waawul, Worl (Kwini) (Cheinmora et al., 2017).

Field Notes Silky Grevillea grows as a tree or shrub to 10 m in height. It has pinnatisect (deeply lobed) leaves up to 210 mm long and 5 mm wide and bright orange flowers on racemes up to 200 mm long that appear between April and July, or in December. Silky Grevillea occurs in yellow sand over sandstone across the top end of Australia from the Kimberley region of Western Australia

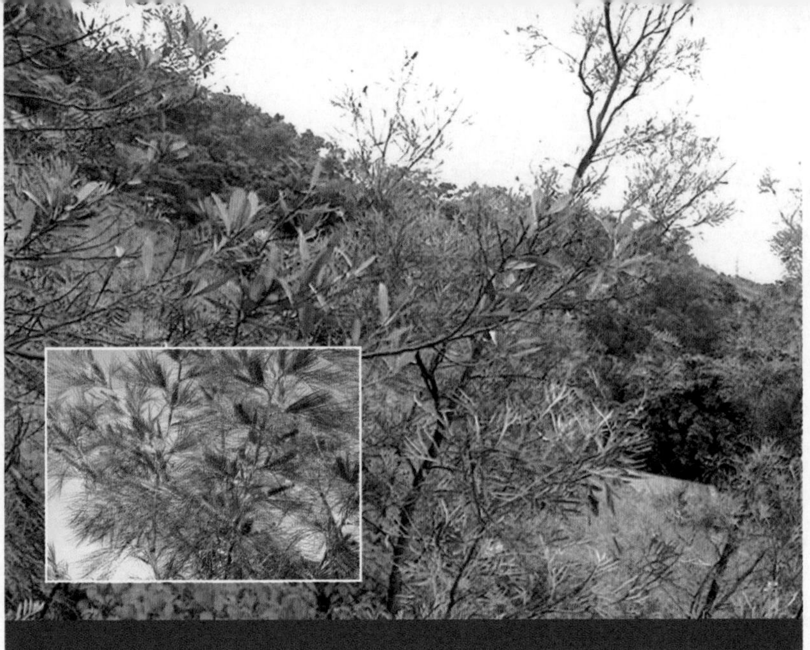

through to central Queensland (ALA, 2022; WAH, 2022).

Medicinal Uses Decoctions of mashed-up leaves of Silky Grevillea were used externally as a body wash to treat general malaise and were applied to the head to treat headaches. Crushed leaves were held under the nose and the vapours inhaled for the relief of the symptoms of colds and influenza. Nectar was sucked straight from the flowers to relieve sore throats (Edwards, 2005).

Other Uses The flowers of Silky Grevillea are full of nectar that Aboriginal people either sucked directly from the flowers or steeped in water to make a sweet drink (ANPSA, 2022; DBCA, 2019; Edwards, 2005; Fox & Garde, 2018; Hiddins, 2001; Karadada et al., 2011; Purdie et al., 2018; Vigilante et al., 2013; Wightman, 2003). The Kwini and others use the leaves to flavour emu, kangaroo and wallaby meat as it is cooked in ground ovens (Cheinmora et al., 2017; Edwards, 2005). The trunks of Silky Grevillea have often been used for spear shafts after they were straightened by fire (El Questro, n.d.). The timber was also used for making boomerangs. The burnt bark produces a fine black ash, which the Gija rubbed into their hair to make it grow and keep it black (Wightman, 2003).

Silkyheads

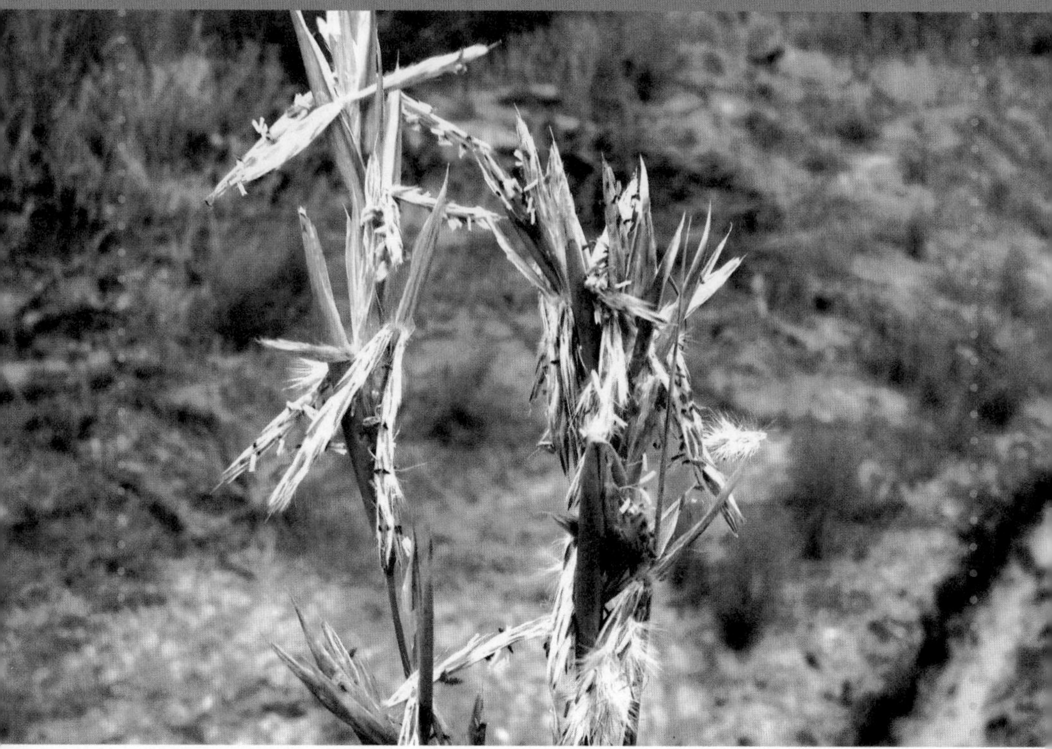

Scientific Name *Cymbopogon obtectus* S.T.Blake.

Common Name Silkyheads, Silky Heads.

Aboriginal Names Karltu-karltu (Kukatja) (Valiquette, 1993), Karrinyarra (Walpiri) (Northern Tanami IPA, 2015).

Field Notes Silkyheads are a fragrant, tufted, perennial grass with culms that grow to around 1 m in height. Its narrow leaves can be flat or folded, tapering to a long, fine point. Its green-purple flowers have long, fluffy hairs. They usually appear in the summer months. Silkyheads occur in a variety of soils, including sand, loam and granite, right across mainland Australia (ALA, 2022; eFlora.SA, 2022; WAH, 2022).

Medicinal Uses Decoctions of crushed leaves were drunk to relieve coughs and the other symptoms of colds and influenza. They were also used externally as liniment to ease sore muscles and headaches and as antiseptic wash on sores and wounds to

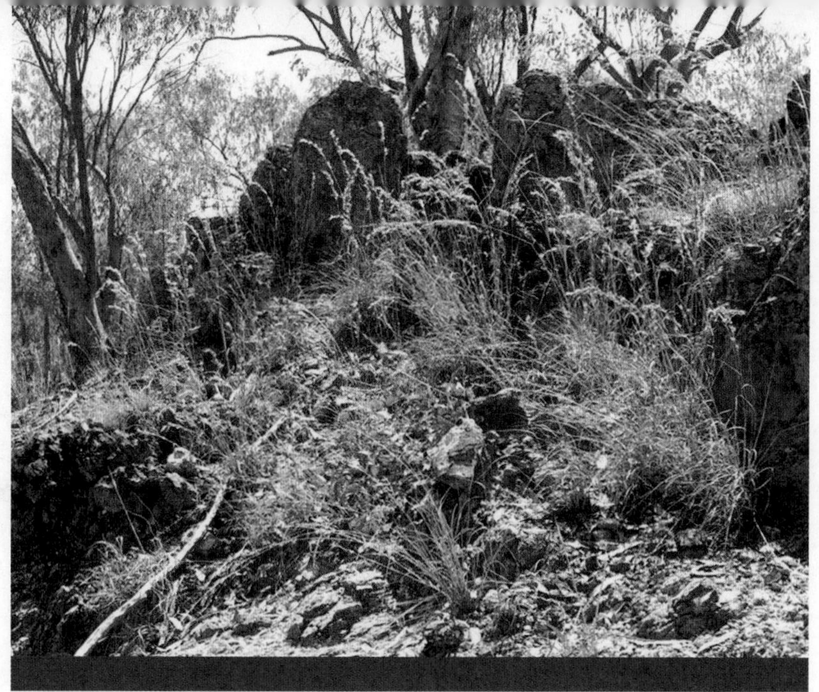

aid the healing process. Colds were treated with the crushed leaves held under the nose or placed in the nostrils. Decoctions of the roots were poured into the ear to relieve earache (Cock, 2011; Fern, 2021).

Silky Oilgrass

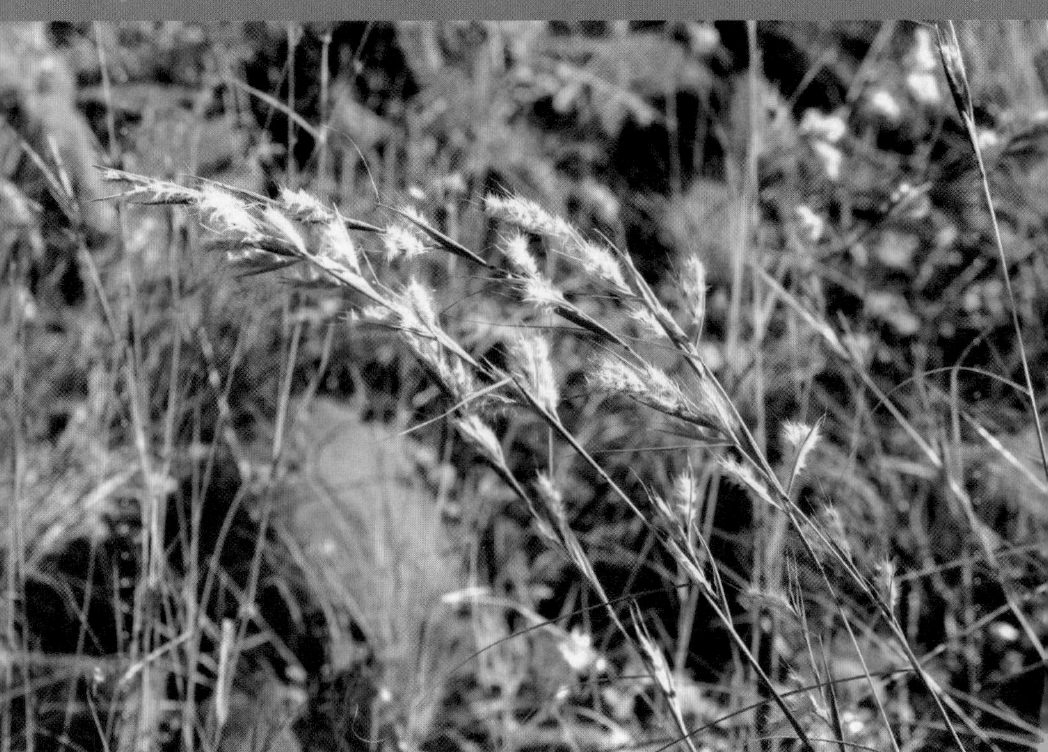

Scientific Name *Cymbopogon bombycinus* (R.Br.) Domin.

Common Names Silky Oilgrass, Little Lemon Grass, Citronella Grass.

Aboriginal Names Janjani (Bunuba) (Oscar et al., 2019), Malorr, Lerawardie (Nyikina) (Young et al., 2012), Ngarrngarrji, Malmalji (Gija) (Purdie et al., 2018), Giwiri, Guwuru (Jaru) (Wightman, 2003), Majal (Kwini) (Cheinmora et al., 2017).

Field Notes Silky Oilgrass is an aromatic, tufted, perennial grass or herb with culms that grow up to 1.2 m in height. Its basal leaf sheaths are rigid and flat and up to 400 mm long. The flowers look like masses of silk, hence the common name. The flower heads are present between April and August. Silky Oilgrass occurs in red-brown sand over laterite, granite and sandstone around swampy areas in the Pilbara and Kimberley regions of Western Australia, the Northern Territory and Queensland as far south as the border with

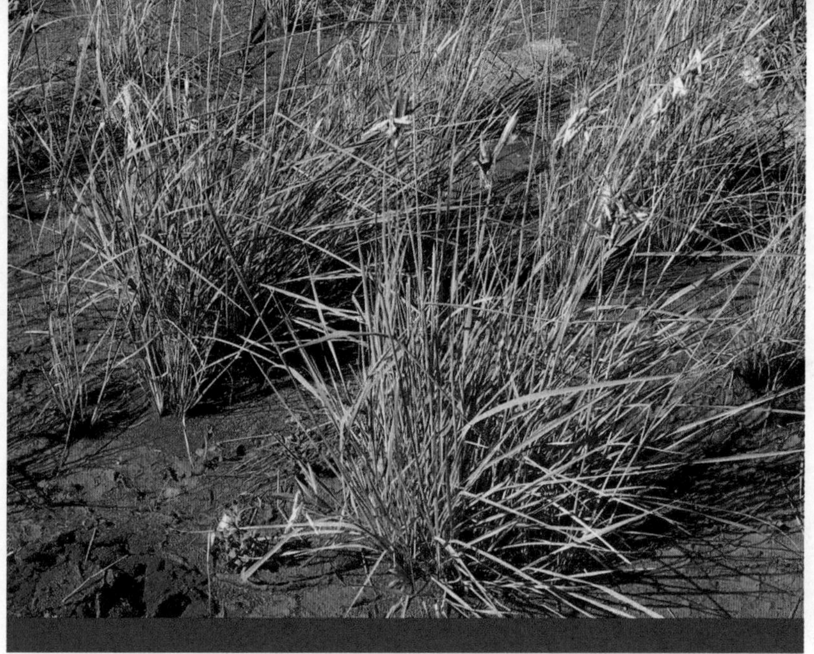

New South Wales (ALA, 2022; Lassak & McCarthy, 2001; WAH, 2022).

Medicinal Uses Some Aboriginal groups used infusions of the whole Silky Oilgrass plant to bathe sore eyes due to conjunctivitis (Lassak & McCarthy, 2001). The plant was also used by some groups as 'smoke medicine' (Young et al., 2012). Decoctions of the stems and leaves were used externally as a wash to relieve the symptoms of colds and influenza and to treat fever and headaches. A small amount of the decoction was also sipped for the same purpose. The vapours inhaled whilst boiling the stems and leaves for the decoction helped clear nasal congestion and chest congestion (Purdie et al., 2018; Smith, 1991; Wightman, 2003). Smith (1991) relates that in parts of the Northern Territory:

> *The leaves and young stems are collected fresh, soaked in water overnight, covered with crushed termitaria (outer casing of termite mounds) and placed in a pit over hot coals. A pregnant mother giving birth lies over the pit for pain relief. Some of the heated mixture can be applied directly over hurting parts for pain relief. The newborn baby can be placed over the pit with the mother to make it quiet and placid. This is an important ritual in the management of infants that is still commonly practised today.*

Silver Cadjeput

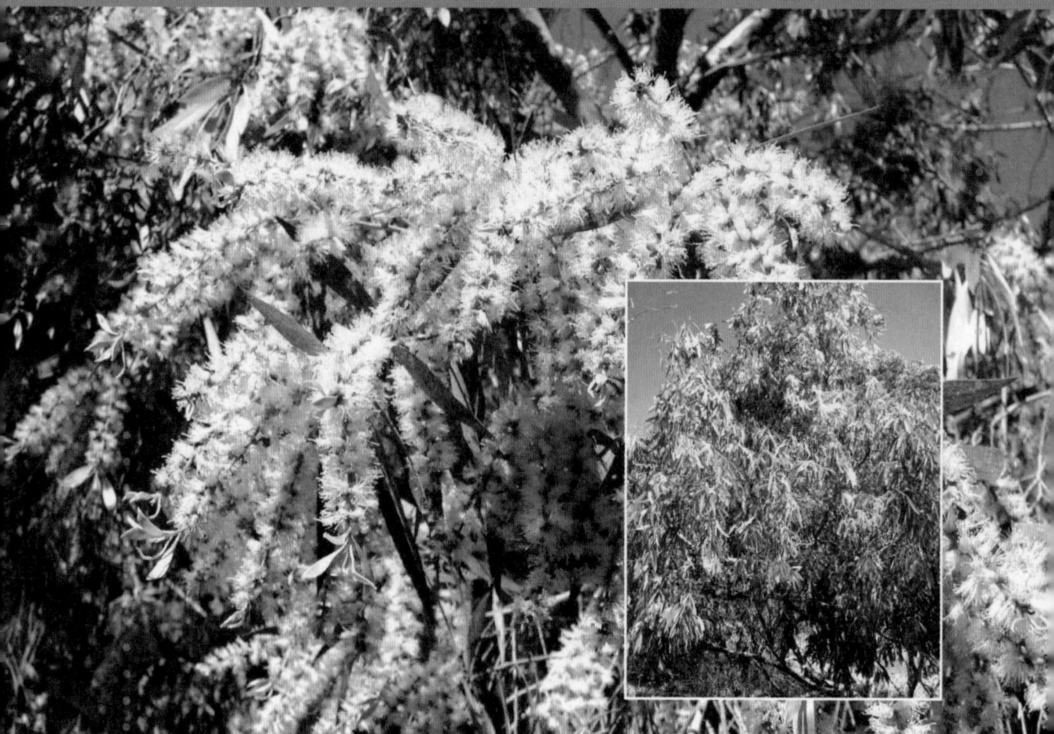

Scientific Name *Melaleuca argentea* W.Fitzg.

Common Names Silver Cadjeput, Silver-leafed Paperbark, Grey Paperbark.

Aboriginal Names Bandiran (Bunuba) (Oscar et al., 2019), Woolegalegang (Miriwoong) (Leonard et al., 2013), Danggai (Wunambal, Gaambera) (Karadada et al., 2011), Kurrumpa, Mawulpirri (Walmajarri) (Richards & Hudson, 2012), Jalkupurta (Nyangumarta), Dimalum (Miwa) (Kimberley Specialists, 2020), Ngarli winya, Bandûran winya (Kwini) (Cheinmora et al., 2017; Crawford, 1982).

Field Notes Silver Cadjeput grows as a shrub or tree up to 18 m in height (it has been known to reach 20 m, but this is rare). Its silvery-green leaves are alternate, elliptic, straight or sickle-shaped and up to 130 mm long and 24 mm wide. Its yellow-cream to white, bottlebrush-type flowers are arranged on the ends of branches.

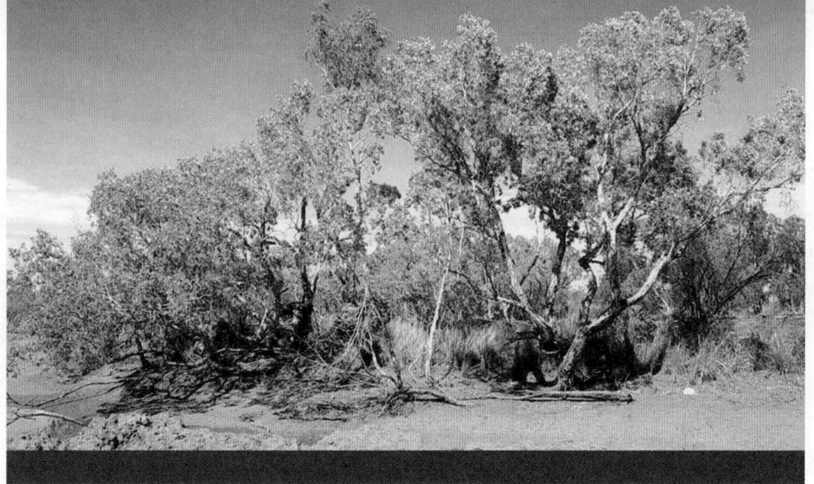

Flowering is between July and November. Its fruit are woody, cup-shaped to cylindrical capsules up to 4 mm in diameter. Silver Cadjeput occurs in alluvium, sand or clay along watercourses and in swamps in the Pilbara and Kimberley regions of Western Australia as well as the Northern Territory, northern Queensland and down along the east coast as far south as Mackay (ALA, 2022; ATRP, 2020; WAH, 2022).

Medicinal Uses Decoctions of fresh leaves of Silver Cadjeput were used externally as a body wash to relieve headaches, the symptoms of colds and influenza, and general malaise (Smith, 1991). The decoctions were also used as an antiseptic wash to treat sores, scabies infestations, itchy skin and skin rashes. Warmed leaves were held under the nose or rubbed on the chest to relieve coughs or other symptoms of colds and influenza. They can also be rubbed on the forehead for headaches or any aching part of the body for pain relief (Williams, 2011).

Other Uses The flowers of the Silver Cadjeput are full of nectar, which was either sucked directly from the flower or the flowers were soaked in water to make a sweet drink (Kimberley Specialists, 2020). The leaves were used by some Aboriginal groups to flavour meats for cooking (Williams, 2011). The bark was used to wrap foods for cooking and to transport food from one camp to another in paperbark coolamons (Cheinmora et al., 2017; Crawford, 1982; Karadada et al., 2011; Kimberley Specialists, 2020; Oscar et al., 2019).

Sleepy Morning

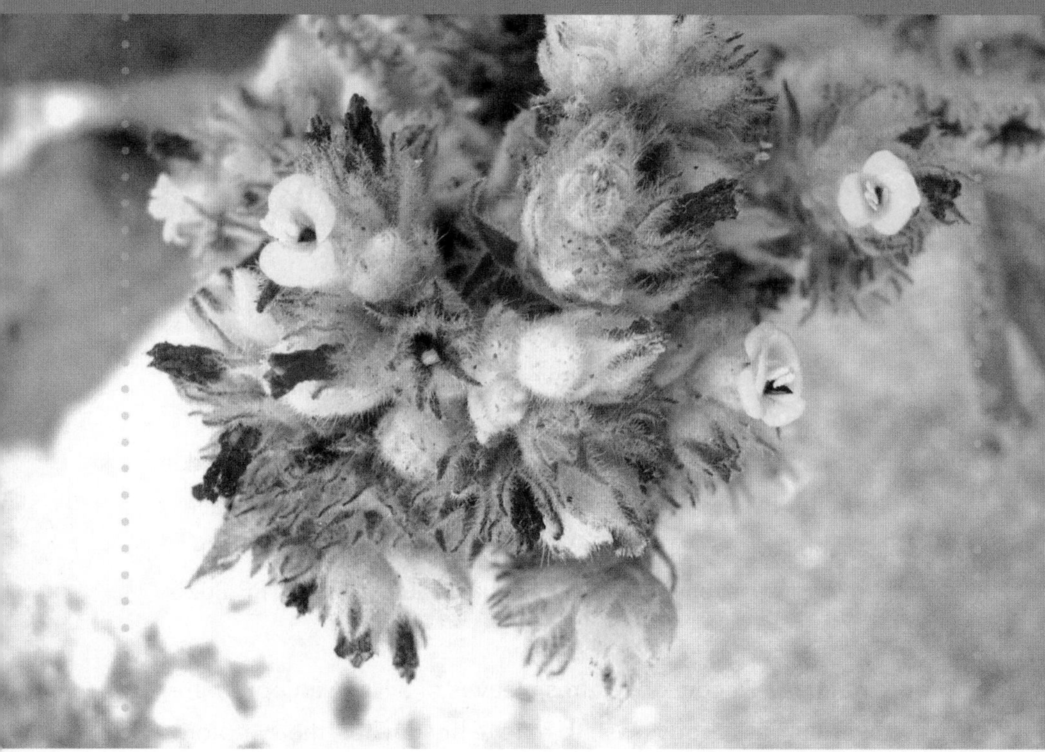

Scientific Name *Waltheria indica* L.

Common Name Sleepy Morning.

Aboriginal Name Ngurnu-ngurnu (Kukatja, Ngardi) (Cataldi, 2004; Valiquette, 1993).

Field Notes Sleepy Morning is an erect, perennial herb or shrub that grows to around 1.5 m in height. Its leaves are alternate, narrowly ovate or oblong, with irregularly serrate edges, and are up to 120 mm long by 70 mm wide. Its small, tube-shaped, yellow-to-orange flowers are present in clusters between March and December. Its fruit are tiny capsules containing one seed. In Australia, Sleepy Morning occurs in a variety of soils, often near watercourses, in the Pilbara and Kimberley regions of Western Australia, the Northern Territory and most of Queensland. Sleepy Morning is widely spread throughout the tropical and sub-tropical areas of the world (ALA, 2022; ATRP, 2020; SMIP, 2022; WAH, 2022).

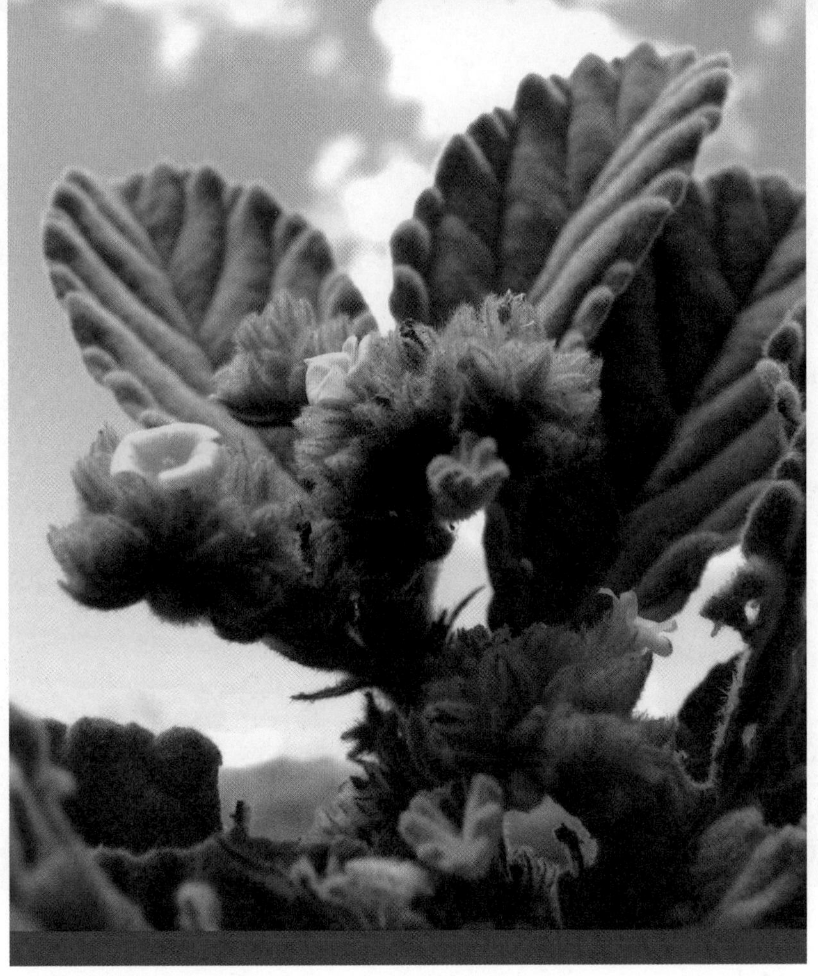

Medicinal Uses Sleepy Morning is used in folk medicine right throughout the tropics where it grows and is cultivated in some countries for its medicinal properties. Decoctions of the leaves and stems are taken internally to relieve fevers, coughs, colds, urinary tract infections, vaginal infections, hypertension, ulcers and haemoptysis (the coughing up of blood). In South-east Asia, decoctions of the root are given to children as an antidiarrhoeal and general tonic, and to adults as a cough suppressant. Decoctions of the roots are used externally as an antiseptic wash for healing sores and wounds. As the common name suggests, the plant is reported to have a slight sedative effect (Fern, 2021). In Hawaii, people chew the roots to ease sore throats (SMIP, 2022). In Australia, the Kukatja chewed the leaves and spat the mash out onto burns, wounds and sores to aid the healing process (Valiquette, 1993).

Smartweed

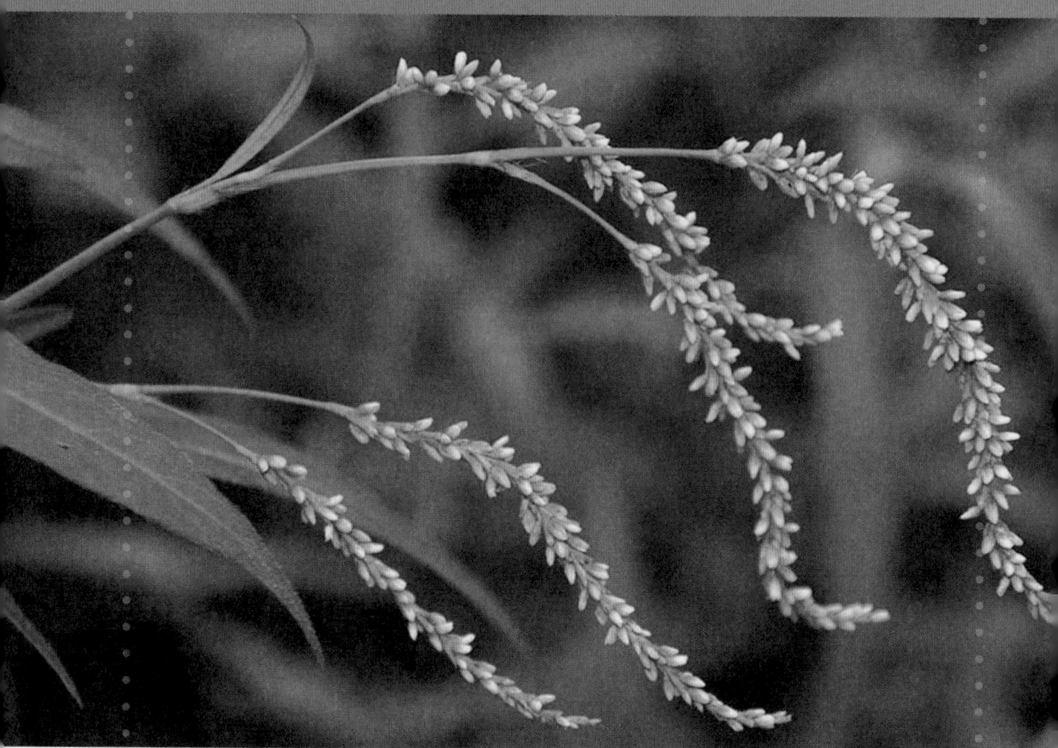

Scientific Name *Persicaria barbata* (L.) H.Hara., previously known as *Polygonum barbatum* L.

Common Names Smartweed, Joint Weed.

Field Notes Smartweed is a terrestrial or aquatic perennial herb that grows to 1 m in height. It has short leaves that are tapered at both ends, and white-cream or green-white-pink flowers that appear on many flowered, branched racemes between March and November. Smartweed is found in or beside creeks and swamps in the Kimberley region in Western Australia, the Northern Territory and down the east coast of Queensland as far as the border with New South Wales. It also occurs in southern China, India, Myanmar, Thailand, Malaysia, Indonesia, Vietnam, the Philippines and New Guinea (ALA, 2022; Fern, 2021; Lassak & McCarthy, 2001; WAH, 2022).

Medicinal Uses Infusions of the leaves were taken internally for colic. In India, decoctions of the leaves have been used as a diuretic

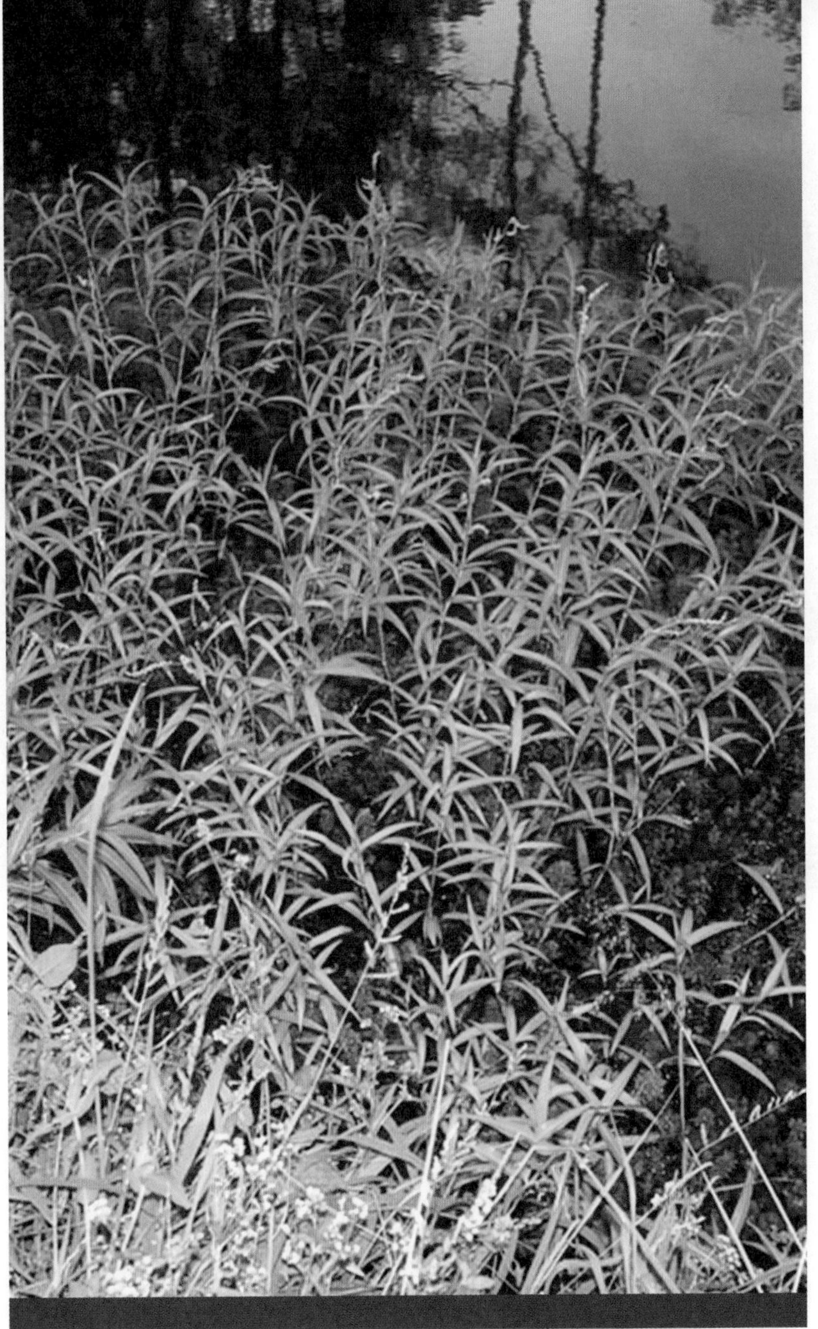

and an astringent (Lassak & McCarthy, 2001). A paste of the root was used externally to treat scabies infestations. Sap from the pounded leaves was applied externally to wounds and sores to aid healing (Fern, 2021).

Smelly Bush

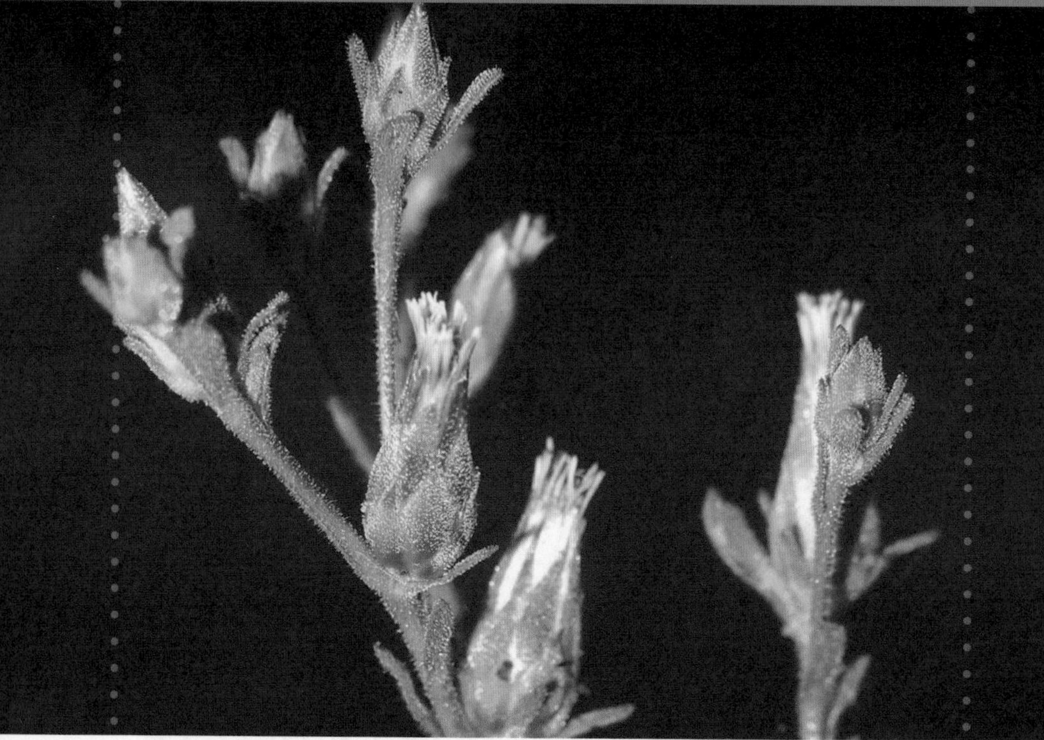

Scientific Name *Streptoglossa odora* (F.Muell.) Dunlop, previously known as *Pterigeron odorus* (F.Muell.) Benth.

Common Names Smelly Bush, Stinking Roger, Smelly Weed, Asters.

Aboriginal Names Manyanyiny (Gija) Purdie et al., 2018), Manyanyi (Jaru) (Wightman, 2003).

Field Notes Smelly Bush is a spreading, strongly aromatic, perennial herb that grows to just under 1 m in height. Its fragrant leaves are stalkless, obviate and tapered at both ends. Its pink or blue-purple globular flower heads appear between April and November. Smelly Bush is found in clay, gravelly or stony soils on claypans, near creeks and on floodplains all over the top half of Australia, including the Pilbara and Kimberley regions of Western Australia (ALA, 2022; Lassak & McCarthy, 2001; WAH, 2022).

Medicinal Uses Infusions or decoctions of crushed leaves of Smelly Bush were taken internally for symptomatic relief of colds, influenza

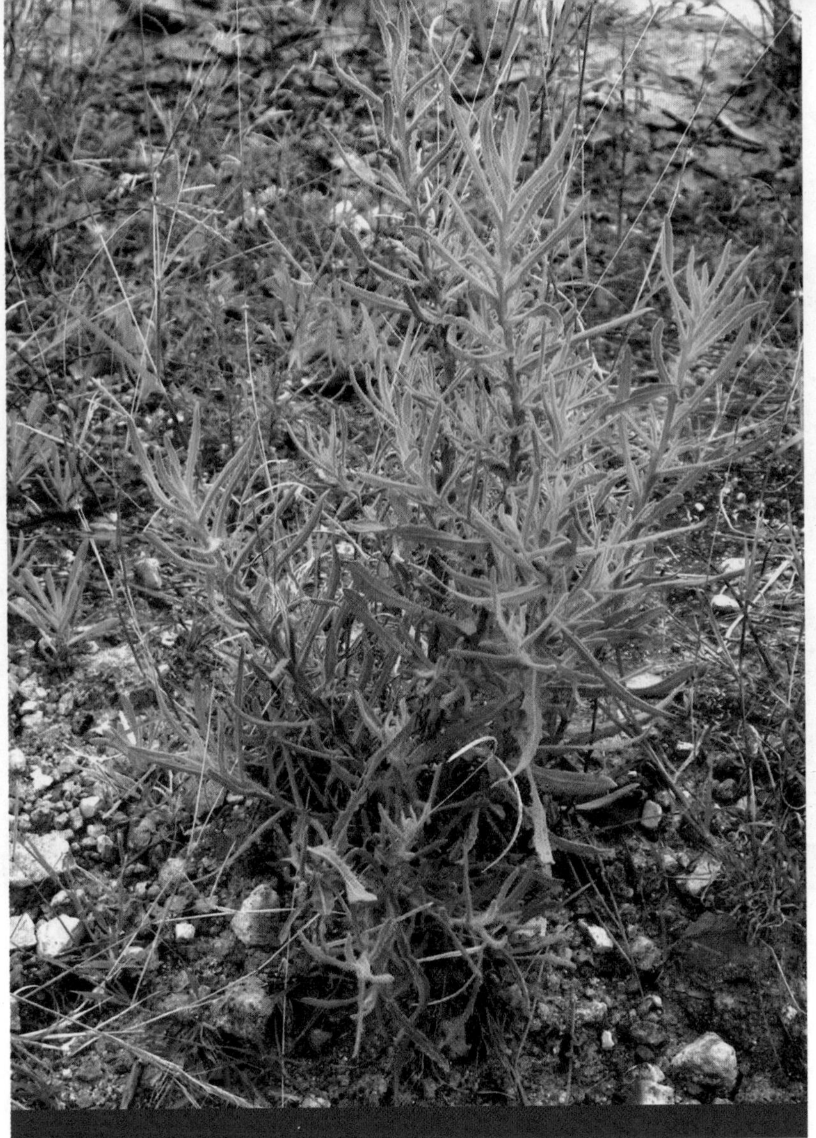

and headaches, and were also used to bathe the head for the same purpose. The decoctions were also used externally as an antiseptic wash for skin disorders, such as sores and scabies infestations (Lassak & McCarthy, 2001; Low, 1990; Reid, 1986; Smith, 1991; Wightman, 2003). Plugs of the crushed leaves were also inserted into the nose or crushed leaves were placed as poultices on the chest to ease the symptoms of colds and influenza (Williams, 2013; Wightman, 2003).

Snakevine

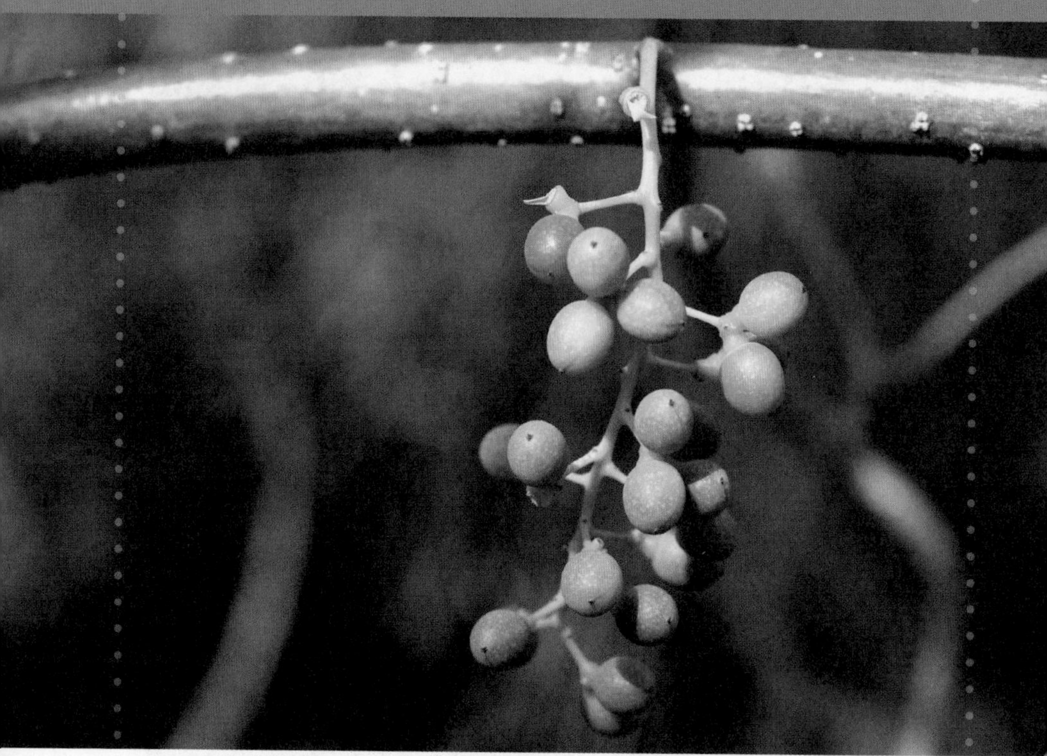

Scientific Name *Tinospora smilacina* Benth.

Common Names Snakevine, Snake Vine.

Aboriginal Names Urndanda (Yawuru), Wilgar (Nyikina) (Reid, 1986), Bandarrang, Bandarragu, Giny, Bandarang (Bardi) (Kane, 2022), Undala (Bardi) (Smith & Kalotas, 1985), Kululungkurr, Wararrkaji (Walmajarri) (Richards & Hudson, 2012), Wirlkaru (Nyangumarta), Waramboorrji (Gija) (Purdie et al., 2018), Waramburr, Manjanu (Jaru) (Wightman, 2003), Jalaroo (Gooniyandi) (Dilkes-Hall et al., 2019), Warakatji, Warampurrpa, Waratji (Kukatja) (Valiquette, 1993), Ngalyipi (Ngardi) (Cataldi, 2004), Wilkara (Nyikina) (Milgin et al., 2009), Waarnburr manya, Kiirun (Kwini) (Cheinmora et al., 2017).

Field Notes Snakevine is a slender, woody, deciduous, climbing plant that twists around trees. Its fleshy leaves vary from triangular to heart-shaped and are up to 120 mm long. Male and female flowers are borne on separate plants and are small, inconspicuous and appear in long, unbranched clusters from March to November. Snakevine occurs in sandy and clay soils, on sand dunes, riverine flats, hills and plateaus all over the tropical and sub-tropical northern parts of Australia, including the Pilbara and Kimberley regions of Western Australia. In New South Wales it is found along the coast as far south as Port Macquarie (ALA, 2022; Lassak & McCarthy, 2001; WAH, 2022).

Medicinal Uses Mashed stems of Snakevine were applied to the head for headaches and to the limbs for rheumatic pain. Decoctions of the stems were used to bathe painful joints and other parts. Boiled stems were used as a ligature around limbs for snakebite or for stonefish stings (Cheinmora et al., 2017; Isaacs, 1987; Lassak & McCarthy, 2001; Purdie et al., 2018; Reid, 1986; Smith, 1991; Webb, 1959; Wightman, 2003). Crushed roots were also applied to stings to relieve pain and itching (Low, 1990). Decoctions of the crushed roots were used as a medicinal wash to help draw out blind boils and carbuncles. Warmed leaves were placed directly over sores, cuts and boils (Smith, 1991; Webb, 1959). The sap was applied to painful sores. The leaves were chewed to relieve the symptoms of bad colds and influenza (Isaacs, 1987). Wightman (2003) relates what the Gija believe about Snakevine:

> *This plant also has magical powers; it can be used by a man to attract a woman and by a woman to attract a man. It can also be used to wrap around kids who are overweight to make them lose weight and become skinny.*

Wightman (2003) also relates that, 'Some Jaru people consider the red fruit to have special powers and that if you brush past them in the bush, they stop your heart from beating'.

Other Uses The arial roots are used by some Aboriginal groups to tie up bundles of wood or food (Wiynjorrotj et al., 2005).

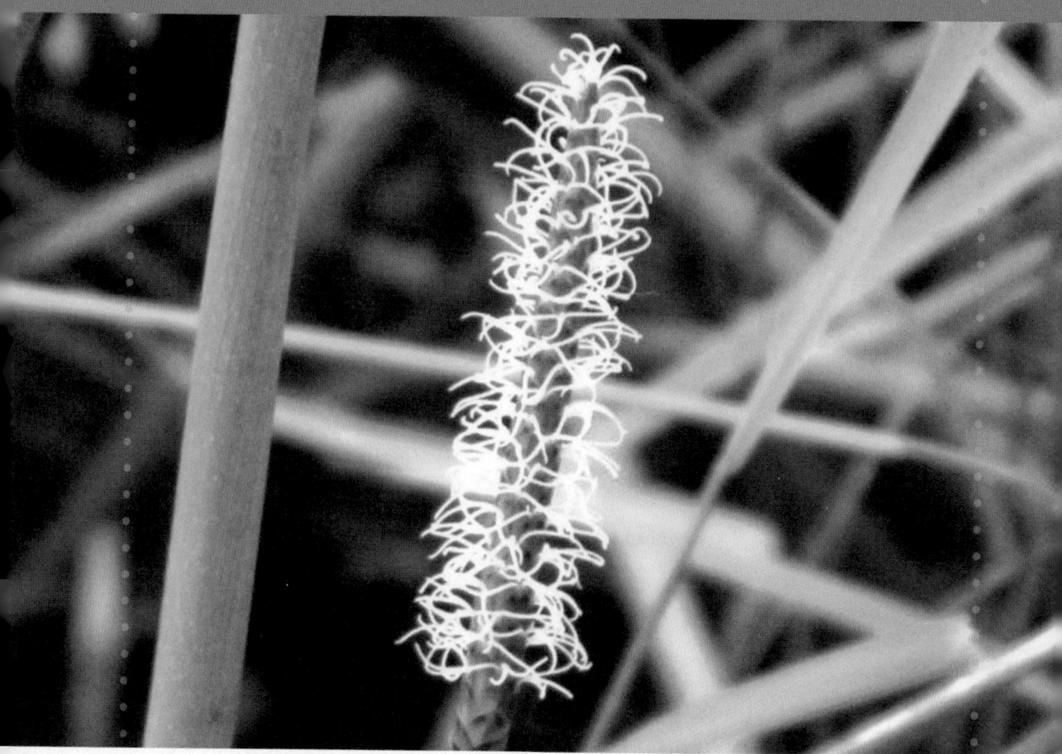

Scientific Name *Eleocharis dulcis* (Burm.f.) Henschel.

Common Names Spike Rush, Chinese Water Chestnut, Water Chestnut.

Aboriginal Name Bilgin (Bardi) (Smith & Kalotas, 1985), Arnuu (Wunambal, Gaambera) (Karadada et al., 2011), Arnu minya, Jabren minya (Kwini) (Cheinmora et al., 2017; Crawford, 1982).

Field Notes Spike Rush is a tuberous (or stoloniferous), partly submerged, tufted, perennial, grass-like sedge that can reach up to 1.5 m in height. Its reddish-brown leaves are reduced to some bladeless basal sheaths up to 200 mm long. Small white flowers appear on spikelets from May to August. The spikelets are cylindrical and broader than the stem. Spike Rush is found in pools, billabongs and lagoons in the Pilbara and Kimberley regions of Western Australia, across the top end to Queensland and as far south on the east coast as Port Macquarie in New South Wales. It also occurs

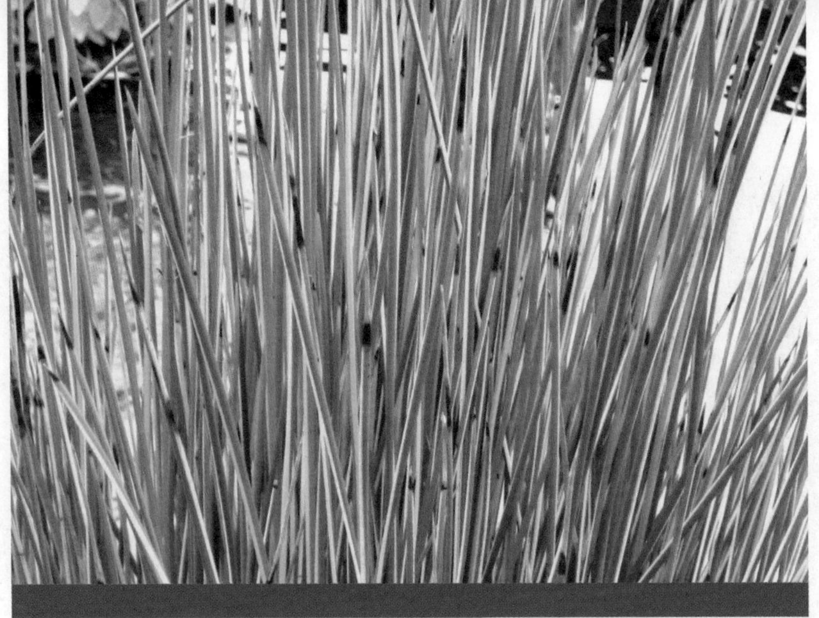

on the Indian subcontinent, in South-east Asia, New Guinea and Polynesia (ALA, 2022; Fern, 2021; Moore, 2008; WAH, 2022).

Medicinal Uses Infusions of the whole Spike Rush plant were poured onto wounds to aid healing. Only the plants that grew in or near salt water were used in Australia (Cock, 2011; Lassak & McCarthy, 2001). Sometimes the decaying plant would be bound to the wound for the same purpose (Low, 1990). In China, the plant is used to treat a number of ailments including abdominal pain, amenorrhoea, hernia and liver problems (Fern, 2021). Moore (2008) informs us that: 'The corms contain an antibiotic principle called "puchin", which acts like penicillin'.

Other Uses The sweet, round Spike Rush corms (small tubers) are edible and were highly valued as a nutritious food by Aboriginal groups. The young corms were eaten raw or roasted but the older ones were best roasted. They were sometimes made into Johnny cakes that, when baked, could be kept for up to two weeks without spoiling (Cheinmora et al., 2017; Fox & Garde, 2018; Isaacs, 1987; Glasby, 2018; Karadada et al., 2011; Low, 1991; Moore, 2008; Smith & Kalotas, 1985; Vigilante et al., 2013). The best time to harvest the corms is during the early dry season (Cheinmora et al., 2017). The corms are used in Chinese cuisine, hence the common name Chinese Water Chestnut (Moore, 2008).

Spinifex

Scientific Name *Triodia microstachya* R.Br.

Common Names Spinifex, Porcupine Grass.

Aboriginal Names Jardang, Gajarrang (Miriwoong) (Leonard et al., 2013).

Field Notes Spinifex is a resinous, tussock-forming, perennial, grass-like plant that grows to 2.5 m in height, with large panicles, racemose and crowded spikelets. Its green-purple to red flowers are present from January to May. Spinifex occurs in white to pink sand and sandstone on coastal beaches and dunes and rocky sandstone hills in the Kimberley region of Western Australia, the Northern Territory and Far North Queensland (ALA, 2022; WAH, 2022).

Medicinal uses Decoctions of the leaves are used as an external medicinal wash to treat the symptoms of colds, influenza and general soreness. Decoctions of the resin from the plant can be used in the same way (Wiynjorrotj et al., 2005).

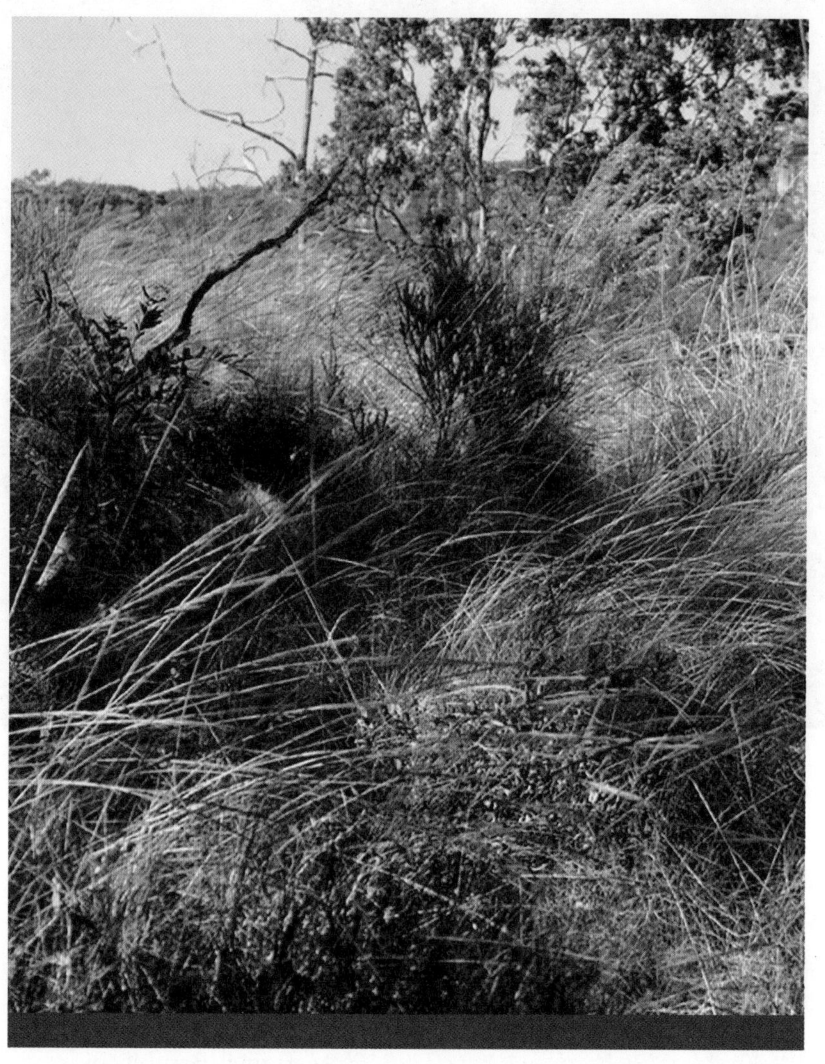

Split Jack

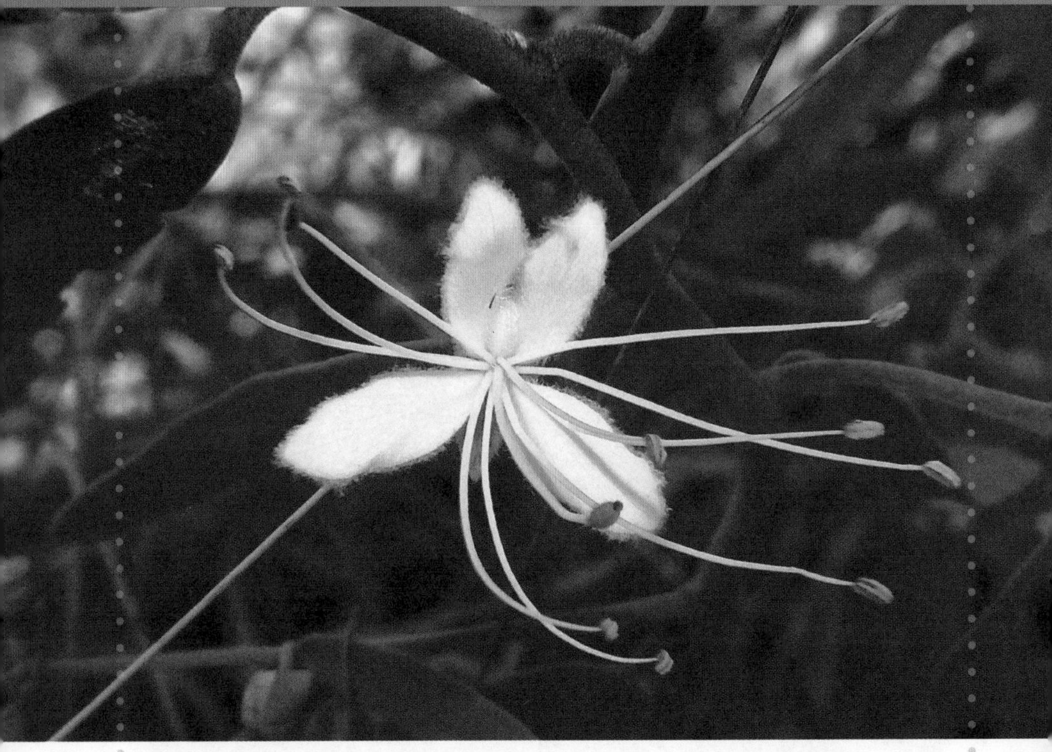

Scientific Name *Capparis lasiantha* DC.

Common Names Split Jack, Splitjack, Wyjeelah, Nepine, Nipang Creeper, Nipan, Native Orange, Bush Caper, Bush Pawpaw, Wild Passionfruit.

Aboriginal Names Ngoorla (Bardi) (Kenneally et al., 1996), Nguli (Bardi) (Smith & Kalotas, 1985), Palkarta, Pampilyi, Yupina (Walmajarri) (Richards & Hudson, 2012), Marranyil, Bambilyiny (Gija) (Purdie et al., 2018), Kakarranyurranpa, Ngirintilpa, Ngirintil-ngirintilpa, Pilkyikaarl-kaarlpa (Kukatja) (Valiquette, 1993), Bambily, Yiringgi, Yidiringgi (Jaru) (Wightman, 2003), Balkarda (Nyikina) (Smith & Smith, 2009).

Field Notes Split Jack is a spiny, twining shrub or climber that is found climbing up to 4 m high. It has long ovate leaves that are up to 50 mm in length. Its white flowers are around 25 mm in diameter with four petals and long, spreading stamens. Flowering is between

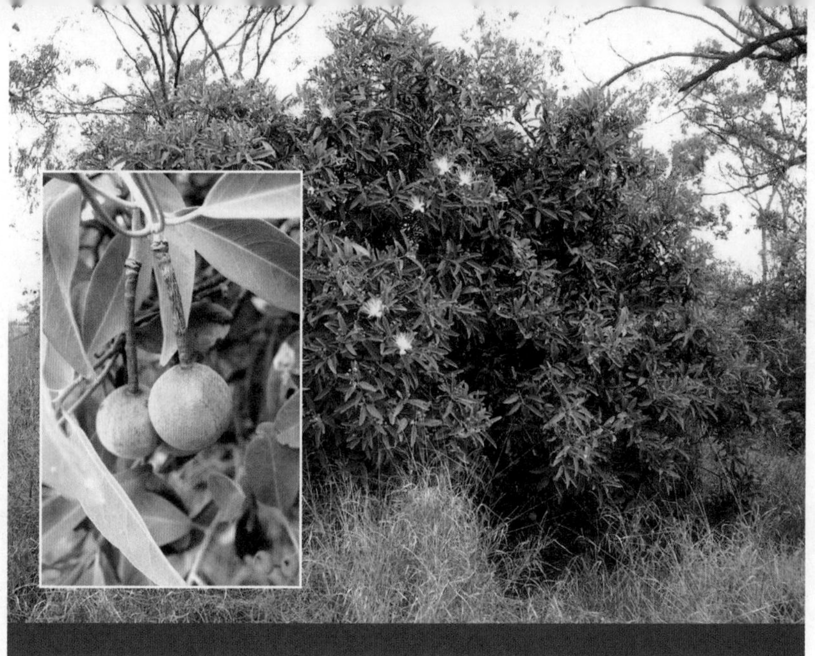

June and September. Its fruit are orange, ellipsoidal berries about 40 mm long and 18 mm in diameter, with a soft pulp and numerous seeds. Split Jack is found in sandy and clayey soils in the Gascoyne, Pilbara and Kimberley regions of Western Australia, the Northern Territory, Queensland and northern New South Wales (ALA, 2022; Lassak & McCarthy, 2001; WAH, 2022).

Medicinal Uses Infusions or decoctions of the whole plant were applied externally to treat swellings, snakebites, insect bites and stings (Cock, 2011; Lassak & McCarthy, 2001; Low, 1990; Reid, 1986; Webb, 1959). Leaves were warmed and applied as a poultice to areas of arthritic and rheumatic pain (Kenneally et al., 1996). Nectar from the flowers of Split Jack was ingested as a cough suppressant (ANPSA, 2022; Webb, 1959).

Other Uses The whole fruit of Split Jack is edible, including the seeds, when the fruit are yellow and have split open. They are reported to be sweet and tasty (ANPSA, 2022; Low, 1991; RFCA, 1993; Reid, 1986; Wheaton, 1994; Wightman, 2003).

Spotted-leaved Red Mangrove

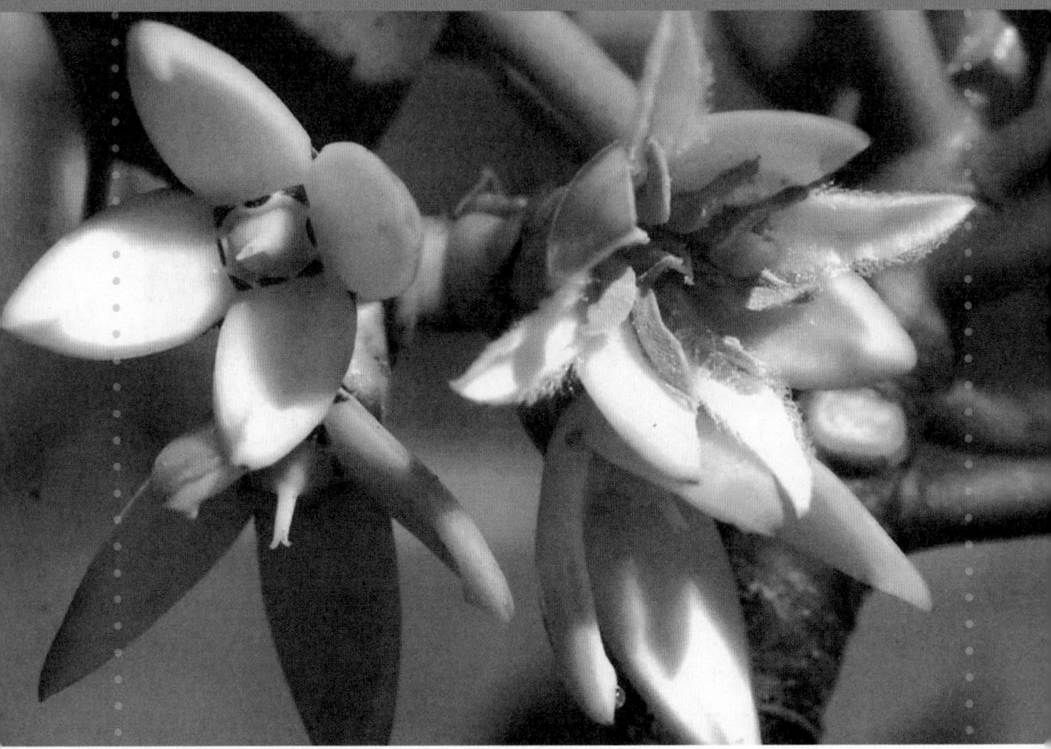

Scientific Name *Rhizophora stylosa* Griff.

Common Names Spotted-leaved Red Mangrove, Spotted Mangrove, Red Mangrove, Small Stilted Mangrove, Stilt-root Mangrove.

Aboriginal Names Jarrgarla (Wunambal, Gaambera) (Karadada et al., 2011), Bindun, Bindurnu (Bardi) (Smith & Kalotas, 1985), Biindoon (Bardi) (Kenneally et al., 1996).

Field Notes Spotted-leaved Red Mangrove is a shrub or tree, with stilt and aerial roots, that can grow to a height of 20 m. Its bark is dark brown to black. Its leaves are obovate, thick and leathery, have a small point projecting at the apex and are up to 110 mm long by 50 mm wide. Its small, white, feathery flowers appear between April and November. Its fruit are smooth, brown, pear-shaped and up to 30 mm in diameter. Spotted-leaved Red Mangrove occurs in mud, on tidal flats, backwaters and the landward edge of

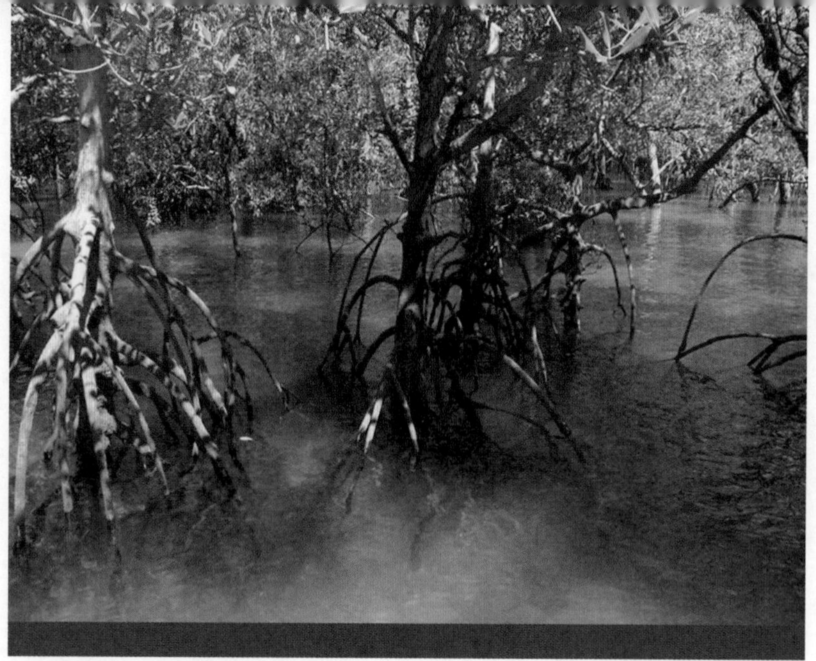

mangroves around the northern coast of Australia, from the Pilbara and Kimberley regions of Western Australia to northern New South Wales. It also occurs in Cambodia, Indonesia, Japan (Ryukyu Islands), Malaysia, the Philippines, New Guinea, Vietnam and some Pacific islands (ALA, 2022; WAH, 2022).

Medicinal Uses Decoctions of the leaves and stems of Spotted-leaved Red Mangrove were used externally as an antiseptic wash to treat chickenpox rash, skin sores and leg ulcers (Lee, 2003; Mangroves Australia, 2022).

Other Uses The fruit of Spotted-leaved Red Mangrove were eaten by some Aboriginal groups across the top end of Australia after some processing. They first cooked the fruit in a ground oven until they were soft. They were then strained with water several times in a dilly bag then squeezed against the knee to remove the excess water (Edwards, 2005). Edible mangrove worms are found in the wood of this tree (Karadada et al., 2011). The Bardi used the wood of Spotted-leaved Red Mangrove to make fishing boomerangs, spears, shields and ceremonial objects (Kenneally et al., 1996; Smith & Kalotas, 1985).

Spreading Sneezeweed

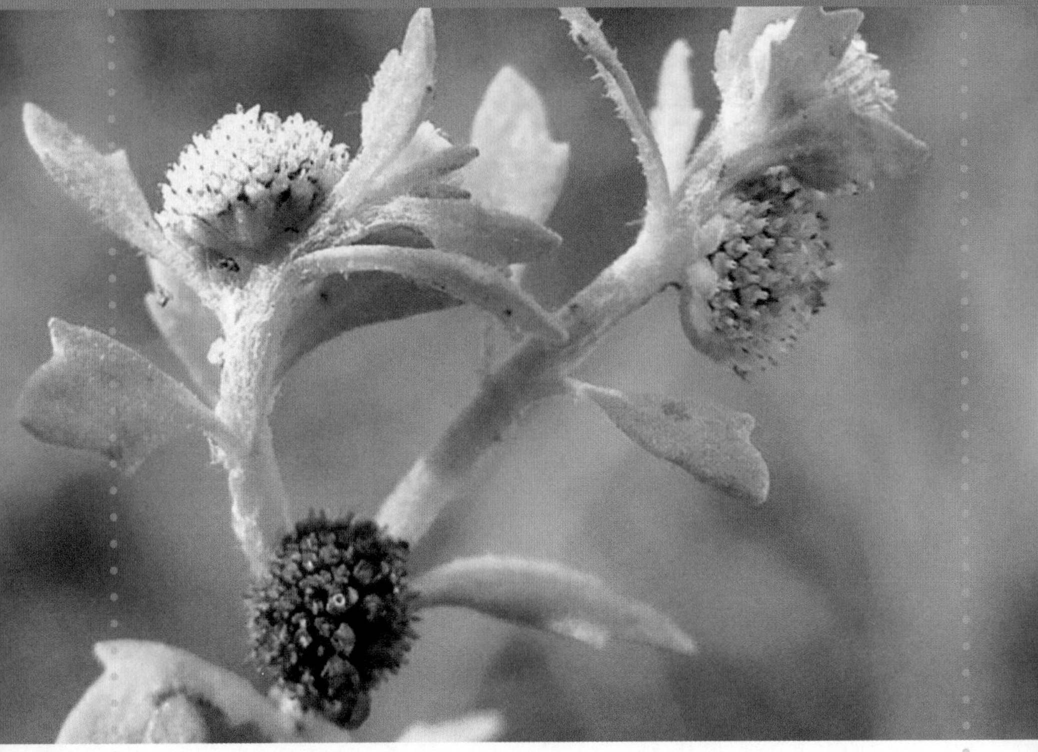

Scientific Name *Centipeda minima* (L.) A.Braun & Asch.

Common Names Spreading Sneezeweed, Desert Sneezeweed.

Aboriginal Names Parntirrminyirrkura, Tjurrtjurrpa (Kukatja) (Valiquette, 1993).

Field Notes Spreading Sneezeweed is a small, erect or spreading, aromatic, annual herb that is seldom found above 200 mm high. It spreads along the ground with stems up to 200 mm long. Its leaves are tapered at both ends, grow up to 27 mm long and have toothed margins. Its small, cream-yellow flowers appear in clusters between May and October. Spreading Sneezeweed is found in sand, red clay, loam, gritty alluvium and gravel around lakes, rivers and pools, on claypans, along drainage lines and in gullies in every state of Australia. In Western Australia it is only found in the Gascoyne, Pilbara and Kimberley regions. Other countries where it occurs include China, India, Indonesia, Japan, New Guinea, the

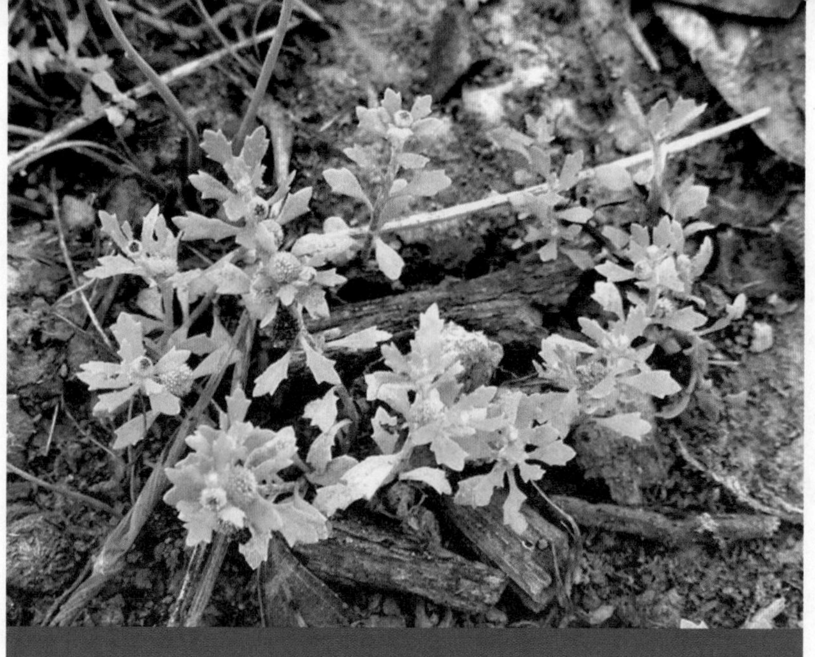

Philippines, Thailand and some Pacific islands (ALA, 2022; Fern, 2021; PFAF, 2022; WAH, 2022).

Medicinal Uses Weak decoctions of the Spreading Sneezeweed plant have been used to bathe purulent eyes due to conjunctivitis and sandy blight (trachoma). The crushed plant can be rubbed on the nose or held under the nose and the vapours inhaled to relieve the symptoms of colds and influenza. (Cock, 2011; Lassak & McCarthy, 2001; Low, 1990; Reid, 1986; Webb, 1959). A paste made from the boiled herb was applied to the cheek to ease toothache and was also used externally as a liniment for swellings and inflammation (Fern, 2021). Crushed leaves were also applied to wounds and sores to aid the healing process (Valiquette, 1993).

Stem-fruit Fig

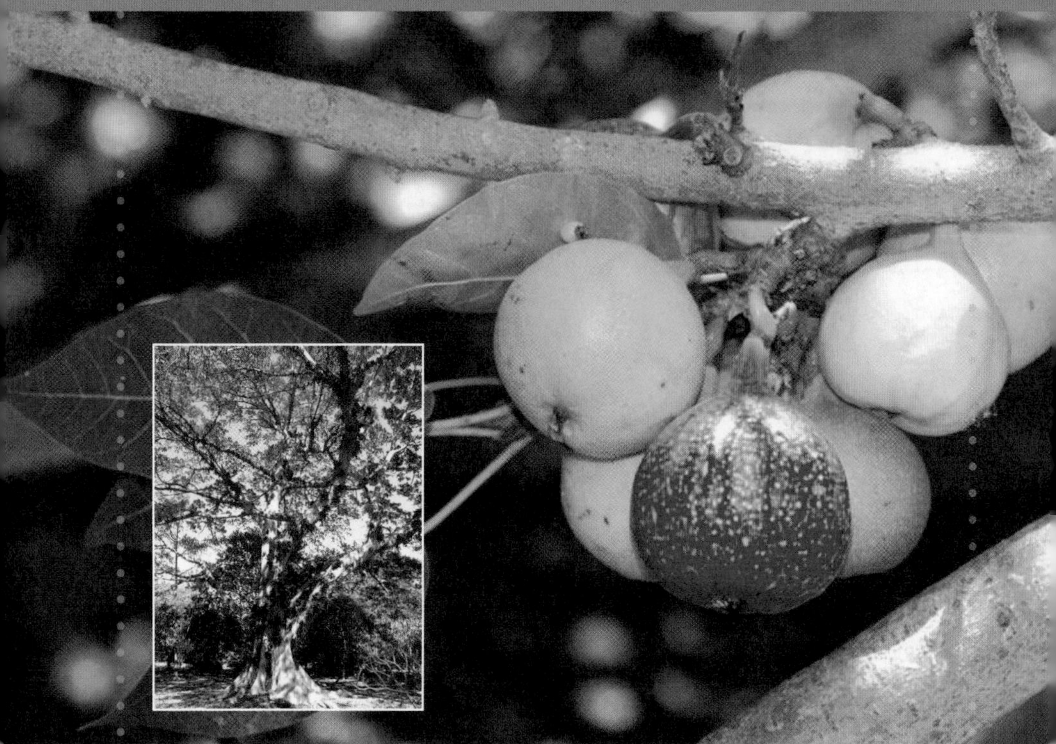

Scientific Name *Ficus racemosa* L.

Common Names Stem-fruit Fig, Cluster Fig Tree, Indian Fig Tree.

Aboriginal Names Jamarndaj (Miriwoong) (Leonard et al., 2013), Jiliwa, Ganjirr (Wunambal, Gaambera) (Karadada et al., 2011), Jamartany, Putinyja (Walmajarri) (Richards & Hudson, 2012), Jawoonany, Ngalalabany, Jamarndaji (Gija) (Purdie et al., 2018), Jamaraj, Jamarndaj, Jalywarr (Jaru) (Wightman, 2003) Kanjûrr minya (tree), Karnjirr minya (tree), Ongu minya (fruit), Uunku minya (fruit) (Kwini) (Cheinmora et al., 2017; Crawford, 1982).

Field Notes Stem-fruit fig is a monoecious (having both male and female parts) tree that grows up to 30 m in height. Its bark is smooth and greyish brown. Its leaves vary in shape and can be up to 140 mm long. Its tiny white flowers appear on the trunk in Australia from April to August. Its fruit are pear-shaped, up to 25 mm in diameter and grow close to the trunk in clusters.

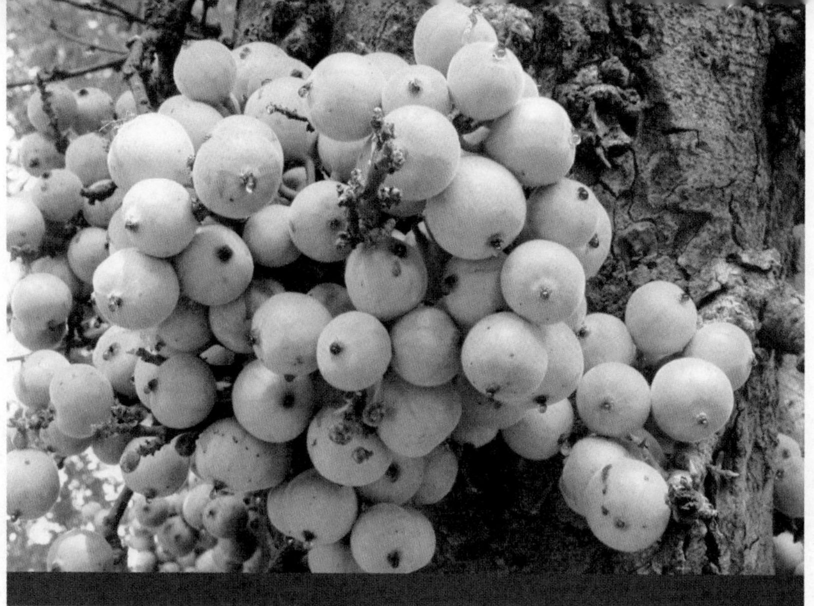

In Australia, the fruit are available from mid-November to February (Crawford, 1982). Stem-fruit Fig occurs in alluvium, sand or basaltic loam beside creeks and rivers in the Kimberley region of Western Australia, the Northern Territory and Queensland as far south as the border with New South Wales. Stem-fruit Fig also occurs in Malaysia, Indonesia, Indochina and on the Indian subcontinent (ALA, 2022; ATRP, 2020; Fern, 2021; WAH, 2022).

Medicinal Uses Infusions of Stem-fruit Fig leaves, inner bark and wood were taken internally to treat diarrhoea. The resin was a specific treatment for dermatophytosis (ringworm and tinea) (Fern, 2021; Low, 1990; Western Australia Now and Then, 2022). The root was chewed as a treatment for tonsillitis. In Asian countries, infusions or decoctions of the bark and fruit were used to stop internal bleeding (Fern, 2021).

Other Uses The large, yellow fruit of Stem-fruit Fig can be eaten raw or cooked and are reported to be very sweet (Cheinmora et al., 2017; Crawford, 1982; Fox & Garde, 2018; Karadada et al., 2011; Maiden, 1889; Smith, 1991; Wightman, 2003). Some Aboriginal groups made dugout canoes from the trunk of this tree (El Questro, n.d.; Karadada et al., 2011).

Sticky Hopbush

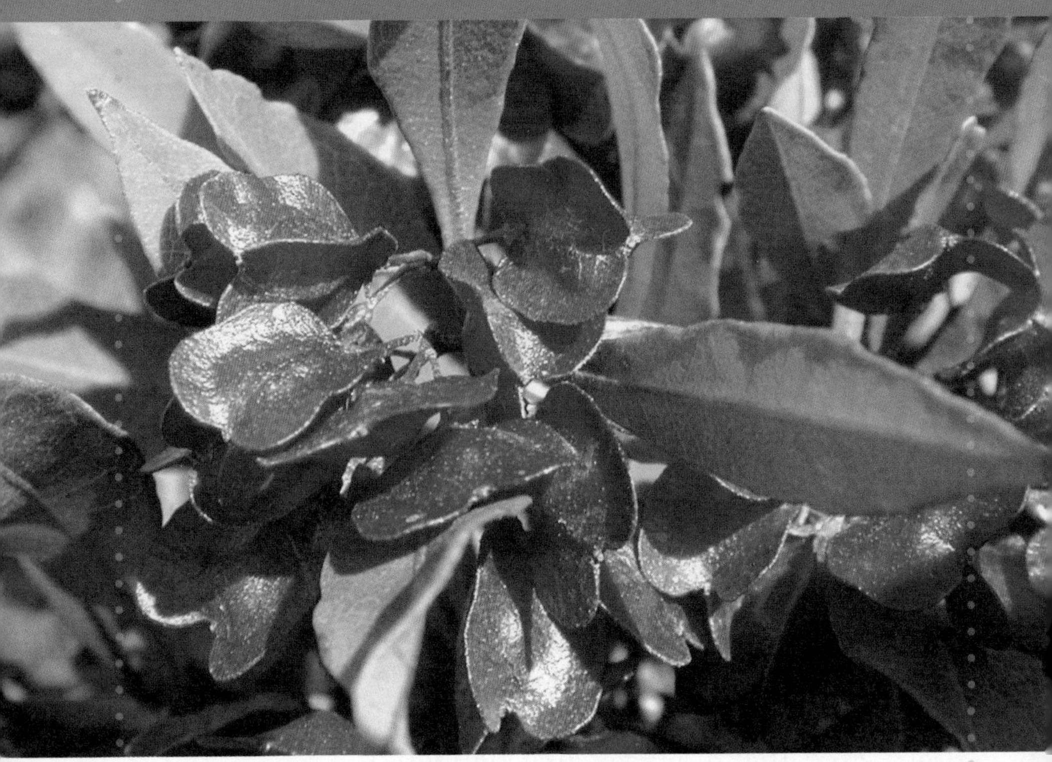

Scientific Name *Dodonaea viscosa* Jacq.

Common Names Sticky Hopbush, Desert Hopbush, Broad Leaf Hopbush, Candlewood, Narrow Leaf Hopbush, Native Hopbush, Soapwood, Switch Sorrel, Wedge Leaf Hopbush, Native Hop, Giant Hopbush, Hopbush.

Aboriginal Name Tjininypa (Kukatja) (Valiquette, 1993).

Field Notes Sticky Hopbush is an evergreen shrub or small tree that grows up to 5 m in height. The sticky leaves are usually spatulate (spoon-shaped) and are reddish or purplish in colour. In Western Australia, its small, inconspicuous, greenish-yellow flowers are less than 10 mm in size and appear from June to August. Its pale brown or coral pink fruit are distinctive capsules with papery wings. Sticky Hopbush is found in sand, loam and clay in arid and semi-arid areas in a variety of habitats throughout mainland Australia, as well as Africa, many countries throughout Europe, the Pacific islands and

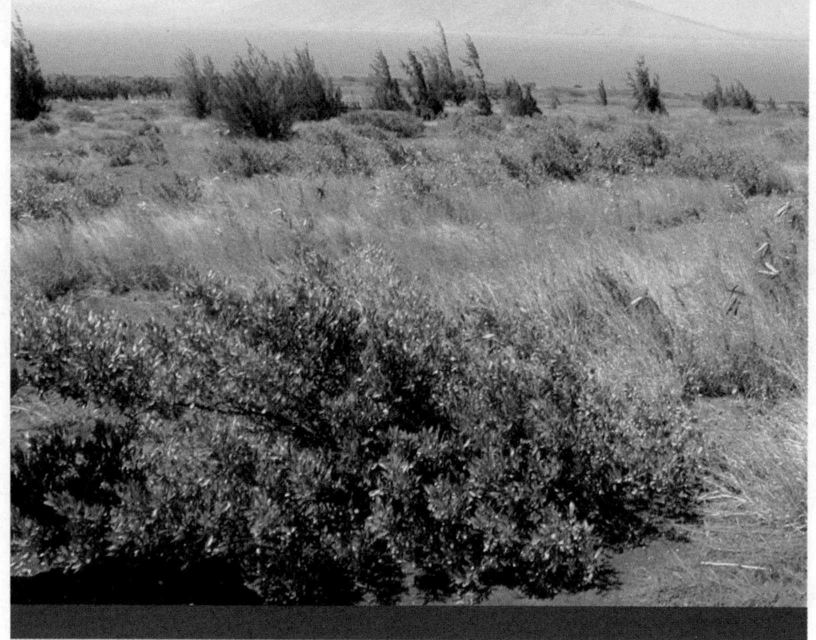

the Americas (ALA, 2022; Cribb & Cribb, 1983; Lassak & McCarthy, 2008; WAH, 2022).

Medicinal Uses The leaves of Sticky Hopbush were chewed to soothe toothache, although the juice was not swallowed (Lassak & McCarthy, 2001). The crushed leaves and the juice were used externally as a poultice to treat stonefish stings and stingray wounds. The juice of the crushed leaves is also reported to have antifungal and anti-inflammatory properties (Venkatesh et al., 2008). Infusions or decoctions of the leaves were rubbed all over the body to reduce fever (Lassak & McCarthy, 2001).

Other Uses The leafy branches produce clean smoke, which was used by some Aboriginal groups to smoke babies in smoking ceremonies 'to keep bad spirits away' and as an insect repellent (Hansen & Horsfall, 2016). The fruit has been used as a substitute for hops for making beer (Fern, 2021).

Stiffleaf Sedge

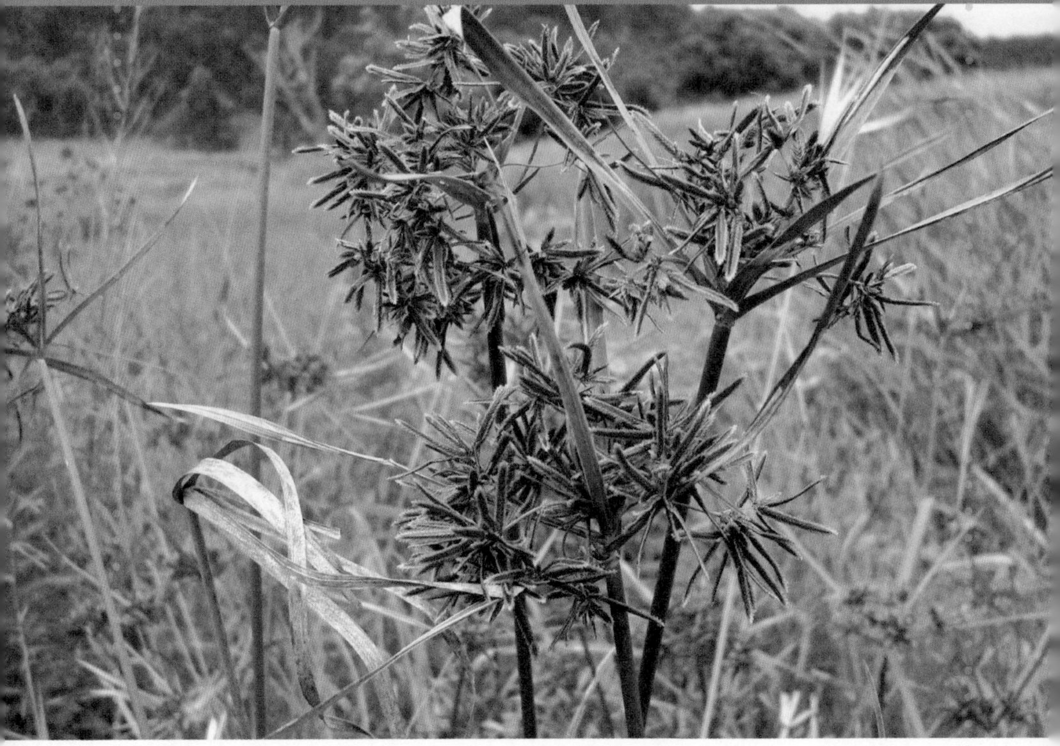

Scientific Name *Cyperus vaginatus* R.Br.

Common Names Stiffleaf Sedge, Stiff-leaf Sedge, Stiff Flat-sedge.

Aboriginal Name Purta-purta (Kukatja) (Valiquette, 1993).

Field Notes Stiffleaf Sedge is a rhizomatous, tufted, perennial sedge with rigid culms (stems) up to 2 m in height. Its leaves are stiff sheaths, except on juvenile plants. Green-brown flower heads can be present any time between February and November. The spikelets are flattened and there are between four and 15 in each cluster. Its small seeds or nuts are trigonous, obovoid to ellipsoid, grey-brown and only 0.8 mm long and 0.5 mm in diameter. Stiffleaf Sedge occurs in sand, clay, alluvium and amongst limestone rocks along watercourses in the Gascoyne, Pilbara and Kimberley regions of Western Australia, the Northern Territory, north-west Queensland and New South Wales (ALA, 2022; eFlora.SA, 2022; WAH, 2022).

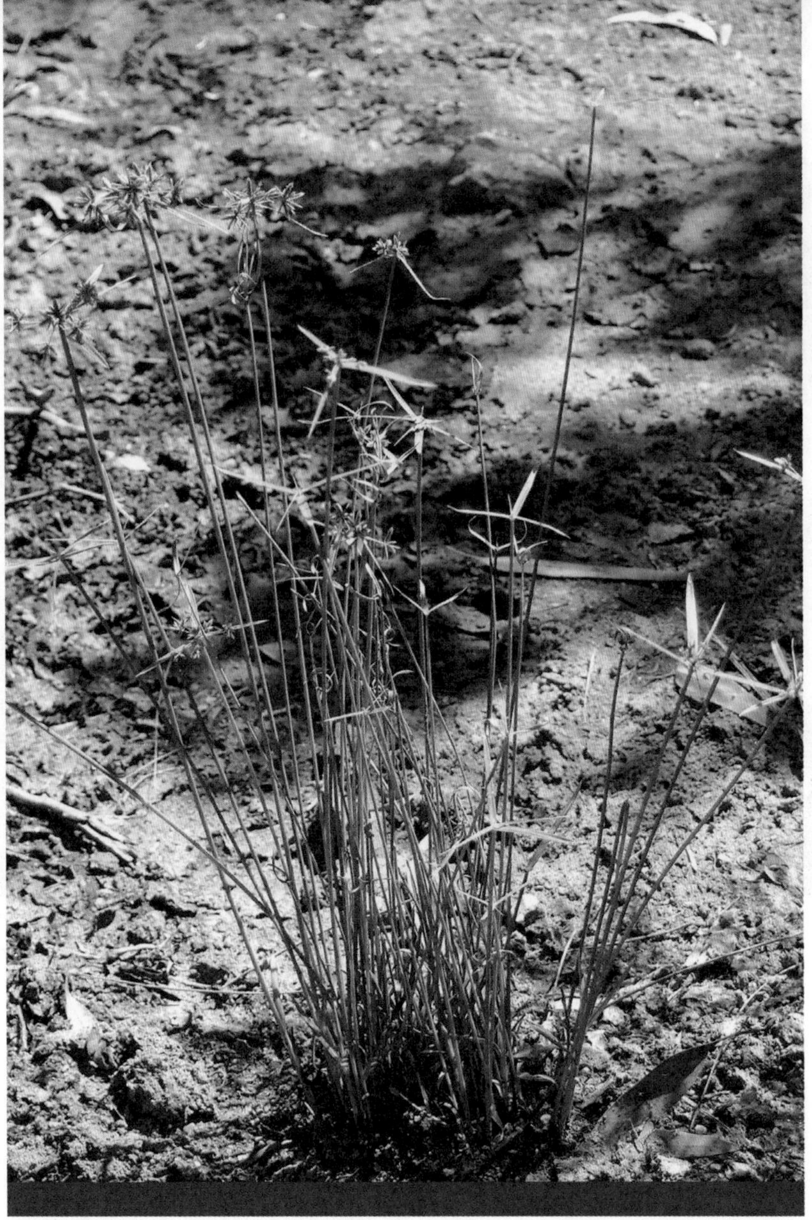

Medicinal Uses Decoctions of the flowers and leaves of Stiffleaf Sedge were sipped to soothe sore throats (Morse, 2005).

Other Uses The fibre that can be extracted from the outer parts of the culms or stems is traditionally used by some Aboriginal groups to make nets and cordage (ALA, 2022).

Stinking Passionflower

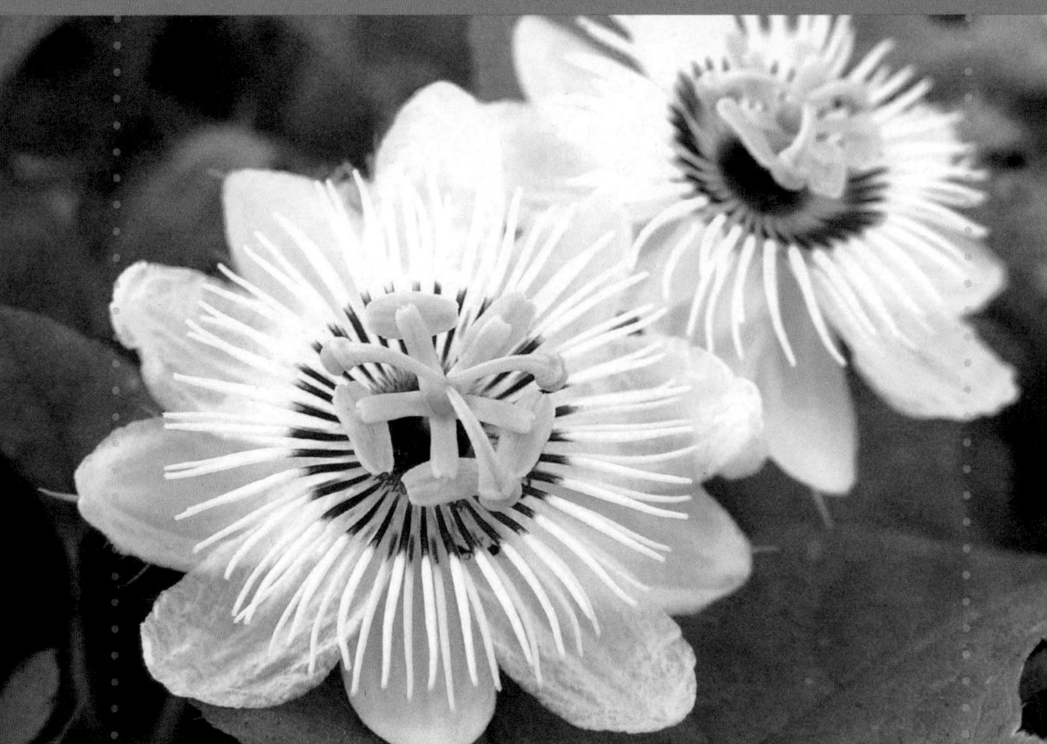

Scientific Name *Passiflora foetida* L.

Common Names Stinking Passionflower, Goat-Scented Passionflower, Love-in-a-Mist, Bush Passionfruit, Wild Passionfruit.

Aboriginal Names Gambu (Bunuba) (Oscar et al., 2019), Yidiringgi (Jaru) (Martin, 2014), Jool Jool (Nyul Nyul), Itiringki, Watakiyi (Ngardi) (Cataldi, 2004), Yirirrinytji (Kukatja) (Valiquette, 1993), Kiilu winya (Kwini) (Cheinmora et al., 2017).

Field Notes Stinking Passionflower was introduced to Australia in the 1880s. It is native to Central and South America. The word *foetida* is a Latin word that means 'stinking' and refers to the strong aroma emitted if the foliage is damaged. It is recognised as a weed in most areas of Australia where it grows. Stinking Passionflower is a climbing, herbaceous, perennial plant with stems growing up to 2.5 m in length. The leaves have three lobes, are arrowhead-shaped and are up to 130 mm long. The flowers are singular, white or light purple with white spots or lines and are up to 30 mm in diameter. The fruit are orange or orange-red, ovoid-globose, glabrous berries covered with a spidery calyx and are up to 30 mm in diameter. The fruit contain many light brown to black, elliptic seeds that are up to 4 mm across. In Australia, flowering occurs between February and November. Stinking Passionflower occurs mainly in coastal areas and on river and creek banks in the Gascoyne, Pilbara and Kimberley regions of Western Australia, the Northern Territory, Queensland and the northern coast of New South Wales. It has been introduced to many other tropical and sub-tropical countries and is now pantropical (ALA, 2022; WAH, 2022).

Medicinal Uses The leaves of Stinking Passionflower have medicinal properties and are used in folk medicine in some countries to treat neurasthenia, insomnia, early menstruation, oedema, itchy skin and coughs. Decoctions of the whole plant are taken internally to treat intestinal parasites (nematodes and flatworms) in children, chesty coughs, tuberculosis and the symptoms of colds and influenza. Infusions or decoctions of the leaves were used as an antiseptic wash to hasten the healing of wounds (Cribb & Cribb, 1981; Fern, 2021).

Other Uses The fruit contain black seeds and a sweet tangy pulp, both of which are edible. The taste is reported to be similar to cultivated passionfruit (*Passiflora edulis*) (Cheinmora et al., 2017; Cribb & Cribb, 1981; Fox & Garde, 2018; Low, 1991). Aboriginal people across the top end of Australia have been eating the fruit with relish since its introduction. The young shoot tips and leaves are a valuable, wild-gathered vegetable in several South-east Asian countries where they are thoroughly cooked by boiling first and then usually consumed in a soup (Fern, 2021).

CAUTION: The young fruit of Stinking Passionflower are cyanogenic and hence poisonous. They are only edible when fully ripe (Cheinmora et al., 2017).

Stinkweed

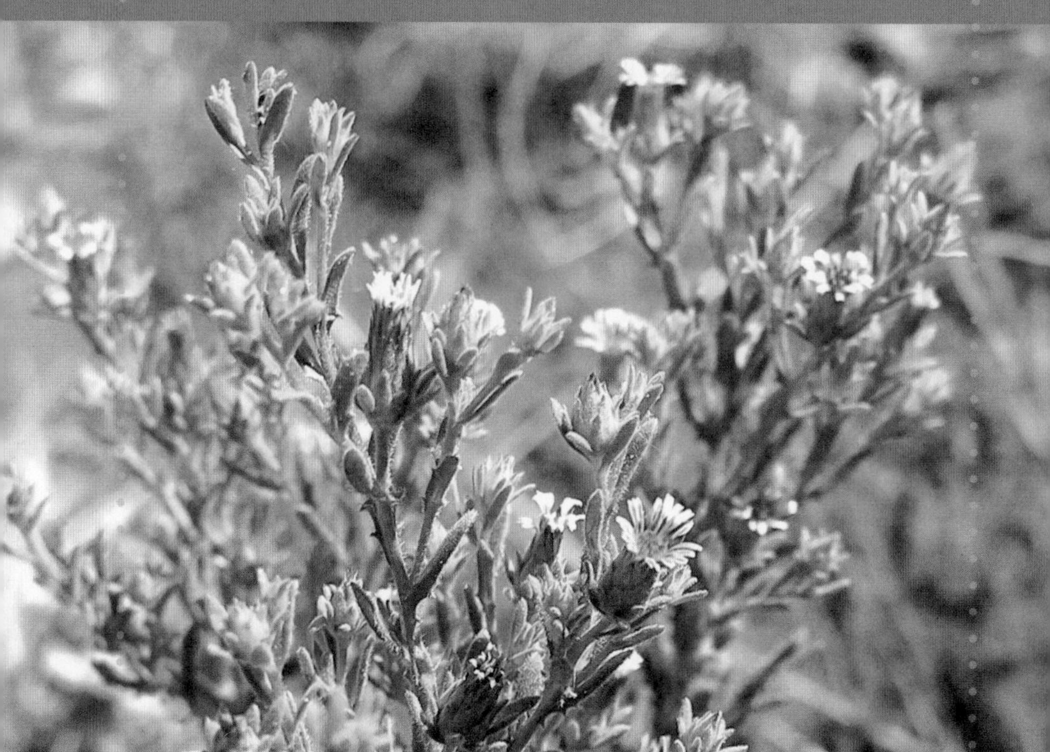

Scientific Name *Streptoglossa bubakii* (Domin) Dunlop.

Common Name Stinkweed.

Aboriginal Names Manyanyi (Gija and Jaru) (Wightman, 2003), Mangani, Wangarti (Kukatja) (Valiquette, 1993).

Field Notes Stinkweed is an erect, much-branched, aromatic, hairy and viscid, perennial herb that grows to 800 mm in height. The leaves are oblanceolate or obovate, up to 70 mm long and 18 mm wide, often with serrated margins. Pink, purple-blue or red-brown flowers with tiny petals are present between May and October. Stinkweed occurs in sandy and clayey soils, on rocky grounds, saline flats and along creek lines in the Pilbara and Kimberley regions of Western Australia, the Northern Territory and central Queensland (ALA, 2022; WAH, 2022).

Medicinal Uses Decoctions of the whole plant were used as a medicinal body wash for relief from colds, influenza and skin

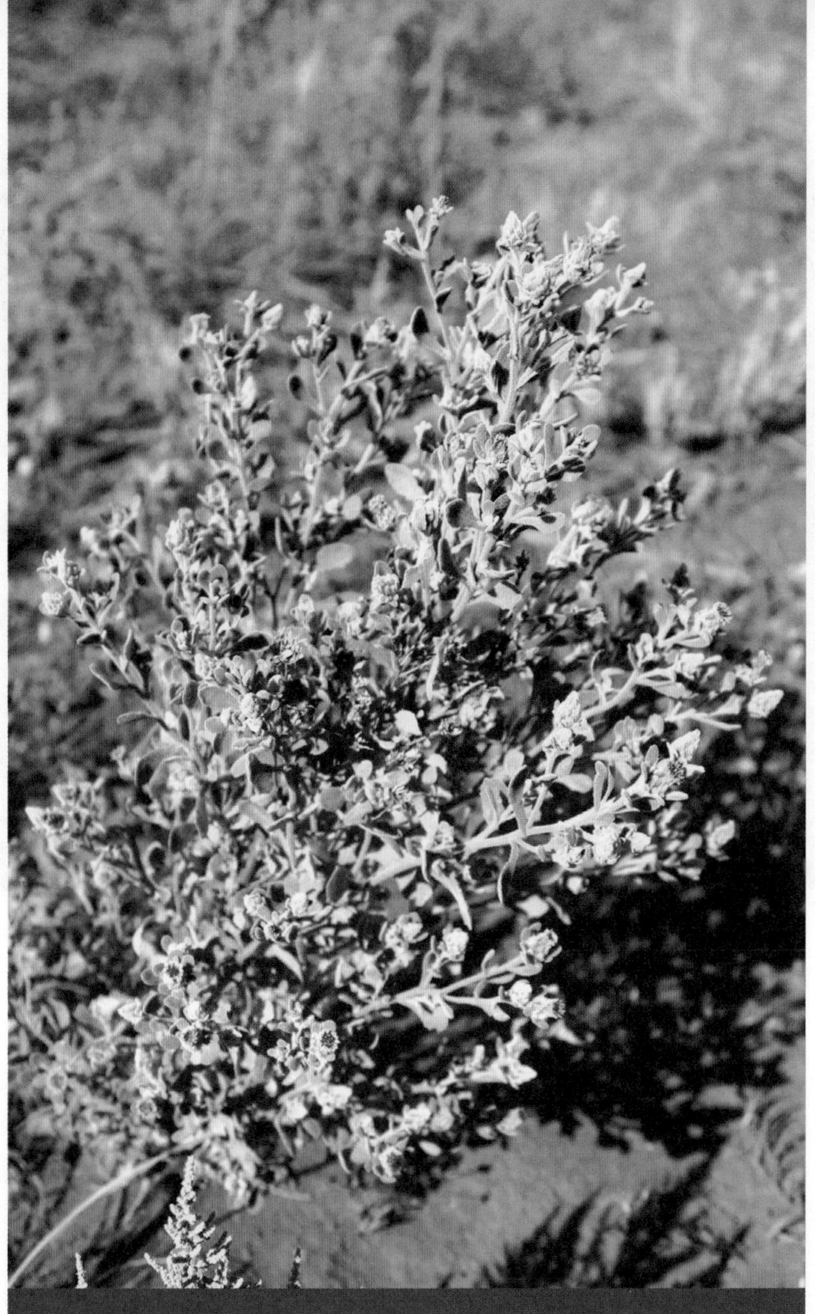

disorders, such as sores and scabies infestations. The decoctions can be stored for up to one week. The leaves were crushed in the hand and the vapours inhaled to relieve the symptoms of colds and influenza. Alternatively, a plug of crushed leaves was inserted and left in the nasal cavities for a lasting effect (Smith, 1991; Williams, 2013; Wightman, 2003).

Strychnine Bush

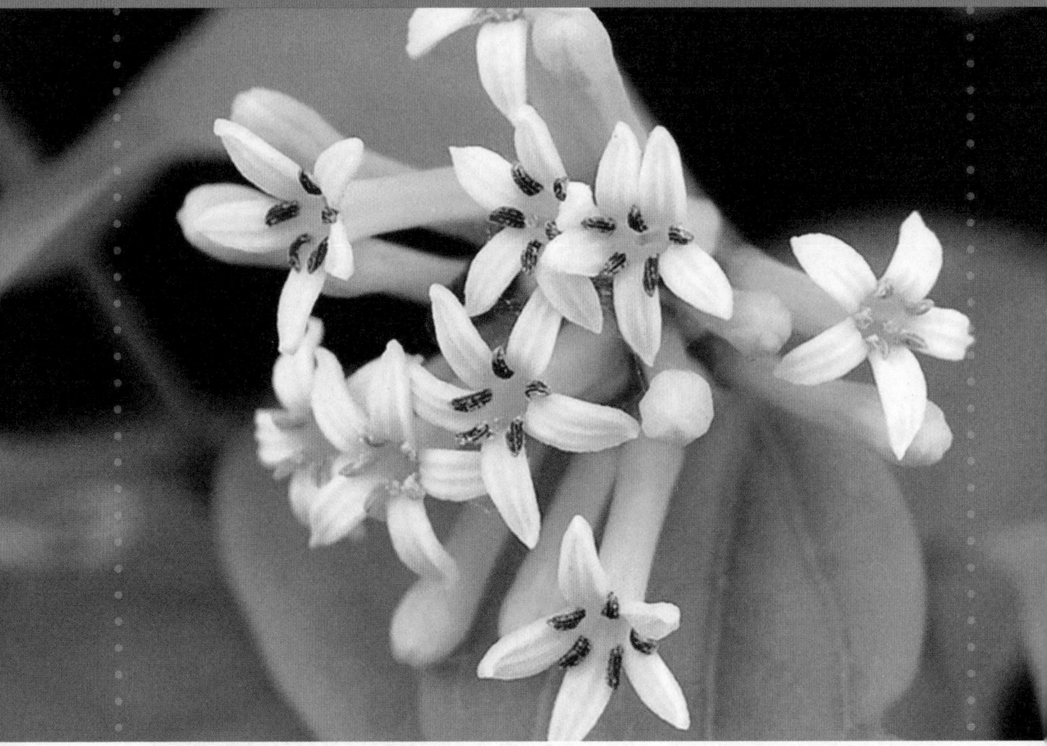

Scientific Name *Strychnos lucida* R.Br.

Common Names Strychnine Bush, Strychnine Tree.

Field Notes Strychnine Bush is a deciduous shrub or tree that can grow up to 12 m in height. It has green, ovate leaves up to 60 mm long and 37 mm wide and white-cream or green-yellow, tubular flowers that appear between September and January. The fruit are globular berries up to 30 mm in diameter. Strychnine Bush is found on rocky sandstone rises and ridges, basalt screes and limestone outcrops in coastal and near-coastal areas across the tropical north of Australia from the Kimberley region in Western Australia to the Cape York Peninsula in Far North Queensland (ALA, 2022; ATRP, 2020; WAH, 2022). It is also endemic to Indonesia, Malaysia and Thailand (Fern, 2021).

Medicinal Uses The white pulp in the fruit of Strychnine Bush was applied directly onto the skin as a treatment for scabies infestations.

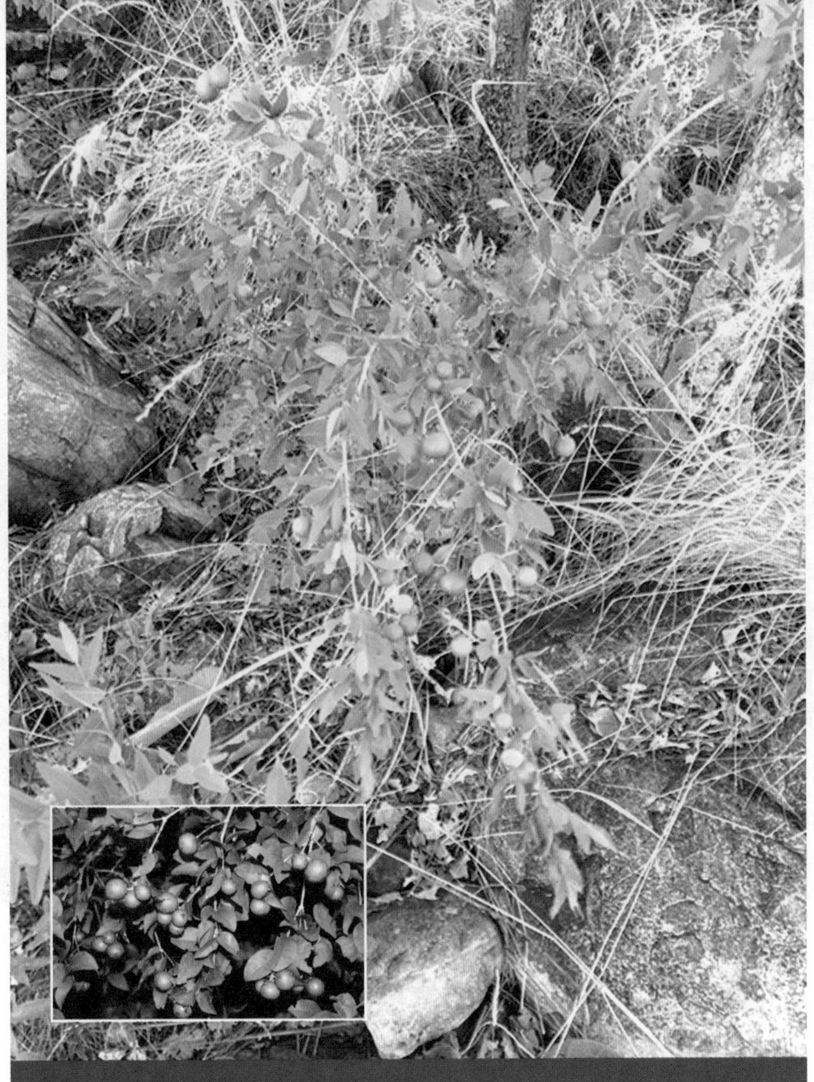

It was also smeared on weeping rashes, burns, leprosy lesions, sores and cuts to dry them and hasten the healing process. It was applied to other parts of the body to treat general malaise (Fern, 2021; Hiddins, 2001; Smith, 1991). In Asia, it has been used in folk medicine for the treatment of ailments such as malaria, diarrhoea, fever, hypertension, cancer, diabetes mellitus and skin infections (Fern, 2021).

Other Uses Crushed leaves and the fruit of Strychnine Bush were used as a fish poison.

CAUTION: The fruit are poisonous and NOT edible. The seeds of the fruit contain strychnine (Hiddins, 2001; Smith, 1991).

Supplejack

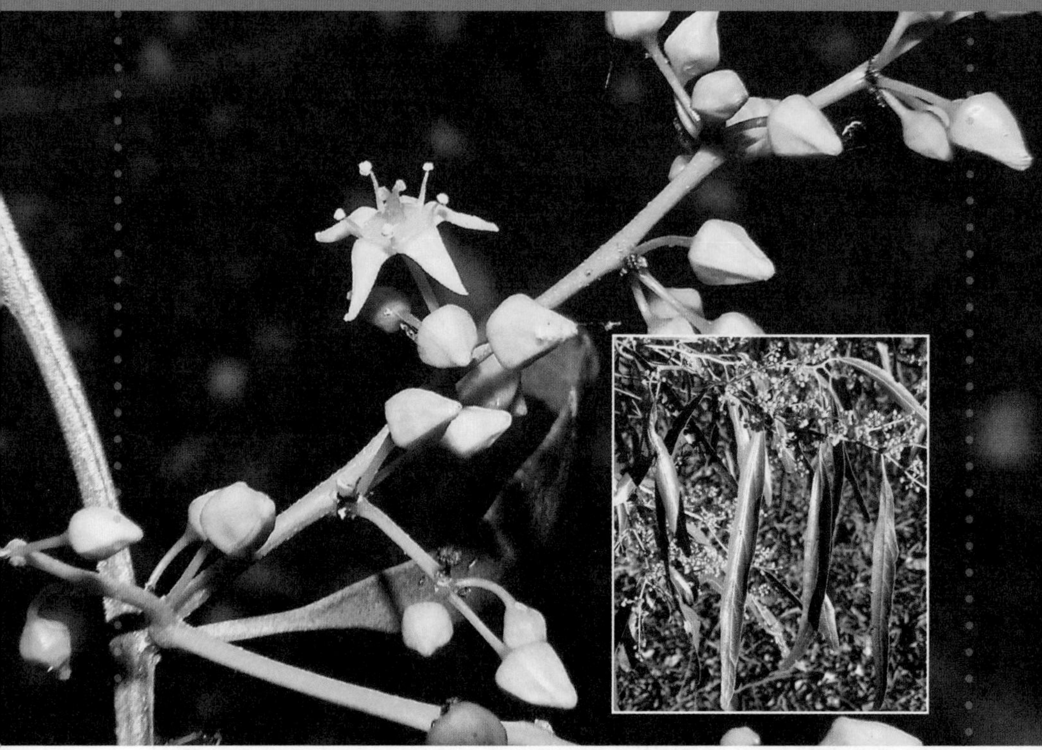

Scientific Name *Ventilago viminalis* Hook.

Common Names Supplejack, Supple Jack, Vine Tree.

Aboriginal Names Bandarrakoo (Nyikina) (Smith & Smith, 2009), Ganayanay (Yuwaalayaay), Bandarang (Bardi) (Smith & Kalotas, 1985), Warlagarriny, Warlakarri (Gija) (Purdie et al., 2018), Walagarri (Jaru) (Wightman, 2003), Nyamalalya, Walakari (Kukatja) (Valiquette, 1993), Walakarri (Walpiri) (Northern Tanami IPA, 2015).

Field Notes Supplejack is a weeping tree that grows to 10 m in height. It has long, lanceolate, bright green leaves and small cream-to-yellow flowers that are present between May and September. Its fruit have a globular base up to 4 mm in diameter and a narrowly oblong wing up to 40 mm long and 7 mm wide. Supplejack is found in red sand or alluvial soils and cracking clay in the Pilbara and Kimberley regions of Western Australia, the Northern Territory, Queensland and northern New South Wales (ALA, 2022; ATRP, 2020; Lassak & McCarthy, 2001; WAH, 2022).

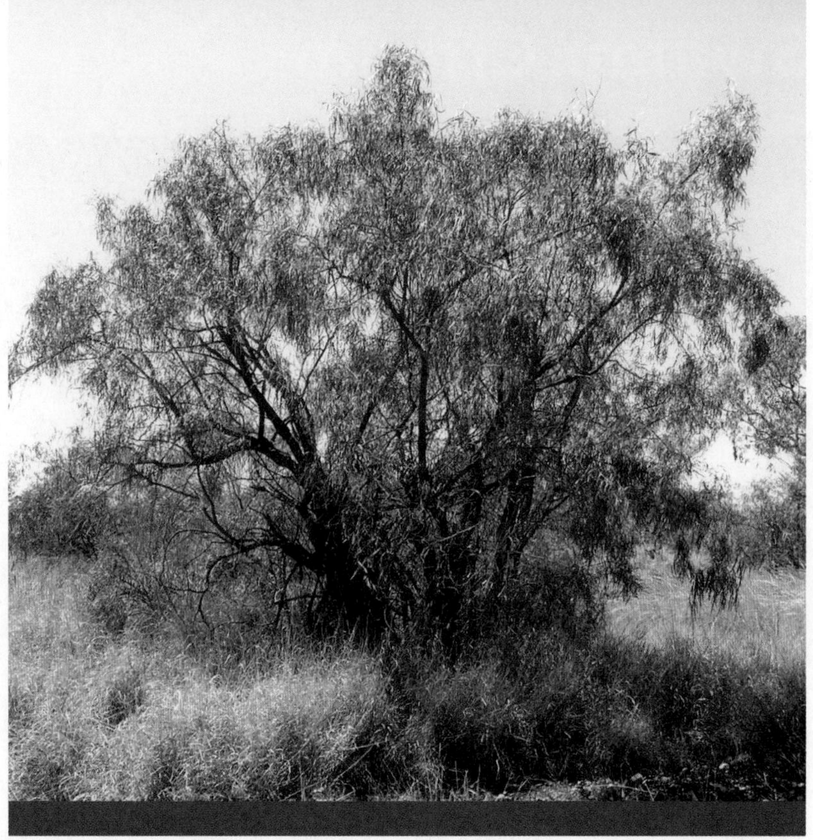

Medicinal Uses Infusions or decoctions of the roots and bark or leaves were used as a mouthwash for toothache, and were applied externally for rheumatic pain, swellings, insect bites, cuts and sores (Cock, 2011; Kenneally et al., 1996; Lassak & McCarthy, 2001; Purdie et al., 2018; Reid, 1986; Webb, 1959; Wightman, 2003).

Other Uses The gum that oozes from the Supplejack tree due to wounds from insect activity is reported to be edible (Fern, 2021; Land for Wildlife, n.d.). The wood is said to be one of the best woods for producing fire by friction (Fern, 2021). The Gija and Jaru make boomerangs, fighting sticks and shields from the wood (Deegan et al., 2010; Purdie et al., 2018). Ash from burnt bark was mixed with native tobacco 'to make it cheeky' (Kenneally et al., 1996).

Swamp Crinum

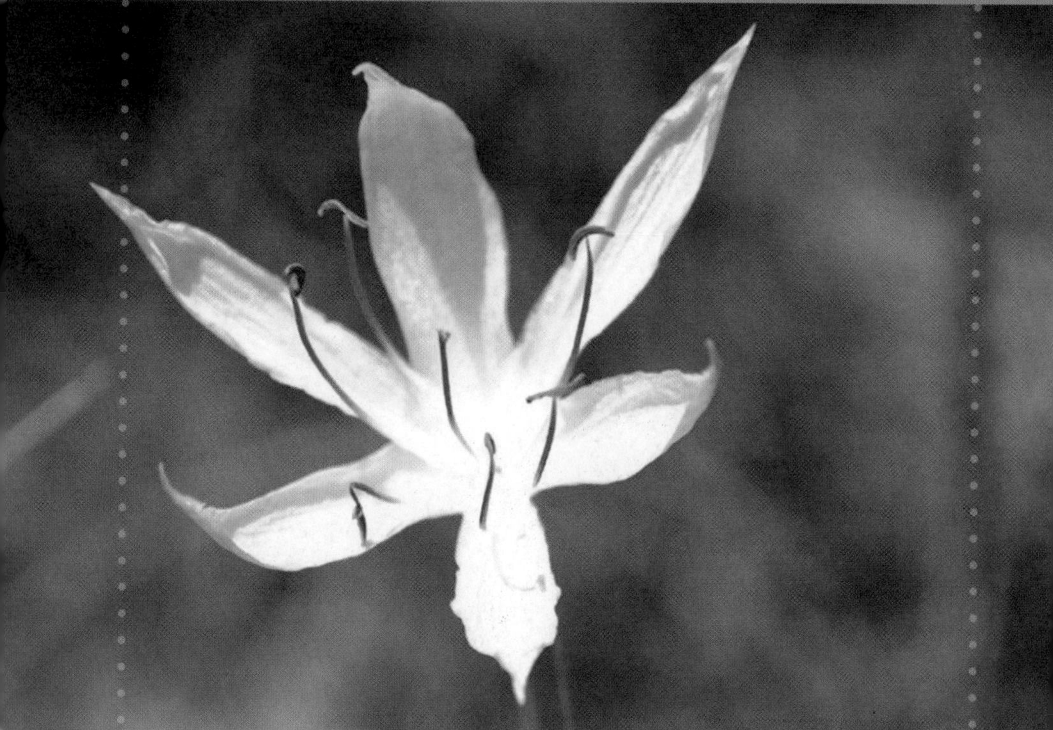

Scientific Name *Crinum uniflorum* F.Muell.

Common Names Swamp Crinum, Bush Lily.

Field Notes Swamp Crinum is a bulbaceous perennial that grows to just under 1 m in height. It has narrow grass-like leaves. The white-pink flowers, usually one flower to a slim stem, have six narrow, pointed petals and long anthers. Flowering begins with the onset of the wet season (December to March). Swamp Crinum occurs in lateritic loam or clay often in swamps in the north of the Kimberley region of Western Australia, the Northern Territory and Far North Queensland (ALA, 2022; Cairns to Cape Tribulation, 2016; WAH, 2022).

Medicinal Uses Decoctions of the whole plant can be used externally as an antiseptic wash on sores and wounds (Cock, 2011) and as a liniment for arthritic and rheumatic pain (Wiynjorrotj et al., 2005).

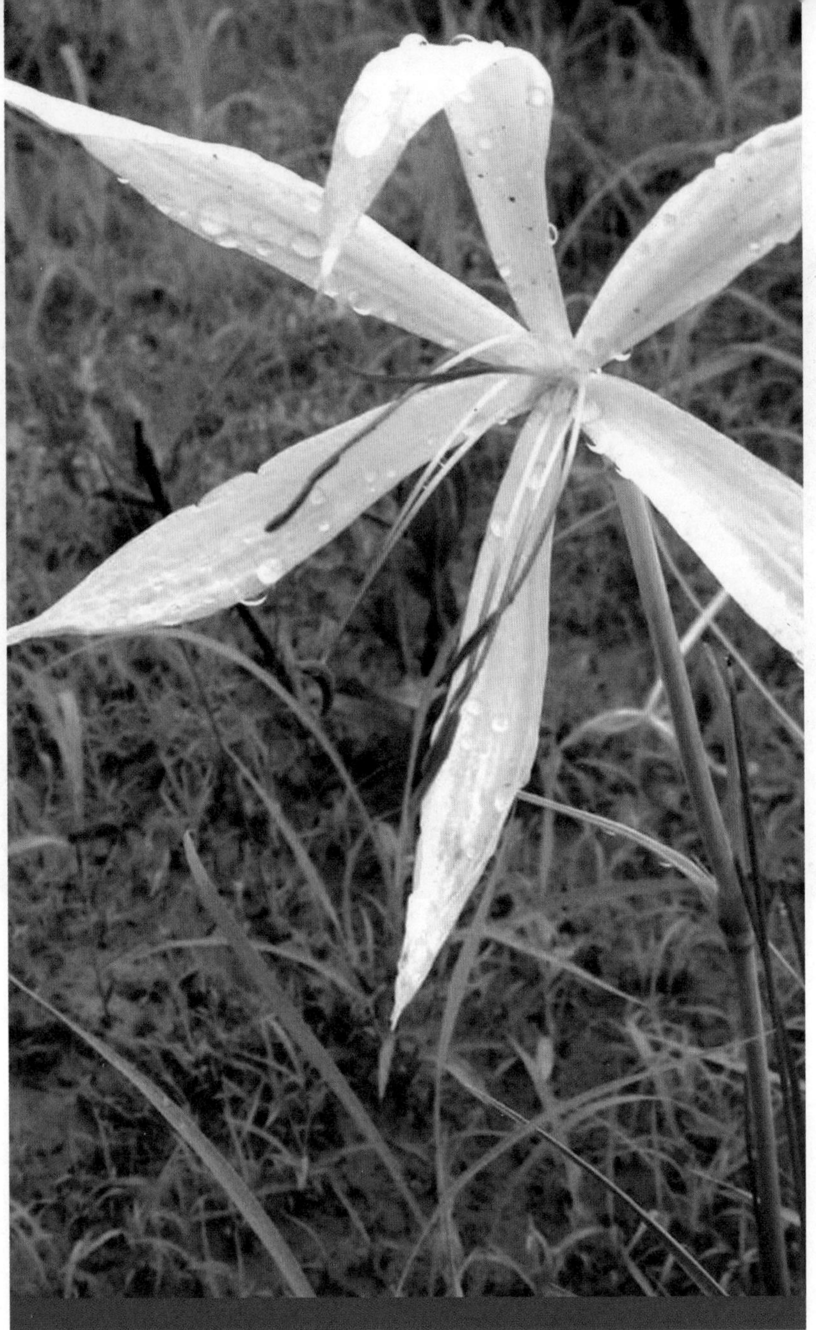

Other Uses The tubers of Swamp Crinum are edible and were scraped, ground into a paste and used like Gandungai (arrowroot). They are reported to be slightly bitter (Bininj Kunwok, 2022; McNiven & Hitchcock, 2015).

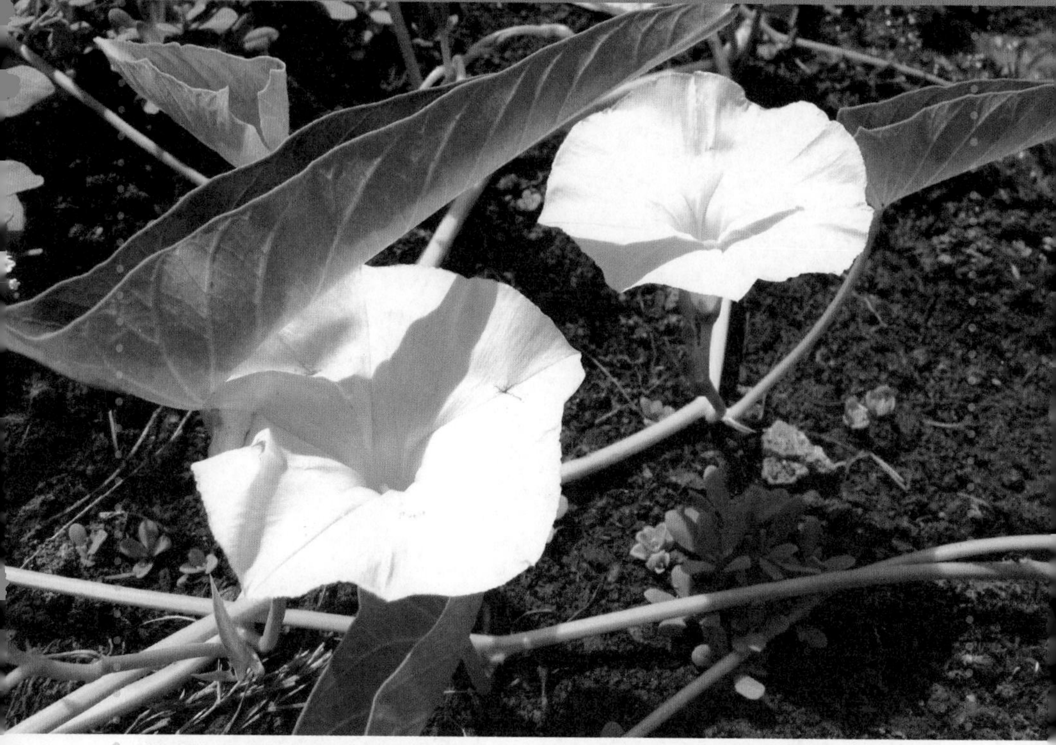

Scientific Name *Ipomoea aquatica* Forssk.

Common Names Swamp Morning Glory, Black Soil Yam, Potato Vine, Chinese Water Spinach, Chinese Watercress, Chinese Convolvulus, Swamp Cabbage, Kangkong.

Aboriginal Names Garndiny, Yoowalany (Gija) (Purdie et al., 2018), Gurulyu (Jaru) (Deegan et al., 2010), Garndi (Jaru) (Wightman, 2003).

Field Notes Swamp Morning Glory grows as a prostrate or climbing, sometimes aquatic, annual or perennial vine with stems that can be as long as 3 m. Its leaves are arrowhead-shaped to lanceolate and up to 150 mm long. Its purple-blue or white trumpet-shaped flowers are up to 50 mm in diameter. In the Kimberley, flowering is between March and May. Swamp Morning Glory is endemic to Australia where it occurs floating in water or on mudflats, often along creeks, in the Kimberley region of Western

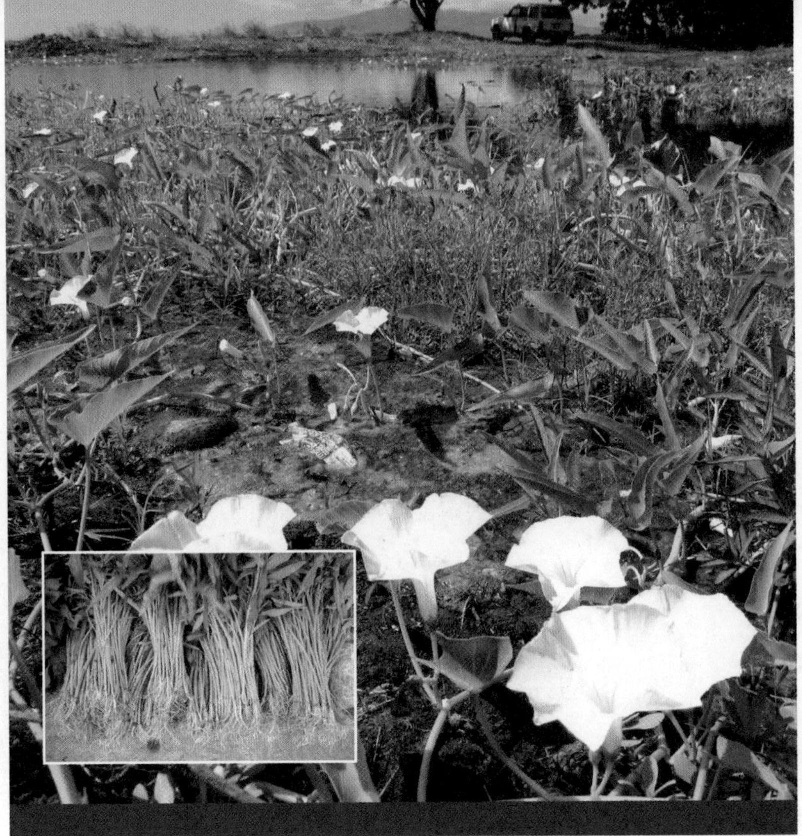

Australia, the Northern Territory and Queensland. It is grown extensively in Asia but has been introduced to many other areas of the world (ALA, 2022; WAH, 2022).

Medicinal Uses The leaves, buds and shoots of Swamp Morning Glory are used in folk medicine in parts of Asia. The young shoots are reported to be mildly laxative and are used to treat diabetes and fever. Crushed leaves are applied as a poultice to treat sores and to draw out boils. Pastes made from the buds are used to treat dermatophytosis (ringworm and tinea) (Fern, 2021; PFAF, 2022). The herb is a rich source of ascorbic acid (vitamin C), iron, calcium and vitamins A, B and E (Williams, 2012).

Other Uses The leaves, shoots, stems and roots of Swamp Morning Glory are all edible. The leaves and stems are widely used in Asia as a vegetable. Aboriginal people all over the top end of Australia ate the tuberous roots, which are roasted in hot ashes before eating (Purdie et al., 2018; Vigilante et al., 2013; Wightman, 2003; Williams, 2012).

Swamp Tea Tree

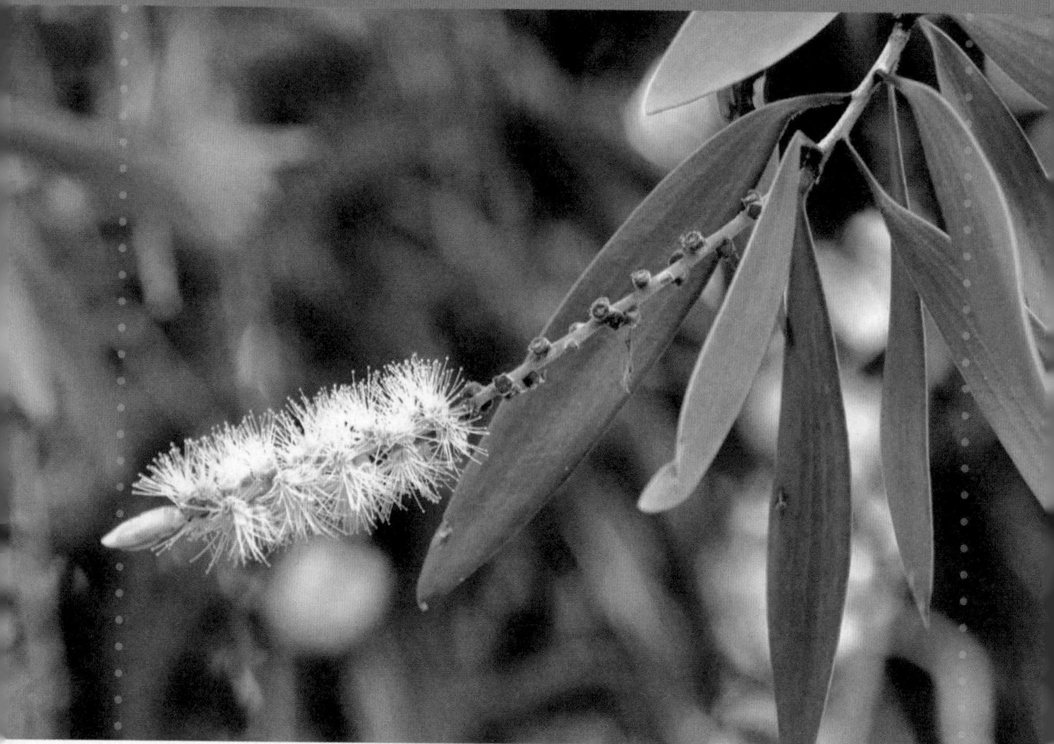

Scientific Name *Melaleuca cajuputi* Powell.

Common Names Swamp Tea Tree, Paperbark Tea Tree, Cajuput, White Samet.

Aboriginal Names Jawoolawoolang (Miriwoong) (Leonard et al., 2013), Ngarli minya (Kwini) (Cheinmora et al., 2017).

Field Notes Swamp Tea Tree is a shrub, or more usually a tree, that grows to 20 m high or more. Its lanceolate leaves are hairy, tapered at both ends and up to 120 mm long. Its white bottlebrush-type flower heads that are up to 90 mm long are present in Australia between April and September. Its fruit are woody capsules that are clustered loosely along the branches. Swamp Tea Tree occurs in black peaty sand or clay in swamps and on tidal flats across the tropical north of Australia from the Kimberley region of Western Australia, the top end of the Northern Territory and the Cape York Peninsula in Queensland. It also occurs in South-east Asia, New

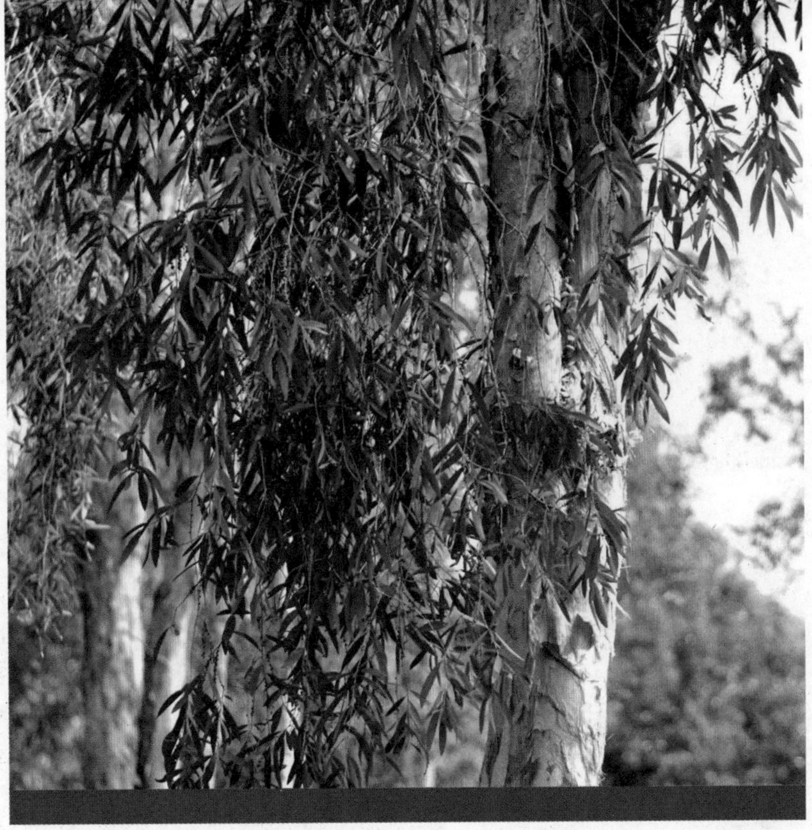

Guinea and the Torres Strait Islands (ALA, 2022; Fern, 2021; Lassak & McCarthy, 2001; WAH, 2022).

Medicinal Uses Crushed leaves from Swamp Tea Tree were rubbed on various parts of the body to relieve aches and pains. Crushed leaves were also held under the nose and the vapours inhaled to relieve the symptoms of colds, influenza and headache. Infusions or decoctions of the leaves and twigs were used as a liniment to treat rheumatic pain. Tea Tree oil (Cajaput oil) is now used internally to treat coughs, colds, stomach cramps, colic and asthma. It is also used externally as a liniment for the relief of neuralgia and rheumatic pain. The oil can also be used like clove oil to relieve toothache (Cock, 2011; Edwards, 2005; Fern, 2021; Lassak & McCarthy, 2001; Smith, 1991; Wet Tropics Management Authority, n.d.; Williams, 2011).

Other Uses The swellings that appear on the trunks of Swamp Tea Tree are a source of a small amount of potable water that can be tapped (Cheinmora et al., 2017).

Tamarind

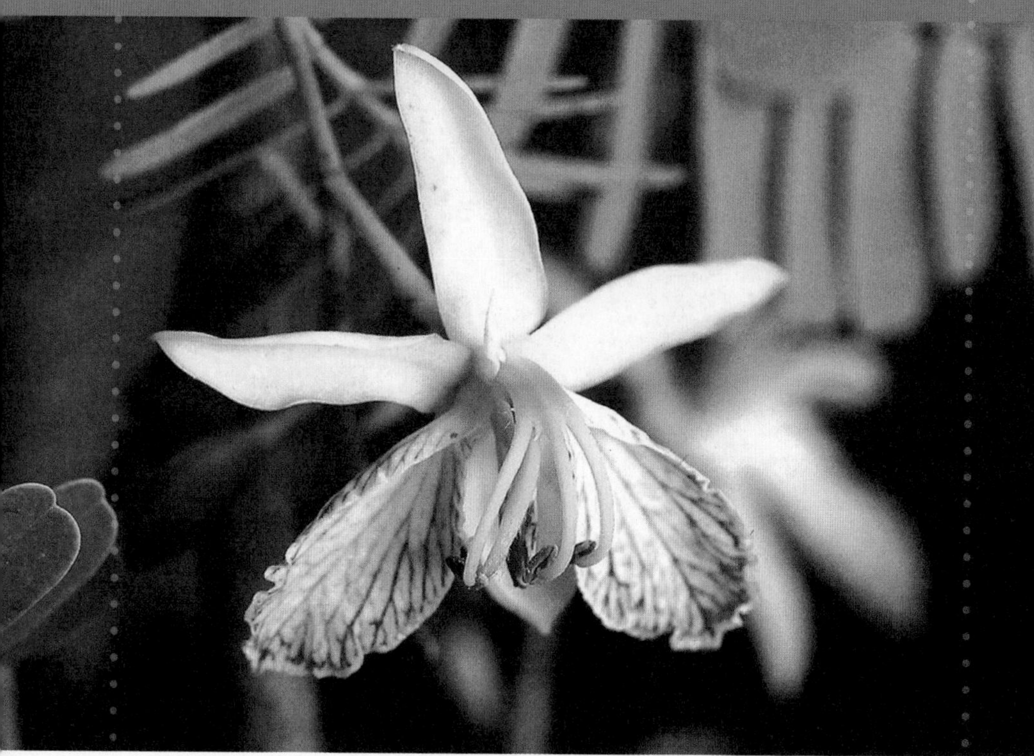

Scientific Name *Tamarindus indica* L.

Common Names Tamarind, Indian Date.

Field Notes Tamarind was introduced by Macassan fishermen from Makassar (now the island of Sulawesi) centuries ago. It was naturalised in Australia long before colonisation, so it is worth a mention in this book. Tamarind is a tree with a dense, spreading crown that grows up to 30 m in height. The bark is dark grey and fissured. Its leaves are pinnately compound with up to 20 pairs of ovate leaflets, each up to 25 mm long. Its small flowers have yellowish petals with orange to red streaks. Flowering in Australia is from December to June. Its fruit or pods are brown, slightly curved and up to 170 mm long and 25 mm wide. Tamarind is thought to have originated in tropical Africa but is now widespread through the tropics and subtropics. In Australia, it occurs in coastal and near-coastal habitats around the top end from the Kimberley region

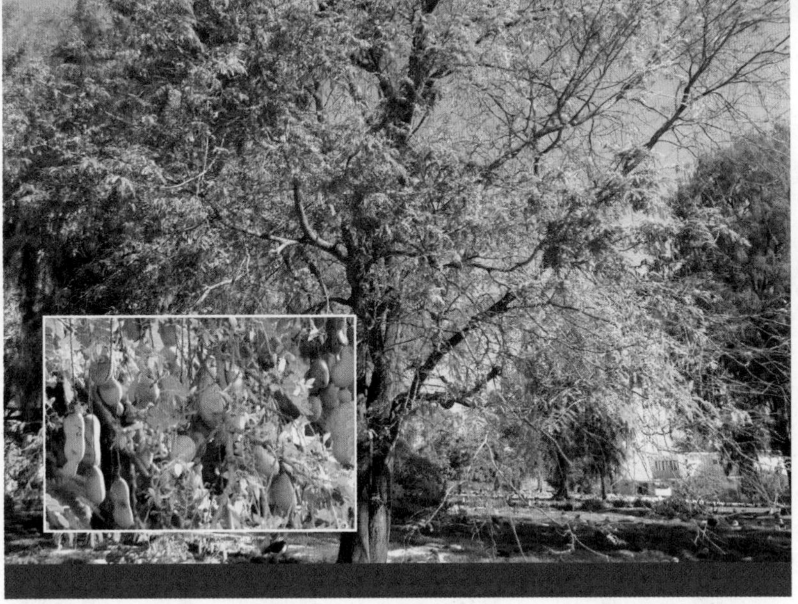

of Western Australia around to the Queensland border with New South Wales (ALA, 2022; WAH, 2022).

Medicinal Uses The Tamarind tree is used in folk medicine in tropical and sub-tropical areas where it is cultivated. The young leaves can be crushed and used as a poultice for sores and wounds or for inflammation of the joints to reduce swelling and relieve pain. Sweetened decoctions of the leaves are used to treat throat infections, coughs, fever and intestinal parasites. Filtered, warmed juice of young leaves, or a poultice of the flowers, is used to treat conjunctivitis. Sweetened infusions of the leaves and flowers are drunk by children to ease the symptoms of measles. Decoctions of the flower buds are used to treat children's bedwetting and urinary tract infections. The flesh of the fruit is eaten to treat fever and as an antacid to control hyperacidity and dyspepsia. Dry seeds are powdered and used to treat dysentery and diarrhoea (Fern, 2021).

Other Uses The flesh of the Tamarind fruit is edible, though slightly tart. It can also be soaked in water to make a tangy drink. The leaves and flowers of young plants can be cooked and eaten as a vegetable (Fern, 2021; Hiddins, 2001). The fruit pulp is mixed with water and used to flavour many Asian dishes. The seeds can be ground to a flour (Fern, 2021).

Taro

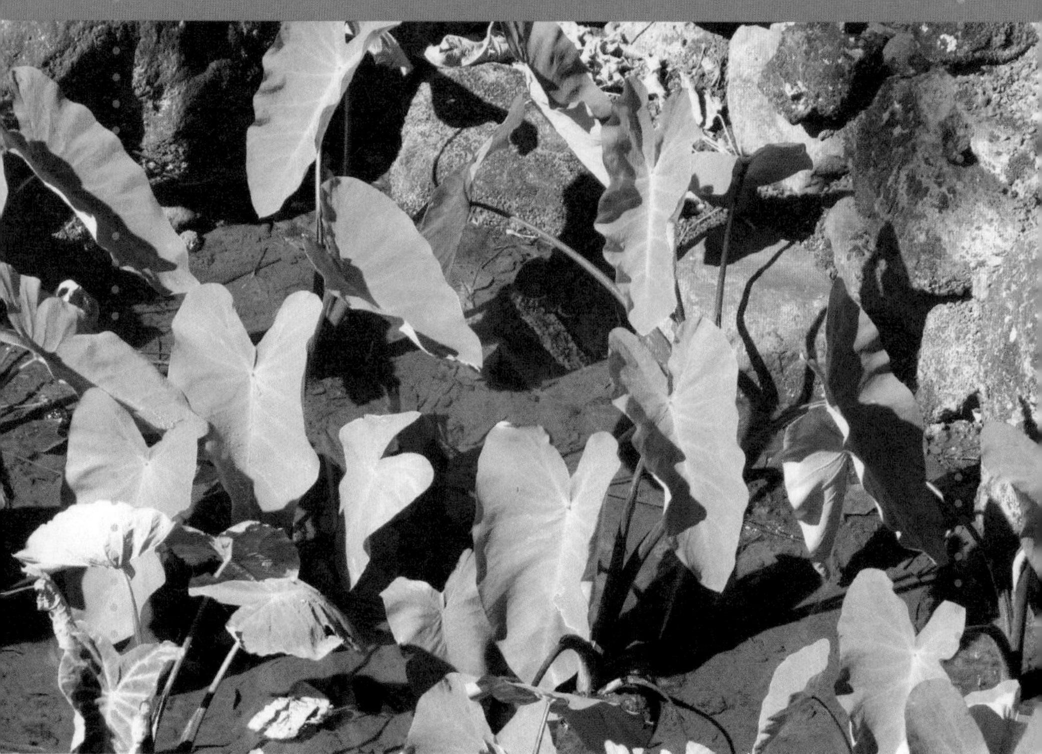

Scientific Name *Colocasia esculenta* (L.) Schott.

Common Names Taro, Elephant Ears.

Aboriginal Names Nhal-nhalng (Miriwong) (Leonard et al., 2013), Walambalambirr (Wunambal, Gaambera) (Karadada et al., 2011), Jemaniny, Jimarniny (Gija) (Purdie et al., 2018), Kinku ninya, Nerrwarl ninya, Neerwal ninya (Kwini) (Cheinmora et al., 2017; Crawford, 1982).

Field Notes Taro is a tuberous perennial herb that grows to 1 m in height. It has elongated, heart-shaped leaves and yellow-green flowers that consist of a spathe and spadix that appear between March and July. Taro occurs in black sand beside creeks and seepage areas in the Kimberley region of Western Australia, the top end of the Northern Territory and along the Queensland and New South Wales coasts, almost to the border with Victoria (ALA, 2022; WAH, 2022).

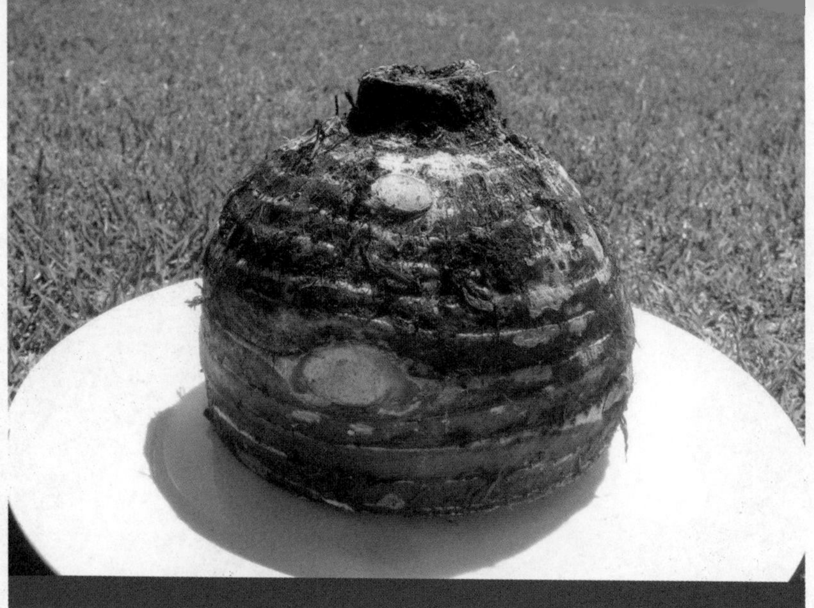

Medicinal Uses Taro has antibacterial and hypotensive properties. In New Guinea, the leaves are heated and applied to boils to draw them out. The sap from the stems has been used to treat conjunctivitis (Fern, 2021).

Other Uses The corms or tubers of Taro are edible but must be cooked as they are caustic when raw. They can be treated the same as potatoes and boiled, baked, fried or cooked in a ground oven. The outer skin is peeled off before they are eaten (Fox & Garde, 2018; Karadada et al., 2011; Purdie et al., 2018; Wightman, 2003; Williams, 2010). The leaves and stems are edible but they must be cooked before they are eaten so the calcium oxalate crystals are destroyed (Crawford, 1982; Maiden, 1889; Williams, 2010). They are sometimes cooked overnight in a ground oven (Isaacs, 1987). The corms are usually harvested from September to November (Crawford, 1982). Wightman (2003) relates that, 'In the past it [a Taro tuber] was used in the traditional welcome to country ceremony to ensure a visitor's safety while on Gija country, it was hit on the back and rubbed on the legs of the visitor'.

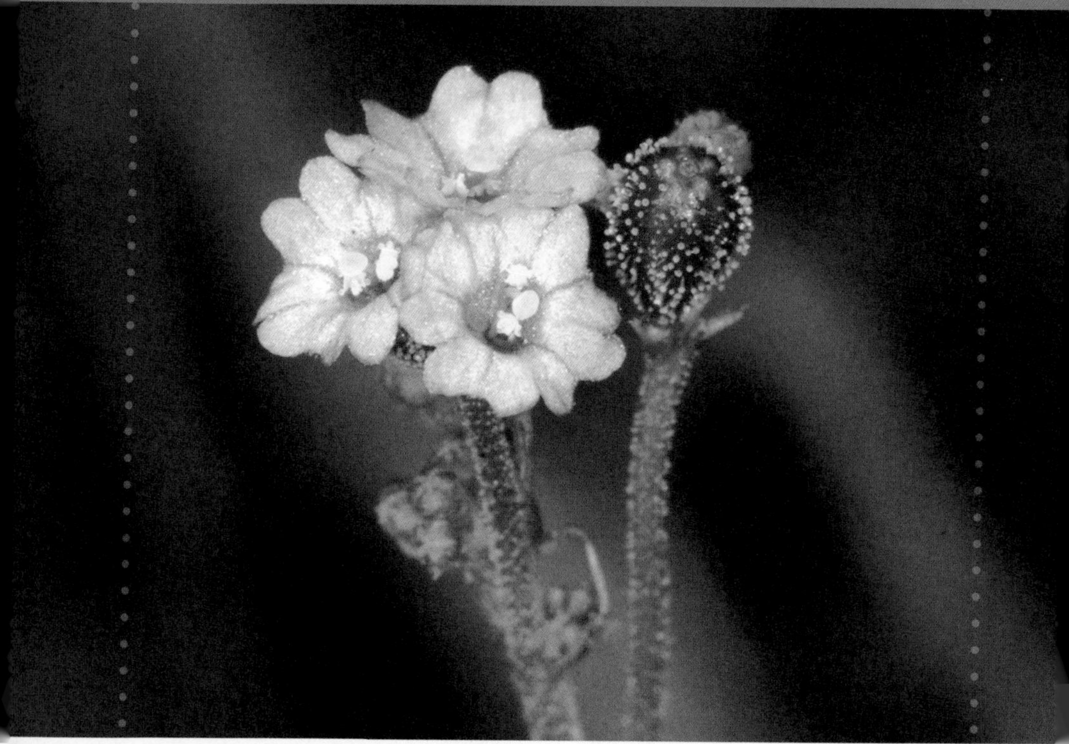

Scientific Name *Boerhavia dominii* Meikle & Hewson.

Common Names Tarvine, Spreading Hogweed, Red hogweed, Tar Vine, Red Spiderling, Wineflower.

Aboriginal Names Noowanyj (Bardi) (Kenneally et al., 1996), Bûrlka minya, Walinyirri winya (Kwini) (Cheinmora et al., 2017).

Field Notes This Tarvine is a prostrate, perennial herb whose stems can reach up to several metres long. Its leaves vary in shape from ovate, heart-shaped or oblong, and are up to 40 mm long. The small, pale pink to lilac flowers appear in the summer. Tarvine is found in every mainland state of Australia, but in Western Australia it is only found in the Pilbara and Kimberley regions. It is also found in the tropical regions of Africa, Asia, America and the Pacific islands (ALA, 2022; Fern, 2021; Lassak & McCarthy, 2001).

Medicinal Uses Decoctions of the roots were applied externally as an antiseptic wash to ulcers and abscesses. In India, the plant is

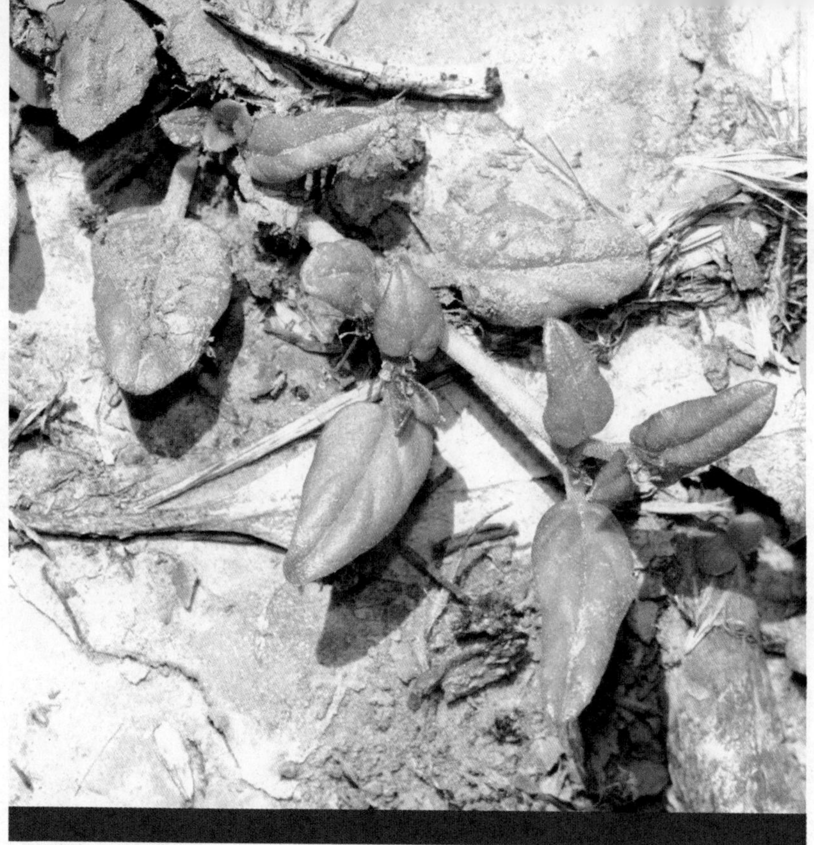

used in Ayurvedic medicine as an emetic and purgative. It is also used in the treatment of various conditions including gastric disturbances, asthma, jaundice, anascara (generalised oedema), anaemia and internal inflammation (Fern, 2021; Lassak & McCarthy, 2001).

Other Uses The tap roots of this Tarvine are edible and were eaten raw or after they were baked in hot ashes or in a ground oven. They are better eaten cooked and peeled, as the bitter skins can irritate the throat. They were usually pounded to break up the fibre and to free the root from the fibrous inner core, which was then discarded. The roots were harvested between January and August (Barker, 1991; Crawford, 1982; Isaacs, 1987; Low, 1991). The leaves and seeds are also edible (Barker, 1991; Fern, 2021).

Three-leaved Cayratia

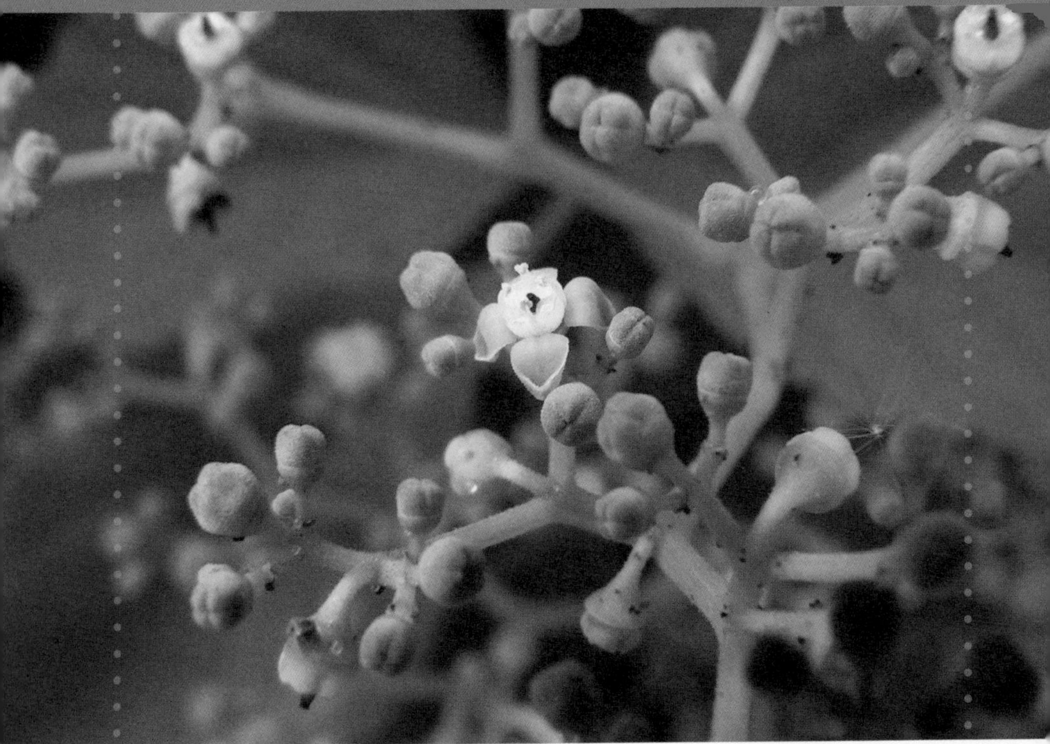

Scientific Name *Causonis trifolia* (L.) Mabb. & J.Wen., previously known as *Cayratia trifolia* Domin.

Common Names Three-leaved Cayratia, Native Grape, Threeleaf Cayratia, Slender Water Vine, Bush Yam.

Aboriginal Names Ngoandj (Bardi) (Smith & Kalotas, 1985), Bigirniny (Gija) (Purdie et al., 2018), Yukuli winya (Kwini) (Cheinmora et al., 2017; Crawford, 1982).

Field Notes Three-leaved Cayratia is a scrambling evergreen, woody vine with stems that can grow to over 20 m in length. It runs along the ground and climbs trees and shrubs, smothering them in time. It has leaves with three ovate or elliptic leaflets up to 60 mm long by 35 mm wide, and small yellow flowers that are leaf-opposed or terminal and about 4 mm in diameter. Its fruit are depressed globose berries, similar to grapes, that are purplish-black when mature. In Australia, Three-leaved Cayratia occurs in

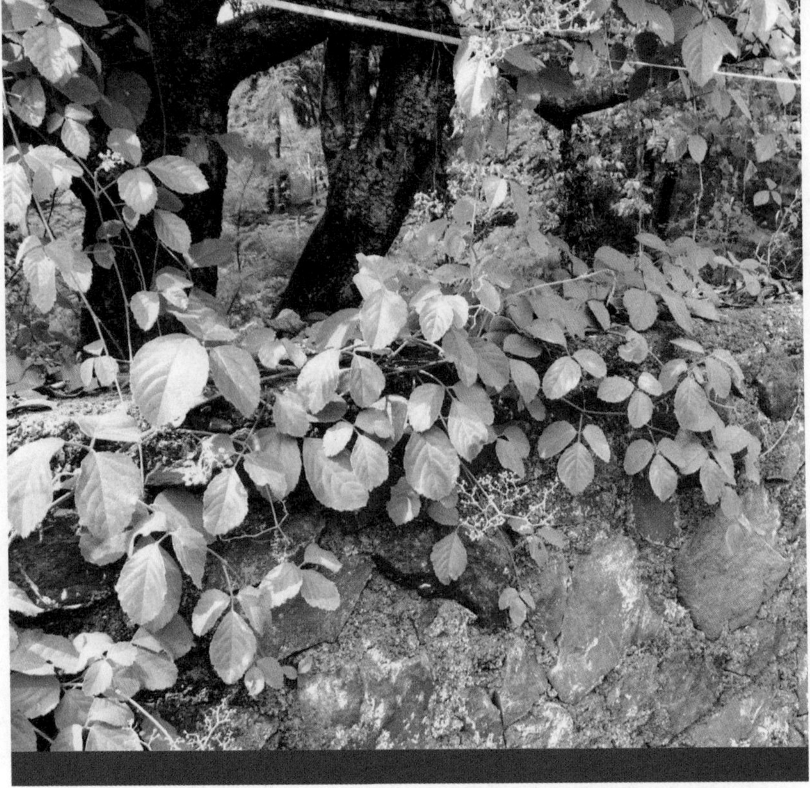

the Kimberley region of Western Australia, the Northern Territory and Far North Queensland. It also occurs in the South Pacific, parts of India and other South-east Asian countries (ALA, 2022; Native Plants Queensland – Townsville Branch, 2022).

Medicinal Uses The juice of the vine was traditionally used by Aboriginal people as a treatment for death adder snakebite (treatment method and efficacy not recorded) (Hiddins, 2001).

Other Uses The tuberous roots of the Three-leaved Cayratia are edible after they have been smashed between two rocks and roasted in hot ashes for about an hour. The roots were harvested between May and November (Cheinmora et al., 2017; Crawford, 1982; DBCA, 2019; Edwards, 2005; Fox & Garde, 2018; Hiddins, 2001; Purdie et al., 2018; Vigilante et al., 2013; Williams, 2012). Crawford (1982) and Cheinmora et al., (2017) warn that, if the tubers are not cooked properly, they will give a person an itchy mouth or throat. The fruit can be eaten raw when ripe and black, but can be slightly bitter (Fox & Garde, 2018; Hiddins, 2001).

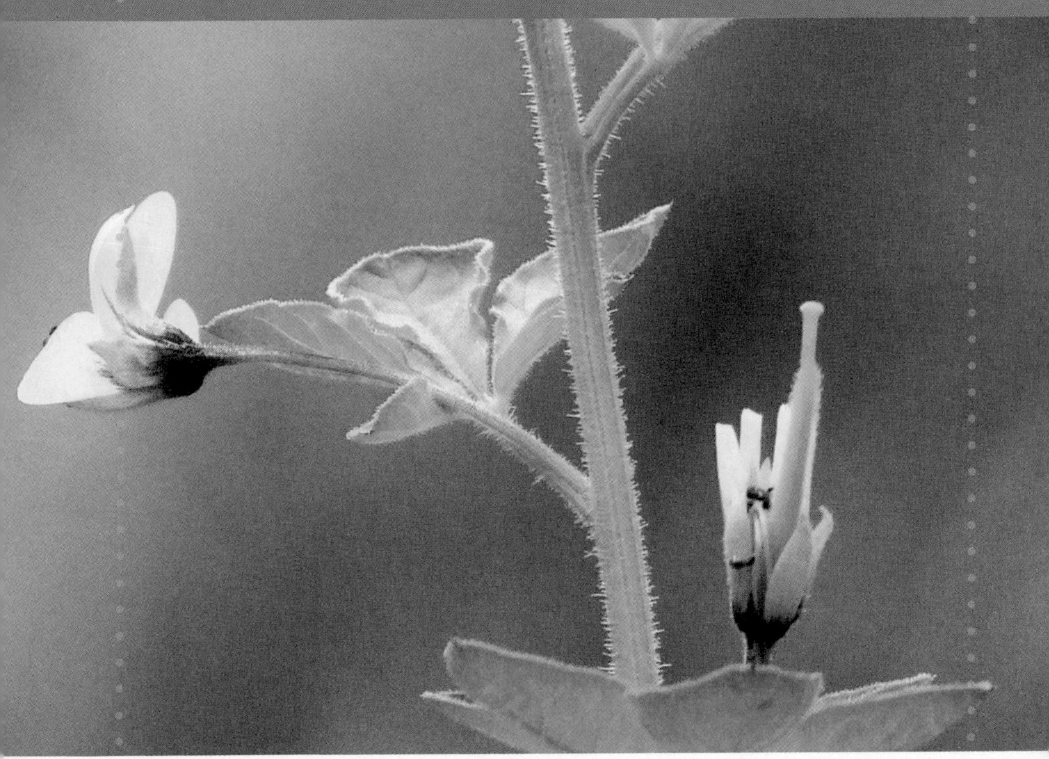

Scientific Name *Arivela viscosa* (L.) Raf., previously known as *Cleome viscosa* L.

Common Names Tickweed, Spider Flower, Asian Spiderflower, Wild Caia, Mustard Bush.

Aboriginal Names Tjinduwadhu (Jindjiparndi), Booloorr-booloorr (Bardi) (Kenneally et al., 1996), Bulur-bulur (Bardi) (Smith & Kalotas, 1985), Purrpurn, Kanturr, Rijijirr, Jirlpirringarni (Walmajarri) (Richards & Hudson, 2012), Tjilpirrinpa, Tjilpirrnganinypa (Kukatja) (Valiquette, 1993), Wijii minya (Kwini) (Cheinmora et al., 2017).

Field Notes Tickweed is a branched, erect, viscid, annual or perennial herb that grows to 1.5 m in height. It has compound, wedge-shaped or spear-shaped leaves and buttercup-like, yellow flowers with four petals that appear any time between February and October. Tickweed occurs in a variety of soils right across the tropical and sub-tropical half of Australia, which includes the Pilbara and

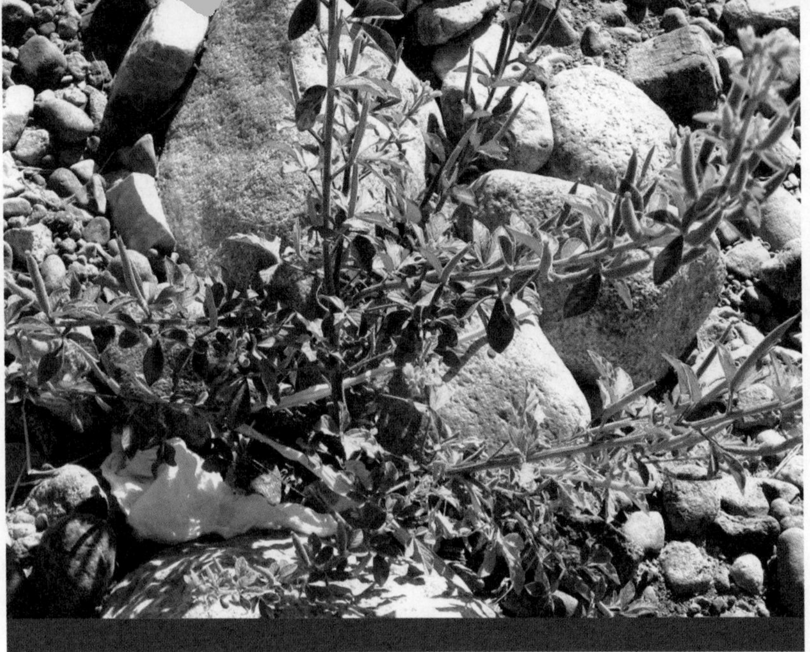

Kimberley regions of Western Australia. The plant is pantropical and is found in many tropical and sub-tropical countries around the world (ALA, 2022; Lassak & McCarthy, 2001; WAH, 2022).

Medicinal Uses The crushed whole Tickweed plant or infusions or decoctions of the crushed whole plant were applied to various parts of the body as a liniment to relieve rheumatic pain, swellings, headache and to heal open sores and leg ulcers. The seeds were chewed to relieve diarrhoea and fever (Cock, 2011; Lassak & McCarthy, 2001; Low, 1990; Reid, 1986; Webb, 1959). The Jaru rubbed the leaves of Tickweed around the inside of the eye socket to treat sore, infected eyes caused by flies (presumably trachoma) (Wightman, 2003). It is also used in traditional medicine in other countries to treat ear infections and intestinal parasites (Lassak & McCarthy, 2001).

Other Uses The seeds of Tickweed are edible (Land for Wildlife, n.d.). The flowers of Tickweed were crushed and rubbed around the eyes as a fly repellent (Kenneally et al., 1996).

Timon Tree

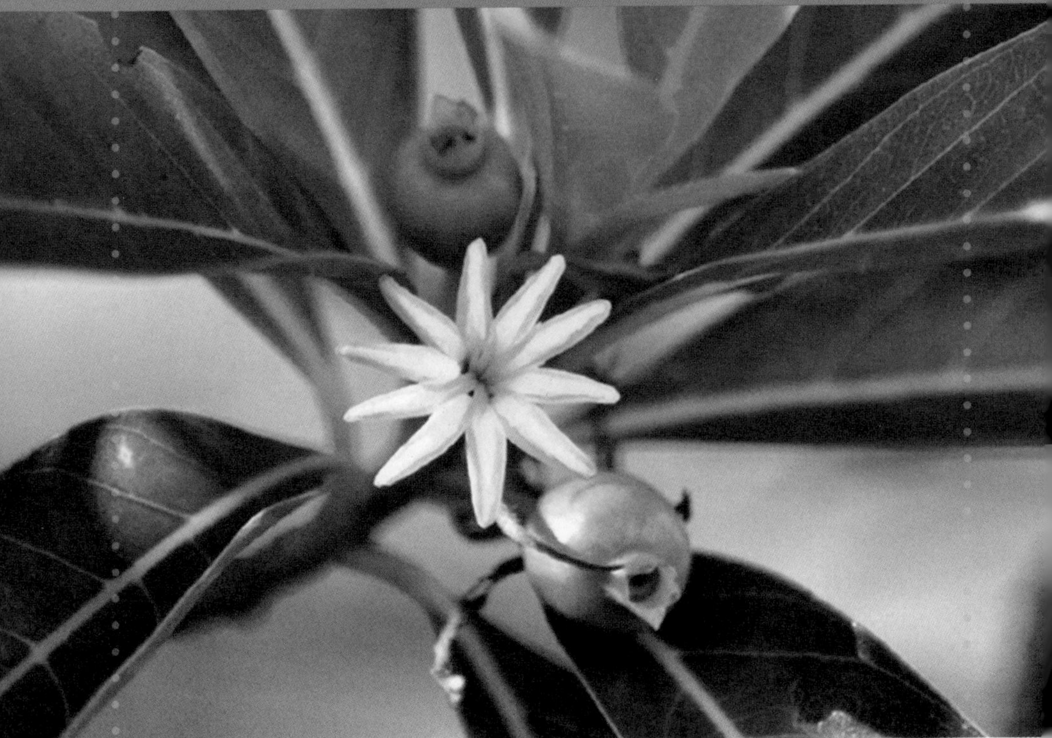

Scientific Name *Timonius timon* (Spreng.) Merr.

Common Names Timon Tree, Tim Tim.

Aboriginal Names Thilnginyi (Bunuba) (Oscar et al., 2019), Garj, Gaaj (Nyul Nyul) (Kenneally et al., 1996), Joonjoonool, Junjunul (Gija) (Purdie et al., 2018; Wightman, 2003), Bandarri minya (Kwini) (Cheinmora et al., 2017).

Field Notes Timon Tree grows as a shrub or tree up to 15 m in height depending on conditions. Its thin, hairy leaves are up to 40 mm long and tapered to a point at the apex. Its white flowers are smaller than the leaves and have two layers of seven petals. The flowers are present between May and November. The fruit are red, globose and about 13 mm in diameter. Timon Tree occurs in sandy, peaty or alluvial soils over rocky sandstone, along watercourses, on tidal flats and riverine flats in the Kimberley region in Western Australia, the Northern Territory and down the east coast of

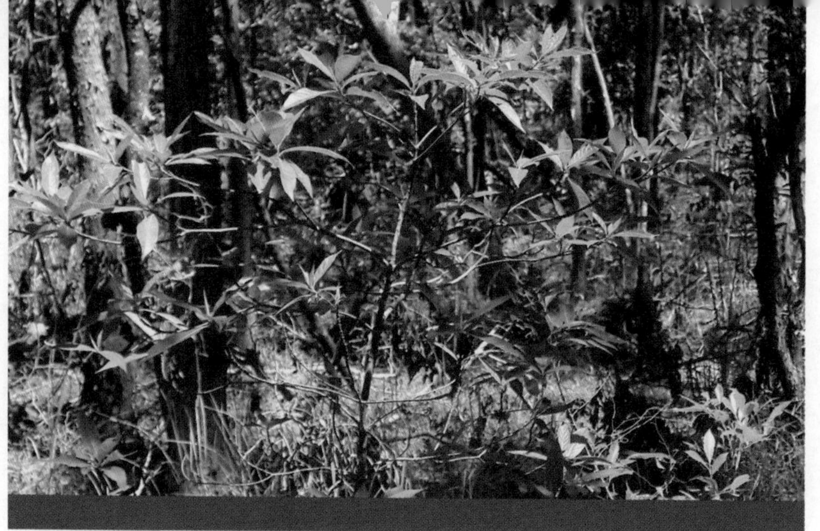

Queensland as far as the border with New South Wales. It also occurs in Indonesia, Papua New Guinea and the Solomon Islands (ALA, 2022; ATRP, 2020; Lassak & McCarthy, 2001; WAH, 2022).

Medicinal Uses Infusions of the dried leaves were used in the treatment of fevers. Fresh leaves were eaten raw or were boiled until soft and eaten as a treatment for coughs, malaria, dyspnoea (shortness of breath), whooping cough and nausea. Juice from fresh leaves that have been heated and squeezed was drunk as a treatment for malaria. Patients with malaria were often bathed in decoctions of the leaves to help reduce fever. Crushed leaves were applied externally as a poultice in the treatment of snakebite. The leaf juice was applied topically as a liniment to relieve arthritic and rheumatic pain. Infusions of the bark were taken internally as a treatment for lung abscesses (Fern, 2021). Decoctions of the crushed wood were used as an eyewash for the treatment of conjunctivitis. Decoctions of the inner bark were drunk to ease the symptoms of colds, influenza and fever (Cock, 2011; Lassak & McCarthy, 2001; Webb, 1959).

Other Uses The fruit of the Timon Tree are edible and are highly esteemed by Aboriginal people wherever the tree grows (Cheinmora et al., 2017; Fern, 2021; Maiden, 1889). The Gija used the wood from the Timon Tree to make boomerangs and woomeras (Purdie et al., 2018).

Tree Orchid

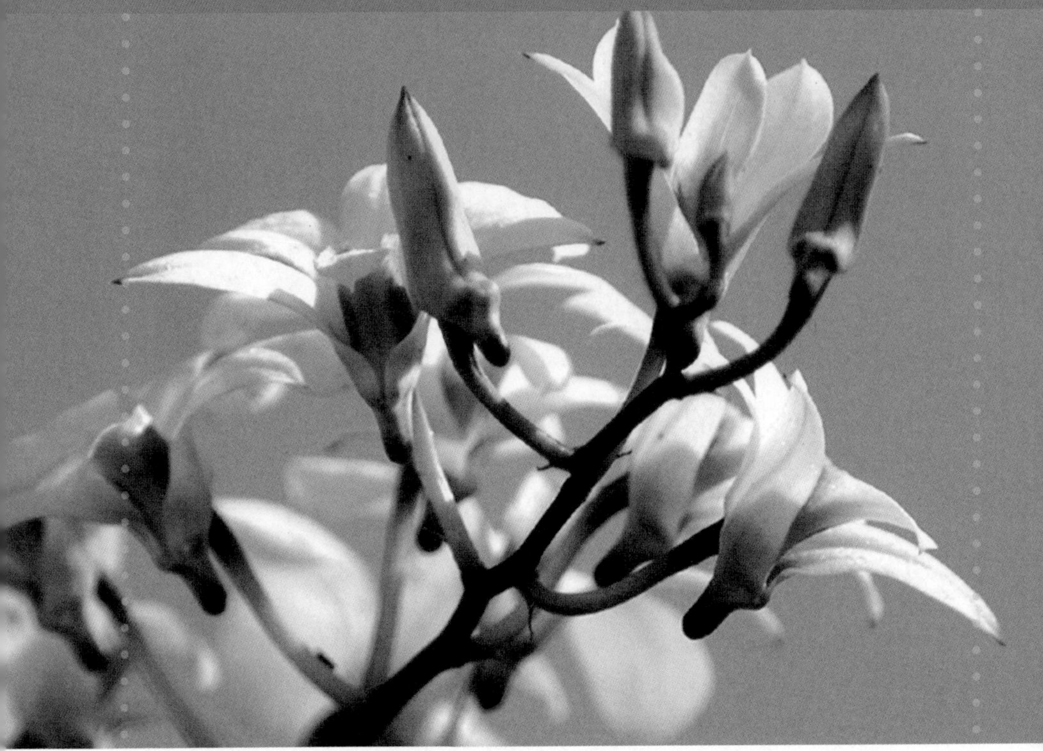

Scientific Name *Dendrobium affine* (Decne.) Steud.

Common Names Tree Orchid, White Butterfly Orchid.

Aboriginal Names Balungguny (Gija) (Gija Bush Food and Medicine, n.d.), Dangilyangal (Kwini) (Cheinmora et al., 2017).

Field Notes Tree Orchid is an epiphytic, perennial herb with tapered to conical pseudobulbs that are up to 700 mm long and 25 mm in diameter. Its leathery, ovate-lanceolate to oblong leaves are up to 200 mm long and 30 mm wide. Its flowers have white sepals and petals with a pink centre and are up to 40 mm wide. Flowering is from May to June. Tree Orchid grows on many species of trees in the far north of the Kimberley region of Western Australia and the Northern Territory. It is also found in New Guinea and on the islands of Timor, Seram and Tanimbar (ALA, 2022; Orchids of New Guinea, 2019; WAH, 2022).

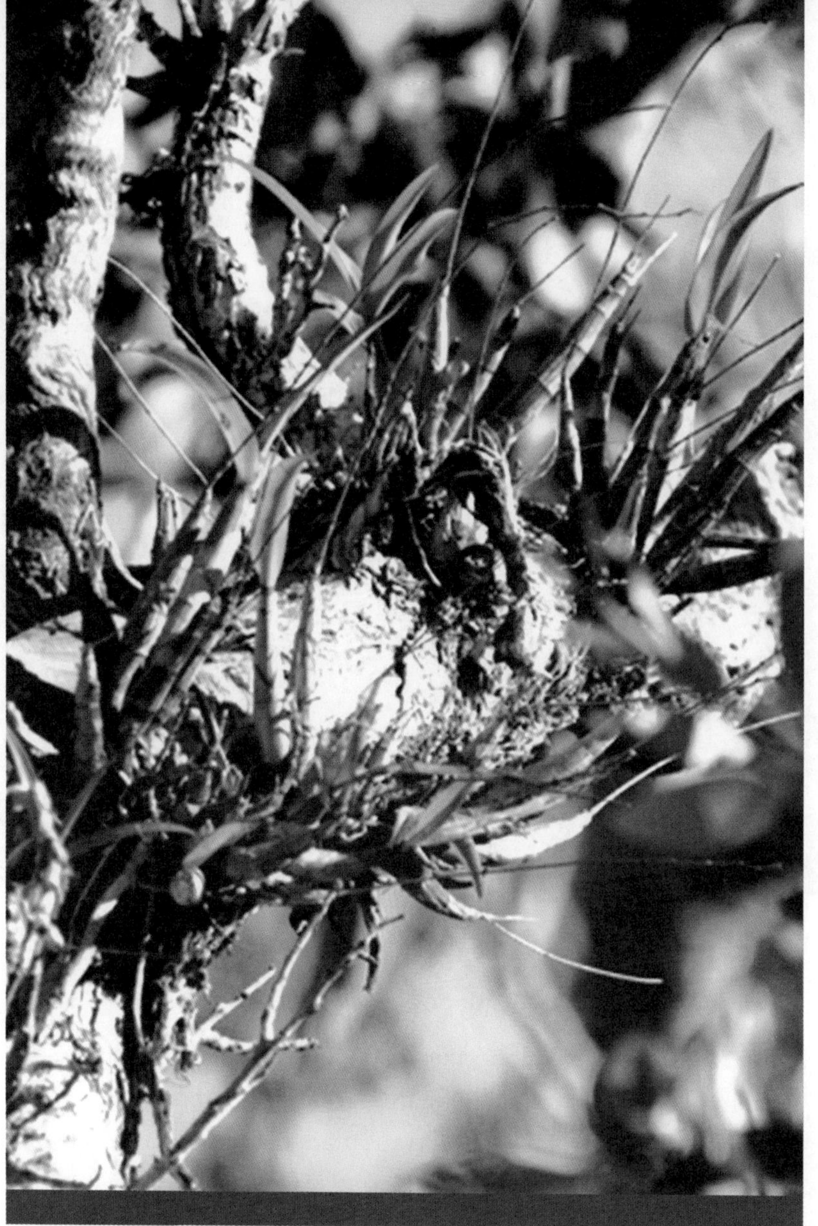

Medicinal Uses Sap or juice from the bulbs of the Tree Orchid was dabbed on wounds, cuts and sores to promote healing (Low, 1990; Smith, 1991; Williams, 2011). The stems were eaten as a cough suppressant (Williams, 2011). The sap from heated leaves was painted on the skin to treat scabies infestations (Wiynjorrotj et al., 2005).

Trefoil Rattlepod

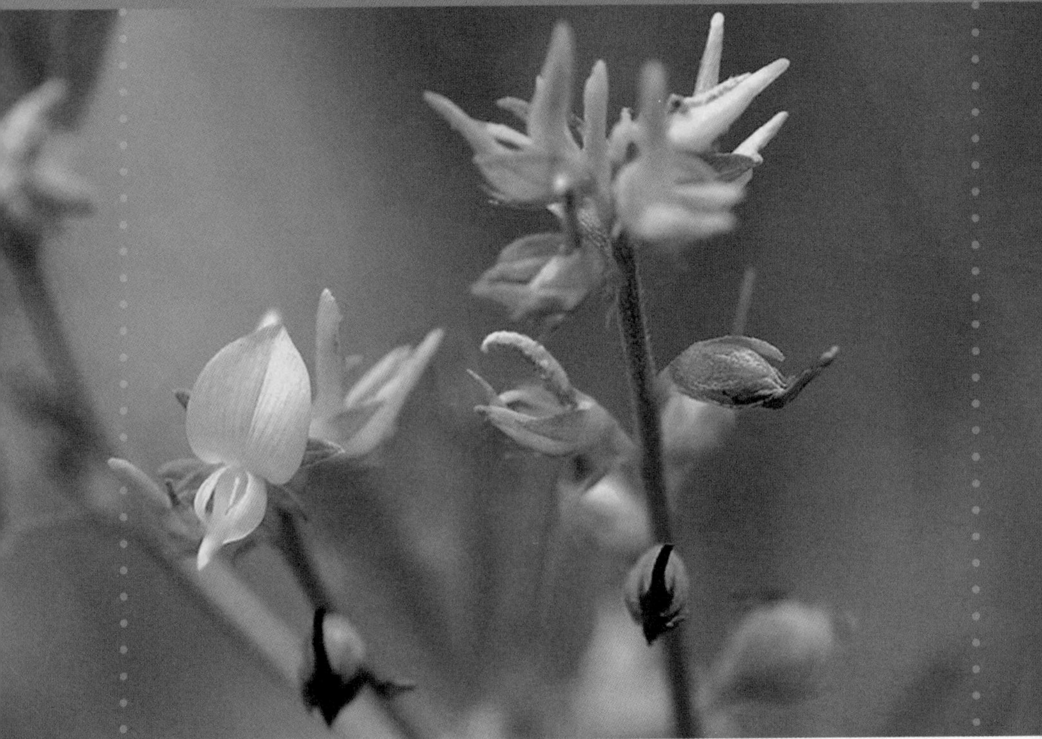

Scientific Name *Crotalaria medicaginea* Lam.

Common Name Trefoil Rattlepod.

Field Notes Trefoil Rattlepod grows as an erect, ascending annual or perennial up to 1 m in height. Its leaves are in groups of three leaflets, the terminal leaflet being subtriangular to narrow-obovate and up to 20 mm long by 7 mm wide. Its yellow flowers are 8 mm long, in few to many (20 or more) terminal erect racemes on peduncles up to 100 mm long. In Australia, the flowers can be present all year round. Its small seed pods are less than 10 mm long and contain only one or two seeds. Trefoil Rattlepod occurs in a variety of soils on sand dunes, hillsides, creekbanks and in gullies across the top half of Australia, including the Pilbara and Kimberley regions of Western Australia. It also occurs in southern China, Afghanistan, the Indian subcontinent, Indonesia, Laos, Myanmar, New Guinea, the Philippines, Thailand and Vietnam (ALA, 2022; eFlora.SA, 2022; Fern, 2021; WAH, 2022).

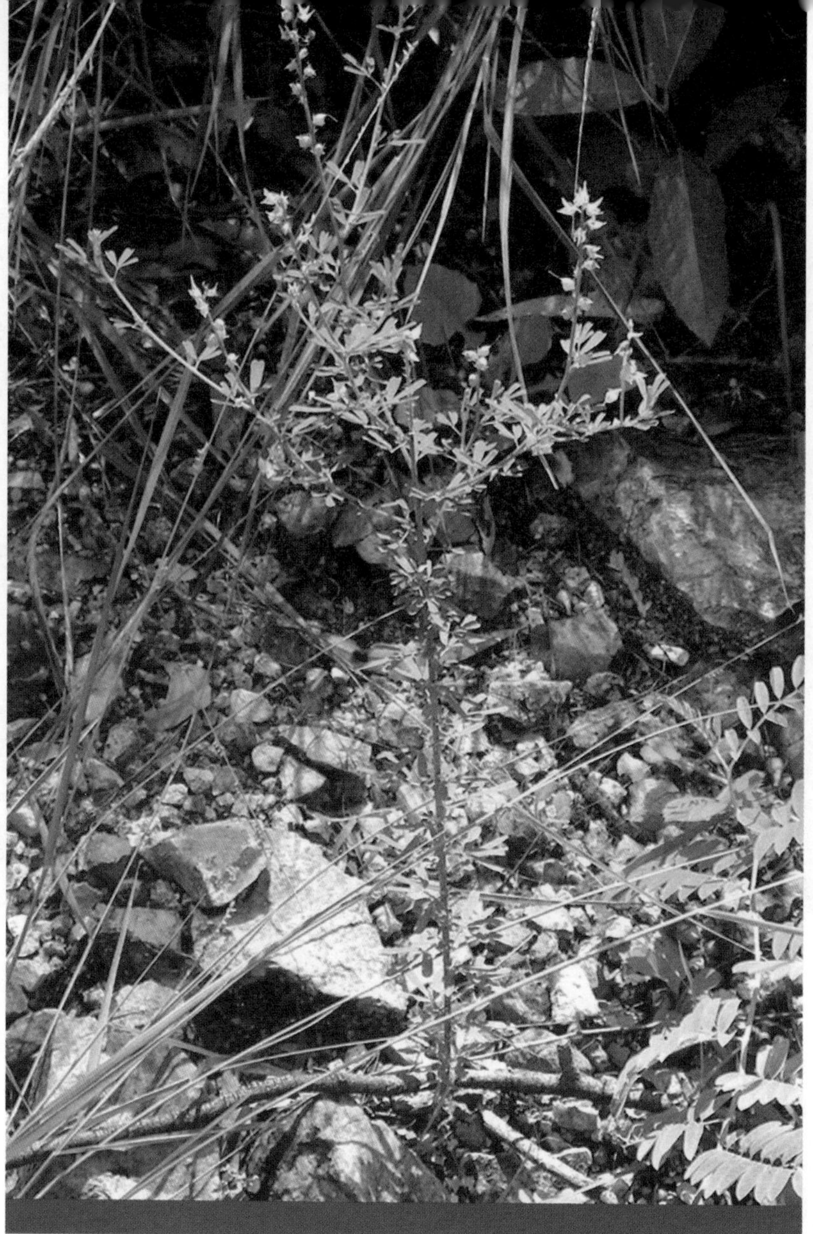

Medicinal Uses Trefoil Rattlepod is used in folk medicine in Africa and Asia where it was taken internally as an expectorant to help expel phlegm. The juice of the leaves is said to reduce excessive salivation. It is used both internally and externally in the treatment of scabies infestations and impetigo. A paste of the leaves is mixed with milk to treat leucorrhoea (white discharge from the vagina) (Fern, 2021).

Tropical Reed

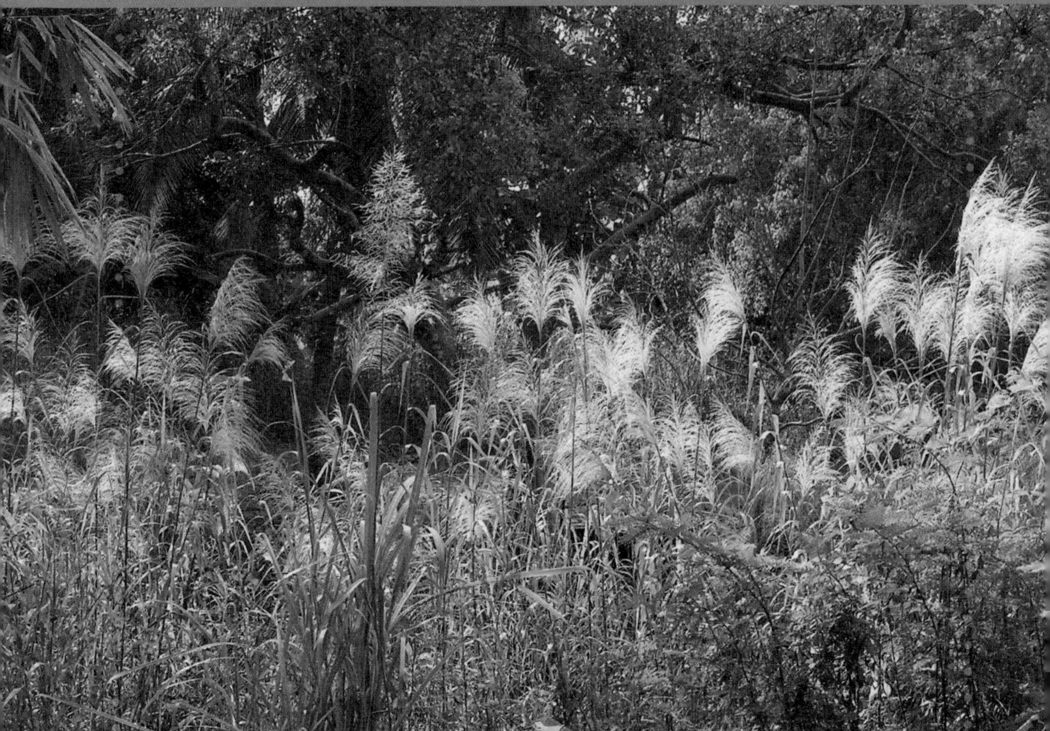

Scientific Names *Phragmites karka* (Retz.) Steud., also known as *Phragmites vallatoria* (Pluk. ex L.) Veldkamp.

Common Names Tropical Reed, Flute Reed, Tall Reed, Nodding Reed.

Aboriginal Names Gamagurd (Kwini) (Crawford, 1982), Kamangkirr (Walmajarri) (Richards & Hudson, 2012).

Field Notes Tropical Reed is a robust, herbaceous perennial grass with woody culms, similar to Bamboo, that can grow up to 10 m in height from an extensive creeping rhizome. Its erect culms can reach 25 mm in diameter. In good conditions, the plant produces large areas of dense growth that excludes most other plant growth. Its leaves are linear and grow from loose sheaths on the culms up to 800 mm long and 40 mm wide. The inflorescences are compound panicles, bearing juvenile spikelets as they emerge, with up to 500 peduncles per sheath. Its fertile spikelets are many flowered,

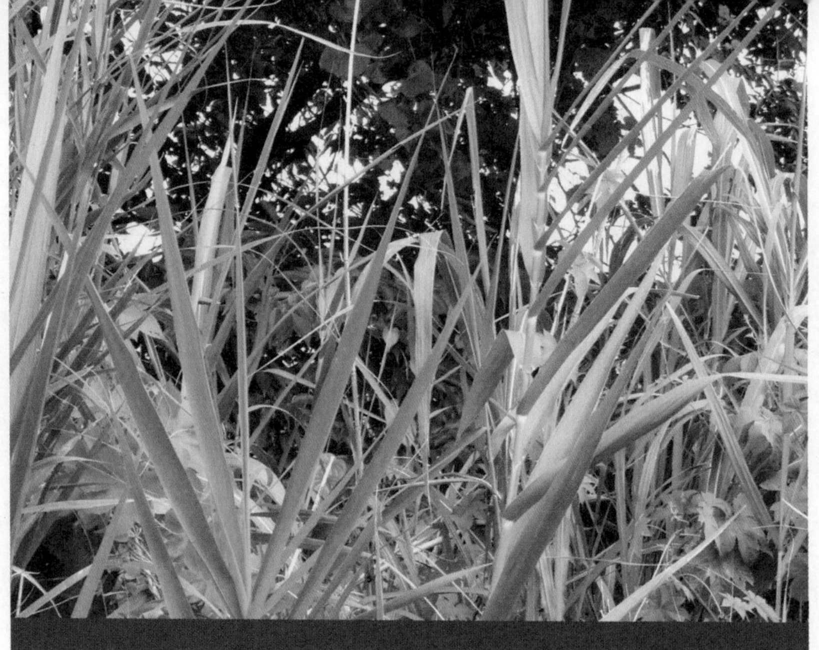

comprising up to 11 fertile florets. Its lower glumes are elliptic and up to 4.5 mm long with the upper glumes being up to 6 mm long. Tropical Reed occurs in the Pilbara and Kimberley regions of Western Australia, the Northern Territory, Queensland and South Australia. It also occurs in Africa, temperate Asia, tropical Asia and on some Pacific islands (ALA, 2022; AusGrass2, 2022).

Medicinal Uses Tropical Reed is used in Ayurvedic medicine in India where the roots were used to treat broken bones. Decoctions of the whole plant are used externally as a liniment to treat arthritic and rheumatic pain. The rhizomes and roots have anti-emetic and diaphoretic properties and were used to treat diabetes. In China, preparations of the rhizomes are regarded as cooling and diuretic (SMIP, 2022).

Other Uses The young shoots of Tropical Reed are edible cooked and can be eaten like asparagus or bamboo shoots. In China, the young shoots are preserved with a coating of salt then dried for later use (Fern, 2021). The Kwini use the culms for spear shafts (Crawford, 1982).

Tropical Speedwell

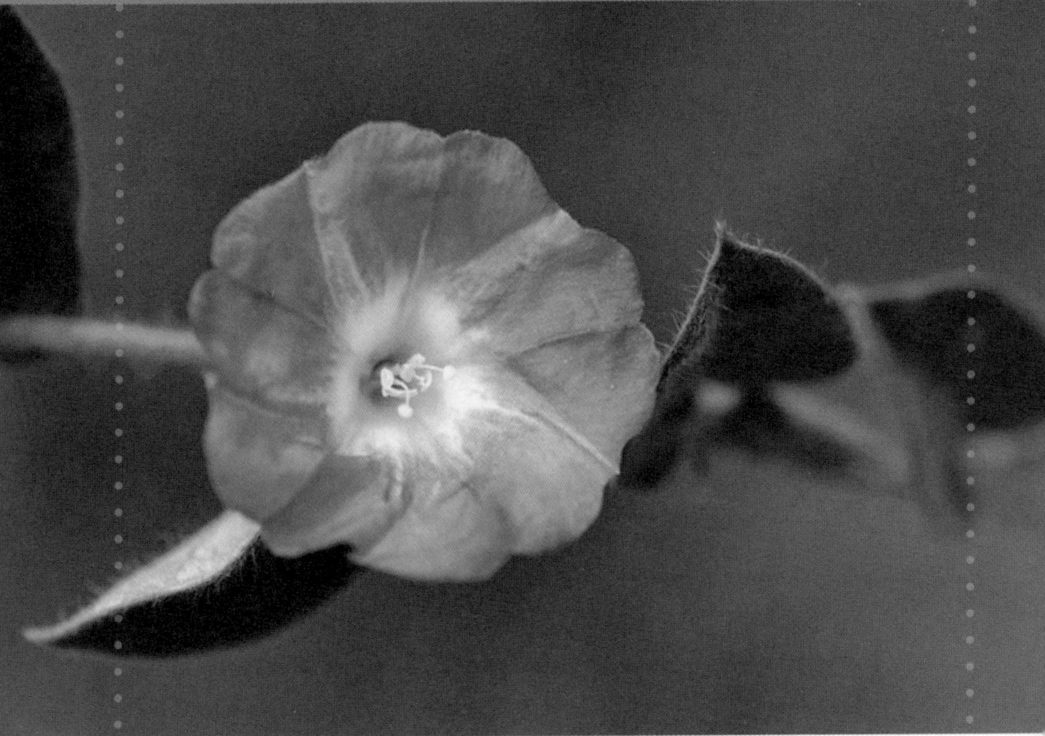

Scientific Name *Evolvulus alsinoides* (L.) L.

Common Names Tropical Speedwell, Dwarf Morning Glory.

Field Notes Tropical Speedwell is a perennial, usually extremely hairy herb that only grows to around 500 mm in height. Its leaves are lanceolate to ovate and up to 10 mm in length or larger. Its round, blue or white flowers appear either solitary or in pairs on a long stalk. Flowering is from January to August. Its fruit are globose capsules, which contain four seeds. Tropical Speedwell occurs in sand, loam or clay, on dunes, plains and amongst boulders, along watercourses and drainage lines in the Pilbara and Kimberley regions of Western Australia, the Northern Territory, Queensland and New South Wales. The true origins of the plant are unknown, but it is now widely spread through most dry tropical and sub-tropical regions of the world (ALA, 2022; Fern, 2021; Flowers of India, 2022; Lassak & McCarthy, 2001; WAH, 2022).

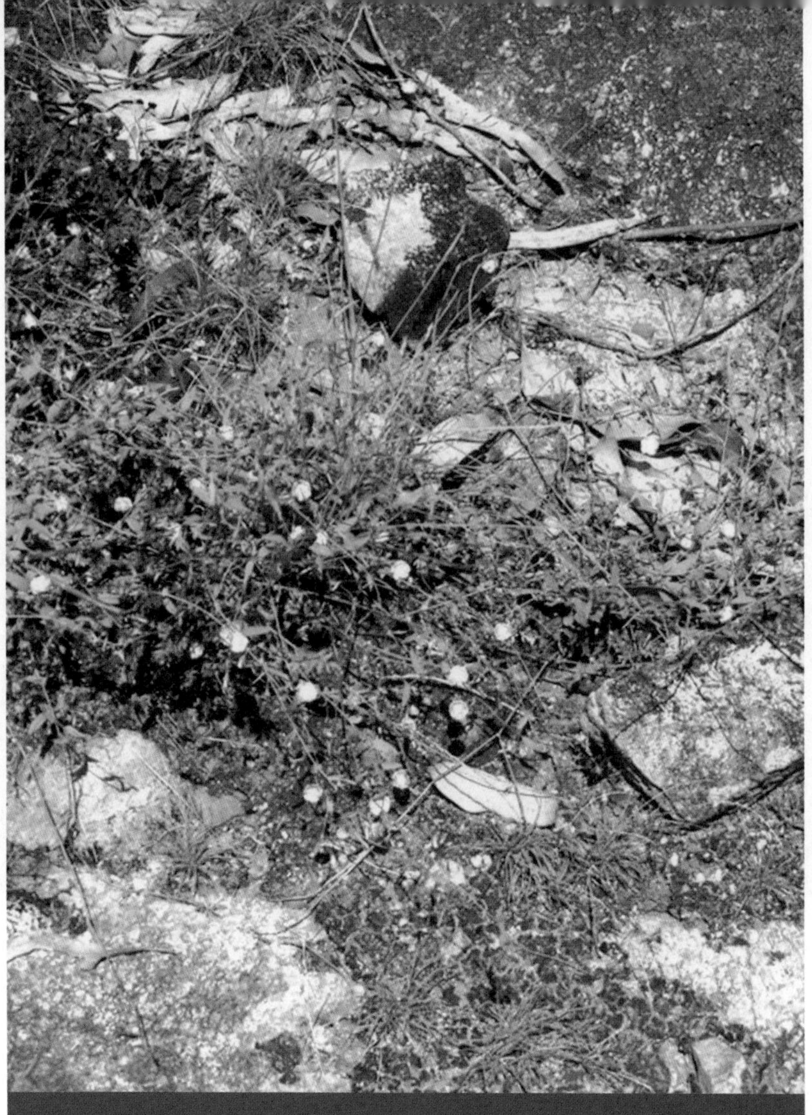

Medicinal Uses Decoctions of the stalks, leaves and roots of Tropical Speedwell were taken internally for diarrhoea, dysentery, intestinal parasites and fever (Cock, 2011; Fern, 2021; Lassak & McCarthy, 2001). Tropical Speedwell is also used in folk medicine in other countries. A powder made from dried leaves was applied topically to treat wounds and sores. Mashed leaves were applied as a poultice on enlarged glands in the neck. Cigarettes were made from the leaves and were smoked to relieve bronchitis and asthma (Fern, 2021).

Turpentine Wattle

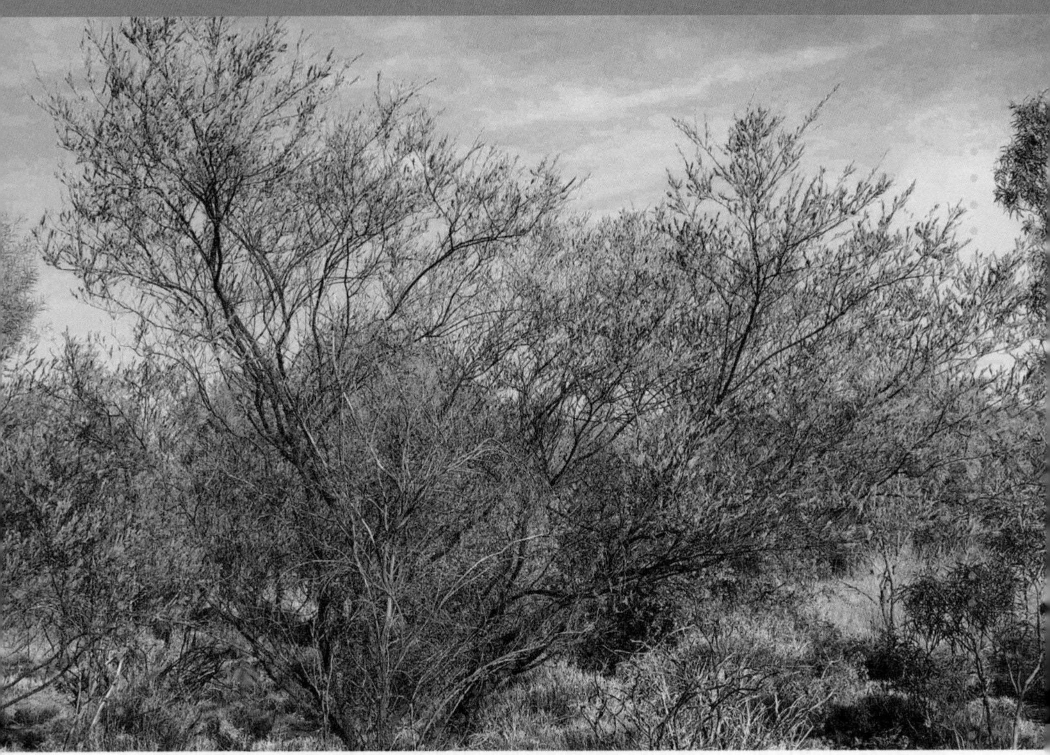

Scientific Name *Acacia lysiphloia* F.Muell.

Common Names Turpentine Wattle, Turpentine, Turpentine Bush.

Aboriginal Names Kanturrpa, Kawarrpa, Pirrpinpa, Purrpurnpa (Kukatja) (Valiquette, 1993), Baalinyji (Gija) (Purdie et al., 2018), Jiwi (Jaru) (Deegan et al., 2010), Burrurn, Burrirn (Jaru) (Wightman, 2003).

Field Notes Turpentine Wattle is a spreading, viscid shrub that grows up to 4 m in height. It has minni-ritchi (curly) bark, and linear-obovate phyllodes that have an angled arrangement and are typically 50 mm long and 7 mm wide. Its yellow flower spikes are axillary, dense and up to 50 mm long. Flowering is from May to September. The fruit or seed pods are straight to strongly curved, flat and up to 100 mm long and 12 mm wide. Turpentine Wattle occurs in red sand, loam, clay or ironstone soils on plains, stony hills, low-lying areas, along streams, in open mixed eucalypt and

Acacia woodland, low scrub and spinifex grassland in the east Pilbara and Kimberley regions of Western Australia, the Northern Territory and north-west Queensland (ALA, 2022; Maslin et al., 2010; WAH, 2022).

Medicinal Uses Crushed phyllodes and branches of Turpentine Wattle were heated over hot coals then used as a poultice on sore muscles and joints for pain relief. Decoctions of the leaves were used externally as a wash to relieve the symptoms of colds, influenza, headaches and itchy skin. Young children were 'smoked' by passing them over a pit of smoking leaves and branches of Turpentine Wattle, which had been mixed with a little powdered termite nest, to promote their health (Morse, 2005; Smith, 1991; Williams, 2011).

Other Uses The seeds of Turpentine Wattle are edible and were ground into flour to make damper or Johnny cakes or used as a tasty additive (Fern, 2021). The roots of this tree often contain Witchetty Grubs, which the Gija and Jaru call 'lagan' or 'laju', that are excellent food (Wightman, 2003). The Gija use long, straight stems from the Turpentine Wattle to make spear shafts (Purdie et al., 2018).

Umbrella Bush

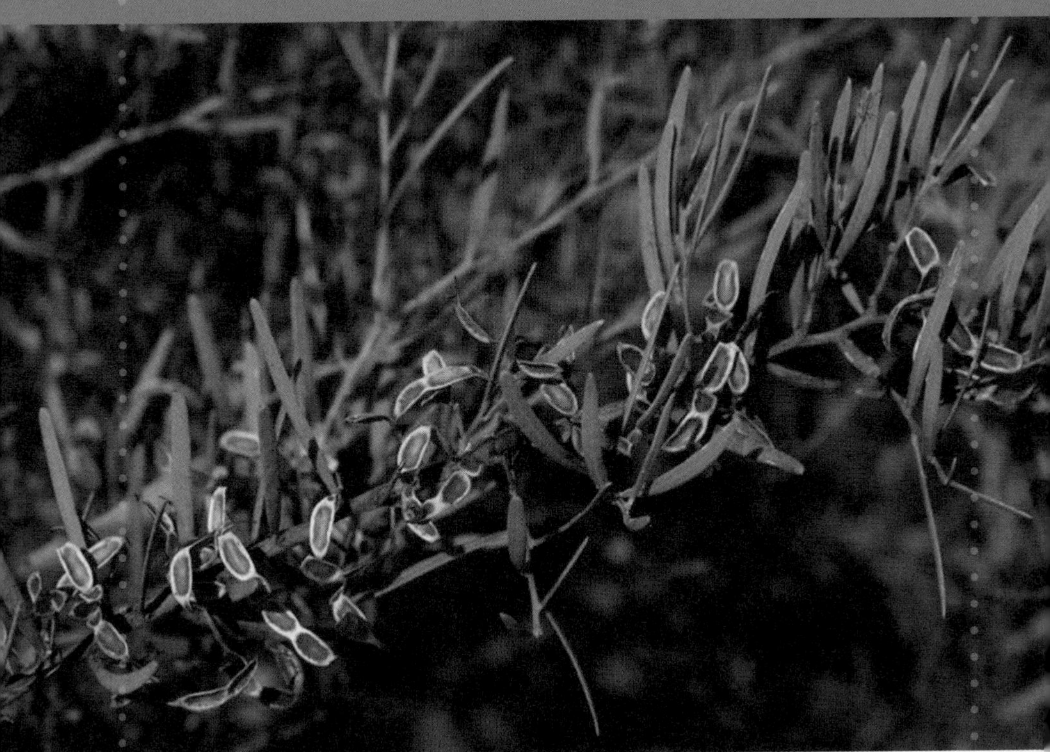

Botanical Name *Acacia ligulata* Benth.

Common Names Umbrella Bush, Small Cooba, Sandhill Wattle, Marpoo, Dune Wattle, Small Coobah, Wirra.

Aboriginal Names Mulkurru, Murlupuka, Putarrpa, Wartarrka (Kukatja) (Valiquette, 1993), Mulkuru, Warlumarti (Ngardi) (Cataldi, 2004).

Description Umbrella Bush is a Wattle that grows as a shrub or small tree to around 4 m in height. It is sometimes dome-shaped but often branches from the ground. The bark is usually grooved at the base but smooth further up. The narrow, oblong-shaped phyllodes are light green to blue-green in colour and grow to around 100 mm long. The yellow to orange, globular flower heads appear along the stems between the leaves from May to October. The curved seed pods are light brown and grow to around 100 mm in length. Umbrella Bush occurs in dry, alkaline soils on coastal

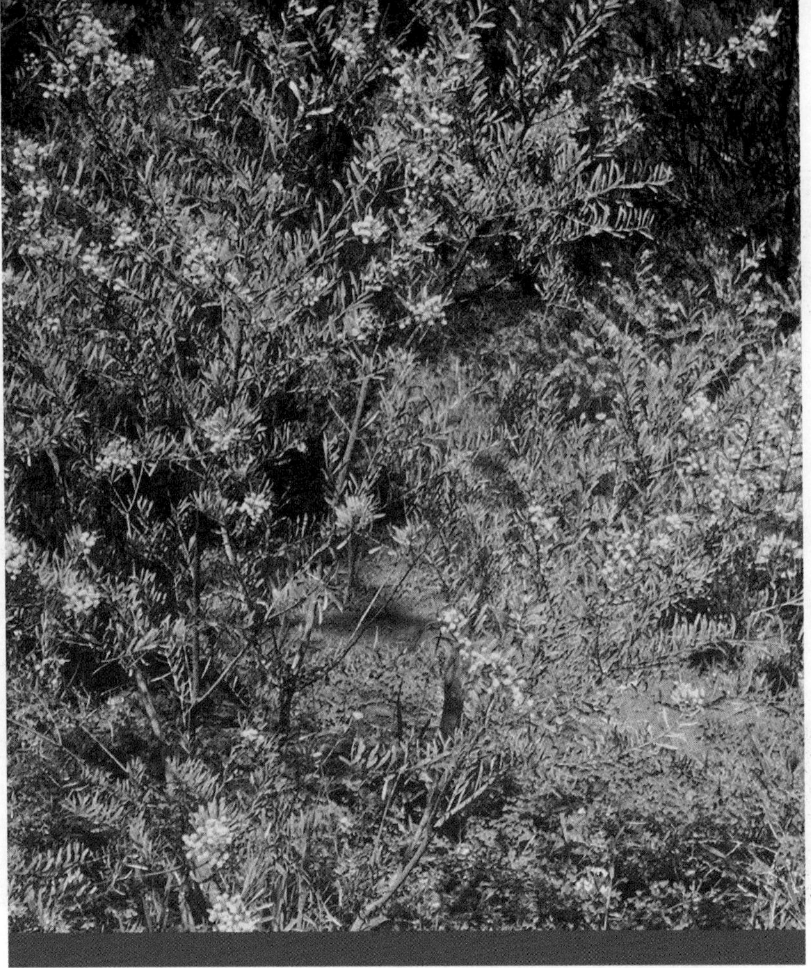

sand dunes over most of Western Australia, South Australia and in the drier regions of southern Queensland, New South Wales and Victoria (ALA, 2022; Bindon, 1996; WAH, 2022).

Medicinal Uses Infusions or decoctions of the bark were used as a cough suppressant and as an antiseptic wash for burns. Decoctions of the bark were also used as general treatment for dizziness, anxiety and seizures. The branches were used as 'smoke medicine' to smoke people suffering from general sickness and women following childbirth (Bindon, 1996; Williams, 2011).

Other Uses The seeds of Umbrella Bush are edible and were ground to a paste and eaten (Bindon, 1996). Witchetty Grubs that inhabited the root system were eaten raw or roasted. The shrub was burnt and the ash mixed with the Native Tobacco or Pituri (*Duboisia hopwoodii*) for chewing (Lassak & McCarthy, 2008).

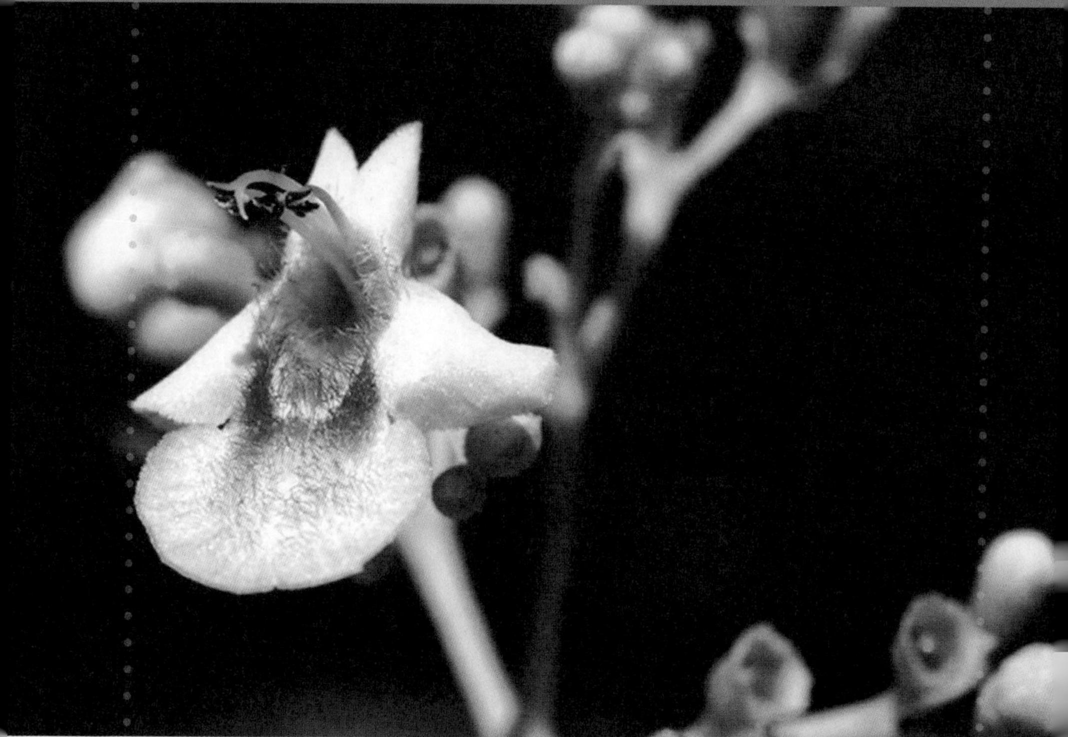

Scientific Name *Vitex glabrata* R.Br.

Common Names Vitex, Smooth Chastetree, Black Plum, Gentileng, Bihbool.

Aboriginal Names Maina (Bunuba) (Oscar et al., 2019), Mejerren (Miriwoong) (Leonard et al., 2013), Girndiyi (Jaru) (Deegan et al., 2010), Inger (Bardi) (Smith & Kalotas, 1985), Ingiirrii (Bardi) (Kenneally et al., 1996), Kukulangi or kulangi (Balanggarra), Gulangi (Wunambal, Gaambera) (Karadada et al., 2011; Vigilante et al., 2013), Minyjiwarrany, Minyjaarrany, Minyjoowarrany, Jawoolji (Gija) (Purdie et al., 2018; Wightman, 2003), Girndi (Gooniyandi) (Dilkes-Hall et al., 2019), Manjarra minya, Kulangi minya (Kwini) (Cheinmora et al., 2017; Crawford, 1982).

Field Notes Vitex is a tree that grows up to 20 m in height. The bark is finely fissured. Its leaves are ovate, have a pointed apex and are up to 60 mm long. Its small white to white-blue-purple flowers

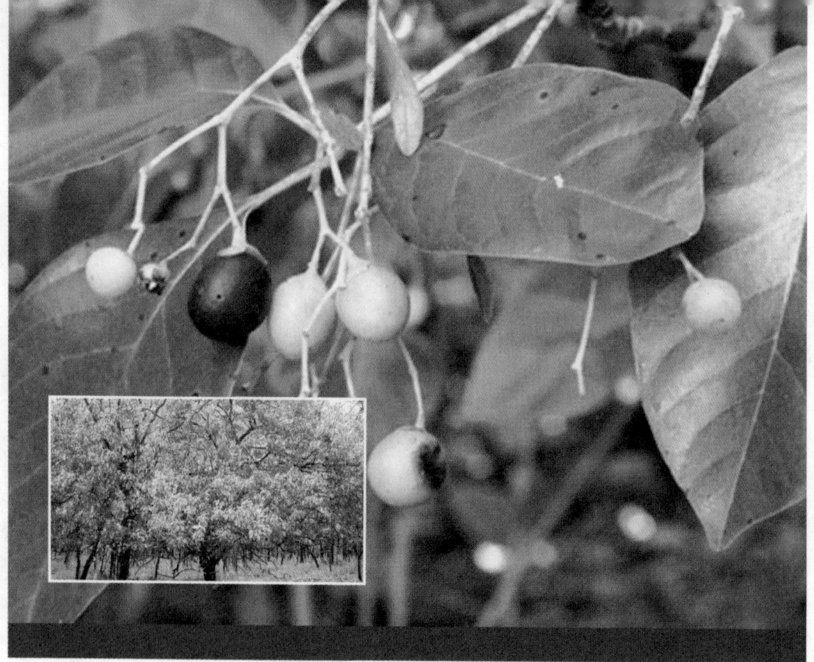

are tubular or cup-shaped. Flowering in Australia is between June and December. The fruit are obovoid to ellipsoid and up to 9 mm in diameter, turning black when ripe. Vitex occurs in sand or laterite in gullies, on floodplains, on rocky hills and along ridges in the Kimberley region of Western Australia, the Northern Territory and Far North Queensland (ALA, 2022; ATRP, 2020; WAH, 2022). It also occurs in Assam, Bangladesh, India, through tropical Asia to Indonesia, the Philippines, Papua New Guinea and the Mariana Islands (Fern, 2021).

Medicinal Uses Decoctions of the bark of Vitex were taken internally in some countries to treat intestinal parasites and as a remedy for gastrointestinal disorders (Fern, 2021).

Other Uses The fruit of the Vitex tree are edible when black and ripe, which in Australia is from late February through March (Crawford, 1982; Isaacs, 1987; Karadada et al., 2011; Wightman, 2003). Sugarbag honey hives are often found in this tree (Oscar et al., 2019).

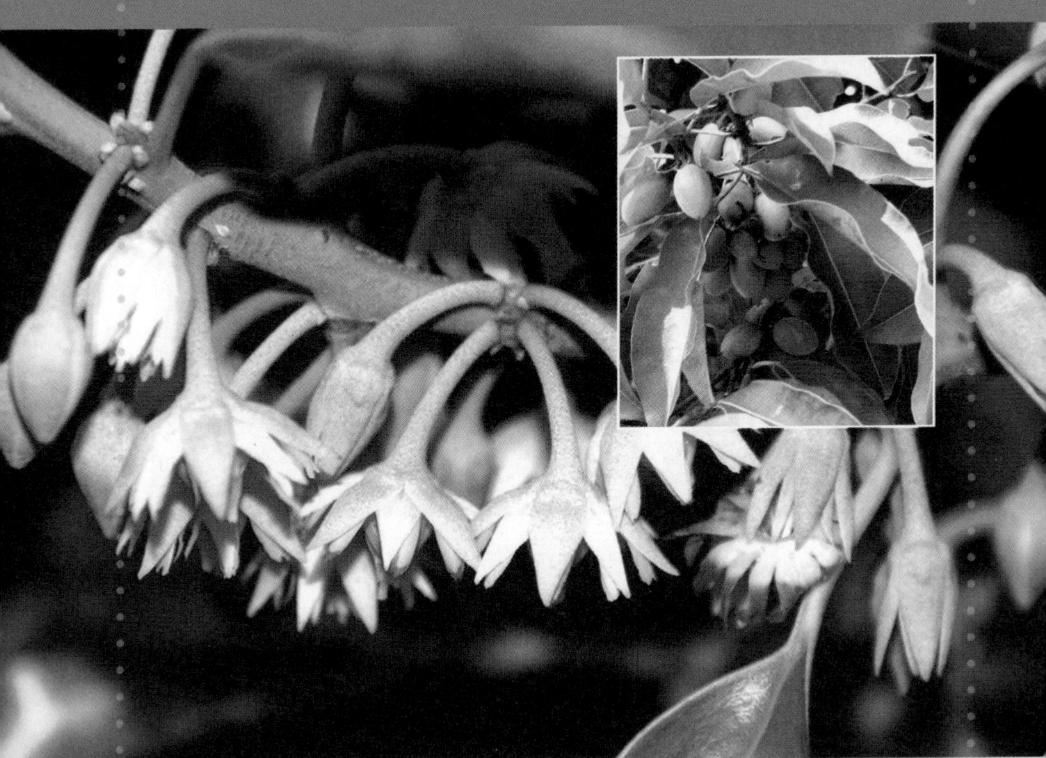

Scientific Name *Mimusops elengi* L.

Common Names Walara, Medlar, Bullet Wood, Bush Jaffa, Spanish Cherry.

Aboriginal Names Mamajen (Nyul Nyul) (Kenneally et al., 1996), Djungun (Bardi (Smith & Kalotas, 1985), Joongoon (Bardi) (Environs Kimberley, n.d.), Yangkowii (Wunambal), Walarra (Wunambal, Gaambera) (Karadada et al., 2011), Walarra minya (Kwini) (Cheinmora et al., 2017; Crawford, 1982).

Field Notes Walara grows as a shrub or tree up to 16 m in height. Its green, ovate leaves are pointed at the end and up to 110 mm long. Its small white or cream, star-shaped flowers appear between January and September. Its fruit are globular to ellipsoid, about 15 mm in diameter and turn red when ripe. Walara occurs in sandy soils, over sandstone and basalt in coastal and near-coastal areas in the Kimberley region of Western Australia, the Northern Territory,

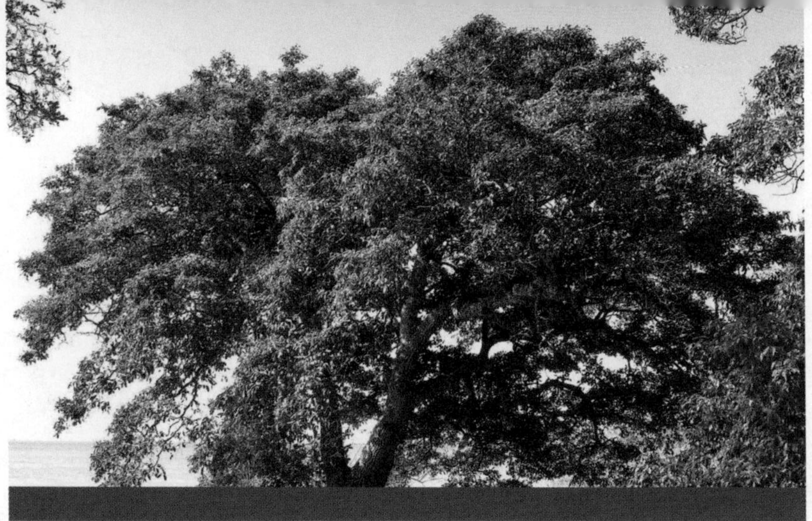

Cape York Peninsula and southwards as far as coastal central Queensland. It is also endemic to India, Indonesia, Malaysia, New Caledonia, New Guinea, the Philippines, Sri Lanka, Thailand and Vanuatu (ALA, 2022; ATRP, 2020; Flowers of India, 2022; WAH, 2022).

Medicinal Uses Walara is used in traditional medicine in South-east Asian countries, especially in India and Sri Lanka where it is used in Ayurvedic medicine. Decoctions of the bark were taken internally to treat diarrhoea and dysentery. Decoctions of the bark and flowers were used as a gargle to treat periodontitis (gum inflammation) and toothache, and externally as a wash to treat snakebite, fever, wounds, scabies infestations and eczema. Infusions or decoctions of the crushed leaves were used externally to treat headache, toothache, wounds and conjunctivitis. The seeds are pounded to a powder and the powder ingested to treat constipation (ALA, 2022; Fern, 2021; Flowers of India, 2022).

Other Uses The fruit of the Walara tree are edible when ripe and are a bright red-orange in colour. They are eaten either raw or warmed in hot sand or ashes. The fruit are available from May to August in Australia (Cheinmora et al., 2017; Crawford, 1982; Edwards, 2005; Fern, 2021; Karadada et al., 2011; Maiden, 1889; Smith & Kalotas, 1995; Vigilante et al., 2013).

CAUTION: SKIPA (2022) warns that eating too many of this fruit can cause constipation.

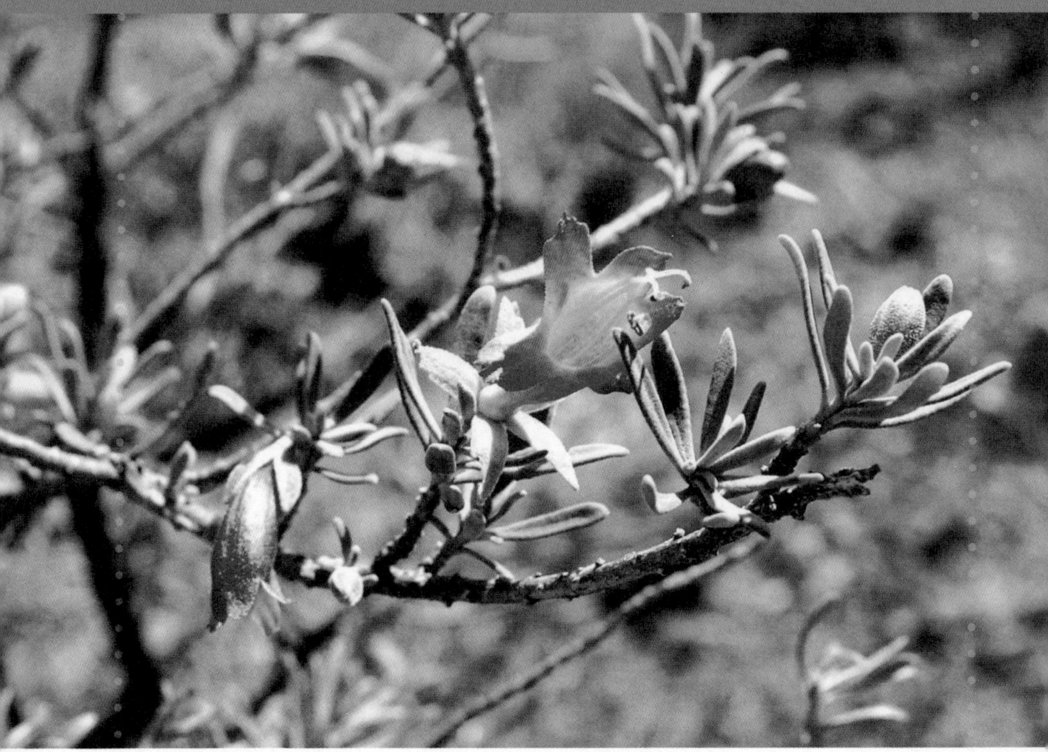

Scientific Name *Eremophila latrobei* F.Muell.

Common Names Warty Fuchsia Bush, Warty-leaf Eremophila, Poverty Bush, Native Fuchsia, Crimson Turkey Bush.

Aboriginal Names Marlupirna, Miinypa, Ngularnpa, Pinytjalpa (Kukatja) (Valiquette, 1993), Miyinypa, Yalnyilingi (Ngardi) (Cataldi, 2004).

Field Notes Warty Fuchsia Bush is a green to silver-green shrub that grows to 2 m tall, but may be as low as 800 mm when in open areas. Its leaves are lanceolate to ovate, finely hairy and up to 40 mm long. The upper surface of the leaf usually has a warty appearance. Its flowers are tubular, orange to red and up to 35 mm long, with stamens extending up to 20 mm beyond the flower tube. Flowering is from April to October. Its fruit are up to 10 mm long with a pointy end. Warty Fuchsia Bush occurs in stony red clay, loam or sandy soils over sandstone, granite and ironstone on gibber

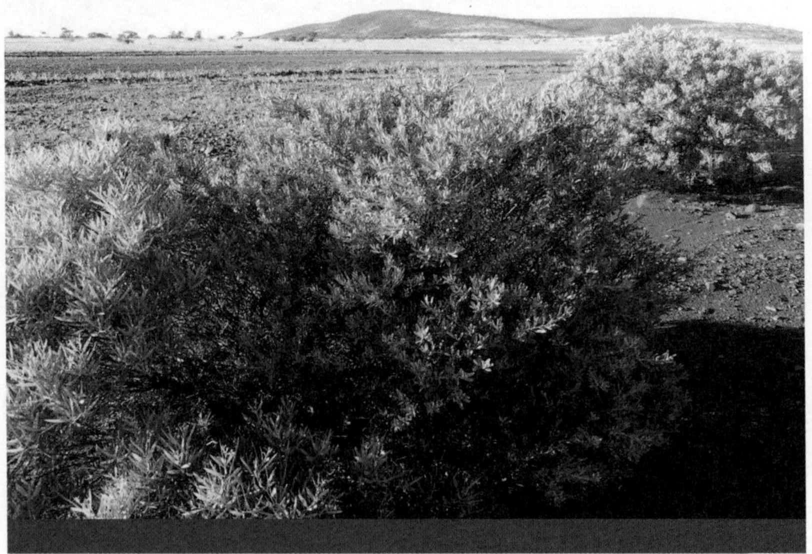

plains, rocky ridges, hillslopes and along creek lines all over the Gascoyne, Mid-west, Goldfields–Esperance and Pilbara regions of Western Australia and the southern reaches of the Kimberley region. Its range extends through all the other mainland states and territories, except Victoria (ALA, 2022; Department Of Primary Industries and Regional Development, 2022; WAH, 2022).

Medicinal Uses The juice from leaves of Warty Fuchsia Bush was used as a 'rubbing medicine' (liniment) to treat arthritic and rheumatic pain. Infusions or decoctions of the leaves were taken internally to treat the symptoms of colds, influenza, headaches and infections. Fresh stems were crushed and put near a decaying tooth to treat toothache. Nectar was sucked straight from the flowers to soothe sore throats (Smith, 1991; Williams, 2013). Decoctions of the leaves were used to treat scabies infestations. The leaves were also added to a smouldering fire for 'smoke medicine' to strengthen babies and to treat diarrhoea (Morse, 2005; Williams, 2013).

Other Uses The sweet nectar was sucked directly from the flowers of Warty Fuchsia Bush as a quick treat (Smith, 1991; Williams, 2013).

Weeping Denhamia

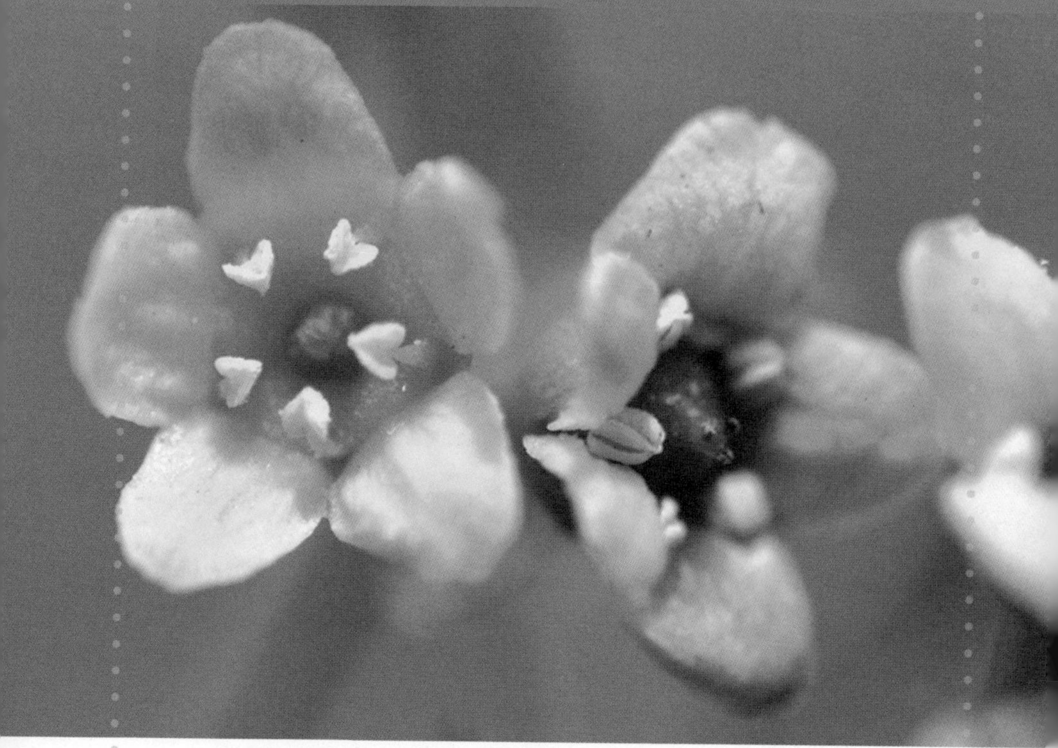

Scientific Name *Denhamia obscura* (A.Rich.) Walp.

Common Names Weeping Denhamia, Denhamia.

Field Notes Weeping Denhamia grows as a shrub or tree up to 9 m in height. It has dense weeping foliage with ovate leaf blades up to 120 mm long, and small, star-shaped, cream to yellow-green flowers that are present from April to August. Its attractive pale-yellow fruit are capsules about 40 mm long with red seeds. Weeping Denhamia occurs in sand and rocky sandstone soils in open forest, monsoon forest, on screes and cliffs in the Kimberley region of Western Australia and the Northern Territory. It has also been sighted in a few places in Queensland (ALA, 2022; ATRP, 2020; WAH, 2022).

Medicinal Uses Some Aboriginal groups plugged cavities in their teeth with the inner bark of Weeping Denhamia to ease toothache (Low, 1990).

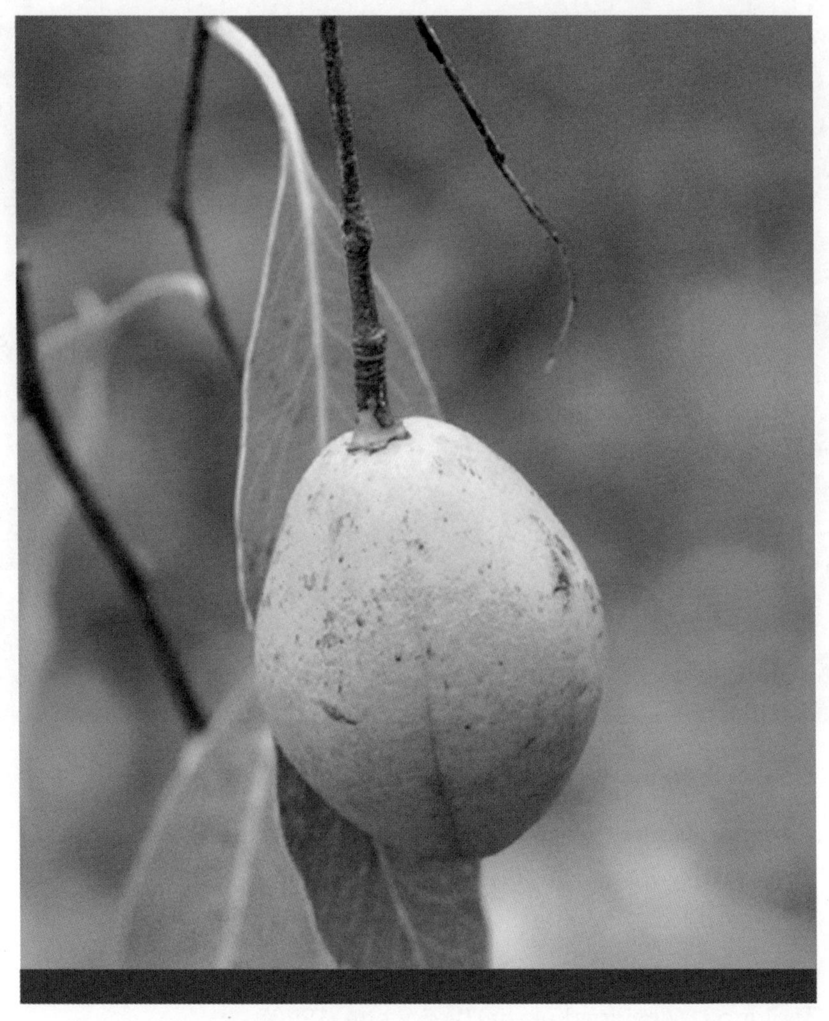

Weeping Pittosporum

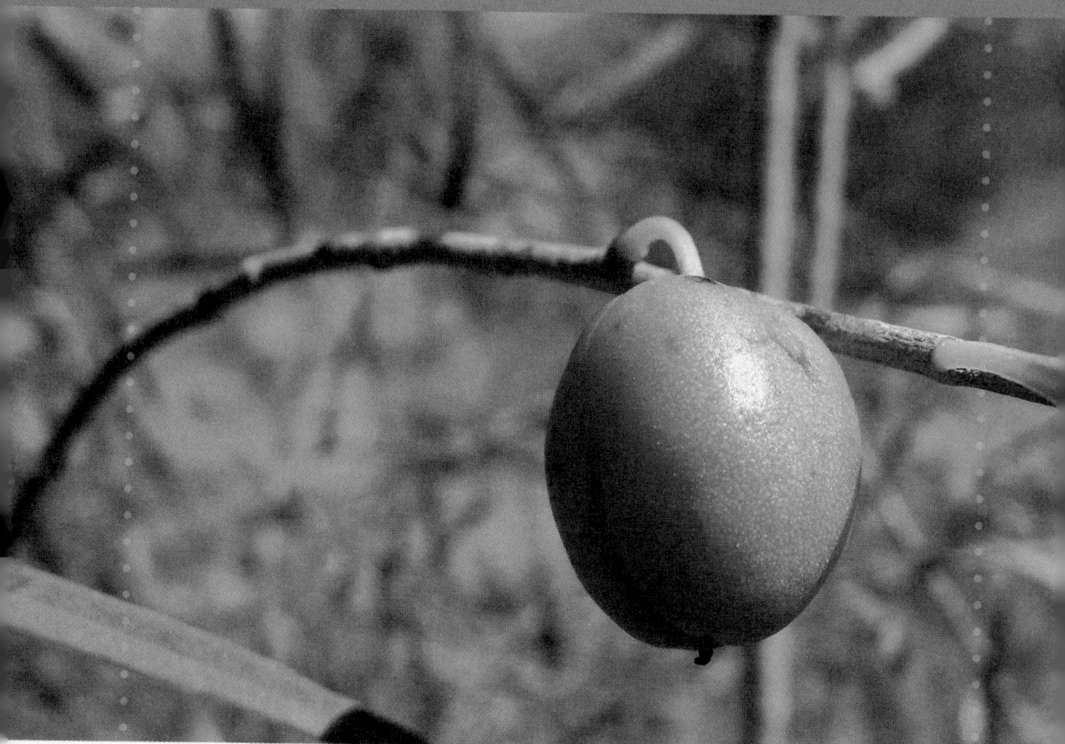

Scientific Name *Pittosporum angustifolium* Lodd.

Common Names Weeping Pittosporum, Butterbush, Native Willow, Poison Berry Tree, Gumbi Gumbi, Gumby Gumby, Cattle Bush, Native Apricot.

Aboriginal Names Karlayin, Katarrpuka, Kuwarrpa, Tipinpa, Tjipirinpa, Winyirirri (Kukatja) (Valiquette, 1993).

Field Notes Weeping Pittosporum grows as a weeping shrub or tree to around 8 m in height. The leaves vary in shape from ovate to elliptic and grow to 85 mm in length. White or cream bell-shaped flowers are present from June to October. The flowers are followed by smooth, yellow to orange, globose fruit about 10–15 mm in diameter. Weeping Pittosporum occurs over most of Western Australia, including the southern reaches of the Kimberley. It also occurs in all other mainland states and territories (ALA, 2022; Cribb & Cribb, 1981; Rippey & Rowland, 1995; WAH, 2022).

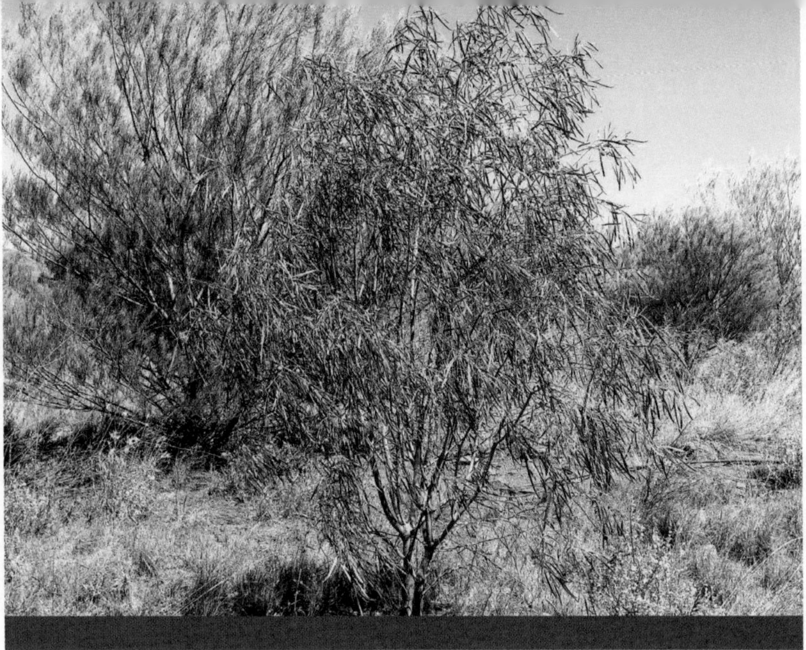

Medicinal Uses Infusions or decoctions of the seeds, fruit pulp, leaves or wood were taken internally for the relief of pain and cramps. Decoctions of the fruit pulp were drunk and applied externally for eczema and pruritus. Compresses of warmed leaves of Weeping Pittosporum were placed on the breasts of new mothers to induce lactation (Peile, 1997). Recent research has shown Weeping Pittosporum to have antibacterial, antifungal, antiinflammatory, antipruritic, antispasmodic, antiviral and antioxidant properties. Studies in Germany have revealed that it could also have anti-cancer properties (Eager, 2020).

Other Uses The seeds of the Weeping Pittosporum tree are edible and were ground into flour to make damper by some Aboriginal groups. The seeds are reported to taste a bit bitter (Cribb & Cribb, 1981; Gott, 2010; Low, 1991; Maiden, 1889). The tree is reported to have a 'good, edible gum'. The fruit flesh is not eaten (Cribb & Cribb, 1981).

CAUTION: Lassak & McCarthy, 2001 warn that infusions and decoctions of this plant should not be taken internally too frequently as the 'haemolytic saponin present may prove injurious'.

Weeping Tea-tree

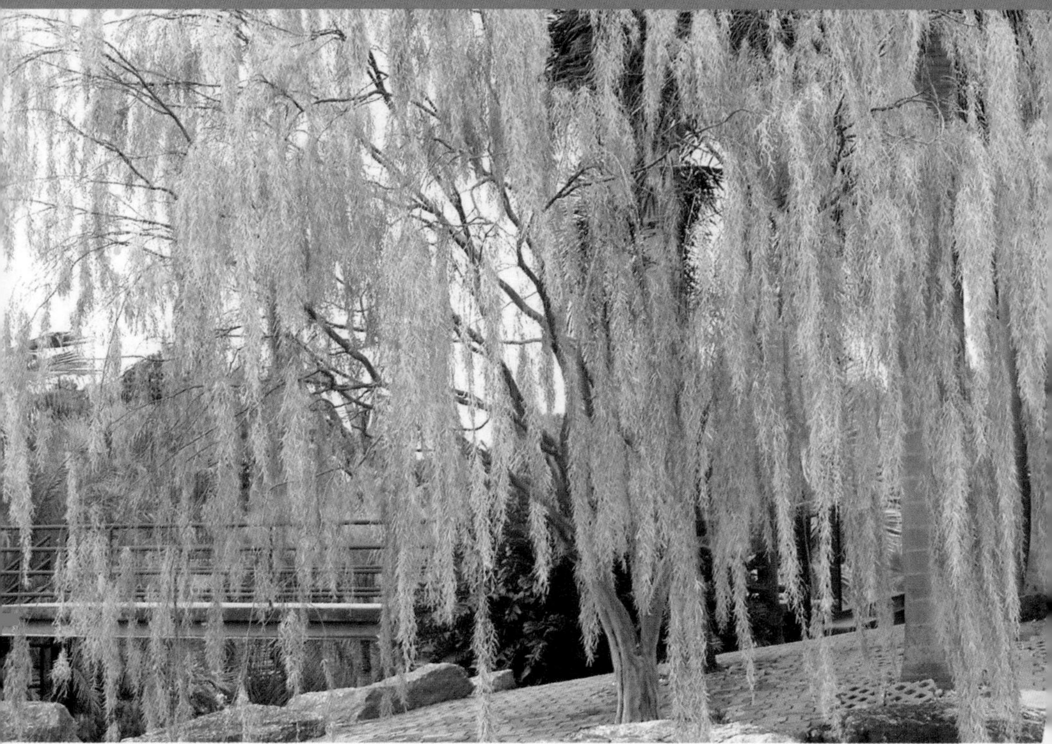

Scientific Name *Leptospermum madidum* subsp. *sativum* A.R.Bean, also known as *Leptospermum parviflorum* Valeton (misapplied).

Common Names Weeping Tea-tree, Whitewood.

Aboriginal Name Wungenji (Gija) (Wightman, 2003).

Field Notes Weeping Tea-tree grows as a weeping shrub or tree to a height of 8 m in good conditions. It has smooth, brownish-pink bark that peels off in curly strips and later becomes white. Its linear leaves are up to 70 mm long. The flowers are small and white and appear around July. Its fruit is thin-walled and only 3.5 mm in diameter. Weeping Tea-tree occurs in sandy soils, along watercourses and in sandstone gorges and is endemic to the Kimberley region of Western Australia, the Northern Territory and Far North Queensland (ALA, 2022; James Cook University, 2022; SMIP, 2022; WAH, 2022).

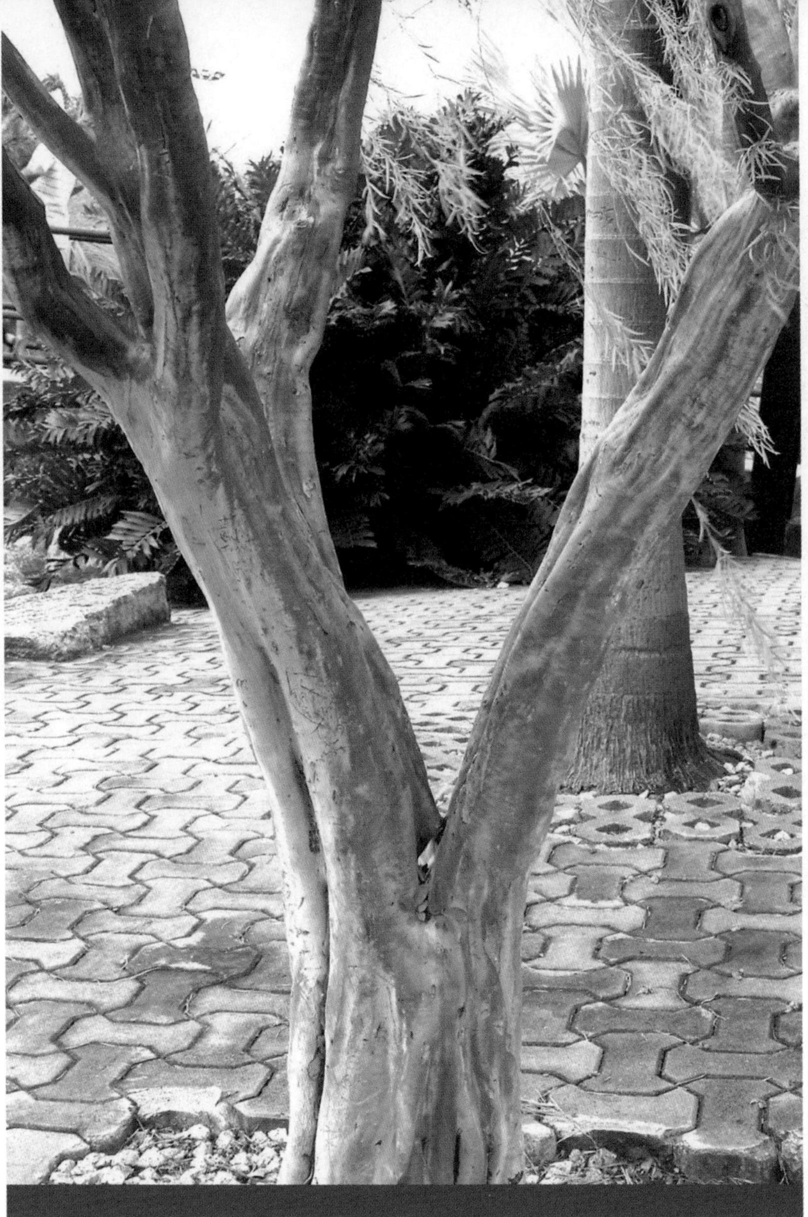

Medicinal Uses Aboriginal groups in Far North Queensland used infusions of crushed leaves of Weeping Tea-tree externally as a wash to treat fevers and general malaise. The vapours from crushed leaves held under the nose were inhaled to relieve the symptoms of colds and influenza (Edwards, 2005).

Other Uses The Gija use the forks in the stem of Weeping Tea-tree to make the hook part of a throwing stick or woomera as the wood is reported to be very strong (Wightman, 2003).

Whipstick Wattle

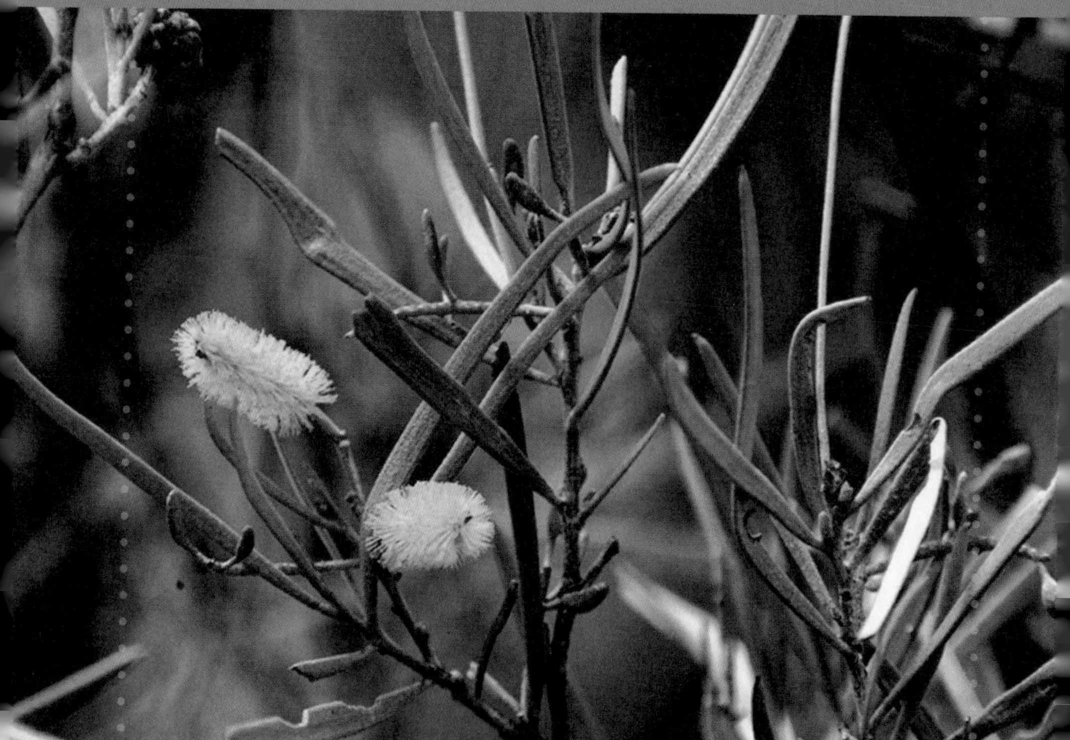

Scientific Name *Acacia adsurgens* Maiden & Blakely.

Common Names Whipstick Wattle, Sugar Brother.

Field Notes Whipstick Wattle is an erect, bushy shrub that grows up to 4 m in height. Its bark is grey to reddish brown, mostly smooth, but sometimes rough around the base. Its pale, yellowish-green phyllodes are long, straight or upwardly curved and up to 180 mm long and 4.5 mm wide. Its yellow flowers are held on spikes up to 25 mm long and occur from March to July. Its long seed pods are straight or slightly curved, and up to 120 mm long and 3.5 mm wide. Whipstick Wattle occurs in red sandy or loamy, often stony soils in the Pilbara and southern Kimberley regions of Western Australia, the Northern Territory and Queensland (ALA, 2022; Maslin et al., 2010; WAH, 2022).

Medicinal Uses Decoctions of the phyllodes were used externally as a wash for general malaise. The phyllodes were also used for

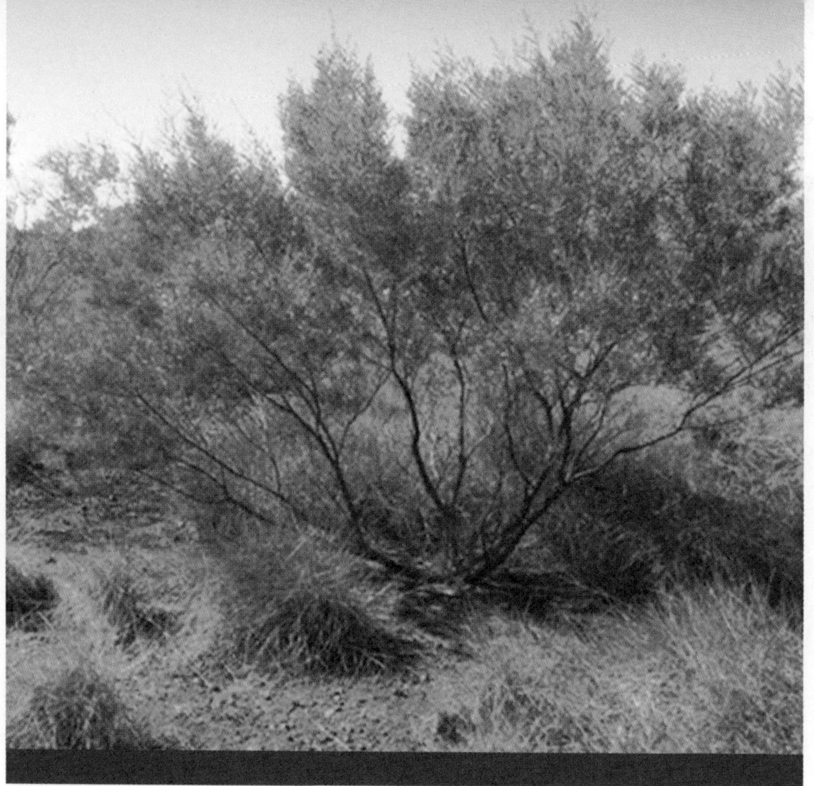

'smoke medicine' to smoke babies as a treatment for diarrhoea (Fern, 2021; Morse, 2005; Williams, 2011).

Other Uses The seeds of the Whipstick Wattle are edible and were usually roasted and ground to a paste prior to consumption. In some places, the tree is a good source of edible Witchetty Grubs that inhabit the roots (Bindon, 2014; Lister et al., 1996; Maslin et al., 2010).

White Apple

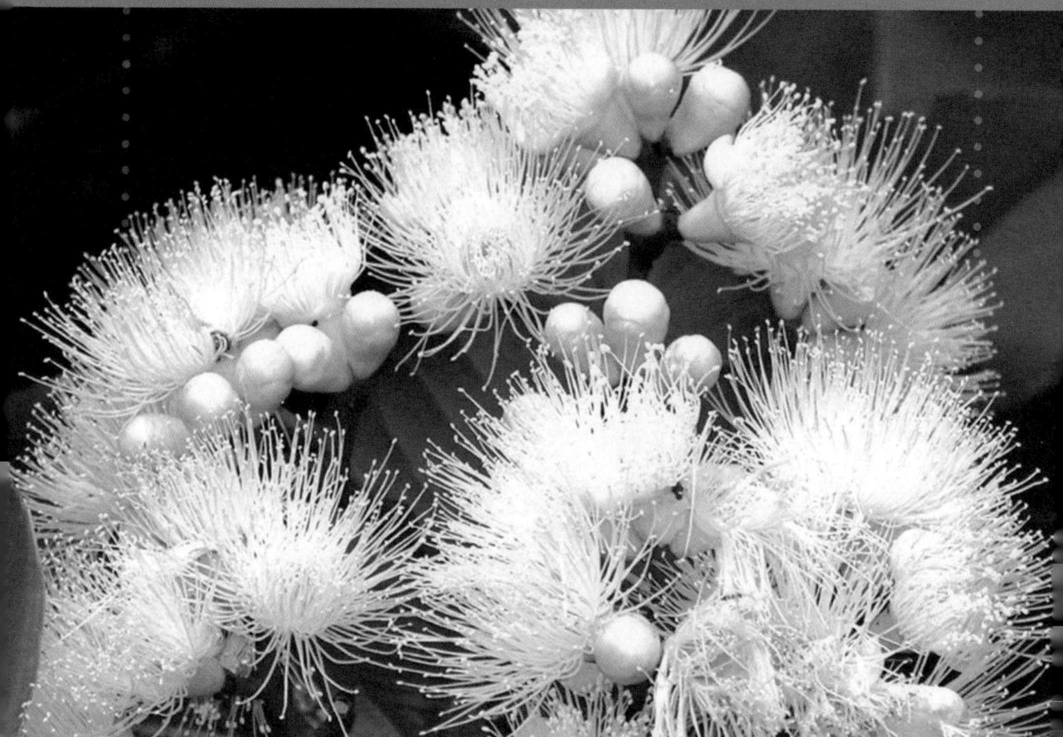

Scientific Names *Syzygium forte* (F.Muell.) B.Hyland, and *Syzygium forte* subsp. *potamophilum* B.Hyland, previously known as *Eugenia grandis* (Blume) Wight (misapplied).

Common Names White Apple, White Bush Apple, Bush Apple, Flaky-barked Satinash, White River Apple, Brown Satinash.

Aboriginal Names Ngalirrgi (Wunambal, Gaambera) (Karadada et al., 2011), Bandarri minya (Kwini) (Cheinmora, et al., 2017; Crawford, 1982).

Field Notes White Apple is a tree that reaches up to 25 m in height. Its bark is brown to orange and tends to be papery. It has large, elliptical leaves up to 140 mm long and large spikey, white flowers that are present between September and January. Its fruit is dirty white, globular, up to 60 mm in diameter and containing a single seed. White Apple occurs along watercourses in the Kimberley region of Western Australia, the Northern Territory and Queensland

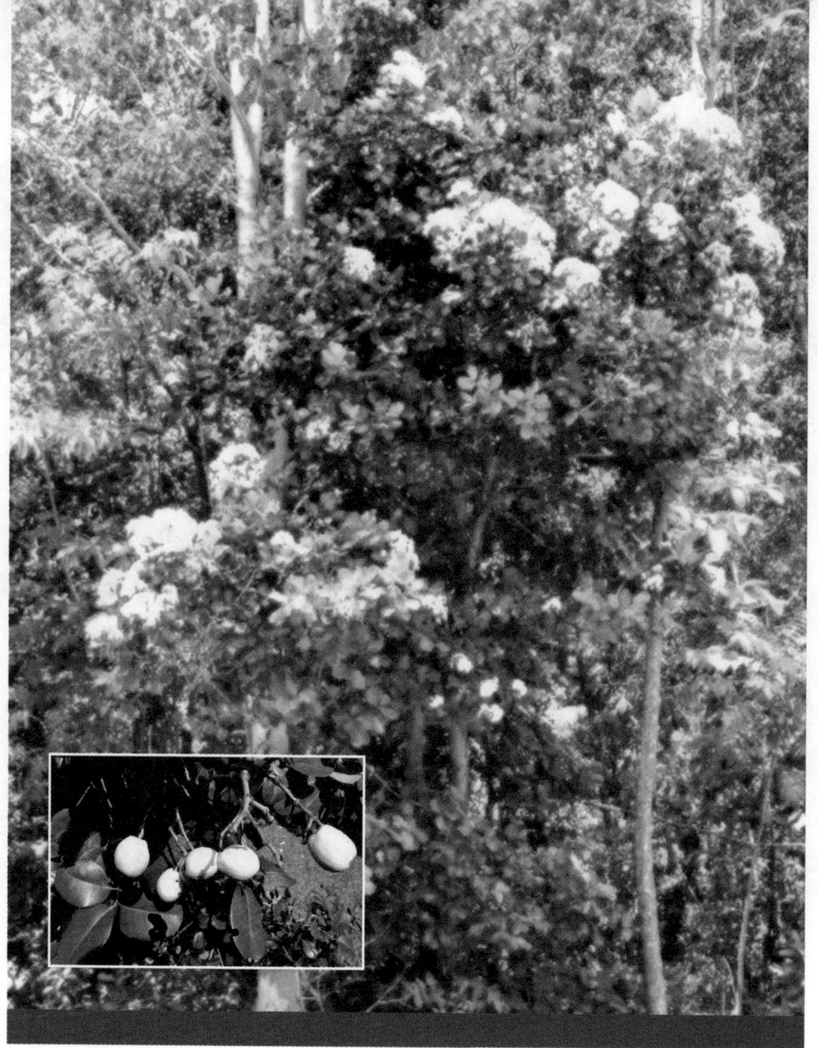

(ALA, 2022; WAH, 2022). It also occurs in Papua New Guinea (Fern, 2021).

Medicinal Uses Decoctions of the red inner bark of White Apple were used as an antiseptic wash to bathe sores and wounds (Edwards, 2005).

Other Uses The fruit of White Apple, which is usually ripe from mid-November to late December, are eaten raw. The flesh is reported to be a bit dry, so the fruit is supposed to be better to eat if it is left to soak in water for a few days (Cheinmora, et al., 2017; Crawford, 1982; Edwards, 2005; Fox & Garde, 2018; Isaacs, 1987; Karadada et al., 2011).

White Berry Bush

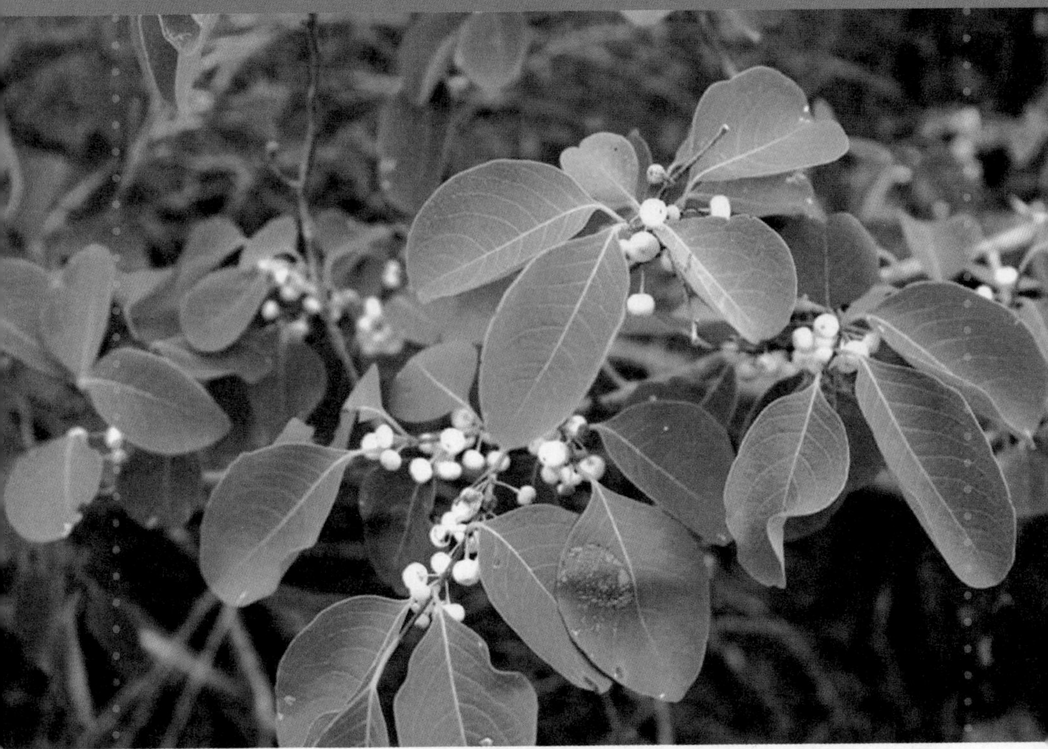

Family **Phyllanthaceae Martinov.**

Scientific Name *Flueggea virosa* (Willd.) Voigt.

Common Names White Berry Bush, White Currant, Snowberry Tree, Common Bushweed.

Aboriginal Names Ngoorrwang (Miriwoong) (Leonard et al., 2013), Gangu (Bunuba) (Oscar et al., 2019), Woolewooleng (Miriwoong) (Leonard et al., 2013), Koowal, Goowaal (Nyul Nyul), Goowal (Yawuru) (Kenneally et al., 1996), Goorralgar (Bardi) (Vigilante et al., 2013), Ngooloorrji, Ngoorrwany, Goowarroolji, Berenggarrji (Gija) (Purdie et al., 2018), Runggu (Jaru) (Wightman, 2003), Garngi (Gooniyandi) (Dilkes-Hall et al., 2019), Arnbarrma ninya, Anbarrma ninya (Kwini) (Cheinmora et al., 2017), Koowal, Koolwal (Nyikina) (Smith & Smith, 2009), Kuwal (Karajarri) (Moss et al., 2021).

Field Notes White Berry Bush grows as an open, spreading shrub or tree to 5 m in height. Its young branchlets are angular and reddish. The leaves are alternate, elliptic to ovate and up to 90 mm

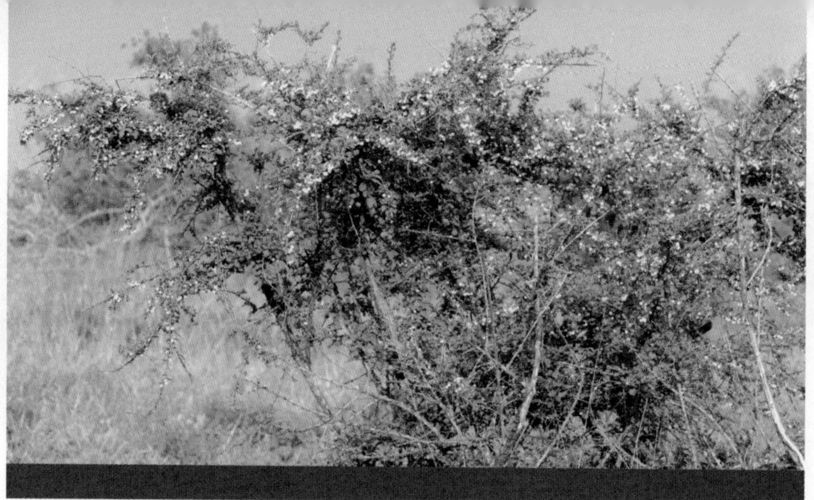

long and 50 mm wide. Its small, creamy-green flowers appear in clusters between August and April. Its fruit are small white berries that are only 5 mm in diameter. White Berry Bush occurs in interdunal grey-brown sand, and alluvium, over limestone, sandstone and basalt on floodplains, hillsides, dunes and around rock pools in the Pilbara and Kimberley regions of Western Australia, the Northern Territory and northern Queensland. It is also endemic to the drier parts of Africa, the Arabian Peninsula, the Indian subcontinent, China and other parts of South-east Asia (ALA, 2022; Fern, 2021; Low, 1991; WAH, 2022).

Medicinal Uses The leaves and bark of White Berry Bush were ground into a paste that was then painted onto sores, rashes and itchy skin. Weak infusions of the leaves were taken internally to treat internal pain and general malaise (Lassak & McCarthy, 2001; Smith, 1991; Webb, 1959). Crushed bark was applied as a poultice to catfish stings to ease the pain (Low, 1990).

Other Uses The fruit of White Berry Bush are edible when mature enough to fall from the bush, which, in Australia, is between December and March. They are reported to be sweet and juicy with a slightly bitter flavour. They were mainly eaten by children (Cheinmora et al., 2017; Fern, 2021; Fox & Garde, 2018; Purdie et al., 2018; Smith, 1991; Low, 1991; Webb, 1959; Wightman, 2003).

White Cheesewood

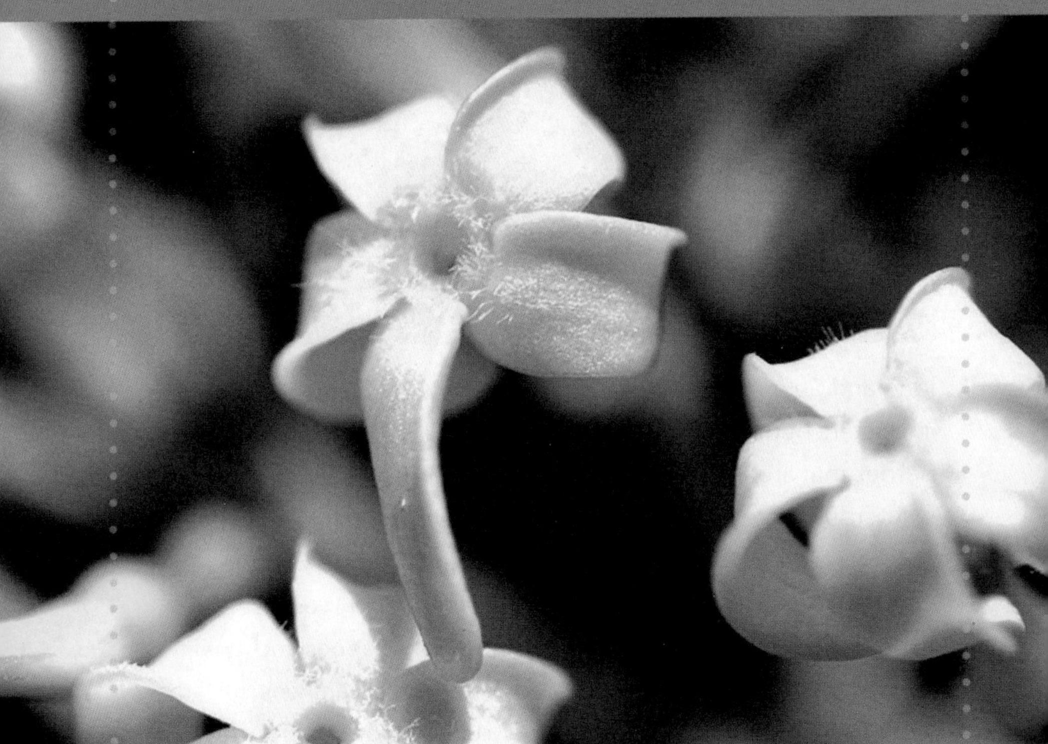

Scientific Name *Alstonia actinophylla* (A.Cunn.) K.Schum.

Common Names White Cheesewood, Milkwood, Cape Cheesewood, Cape Milkwood, Northern Milkwood.

Field Notes White Cheesewood is a shrub or tree that grows up to 25 m in height. Its lanceolate leaves appear in whorls of three to seven and are up to 120 mm long. The small, sweetly scented, white-cream flowers with six petals that are curled backwards appear in clusters from August to October. Its fruit are smooth, cylindrical and up to 200 mm long. White Cheesewood occurs in a variety of soils over sandstone, limestone and basalt on rocky slopes, river and creek banks, outcrops, on ridges and in gorges from the Kimberley region of Western Australia across the tropical north to the Cape York Peninsula in Queensland (ALA, 2022; ATRP, 2020; WAH, 2022).

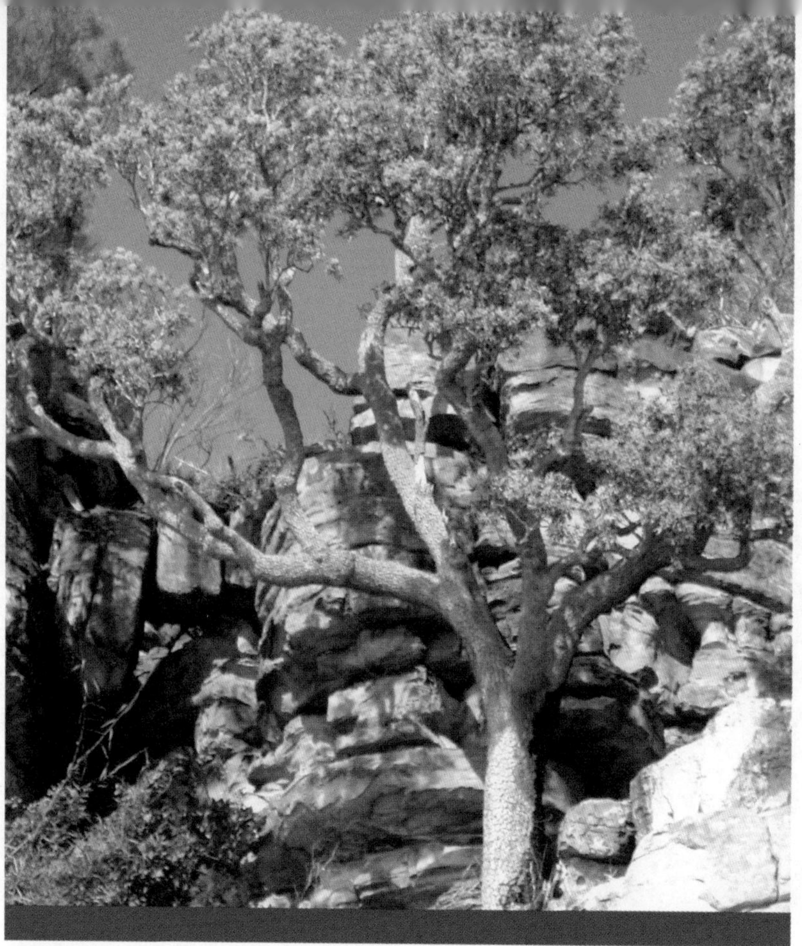

Medicinal Uses The white latex that oozes from the bark of White Cheesewood when cut was thought to promote lactation (the flow of milk) in nursing mothers when painted onto their breasts (Edwards, 2005; Lassak & McCarthy, 2001; Webb, 1959). The milky sap was also applied to wounds and sores to promote healing (Low, 1990).

White Cypress Pine

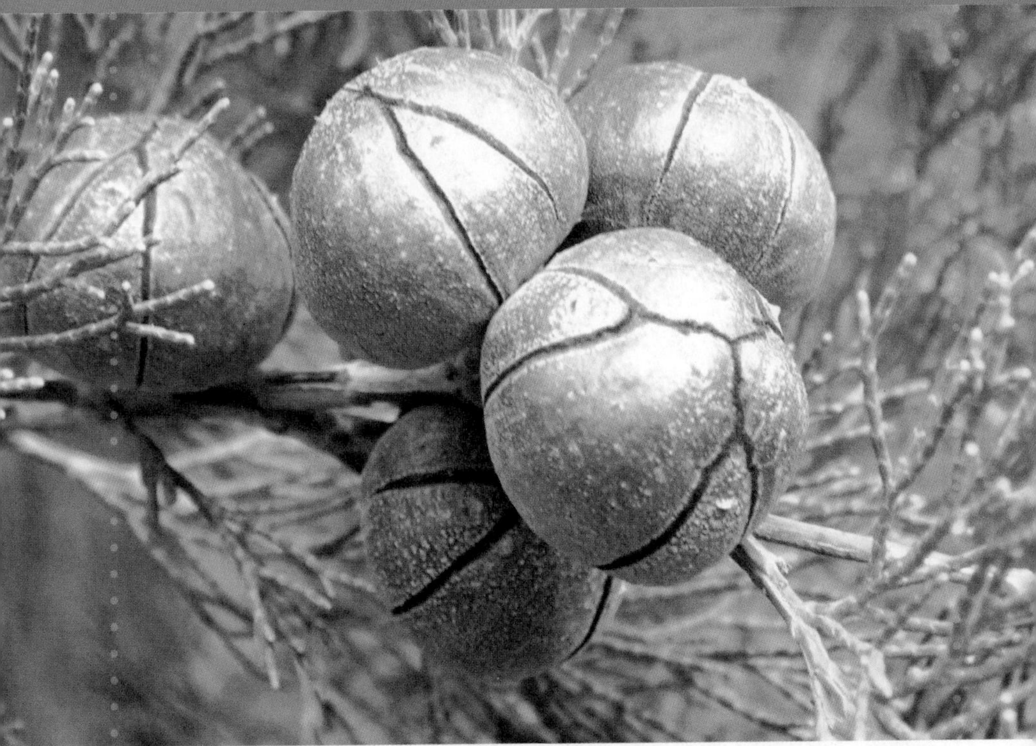

Scientific Name *Callitris columellaris* F.Muell., previously known as *Callitris intratropica* R.T.Baker & H.G.Sm.

Common Names White Cypress Pine, White Pine, Coast Cypress Pine, Murray River Cypress-pine, Northern Cypress-pine.

Aboriginal Names Goowereng (Miriwoong) (Leonard et al., 2013), Guru (Wunambal, Gaambera) (Karadada et al., 2011), Gudigudi (Bardi) (Smith & Kalotas, 1985), Gooweriny (Gija) (Purdie et al., 2018), Kuwuru (Gija) (Wightman, 2003), Kuli (Kukatja) Valiquette, 1993), Krooma mana (Worrorra) (Clendon et al., 2000), Kuru minya, Meiyawarr minya (Kwini) (Cheinmora et al., 2017), Guru (Bunuba) (Moss et al., 2021).

Field Notes White Cypress Pine is a small evergreen, cone-shaped tree that usually grows to around 12 m in height but can be found up to 18 m in some parts of Australia. It has rough, vertically grooved bark and scale-like, blue-green leaves about 6 mm long, which twirl around the branchlets. The dark brown, spherical, woody fruit or cones are roughly 20 mm in diameter. White Cypress Pine occurs in a variety of soils, including sand, clay, loam, gravel and laterite on sandplains, hillsides, in valleys, on clifftops and around salt lakes throughout all of mainland Australia (Lassak & McCarthy, 2008). It grows in most parts of Western Australia, from the northern Kimberley southwards to Esperance (Lassak & McCarthy, 2001; WAH, 2022).

Medicinal Uses The burnt wood of White Cypress Pine was crushed and the ashes were rubbed onto parts of the body to relieve arthritic and rheumatic pain. Ashes were also rubbed on to the head of babies to help close the gap in the bones in the skull called the anterior fontanelle (Purdie et al., 2018; Wightman, 2003). Infusions of the leaves were used as chest rubs to treat coughs and colds, and as an antiseptic wash for burns and insect bites. The leaves, bark and twigs were crushed and mixed with animal fat and rubbed on the chest to relieve congestion (Low, 1990). The leaves, bark and twigs also made a good 'smoke medicine' to relieve congestion in the nose and chest (Karadada et al., 2011). The ashes were sometimes mixed with the ashes of the Conkerberry (*Carissa lanceolata;* p. 138) (Peile, 1997). Decoctions of the red sticky inner bark were applied externally as an antiseptic wash to sores and cuts to aid healing (Smith, 1991; Wightman, 2003) and to strengthen babies (Purdie et al., 2018; Wightman, 2003). Williams & Sides (2008) relate that the Wiradjuri in New South Wales used a piece of bark from the larger roots to treat broken bones. The bark was removed from the tree and, while wet, was bound around the broken limb. The bark dries acting as a splint as it moulds to the shape of the limb thus holding the broken bones in place.

Other Uses The bark and leaves of White Cypress Pine were burnt in campfires to repel mosquitoes (Karadada et al., 2011; Low, 1990; Purdie et al., 2018; Smith & Kalotas, 1985). The timber was used to make paddles, clapsticks and message sticks (Karadada et al., 2011).

White Dragon Tree

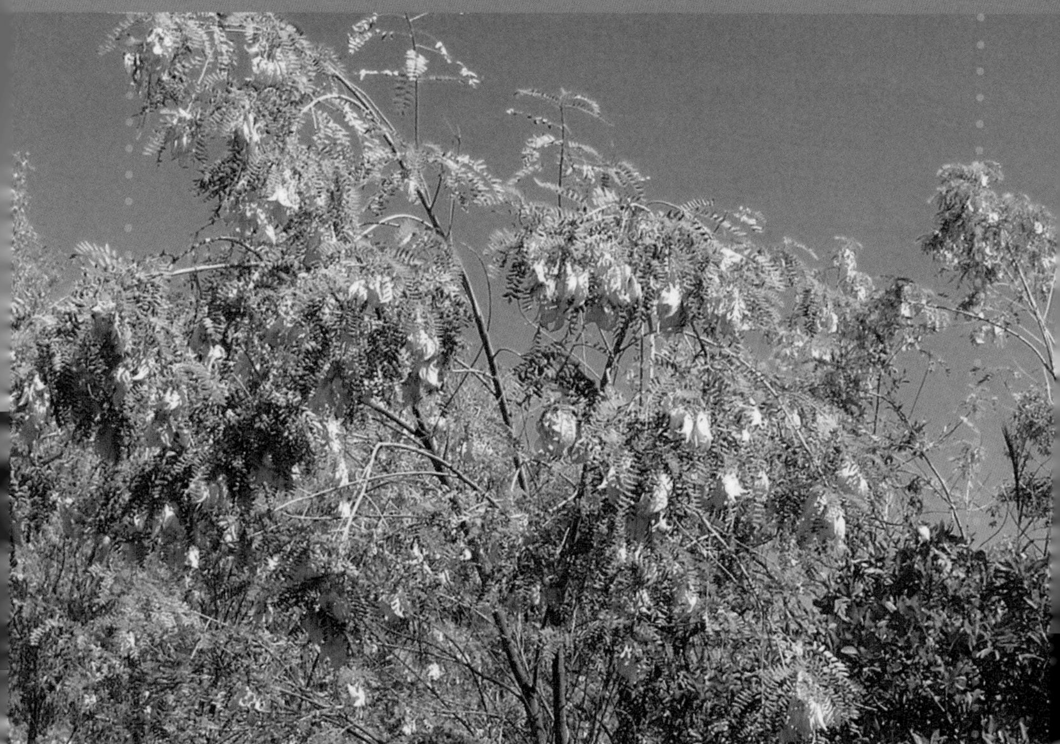

Scientific Name *Sesbania formosa* (F.Muell.) N.T.Burb.

Common Names White Dragon Tree, Swamp Corkwood Tree.

Aboriginal Names Gangarridiadia (Bunuba) (Oscar et al., 2019), Gandiwal (Wunambal, Gaambera) (Karadada et al., 2011), Arninyban, Rirawal (Bardi) (Smith & Kalotas, 1985; Kenneally et al., 2018), Wirarrajartu (Walmajarri) (Richards & Hudson, 2012), Wirrwirrjel, Wirrwirrel (Gija) (Purdie et al., 2018), Rirawal (Yuwuru) (Kenneally et al., 2018), Marriwa, Wirrwirr (Jaru) (Wightman, 2003), Yarnlal ninya (Kwini) (Cheinmora, et al., 2017), Ngalinmarra (Karajarri) (Willing, 2014).

Field Notes White Dragon Tree grows from 2.5 m to 13 m in height depending on conditions. Its bark is pale grey, furrowed and corky. Its green leaf blades are ovate and roughly 30 mm long. It produces white to yellowish-white flowers with variable petals that are distinctly clawed, with the larger petals up to 100 mm long.

The flowers form in clusters of two to seven in the dry season from May to September. The fruit or seed pods are linear, pendulous, and up to 600 mm long and 9 mm wide. White Dragon Tree occurs in alluvium and sand alongside creeks and rivers and around the margins of swamps in the Pilbara and Kimberley regions of Western Australia, the Northern Territory and Queensland (ALA, 2022; ATRP, 2020; Australian Seed, 2022; WAH, 2022).

Medicinal Uses The leaves of the White Dragon Tree were crushed and applied externally as a poultice to sprains, bruises, swellings, areas of rheumatic pain and to itchy skin to stop the itching. Decoctions of the bark were taken internally to treat fever, diarrhoea, dysentery and diabetes. Decoctions of the flowers were drunk to treat sinusitis. A paste made of the ground-up root was applied externally as a liniment to areas of rheumatic pain. The corky bark was burnt and crushed to make an antiseptic powder that was applied to cuts and other wounds to aid healing (Fern, 2021; Willing, 2014).

Other Uses The young leaves of the White Dragon Tree are edible. The flowers are edible and make a pleasant addition to salads. The immature green pods and large fleshy pods are also edible raw or cooked like string beans (Fern, 2021). The wood from the White Dragon Tree was used by the Gija and Jaru to make woomeras, coolamons and fire sticks (Cheinmora, et al., 2017; Purdie et al., 2018; Wightman, 2003).

White Grevillea

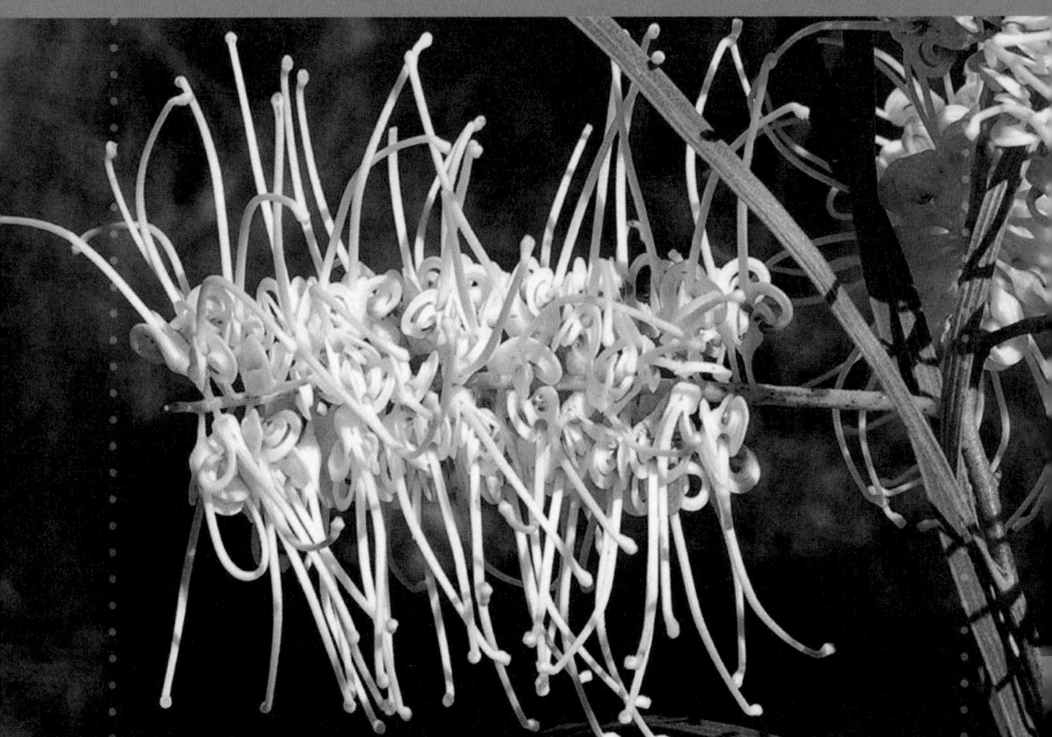

Scientific Name *Grevillea parallela* Knight.

Common Names White Grevillea, Silver Grevillea, Silver Oak.

Field Notes White Grevillea is a tree that grows up to 8 m in height. It has dark-coloured, rough, flaky to tessellated bark over the branches. Its pale green to silvery-grey, linear to linear-lanceolate leaves are pinnatified with up to six lobes and are up to 400 mm long. Its flowers are perfumed, waxy, crowded and held in cylindrical racemes up to 100 mm long forming a crowded terminal panicle. Flowering is between May and July in Western Australia. White Grevillea occurs in sandy soils, on flats and among sandstone rocks in the Kimberley region of Western Australia, the top end of the Northern Territory and northern and central areas of Queensland (ALA, 2022; WAH, 2022).

Medicinal Uses A poultice made from crushed and warmed leaves of White Grevillea was applied to the head to relieve headaches.

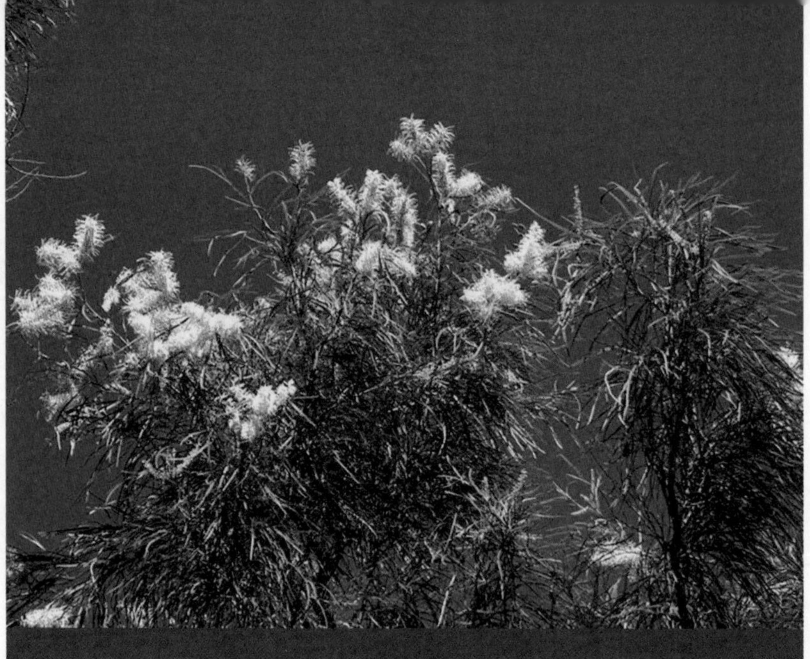

Nectar was sucked directly from the flowers to soothe sore throats. Crushed leaves were held under the nose and the vapours inhaled to relieve the symptoms of colds and influenza. Decoctions of the leaves were used externally as a wash for general malaise and headache, and as eyedrops to treat conjunctivitis (Edwards, 2005).

Other Uses As with other grevilleas, Aboriginal people sucked the sweet nectar directly from the flowers or soaked the flowers in a little water to make a sweet drink. The seeds are also edible and are usually eaten raw. The leaves are often used to flavour meat cooked in a ground oven (Edwards, 2005; SMIP, 2022).

White Mangrove

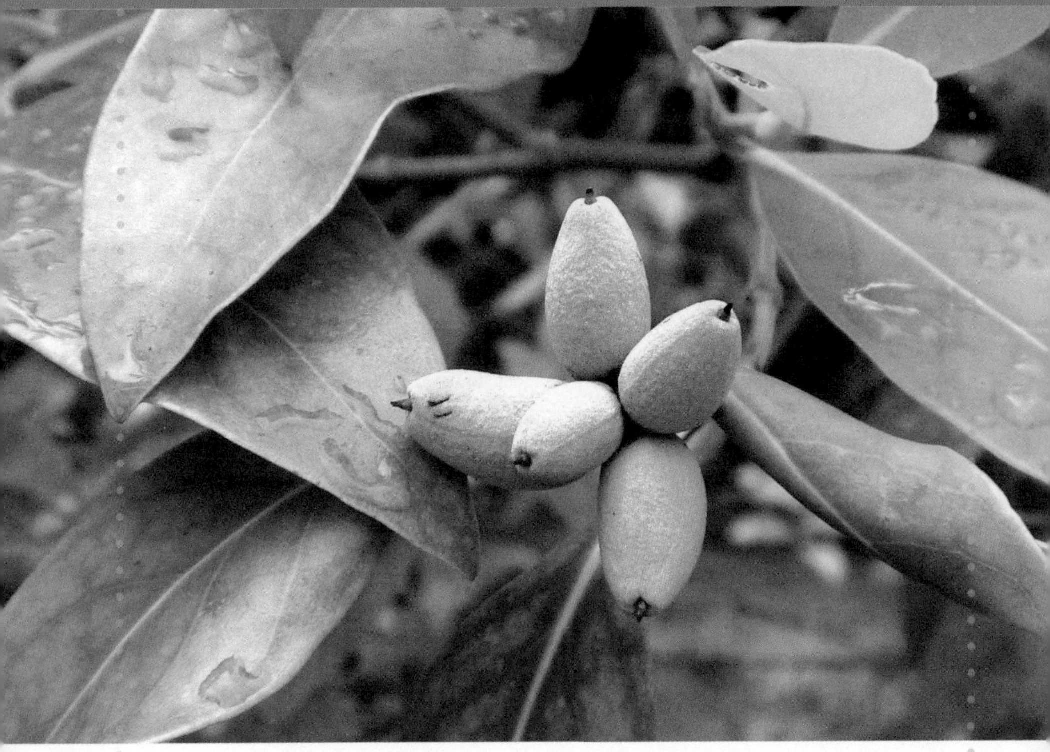

Scientific Name *Avicennia marina* (Forssk.) Vierh.

Common Names White Mangrove, Grey Mangrove, Salt Tree.

Aboriginal Names Biliman (Wunambal, Gaambera) (Karadada et al., 2011), Goorrngool, Ngoorrngool (Bardi), Jamai (Nyul Nyul), Gundurung (Yawuru) (Kenneally et al., 2018), Baru-baruga (Arrawarra), Limil ninya (Kwini) (Cheinmora et al., 2017).

Field Notes White Mangrove grows as a shrub or tree to 16 m or more in height. It has light grey, finely fissured bark and numerous spongy, pencil-like pneumatophores (peg-like roots) that spread out from the base of the trunk. Its glossy, green leaves are ovate, pointed, opposite and up to 80 mm long. It has small, yellow-to-orange flowers that appear in clusters. In Australia, flowering is between November and March. Its pale green flattened fruit are approximately 30 mm long and 20 mm wide. White Mangrove is found in the intertidal zone of muddy or sandy flats, in estuaries

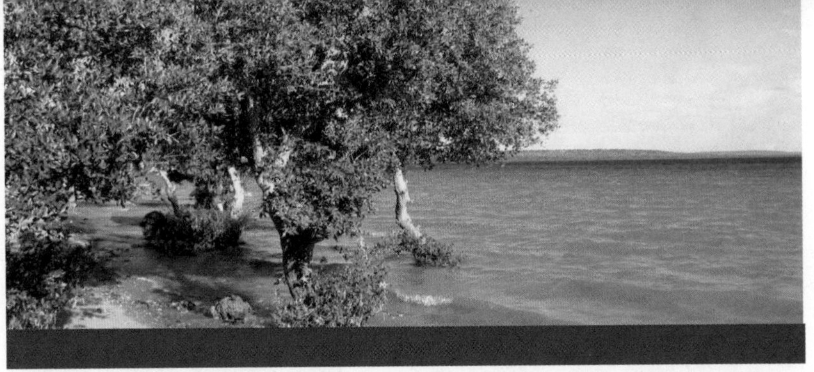

around the coastline throughout the Indian Ocean from Africa through Arabia, Asia to Australia and New Zealand. In Australia, it is found right around the coast north from Dunsborough, just south of Perth, around the top to the Victorian coast with patches along the coast in South Australia (ALA, 2022; Department of Agriculture and Fisheries, 2020; Fern, 2021).

Medicinal Uses The leaves and young shoots were traditionally chewed and used as a poultice on stingray and stonefish stings. The bark can also be rubbed on stings. The wood ash was made into a paste and used to treat skin sores, dermatophytosis (ringworm and tinea), and boils (Fern, 2021; Hiddins, 2001; Low, 1990; Michie, 1993; Smith, 1991). Decoctions of the leaves and bark were used externally to treat scabies infestations (Fern, 2021). In Madagascar, decoctions of the leaves have been used as an antidote for fish poisoning (Fern, 2021). Fern (2022) reports that: 'Research has shown that several medically active components are present in the plant including iridoid glucosides, flavonoids and naphthoquinone derivatives. Some of these have shown strong antiproliferative and moderate cytotoxic activities as well as antibacterial effects.'

Other Uses Northern Aboriginal groups harvested the seeds for eating, but the seeds need special preparation before eating to leach out 'distasteful tannins and bitter substances'. One method of preparation was to place moistened seeds into stone ovens that were sealed with bark and then baked for two hours, after which the baked seeds were placed in a pool and buried in sand for some time before eating. Alternatively, the seeds were baked and crushed and the pulp washed through dillies before eating. After preparation, the seeds are a 'bit bland' but were an important

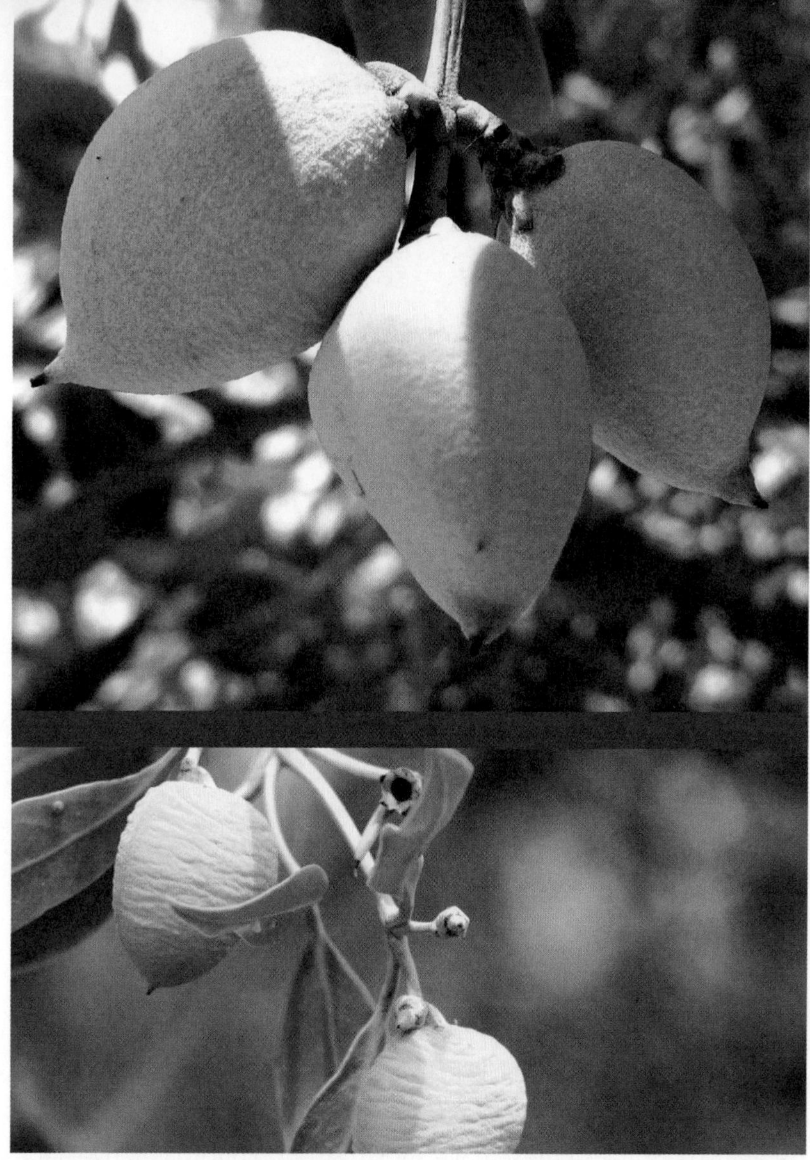

food source for northern Aboriginals in the wet season (Hiddins, 2001; Low, 1991; Michie, 1993; Vigilante et al., 2013). Smith (1991) observed Aboriginal groups in the Northern Territory roasting the fruit in hot ashes before eating them. The Kwini put White Mangrove leaves inside the cavities of dugong and turtle before cooking them in a ground oven, which is supposed to keep the meat moist and add flavour to it (Cheinmora et al., 2017).

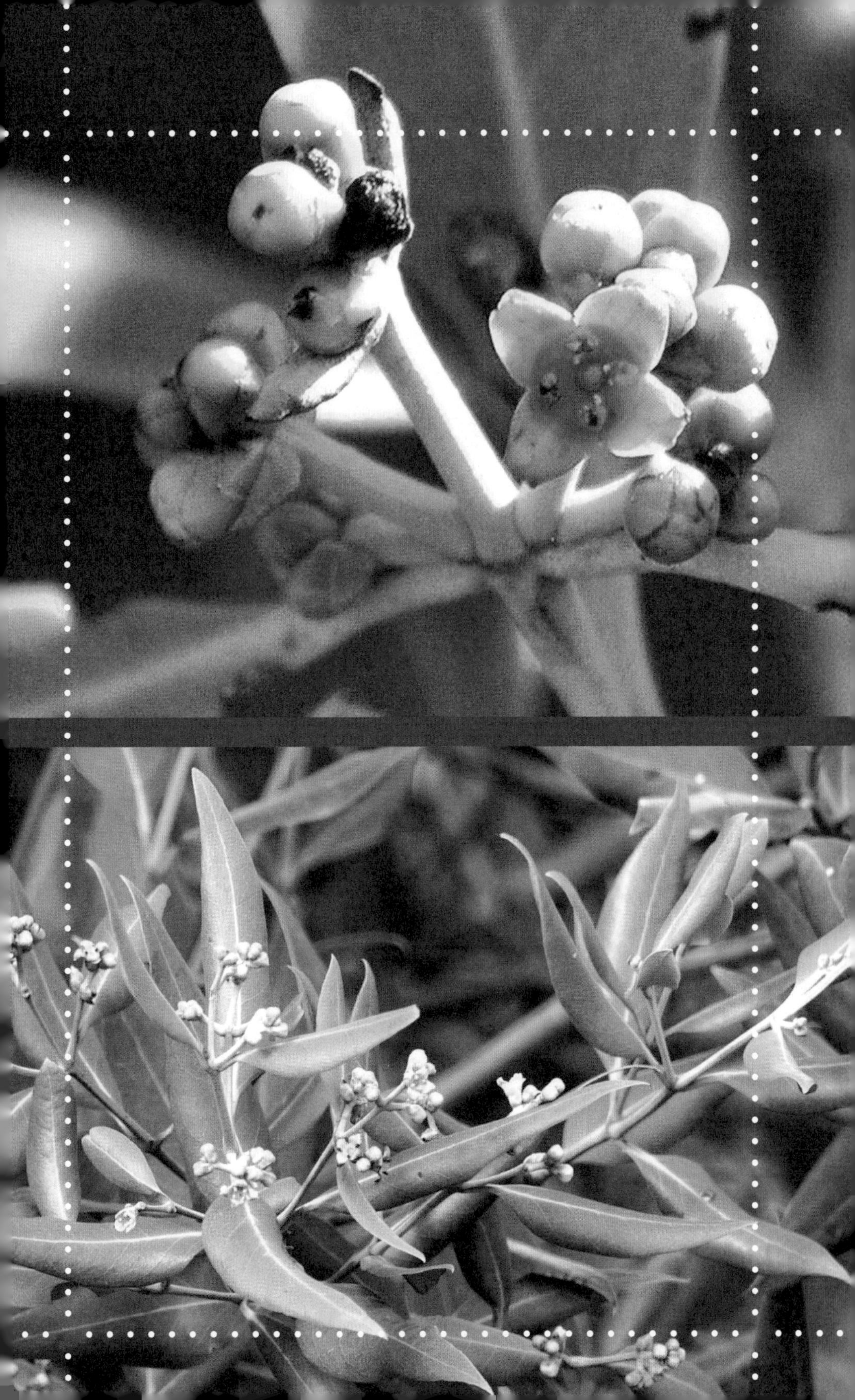

White Nymph Water Lily

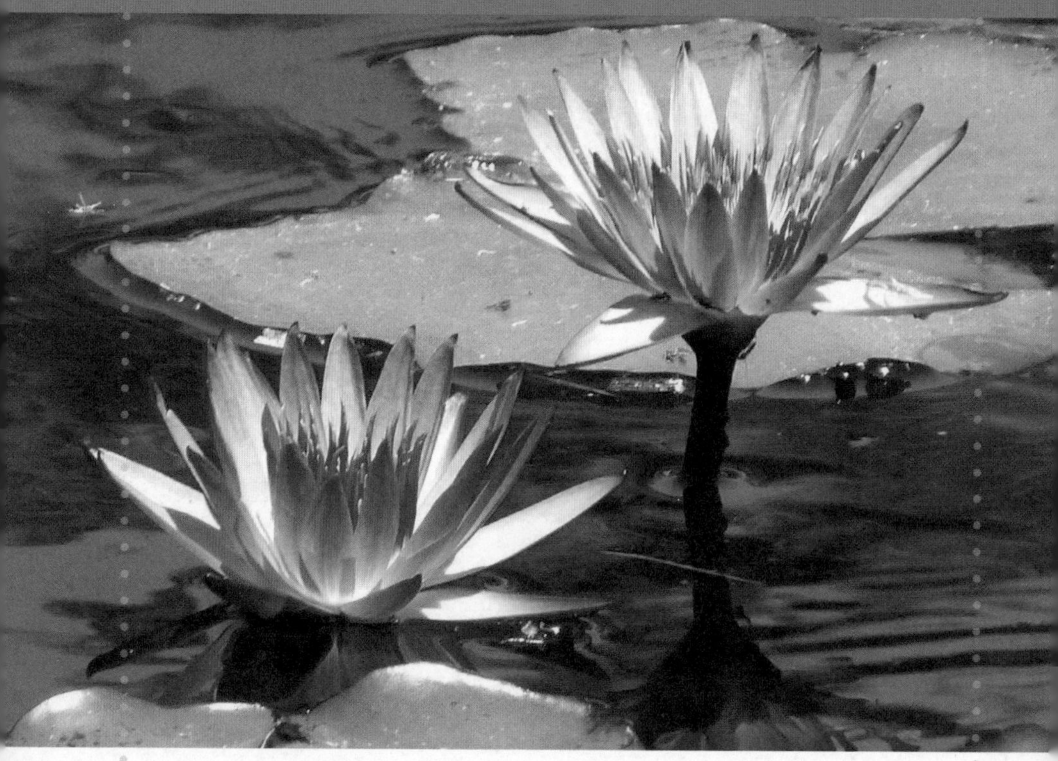

Scientific Name *Nymphaea violacea* Lehm.

Common Names White Nymph Water Lily, Water Lily, Waterlily,Blue Water Lily, Miani.

Aboriginal Names Gajari (Bunuba) (Oscar et al., 2019), Wirdamunga (Nyul Nyul) (Dobbs et al., 2015), Milyani (Wunambal, Gaambera) (Karadada et al., 2011), Arnu (Kwini) (Crawford, 1982), Jamungany, Kukaja, Lukarri (Walmajarri) (Richards & Hudson, 2012), Garrjany, Geloowoorrji (Gija) (Purdie et al., 2018), Garringarri (Gooniyandi) (Dilkes-Hall et al., 2019), Binanyi, Garrja (Jaru) (Wightman, 2003), Miyeeni manya, (Kwini) (Cheinmora et al., 2017).

Field Notes The White Nymph Water Lily is a floating-leaved, aquatic, rhizomatous, perennial plant. Its leaves are broadly oval to circular in shape and up to 290 mm in diameter. The beautiful violet, blue or white flowers have many petals and yellow stamens and are borne on long stalks, growing up to 160 mm in diameter.

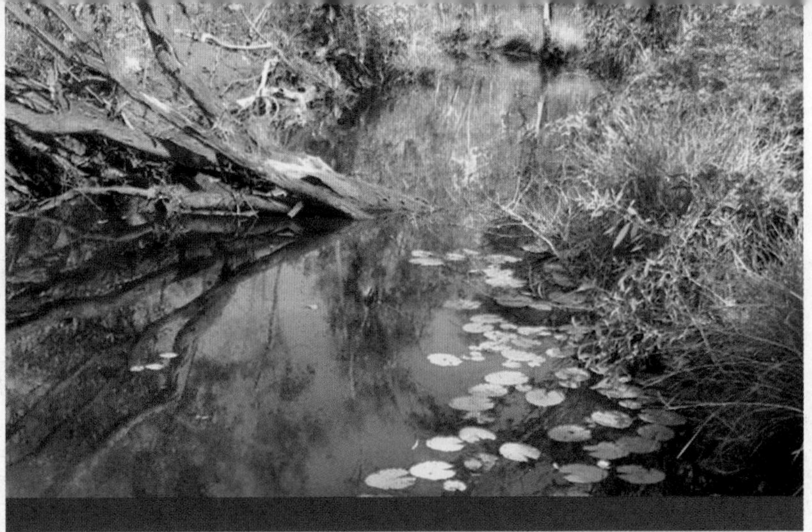

Its flowers can be present at any time of the year. Its fruit are round and spongy berries with many small seeds and are found underwater. The fruit are available from January to July. White Nymph Water Lily occurs in ephemeral or perennial pools, billabongs and rivers in the Kimberley region of Western Australia, the Northern Territory, Far North Queensland and down the east coast as far as the north of New South Wales (ALA, 2022; ANPSA, 2022; WAH, 2022).

Medicinal Uses The seeds and tubers are reported to be a good treatment for diarrhoea (McMahon, 2006). Edwards (2005) relates that, 'Eating this plant is good for diabetics as it is believed it evens out blood sugar levels'.

Other Uses The tubers and flower stems of the White Nymph Water Lily are edible and are traditionally cooked in hot ashes before eating, but the stems can be eaten raw. The tubers are harvested between May and November (Cheinmora et al., 2017; Crawford, 1982; Fox & Garde, 2018; Karadada et al., 2011; McMahon, 2006; Purdie et al., 2018; Vigilante et al., 2013; Wightman, 2003). The seeds are also edible and are eaten raw or roasted, or ground into flour to make damper or Johnny cakes. The fruit are edible too (Fox & Garde, 2018; Karadada et al., 2011; Purdie et al., 2018; RFCA, 1993; Vigilante et al., 2013; Wightman, 2003).

CAUTION: McMahon (2006) warns that, 'Saltwater crocodiles inhabit many of the waterways where water lilies are found'.

White Turkeybush

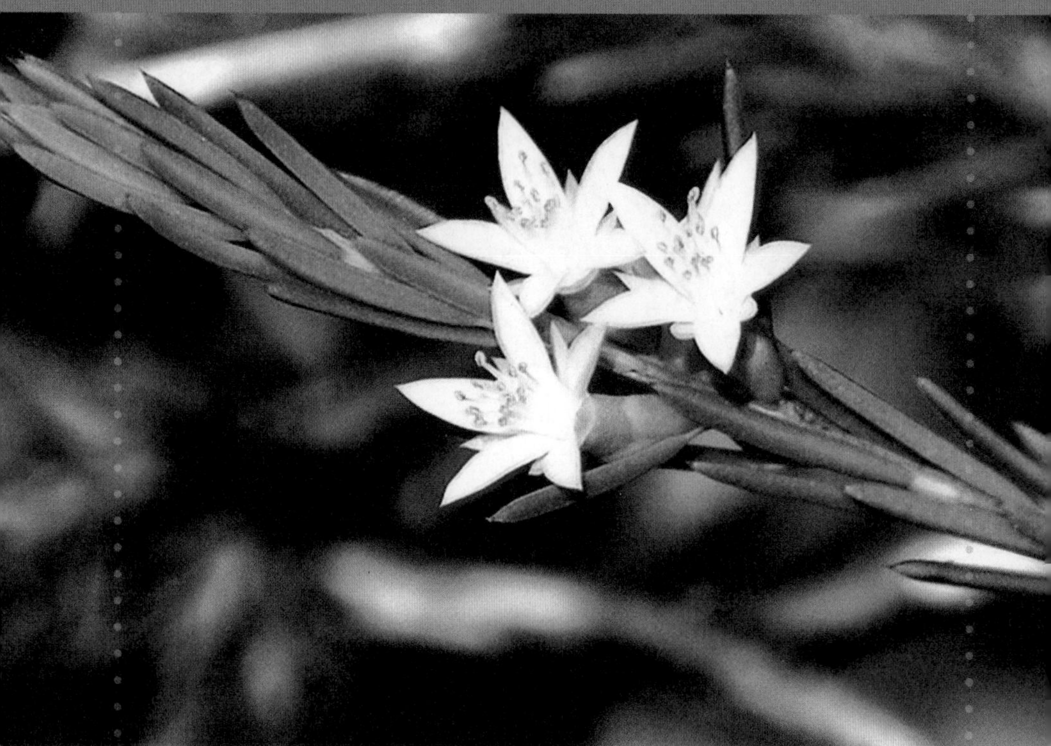

Scientific Name *Calytrix brownii* (Schauer) Craven.

Common Names White Turkeybush, White Turkey Bush.

Aboriginal Names Mangadany (Gija) (Purdie et al., 2018), Wunggun (Jaru) (Wightman, 2003), Mangkada minya, Mangarnda manya (Kwini) (Cheinmora et al., 2017).

Field Notes White Turkeybush is an erect or prostrate shrub that grows up to 4 m in height. Its small green, club-shaped leaves are flattened against the branchlets. Its small, star-shaped, white or cream flowers have five petals. Flowering is from March to August. White Turkeybush is found in skeletal sand or loam over sandstone, quartzite or basalt, along rocky banks of watercourses, on sandstone outcrops and plateaus in the Kimberley region of Western Australia and the Northern Territory (ALA, 2022; WAH, 2022).

Medicinal Uses The vapours given off the crushed leaves or decoctions of the crushed leaves were inhaled to treat sinusitis

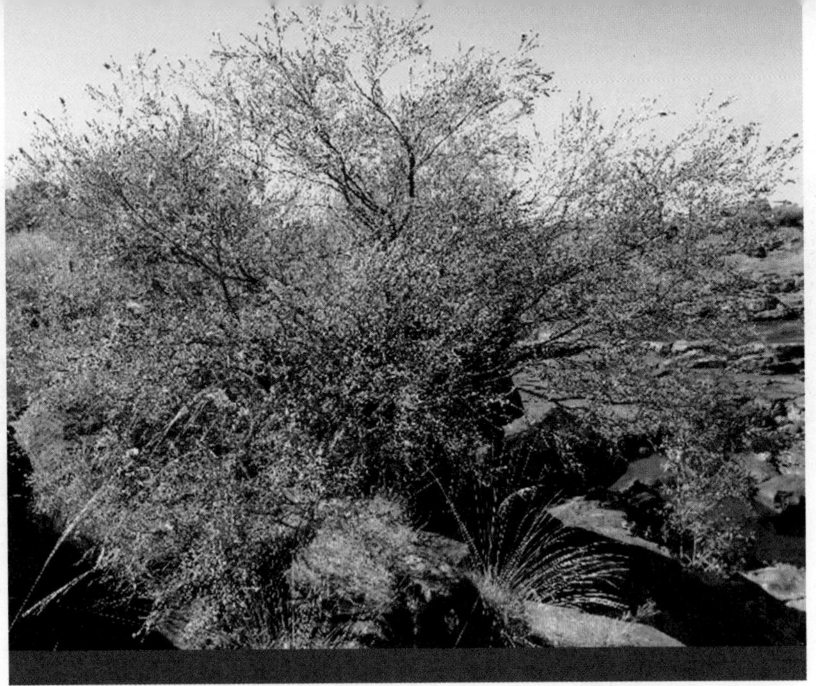

and to relieve the symptoms of colds and influenza. A little of the mixture was sipped to help relieve any internal pain associated with influenza (Smith, 1991; Wightman, 2003). The leaves were crushed and the juice applied as a liniment for arthritic and rheumatic pain. The crushed leaves were also applied as a poultice to wounds and sores to aid healing. The leaves are reported to contain an antiseptic substance called alpha-pinene (Low, 1990).

White Wild Musk Mallow

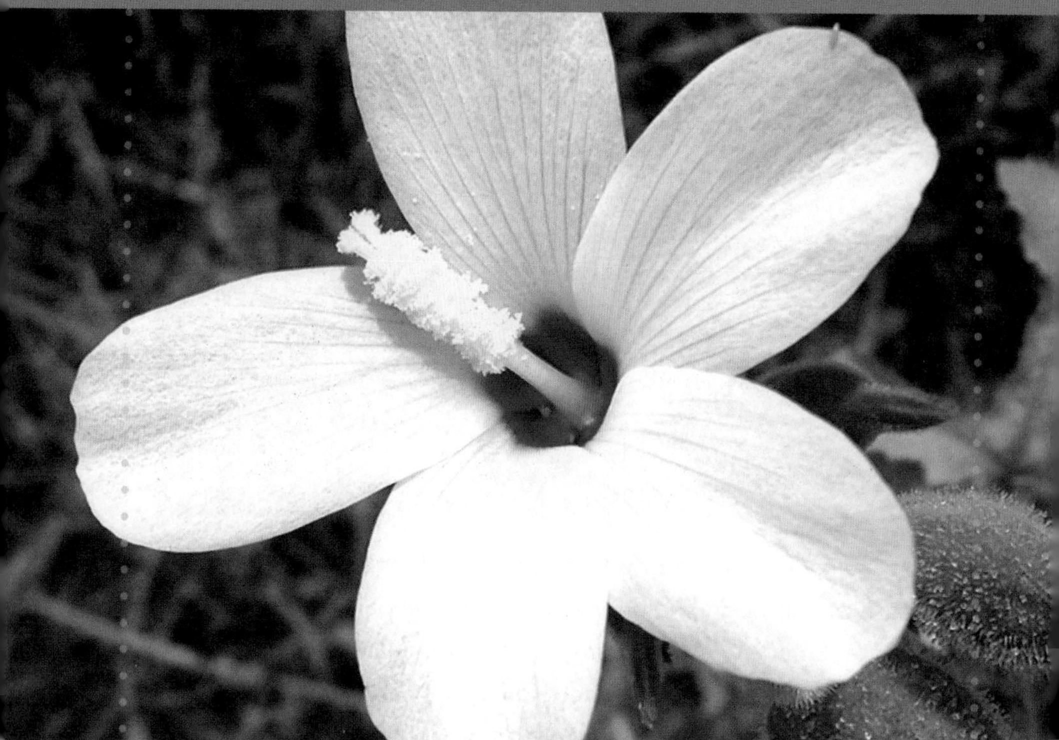

Scientific Name *Abelmoschus ficulneus* (L.) Wight.

Common Names White Wild Musk Mallow, Rosella Yam, Native Rosella.

Aboriginal Names Goornoogal (Gija) (Purdie et al., 2018), Gunuga (Jaru) (Wightman, 2003).

Field Notes White Wild Musk Mallow is a small, erect annual shrub that grows up to 2.5 m or more in height. Its leaves are generally ovate, heart-shaped near the base and up to 80 mm long and 70 mm wide. Its white flowers with pink and red tinges have five ovate petals and are present between March and July. Its fruit or seed capsules are five angled. The plant has small hairs that can cause itching. White Wild Musk Mallow occurs in black soils or clay, on alluvial flats and in irrigation ditches in the Pilbara and Kimberley regions of Western Australia, the Northern Territory and Queensland. It also occurs in tropical Africa, India, Indonesia,

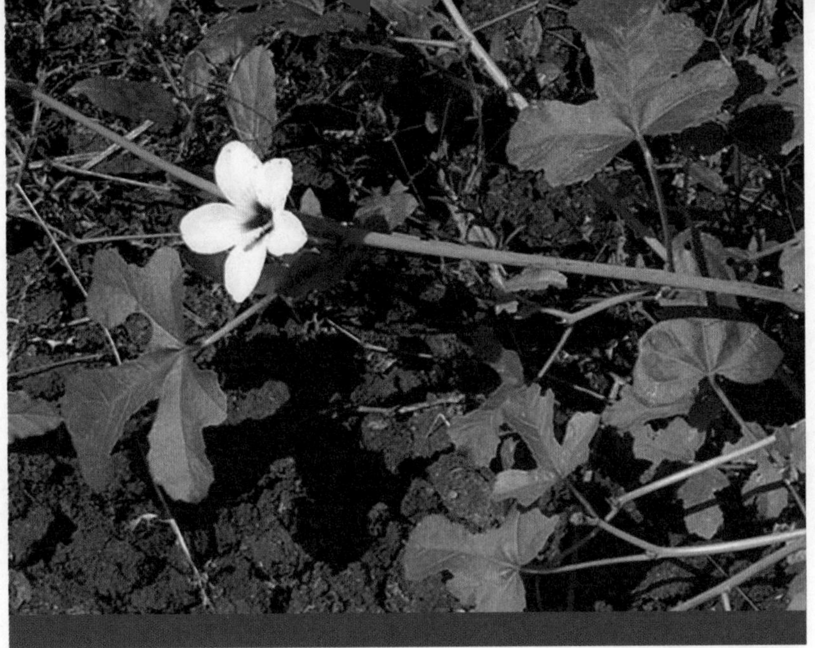

Malaysia, Pakistan and Sri Lanka (ALA, 2022; Flowers of India, 2022; WAH, 2022).

Medicinal Uses Parts of the White Wild Musk Mallow plant are used in folk medicine in Africa. Infusions of crushed leaves and salty water were used to treat diarrhoea. Decoctions of the crushed fresh roots were taken internally to treat calcium deficiency. A paste made of the roots was ingested and applied to scorpion stings (Fern, 2021).

Other Uses The roots and stems of White Wild Musk Mallow are edible and are usually eaten after they have been roasted in hot ashes (Barker, 1991; Cribb & Cribb, 1981; Fern, 2021; Purdie et al., 2018; Wightman, 2003). The yams are available during the wet season and for a short time after (Wightman, 2003). The young mucilaginous pods are also edible (Ewart & Davies, 1917). The leaves were fruit are eaten in Africa in times when food was scarce and may have been eaten in Australia for the same reason (Fern, 2021).

Wickham's Wattle

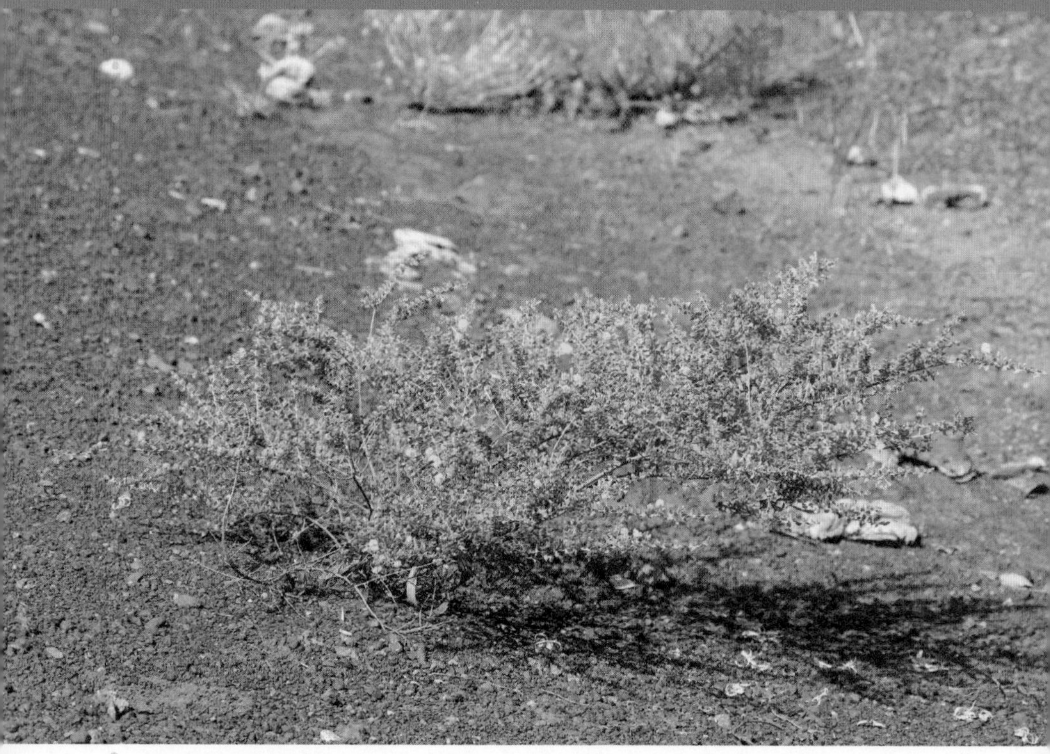

Scientific Name *Acacia wickhamii* Benth.

Common Name Wickham's Wattle.

Aboriginal Names Balalagudu (Bardi) (Keneally et al., 1996), Balalagoord (Bardi) (Paddy et al., 1993).

Field Notes Wickham's Wattle is an erect to low spreading shrub that grows up to 2.5 m in height. Its phyllodes come in many shapes, including narrowly lanceolate to broadly ovate, narrowly elliptic to broadly elliptic and oblong or orbicular. They are straight or curved and up to 30 mm long and 10 mm wide. Its yellow, globular flower heads can be present any time from January to September. Its fruit or seed pods are narrowly oblanceolate, sometimes very narrowly elliptic to linear, basally tapered, straight-sided, flat and up to 90 mm long and 10 mm wide. Wickham's Wattle occurs in a variety of soils, including sandstone and shale, on stony plains and creek banks in the East Pilbara and Kimberley

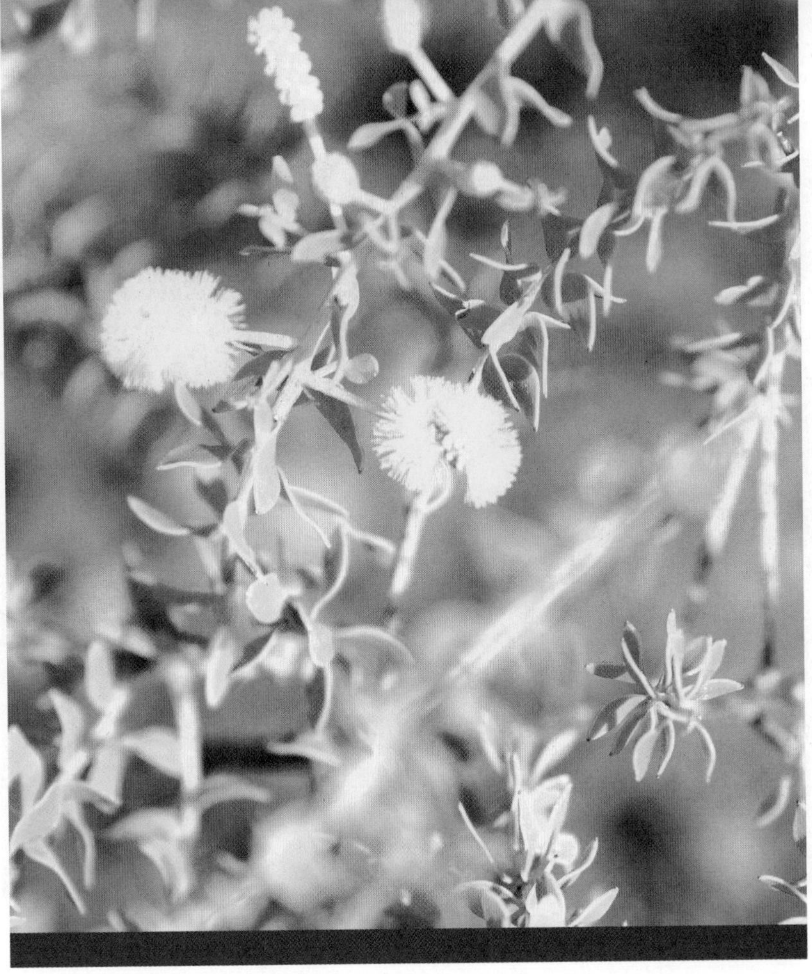

regions of Western Australia, the Northern Territory and Far North Queensland (ALA, 2022; WAH, 2022; World Wide Wattle, 2022).

Medicinal Uses Decoctions of the seeds and leaves of Wickham's Wattle were used as an antiseptic wash to bathe wounds and sores, and as a liniment to treat areas of arthritic and rheumatic pain (Kenneally et al., 1996). Poultices of warmed phyllodes (leaves) were applied to areas of arthritic and rheumatic pain (Paddy et al., 1993).

Other Uses Branches of Wickham's Wattle were tied to a belt made with hair that was worn as a shark repellent when swimming to recover food, such as turtle and dugong, from the water (Kenneally et al., 1996).

Wild Gardenia

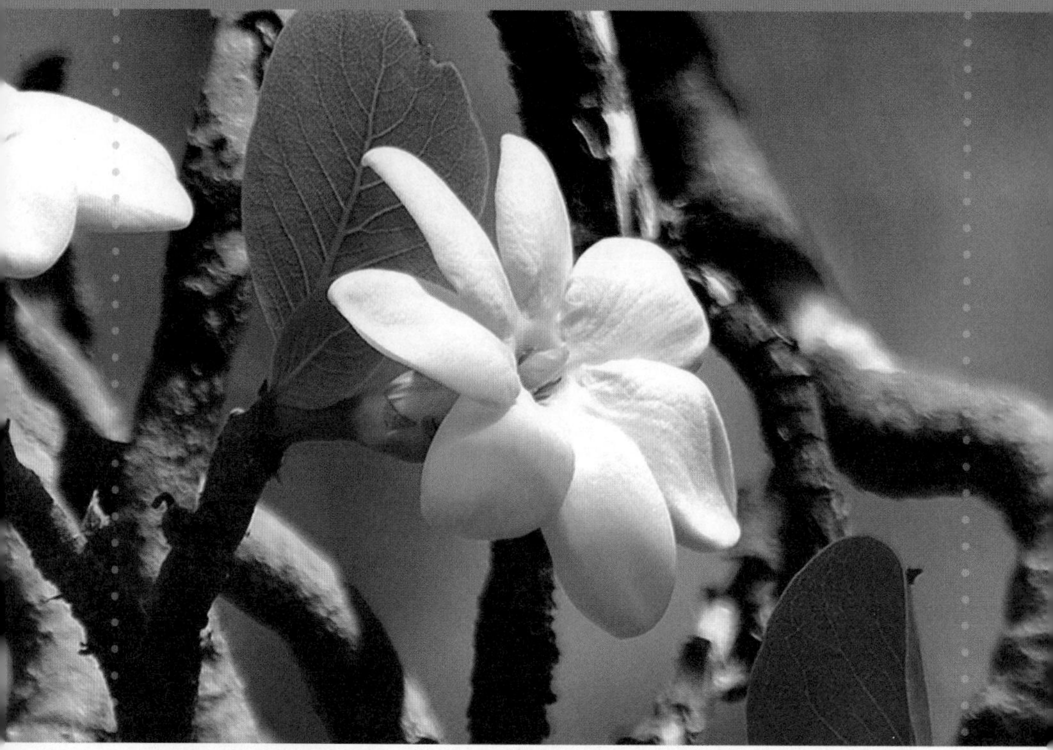

Scientific Name *Gardenia megasperma* F.Muell.

Common Name Wild Gardenia.

Aboriginal Names Wurtarr (Walmajarri) (Richards & Hudson, 2012), Martany (Gija) (Wightman, 2003), Malarra winya (Kwini) (Cheinmora et al., 2017; Crawford, 1982).

Field Notes Wild Gardenia is a tree that grows up to 9 m in height. It has mottled light grey and yellow bark, and large, broadly elliptic leaves that are up to 130 mm long and 18 mm wide. Its large, fragrant, white flowers have ovate petals arranged in whirls, and are up to 50 mm across. They appear at ends of branches between June and November. Green, ovoid fruit approximately 60 mm long and 40 mm in diameter appear after flowering. Wild Gardenia occurs in sandy soils over sandstone, all over the central and northern Kimberley region of Western Australia and the northern half of the Northern Territory (ALA, 2022; WAH, 2022).

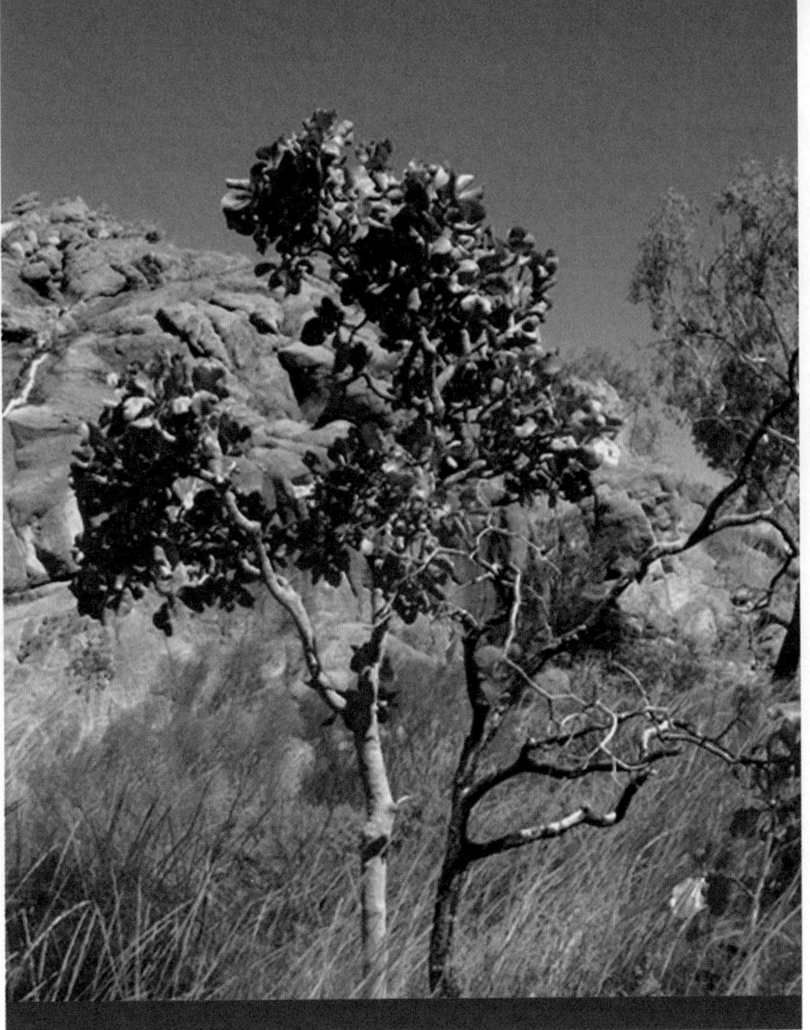

Medicinal Uses Decoctions of the bark of Wild Gardenia were used as a wash to treat skin disorders and itchy skin. A growing tip was broken off and the clear sticky sap that exuded from the break was applied directly to sores and cuts to dry them up and to hasten the healing process (Smith, 1991).

Other Uses The fruit of Wild Gardenia are edible when ripe from October to November (Bindon, 2014; City of Darwin, 2013; Fox & Garde, 2018; RFCA, 1993). The small apical buds between the outer, opposite leaves are edible and were chewed like chewing gum (Wiynjorrotj et al., 2005). The Kwini used the leaves to wrap food that was cooked in a ground oven to give it some flavour (Cheinmora et al., 2017).

Wild Mango

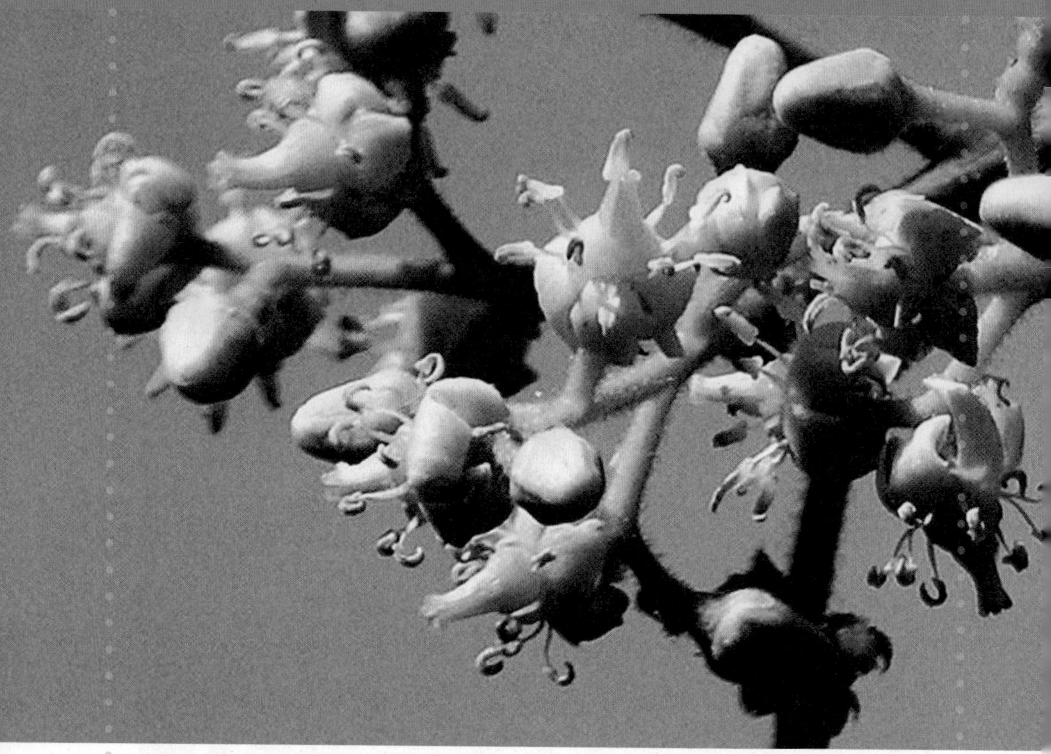

Scientific Names *Buchanania obovata* Engl., also known as *Buchanania oblongifolia* W.Fitzg., previously known as *Buchanania florida* Schauer.

Common Names Wild Mango, Mangkarrba, Green Plum.

Aboriginal Names Laani (Bunuba) (Oscar et al., 2019), Murriya, Gulay (Wunambal, Gaambera) (Karadada et al., 2011), Mangkarrba, Ngauwingai, Glai (tree), Walangga (root) (Kwini) (Crawford, 1982), Gorola, Koroll (Bardi) (Smith & Kalotas, 1985), Kuleyi (Balanggarra) (Crawford, 1982), Daaloony, Taaluny (Gija) (Purdie et al., 2018; Wightman, 2003), Darlung (Miwa) (Kimberley Specialists, 2020), Daloong (Miriwoong) (Leonard et al., 2013), Kulei ninya, Kûlei ninya, Ngawingei ninya (Kwini) (Cheinmora et al., 2017; Crawford, 1982).

Field Notes Wild Mango grows as a shrub or tree up to 15 m in height depending on conditions. It has grey, scaly fissured bark and stiff, light green ovate leaves that are up to 250 mm long and 80 mm

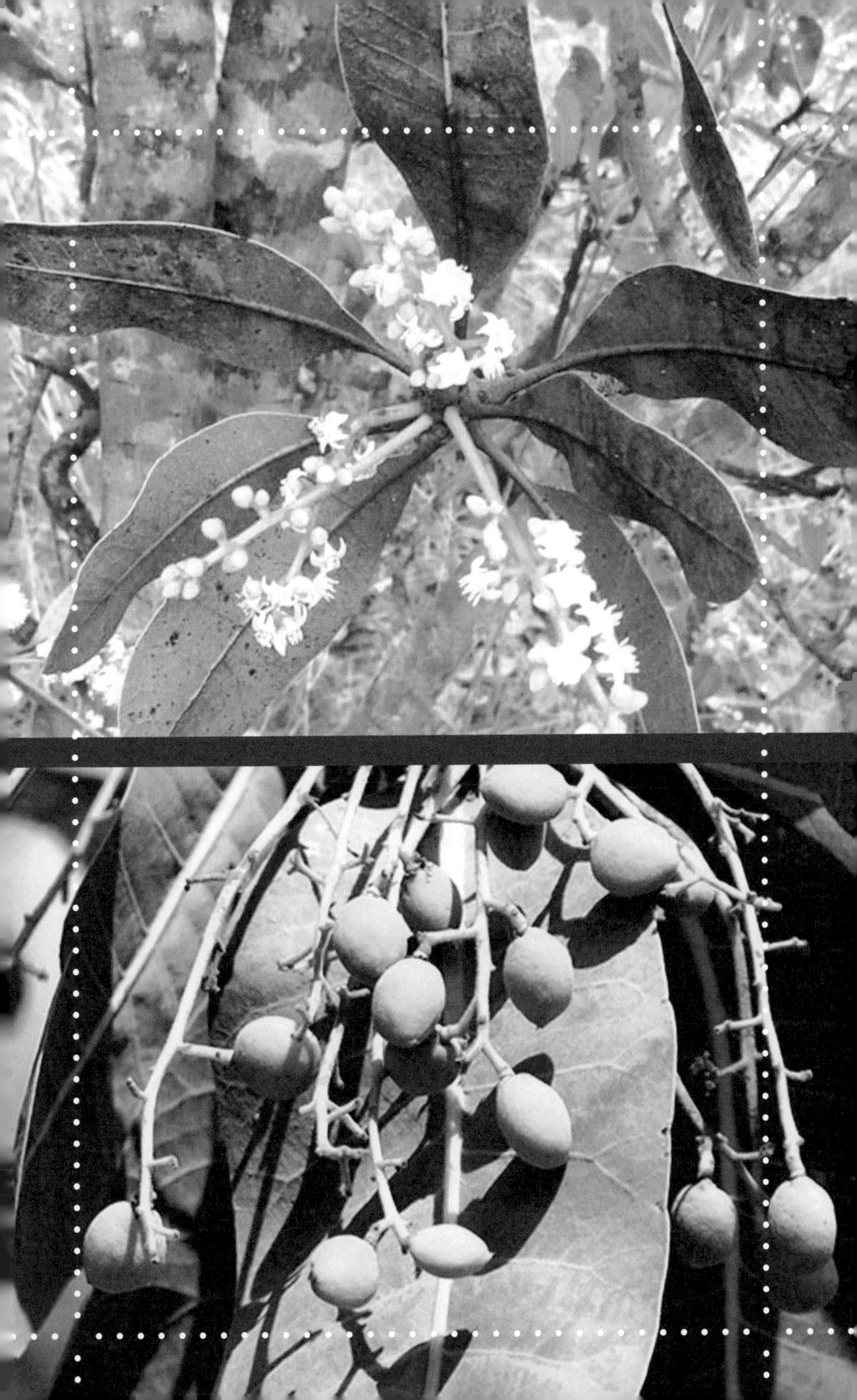

wide. Its white-cream-yellow flowers are about 9 mm in diameter and are present between May to October. Its green fruit are about the size of grapes and hang in clusters. Wild Mango is found in skeletal soils, on rocky sandstone hills and in gorges in the Kimberley region of Western Australia and the northern end of the Northern Territory (ALA, 2022; ATRP, 2020; Lassak & McCarthy, 2001; WAH, 2022).

Medicinal Uses Decoctions of the wood, inner bark and leaves of the Wild Mango were used to treat toothache. Small wood shavings were used to plug the affected tooth (Hiddins, 2001; Western Australia Now & Then, 2022). Infusions of the inner bark and sapwood were used as a mouthwash for toothache and as an eyewash to treat conjunctivitis (Low, 1990). Cavities in aching teeth were plugged with the leaves to relieve toothache. When the leaves were removed, the mouthwash was used to rinse out the mouth (Lassak & McCarthy, 2001; Smith, 1991). Sometimes the leaves were heated and applied as a poultice to wounds and sores to aid healing (Low, 1990). The fruit have mild laxative properties and were used to treat constipation (Hiddins, 2001; Martin, 2014).

Other Uses The 'green plums' are edible and were eaten fresh or dried for later use. They are reported to have a pleasant flavour and are high in ascorbic acid (vitamin C). The fruit are usually collected from mid-November to late December (Cheinmora et al., 2017; Crawford, 1982; DBCA, 2019; Fern, 2021; Fox & Garde, 2018; Hiddins, 2001; Karadada et al., 2011; Low, 1991; McMahon, 2006; RFCA, 1993; Smith, 1991). Wightman (2003) relates that, 'The fruit are often available in large amounts and the flesh and seed can be pounded and smashed up and formed into a large ball, wrapped in paperbark and stored for later use'. The roots of young plants are also edible after being roasted in hot ashes and pounded to soften them. The roots are harvested all year round (Cheinmora et al., 2017; Crawford, 1982; DBCA, 2019; Karadada et al., 2011; Vigilante et al., 2013). The wood of this tree has traditionally been used to make shields (Cheinmora et al., 2017; Crawford, 1982).

Wild Melon

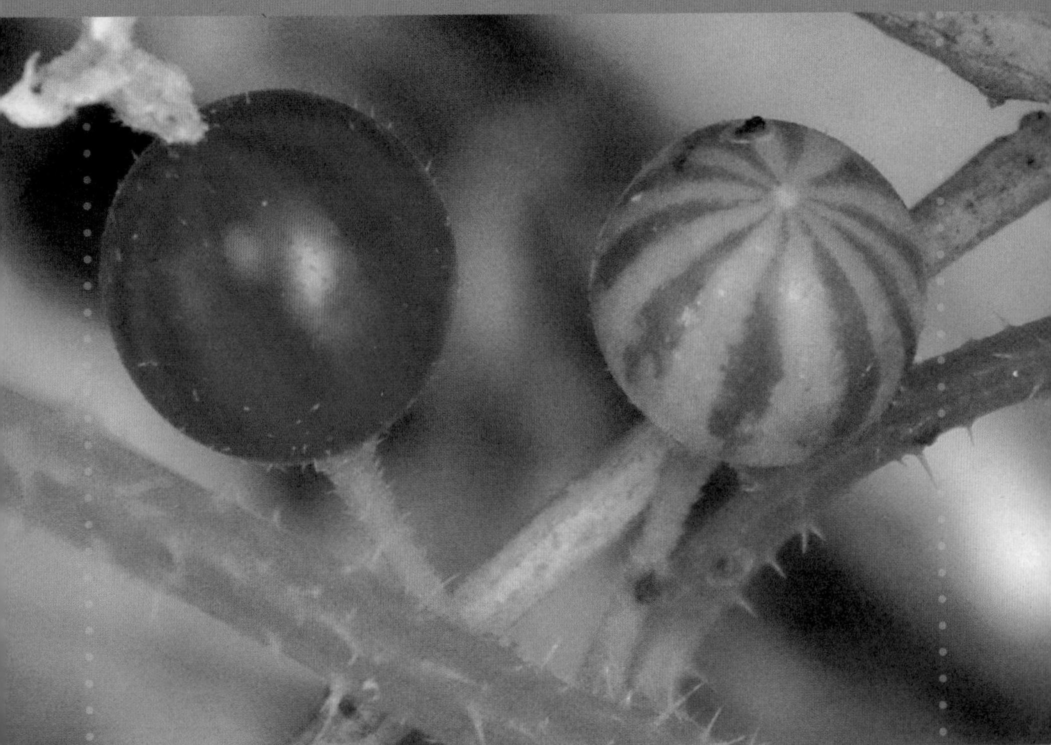

Scientific Name *Cucumis variabilis* P.Sebastian & I.Telford, previously known as *Mukia maderaspatana* (L.) M.Roem (misapplied).

Common Name Wild Melon.

Field Notes Wild Melon is a decumbent or climbing, twining vine in the cucumber family that only grows in the Pilbara and Kimberley regions of Western Australia. It has thin, striped, hairy stems, arrowhead-shaped leaves with three lobes, trumpet-like, yellow flowers and globose, striped, green fruit that eventually turn red. The fruit are about the same size as an apple cucumber. (ALA, 2022; eFlora.SA, 2022).

Medicinal Uses Decoctions of the whole plant were used by some Aboriginal groups as an antiseptic wash to bathe skin sores, cuts, wounds and the eyes to treat conjunctivitis (Cock, 2011; Cancilla & Wingfield, 2017).

Wild Nutmeg

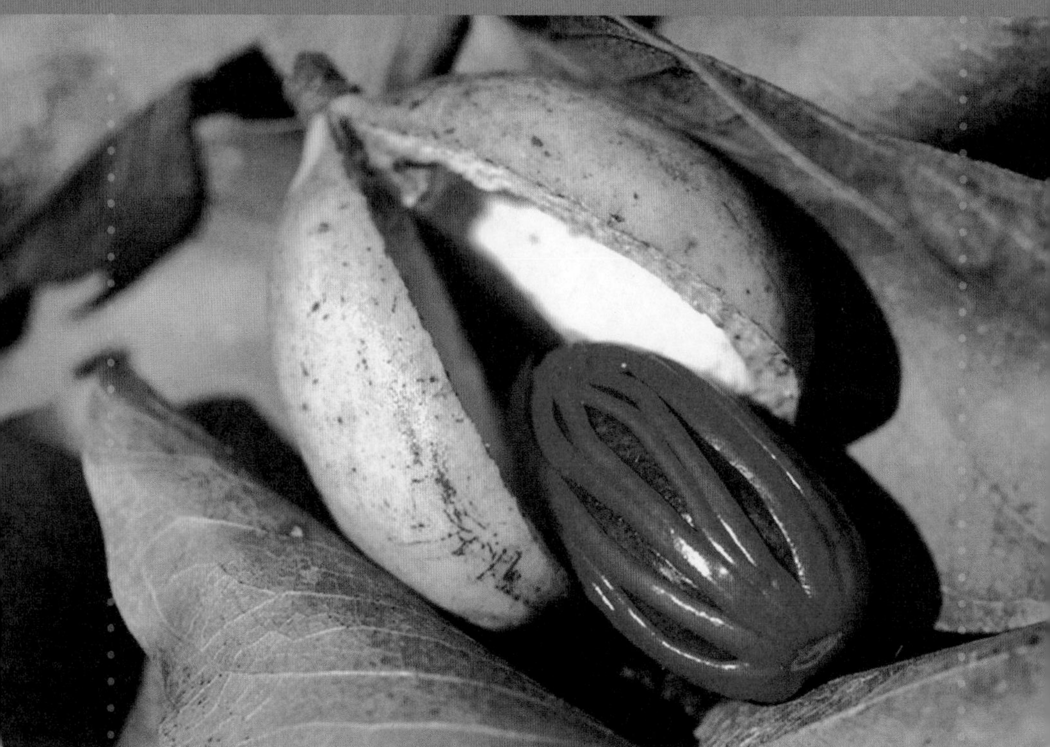

Scientific Name *Myristica insipida* R.Br.

Common Names Wild Nutmeg, Native Nutmeg, Queensland Nutmeg.

Field Notes Wild Nutmeg has separate male and female trees that grow to around 16 m tall. Its leaf blades are ovate with a hairy under surface and are up to 200 mm long by 100 mm wide. Its male inflorescences are terminal with a sub-umbel of two to ten flowers. Its female inflorescences are also terminal with a sub-umbel of only one to four flowers. Its fruit are ellipsoidal and green measuring up to 45 mm long and 25 mm wide and turning brown and hairy as they age. Wild Nutmeg occurs right across the top end of Australia, from the Kimberley region in Western Australia through to Cairns in Queensland. It also occurs on the Torres Strait Islands (Lake, 2015; Lassak & McCarthy, 2001).

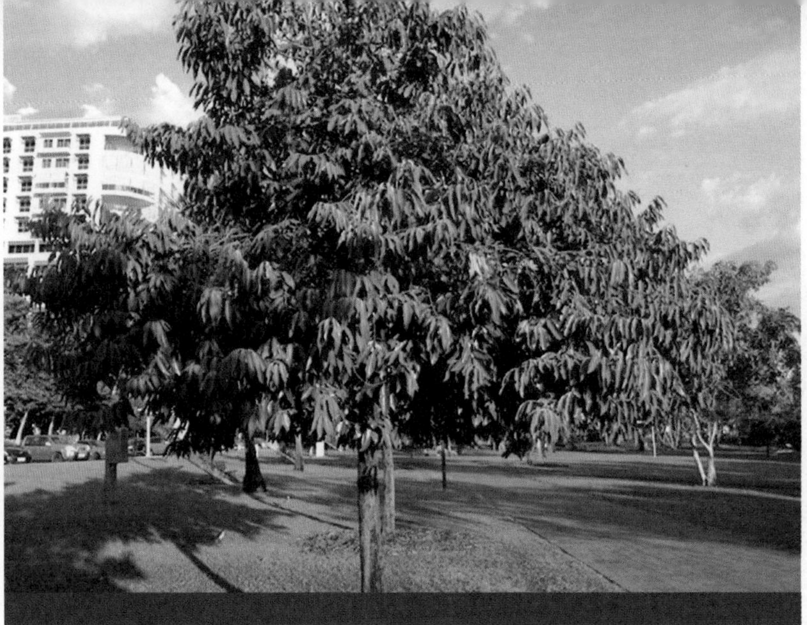

Medicinal Uses Resin oozing from cuts in the bark is thought to have antifungal properties and was used to treat dermatophytosis (ringworm and tinea) (Cock, 2011; Lassak & McCarthy, 2001; Low, 1990).

Other uses The seeds and aril of Wild Nutmeg are edible. The kernel can be grated and used as a substitute for True Nutmeg (*Myristica fragrans*) (Bindon, 2014; Hiddins, 2001; Territory Native Plants, 2022). The red netting or 'mace' surrounding the seeds is also edible and requires no preparation. The trunk of the tree was used by some Aboriginal groups to make dugout canoes (Hiddins, 2001).

Wild Orange

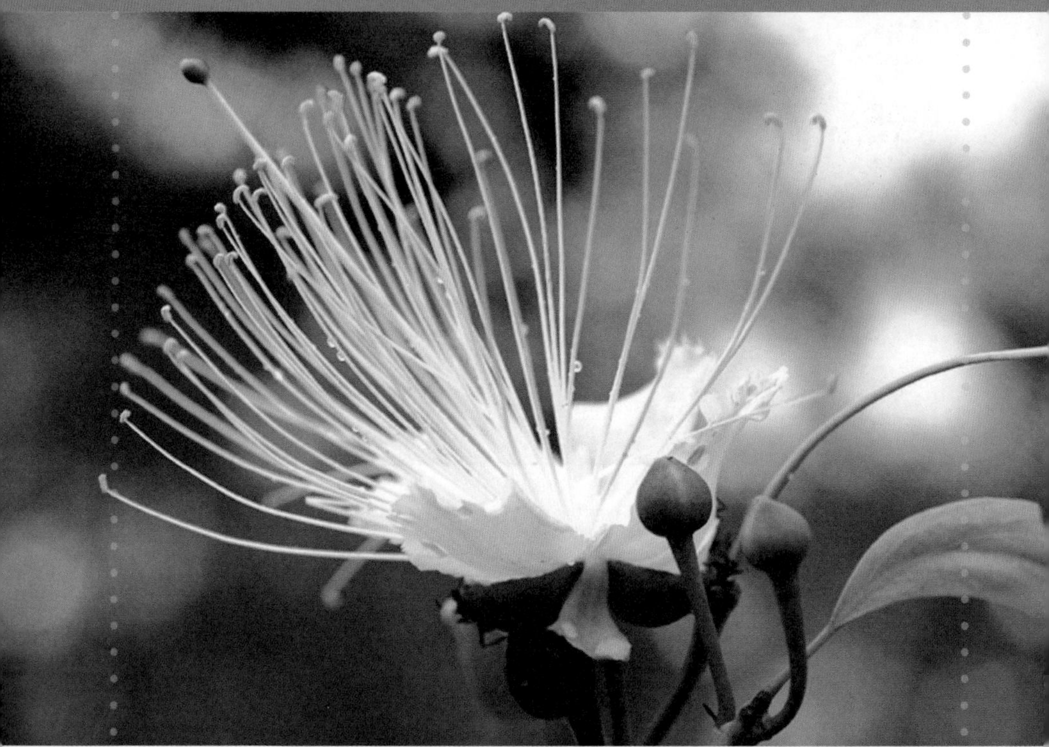

Scientific Name *Capparis umbonata* Lindl.

Common Names Wild Orange, Northern Wild Orange, Bush Orange, Native Guava.

Aboriginal Names Gudida (Bunuba) (Oscar et al., 2019), Joogoorroong (Miriwoong) (Leonard et al., 2013), Minggarra (Wunambal, Gaambera) (Karadada et al., 2011), Djuggurung (Kwini), Joogoorrool, Jugurrul, Jukurrul, Goordidal, Kurtital (Gija) (Purdie et al., 2018; Wightman, 2003), Jukurru, Yupuna (Walmajarri) (Richards & Hudson, 2012), Yuwunar, Yumali, Jugurru (tree form) (Jaru) (Wightman, 2003), Yiringgi, Yidiringgi (shrub form) (Jaru) (Deegan et al., 2010), Nangkulu winya (Kwini) (Cheinmora et al., 2017; Crawford, 1982), Tjukuru (Kukatja) (Valiquette, 1993), Nganybarl (Kyikina) (Milgin, 2009), Jukurru (Walpiri) (Northern Tanami IPA, 2015), Jamparr (Karajarri) (Moss et al., 2021).

Field Notes Wild Orange grows as a shrub or tree up to 10 m in height. It has dark rough bark and long, dull green, leathery leaves that are up to 200 mm long by 40 mm wide. Its white-cream-yellow, upright flowers with long white stamens appear from January to March or from May to September, depending on conditions. Its round fruit appear on long stalks and are approximately 50 mm across. They turn from green to red when ripe. The ripe fruit are usually available between mid-November and December. Wild Orange occurs in alluvium, loam clay or pindan sand on sandstone ridges and floodplains in the Pilbara and Kimberley regions of Western Australia, the Northern Territory and in Queensland as far south as Townsville (ALA, 2022; WAH, 2022).

Medicinal Uses The leaves of Wild Orange were used as a 'steaming medicine', similar to Vicks inhalations, to treat the symptoms of colds and influenza. Smoke from the leaves was inhaled and decoctions of the leaves were used as a wash for the same purpose (Purdie et al., 2018; Wightman, 2003). Infusions of the inner bark were taken internally to treat diarrhoea (Low, 1990) or used externally as an eyewash to treat conjunctivitis. Decoctions of the bark and leaves were used externally as a liniment for rheumatic pain and as an antiseptic wash for skin conditions, such as scabies infestations, sores, boils, wounds and cuts (Smith, 1991).

Other Uses The pink pulp of the fruit is edible when the fruit are ripe, green and soft to touch. The pulp is reported to be quite sweet (Crawford, 1982; Fox & Garde, 2018; Isaacs, 1987; Karadada et al., 2011; Smith, 1991; Wheaton, 1994; Wightman, 2003). The fruit are sometimes buried in hot sand next to a fire to ripen them (Karadada et al., 2011; Wightman, 2003). Smoke from the smouldering leaves of Wild Orange is used by the Jaru 'in funeral ceremonies to cleanse areas where the deceased lived and to keep away bad spirits in the future' (Wightman, 2003).

Wild Parsnip

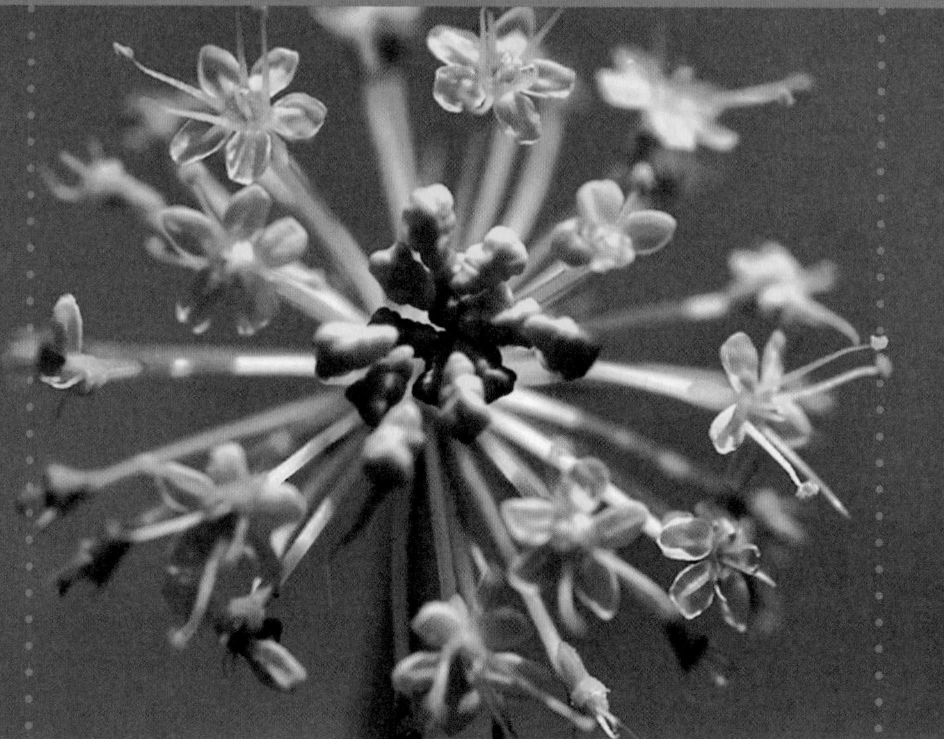

Scientific Name *Trachymene didiscoides* (F.Muell.) B.L.Burtt, previously known as *Trachymene hemicarpa* Benth.

Common Names Wild Parsnip, Wilawanggan, Kangaroo Yam.

Field Notes Wild Parsnip grows as an erect annual, biennial or perennial herb up to 2.5 m in height. Its sparse leaves are wedge-shaped or three lobed with jagged edges. Its small, cream-to-white flowers form umbrella-shaped clusters (umbels) from January to February or April to December. Wild Parsnip occurs in sand or shallow skeletal soils over sandstone, on rocky outcrops, ridges and in gullies in the northern part of the Kimberley region of Western Australia and the Northern Territory (ALA, 2022; Lassak & McCarthy, 2001; WAH, 2022).

Medicinal Uses The green leaves and roots of Wild Parsnip were crushed and rubbed over the body to treat cramps and general

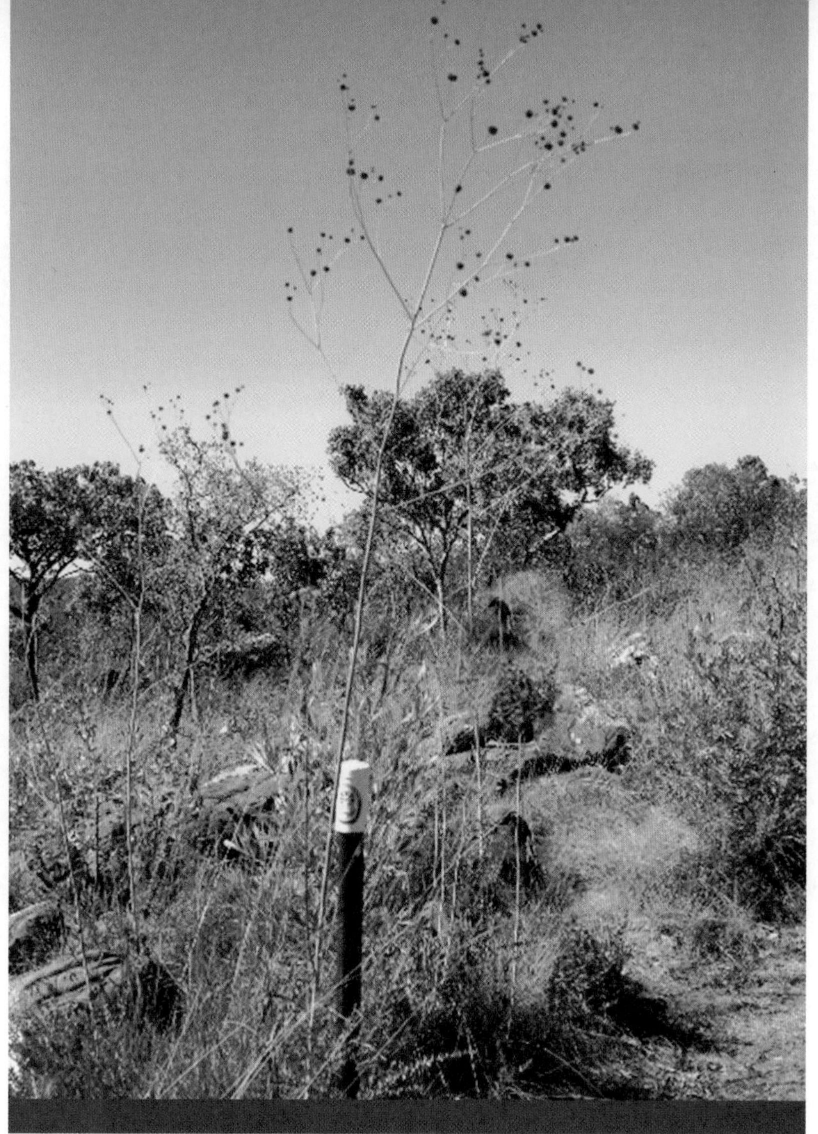

fatigue (Isaacs, 1987; Lassak & McCarthy, 2001; Reid, 1986; Webb, 1959).

Other Uses The roots of Wild Parsnip are edible and were probably roasted in hot ashes before they were eaten (Bradley et al., 2006).

Wild Peach

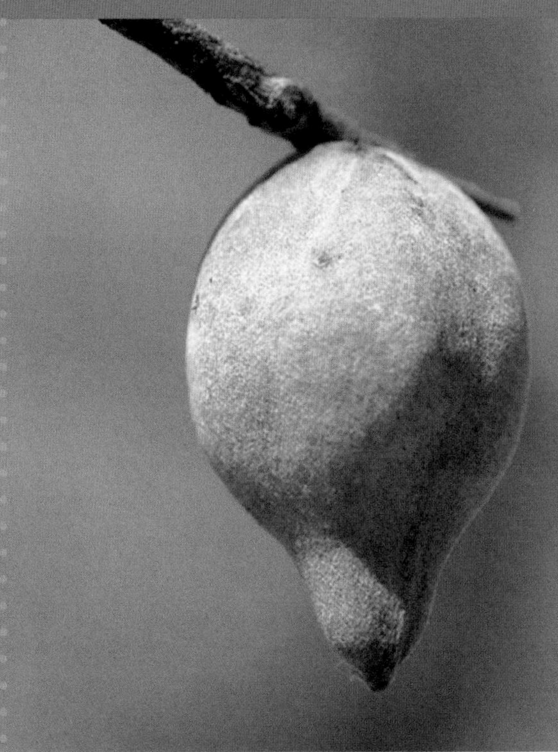

Scientific Names *Terminalia carpentariae* C.T.White, also known as *Terminalia hadleyana* subsp. *carpentariae* (C.T.White) Pedley.

Common Names Wild Peach, Salty Plum, Billy Goat Plum.

Aboriginal Names Mayawu (Wunambal, Gaambera) (Karadada et al., 2011), Juguru (Miwa) (Kimberley Specialists, 2020), Mandarral manya, Mandaraal manya (Kwini) (Cheinmora, et al., 2017).

Field Notes Wild Peach is a spreading shrub or tree that grows up to 10 m in height. It has mottled, yellow, grey, orange and slightly fissured bark. Its simple leaves are roughly 120 mm long by 100 mm wide and vary in shape, including circular, elliptic, oblong, ovate or obovate. Its small cream to light green flowers form on long racemes from October to November. Its ovoid or obovoid, pear-shaped fruit are up to 35 mm long and 17mm in diameter. Fruiting occurs between July and October. Wild Peach occurs in grey sandy clay, brown clay, skeletal alluvial soils, sandstone and limestone on slopes

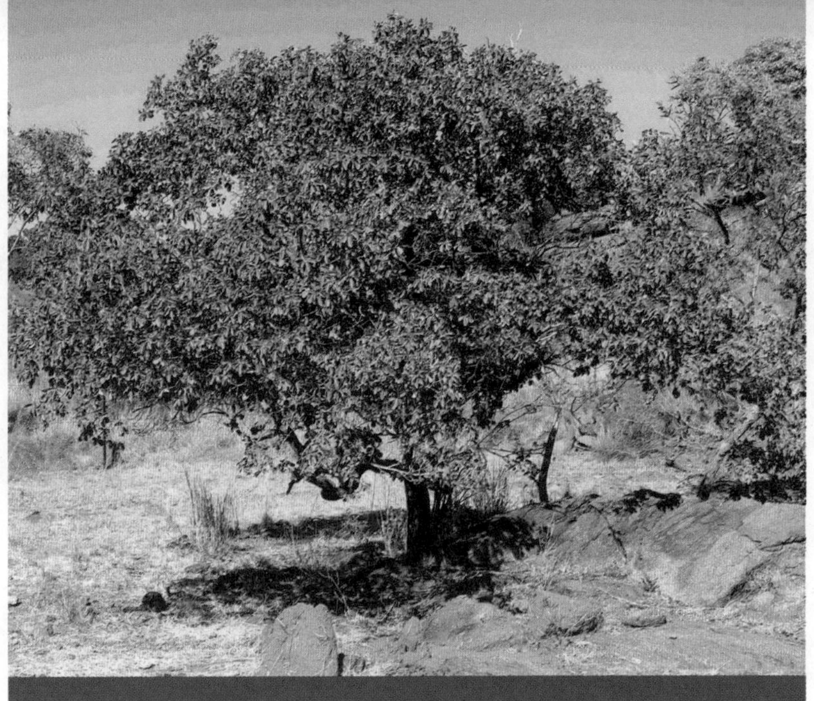

behind beaches, in dry creek beds, on flats between creeks and cliffs, on floodplains and on scree slopes in the northern half of the Kimberley region of Western Australia and the Northern Territory (ALA, 2022; Bininj Kunwok, 2022; WAH, 2022).

Medicinal Uses The red sap of the inner bark was rubbed over parts of the body to strengthen the skin, to improve muscle tone, to ease sore and tired feet, and to improve general well-being. The sticky inner bark is reported to have antiseptic properties and was applied directly to sores, wounds and cuts to aid healing (Devanesen, 2000; Williams, 2011).

Other Uses The fruit of the Wild Peach are edible and are eaten raw when yellow and ripe, usually in the late dry season. They are a sweet and a highly sought-after food in the bush and are reported to have a slight apricot flavour (Cheinmora et al., 2017; Fox & Garde, 2018; Hiddins, 2001; Karadada et al., 2011; Vigilante et al., 2013). The fruit is high in ascorbic acid (vitamin C), having 1995 mg per 100 g of fruit (Flavel, 2018). The gum is also edible and is eaten when fresh or after it has been softened over hot coals if it has gone hard (Fox & Garde, 2018; Hiddins, 2001; McConnell & O'Connor, 1997; Territory Native Plants, 2022).

Wild Pear

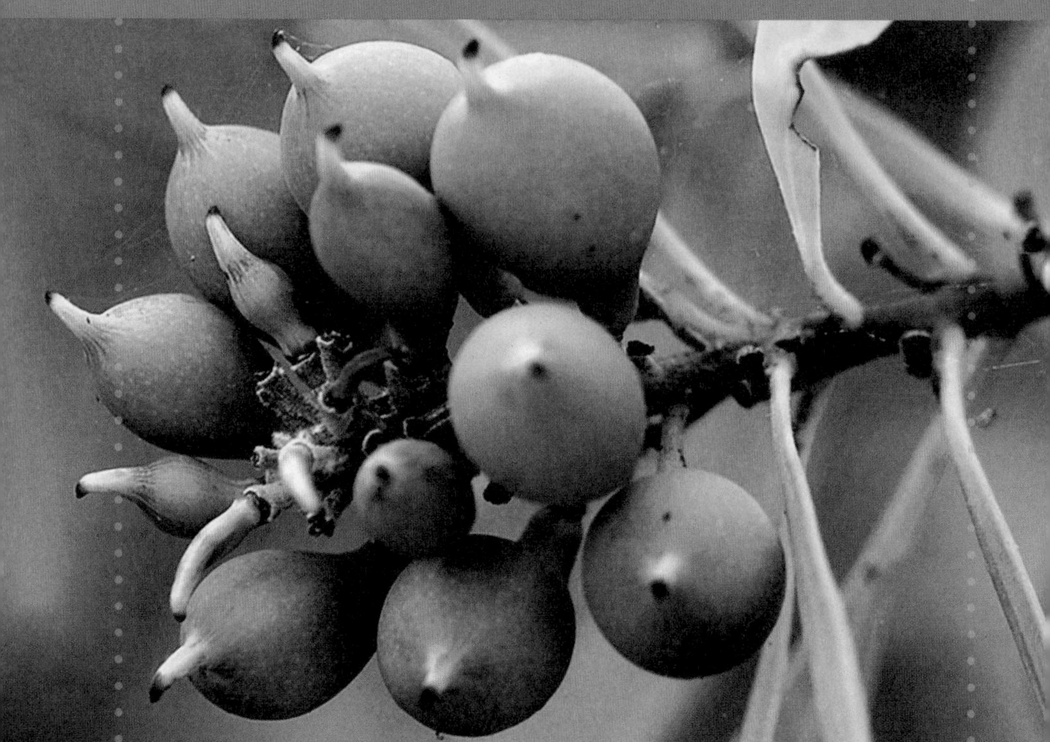

Scientific Name *Persoonia falcata* R.Br.

Common Names Wild Pear, Geebung, Milky Plum, Snottygobble.

Aboriginal Names Galgai, Garndula (Wunambal, Gaambera) (Karadada et al., 2011), Janiya (Walmajarri) (Richards & Hudson, 2012), Ngaliwany (Yawuru), Kamaloon, Gamalun (Bardi) (Smith & Kalotas, 1985), Gamoorloon (Bardi) (Kenneally et al., 1996), Wankid, Wankirr (Nyul Nyul), Ngurrinuy (Nyangumarta), Mirntirrjina (Karajarri, Nyangumarta), Ngurriny (Nyangumarta) (Lands, 1997), Kandala (Balanggarra) (Vigilante et al., 2013), Gantheliny, Kantheliny (Gija) (Purdie et al., 2018), Madjugun (Miwa) (Kimberley Specialists, 2020), Gilayi (Jaru) (Wightman, 2003), Karndala ninya, Kandala ninya, Karndûlû ninya (Kwini) (Cheinmora et al., 2017; Crawford, 1982).

Field Notes Wild Pear grows as an erect shrub or tree to 7 m in height. Its dull green, smooth, leathery leaves are ovate to

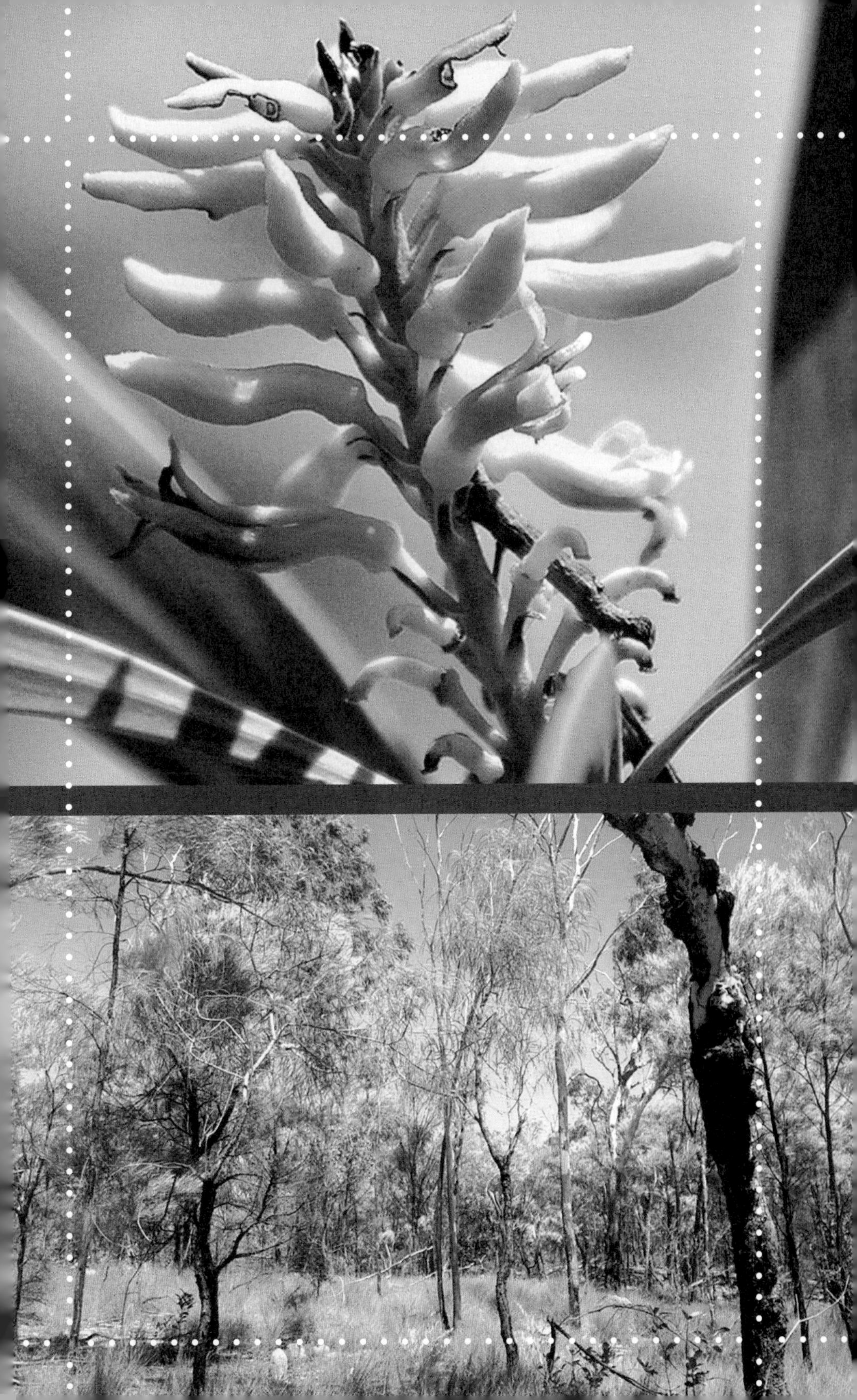

lanceolate and can be up to 200 mm long. Its yellow to cream flowers are tubular, around 15 mm long and borne in dense terminal racemes from June to November. Its green-yellow fruit are ovate drupes with a beaked tip. They are smooth, fleshy, approximately 20 mm long and 10 mm in diameter, with a single seed. Wild Pear occurs in sand and alluvium, along watercourses, on sandstone cliffs, amongst rocks and sometimes in gorges in the Pilbara and Kimberley regions of Western Australia, the Northern Territory and Queensland (ALA, 2022; Lassak & McCarthy, 2001; Native Plants Queensland – Townsville Branch, 2022; WAH, 2022).

Medicinal Uses Infusions or decoctions of the bark and leaves were sipped for sore throats and colds. Infusions of the crushed wood were used as an eyewash to treat conjunctivitis, either straight or mixed with human milk (Cock, 2011; Hiddins, 2001; Lassak & McCarthy, 2001; Smith, 1991; Webb, 1959). Decoctions of the leaves were sipped as a treatment for bad chest infections, sore throats, coughs and diarrhoea. Fresh leaves were dipped into the decoctions and chewed to treat oral thrush (Kane, 2022; Smith, 1991; Wightman, 2003). Crushed leaves were also used as a poultice to treat cuts and other wounds (Kane, 2022). The Gija used infusions of the crushed seeds as a wash to treat sores and the symptoms of influenza (Purdie et al., 2018; Wightman, 2003).

Other Uses The fruit of Wild Pear are edible and are eaten raw when ripe. They are gathered between late November and February. They are reported to taste sweet. The kernel is also eaten by some Aboriginal groups. The whole fruit is sometimes pounded with a stick and sugar added before it is eaten (Cheinmora et al., 2017; Hiddins, 2001; Karadada et al., 2011; Low, 1991; Purdie et al., 2018; Smith, 1991; Wightman, 2003). The kernel can be pounded and mixed with water to make a black custard-like food (Kenneally et al., 2018; Willing, 2014). Crawford (1982) relates that 'the fruit may also be sun-dried, cooked in ashes, hammered and then stored in paperbark' for later use. Case Moth larvae of the

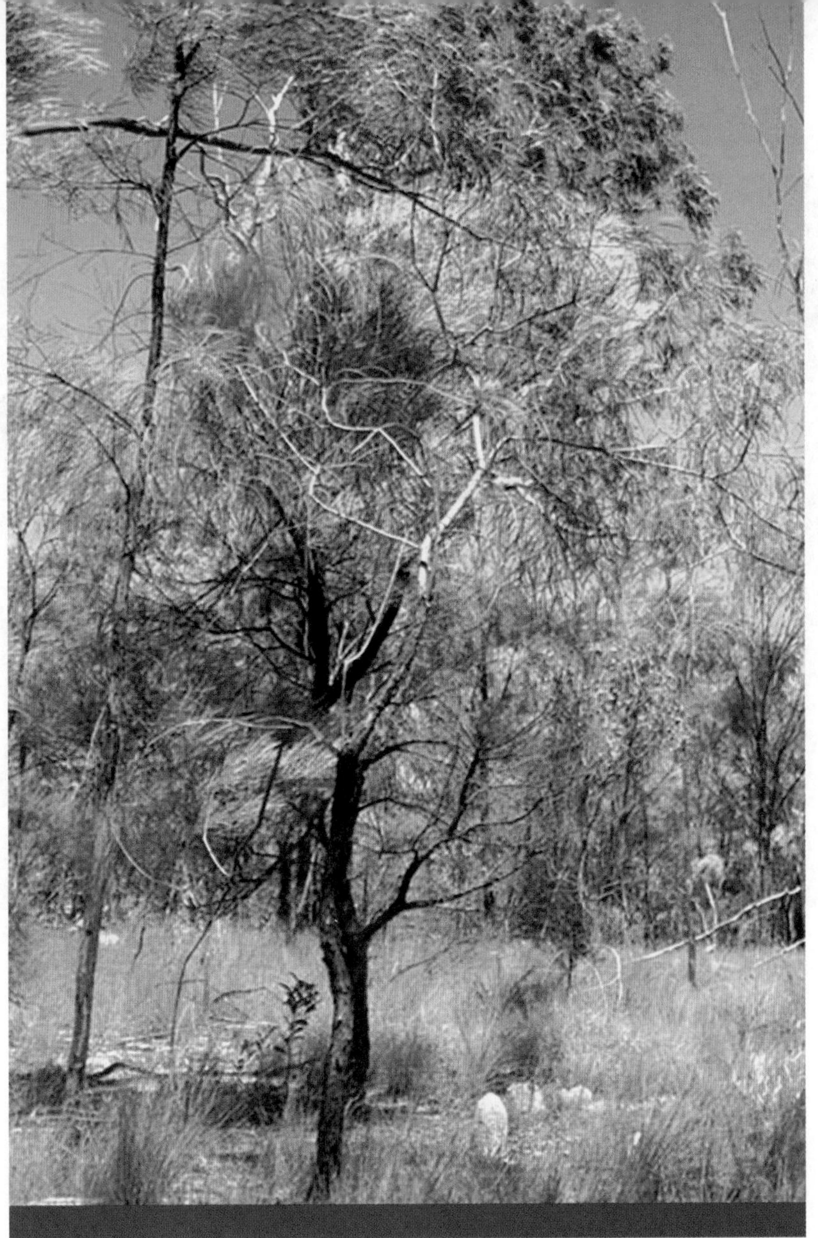

Psychidae family are found in this tree and are eaten raw or slightly roasted (YMAC, 2016). The dense hard wood of the Wild Pear tree is good for making boomerangs (Kimberley Specialists, 2020).

Wild Plum

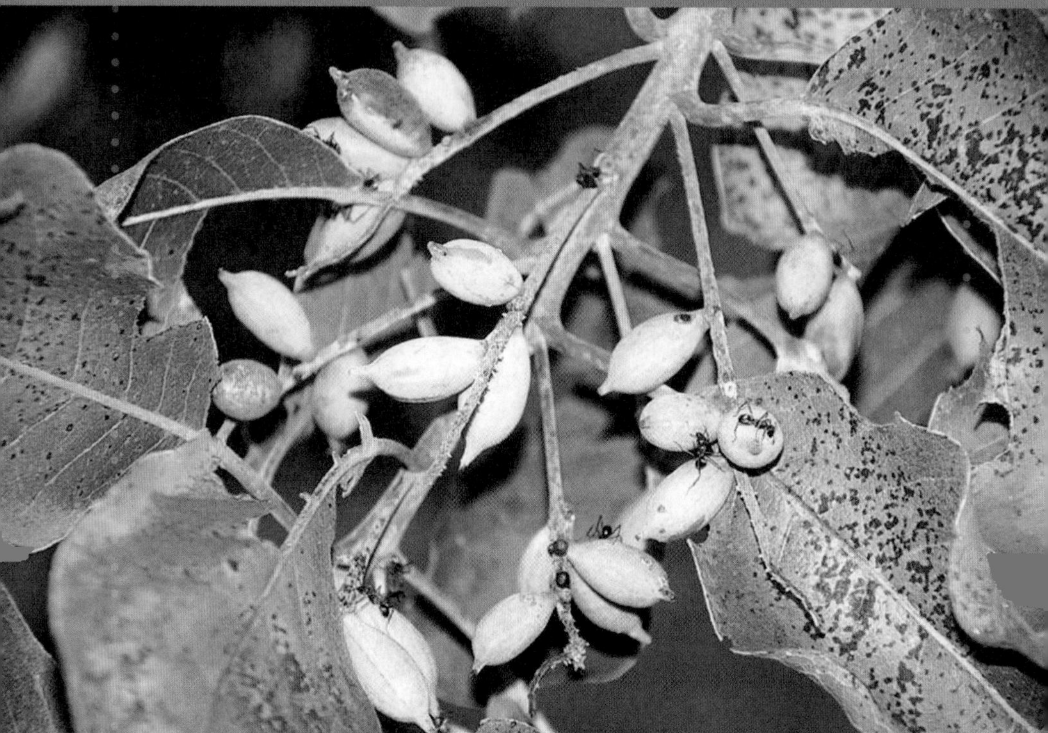

Scientific Name *Terminalia platyphylla* F.Muell.

Common Name Wild Plum.

Aboriginal Names Mandarra (Bunuba) (Oscar et al., 2019), Partinyjal, Marntarra (Walmajarri) (Richards & Hudson, 2012), Nyambarrginy, Thaleginy, Nyarlany (Gija) (Purdie et al., 2018), Marduwa (Jaru) (Wightman, 2003), Mardiya, Mardiwa (Jaru) (Deegan et al., 2010), Midyurung (Miwa) (Kimberley Specialists, 2020), Marrangarr (Kwini) (Cheinmora et al., 2017), Barrakooloo (Nyikina) (Smith & Smith, 2009).

Field Notes Wild Plum is a deciduous or semi-deciduous tree that grows up to 10 m in height. Its large ovate leaves are up to 220 mm long and 140 mm wide. Its small, star-shaped flowers are borne on racemes between January and October. Its fruit are glabrescent, oblong to broadly spindle-shaped with a distinct beak and are up to 40 mm long by 15 mm in diameter. Wild Plum occurs in sandy

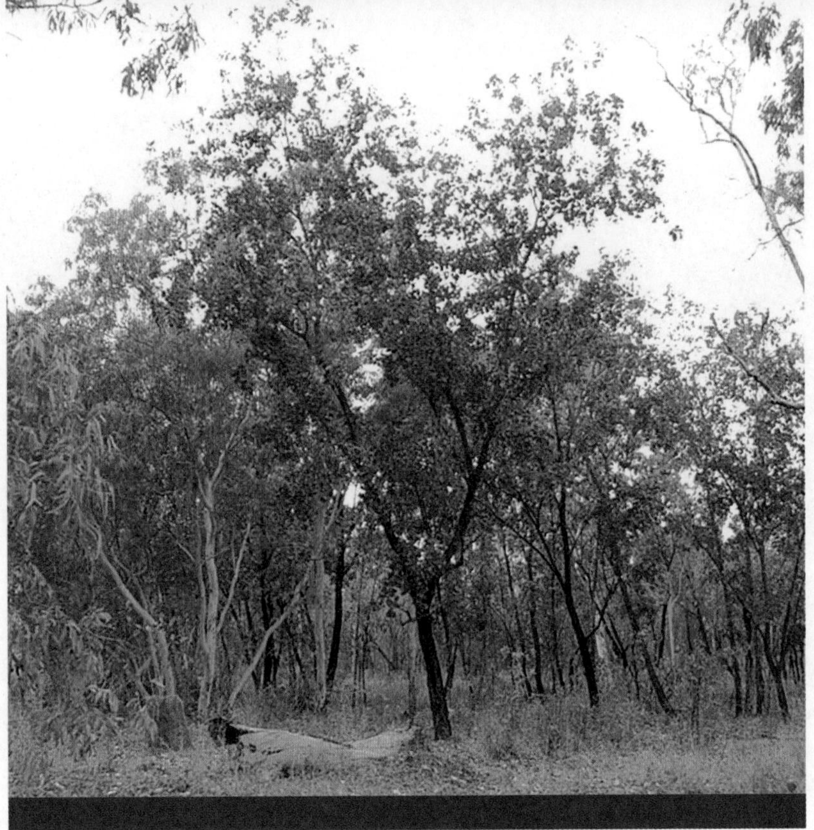

soils, often along creeks, across the top end of Australia from the Kimberley region of Western Australia through the Northern Territory and into Queensland (ALA, 2022; ATRP, 2020; WAH, 2022).

Medicinal Uses The Jaru use the gum from Wild Plum, which they call 'marduwa', for treating stomach upsets and constipation (Wightman, 2003).

Other Uses The fruit of the Wild Plum are edible when purple and ripe in the late wet to early dry season. The gum that oozes from wounds in the tree is edible and can be chewed like toffee (Cheinmora et al., 2017; Oscar et al., 2019; Purdie et al., 2018; Vigilante et al., 2013; Wightman, 2003; Williams, 2011). If the gum is hard, it can be soaked in water to soften it (Wiynjorrotj et al., 2005).

Witchweed

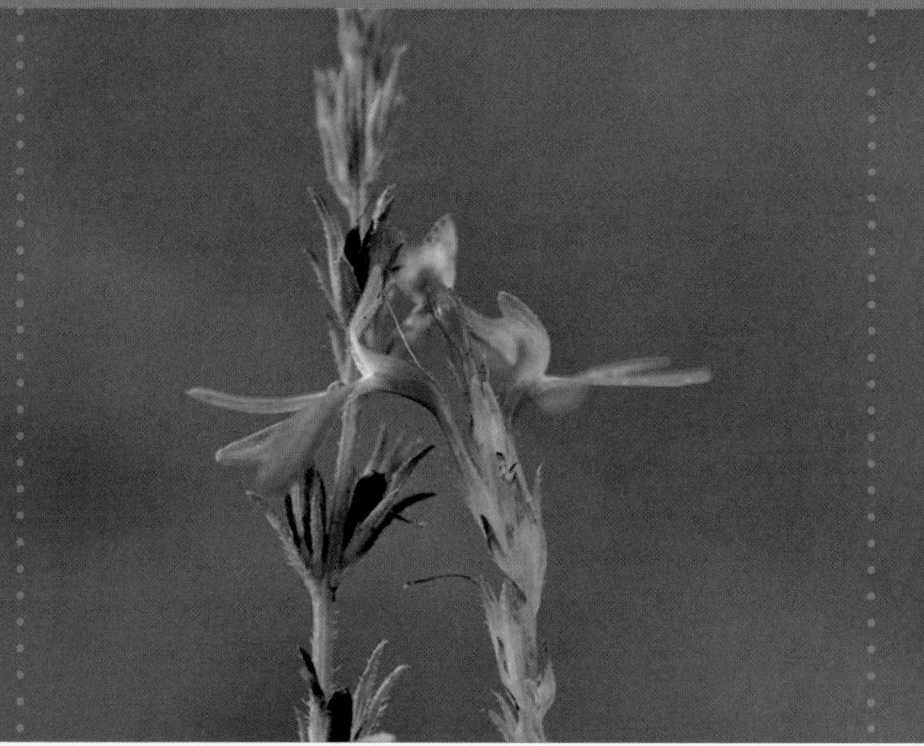

Scientific Name *Striga curviflora* (R.Br.) Benth.

Common Names Witchweed, Witch Weed.

Field Notes Witchweed is a hemiparasitic, erect, annual herb that grows to around 600 mm in height. It has very thin, linear leaves, and pink, blue, purple or white, tubular and bell-shaped flowers that appear between January and October. Its fruit are two-valved capsules. Witchweed is found in sandy, gravelly and clayey soils in the Pilbara and Kimberley regions of Western Australia, the Northern Territory and northern Queensland (ALA, 2022; Lassak & McCarthy, 2001; WAH, 2022).

Medicinal Uses Infusions of the crushed whole Witchweed plant were used externally as an antiseptic wash to bathe wounds, sores and other skin disorders (Cock, 2011; Lassak & McCarthy, 2001).

Other Uses The leaves of Witchweed were used by Aboriginal groups in Queensland as a bush tobacco (Clarke, 2007).

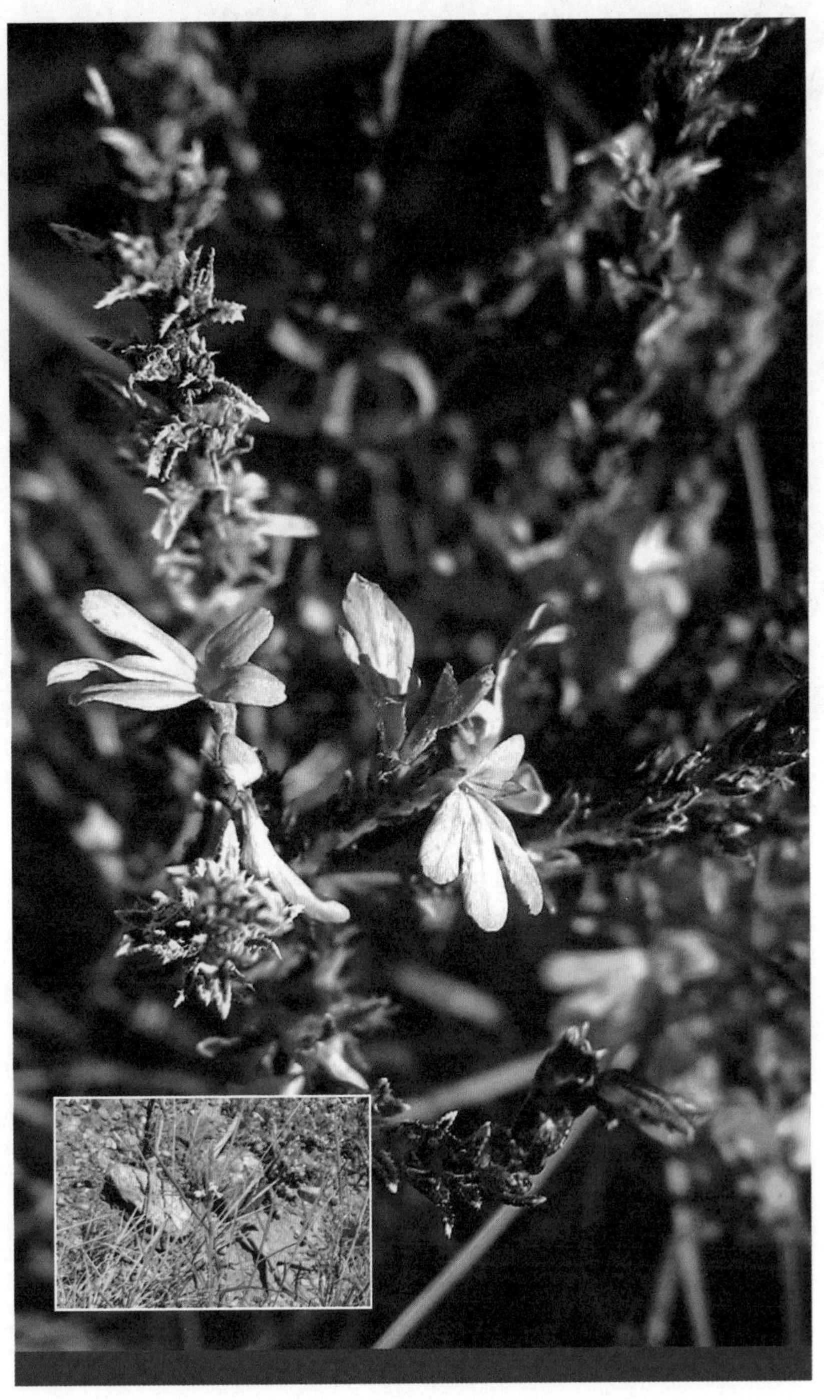

Witinti

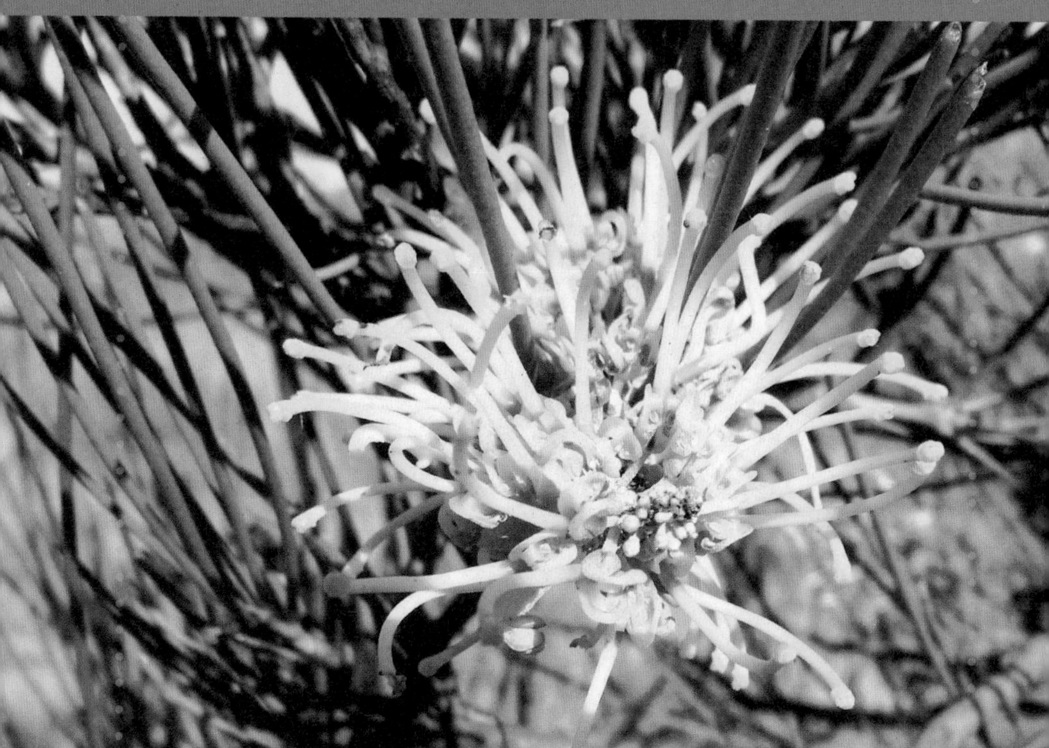

Scientific Name *Hakea lorea* (R.Br.) R.Br. and *Hakea lorea* (R.Br.) R.Br. subsp. *lorea*.

Common Names Witinti, Long-leaved Corkwood, Corkwood, Fork-leaved Corkwood, Honey Hakea.

Aboriginal Names Katapuka (Kukatja) (Valiquette, 1993), Wirarrajartu, Yutuyutu (Walmajarri) (Richards & Hudson, 2012),

Field Notes Witinti is a multi-stemmed shrub or small tree that grows up to 9 m in height depending on conditions. It has thick, corky, deep-fissured grey bark. Its long, thin cylindrical leaves can be up to 680 mm long and 2.3 mm wide. Its bright yellow, spider-like flower heads are very showy and up to 120 mm long. Flowering is from May to October. After flowering, woody pods, slightly curved to 35 mm long, are produced. Witinti occurs in sandy or clayey soils over sandstone, granite or basalt, on plains or in ranges, along drainage lines, claypans and stony sites right across the top

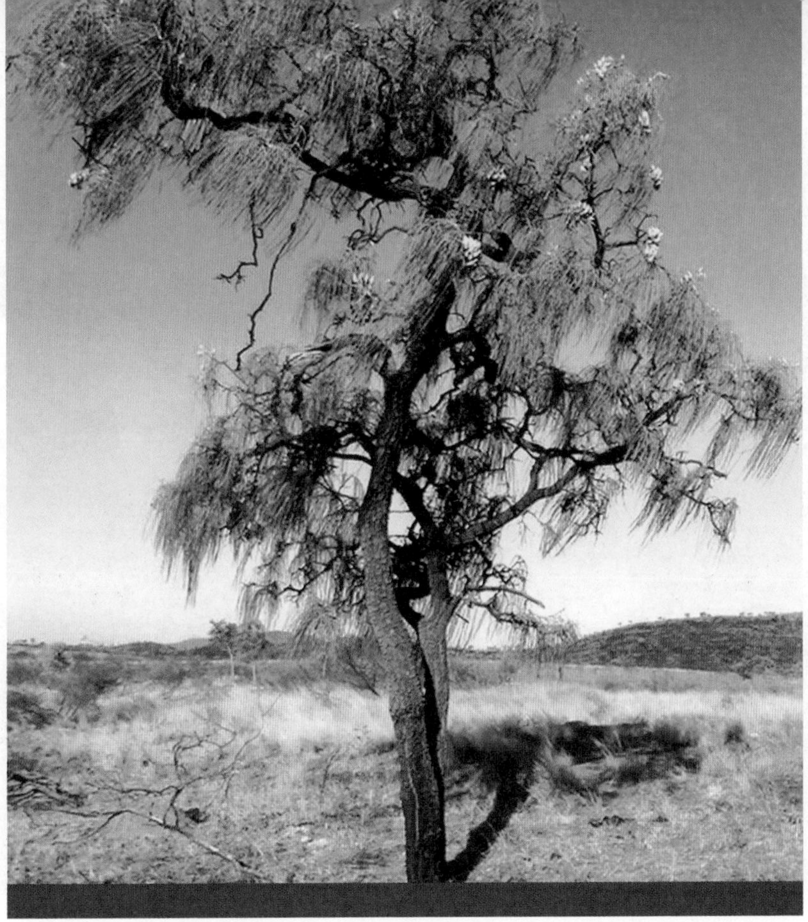

half of Australia, which includes the Gascoyne, Pilbara, Mid-west and Kimberley regions of Western Australia (ALA, 2022; eFlora.SA, 2022; Maiden, 1889; WAH, 2022).

Medicinal Uses Some Aboriginal groups scrape off the outer bark of Witinti and burn it till it is black. The ash is then used as an antiseptic powder to put on sores and wounds to aid healing. The ash is sometimes placed on the forehead of babies to treat fever (Cock, 2011). The Kukatja mix the burnt bark ash with goanna fat and use it as a salve for burns and skin complaints (Valiquette, 1993).

Other Uses The flowers of Witinti drip with nectar, which was sucked straight from the flowers. Alternatively, the flowers were soaked in water to make a sweet drink (Cancilla & Wingfield, 2017; Glasby, 2018). The seeds are edible and are usually eaten raw without preparation (Northern Territory Parks and Wildlife Commission, n.d.).

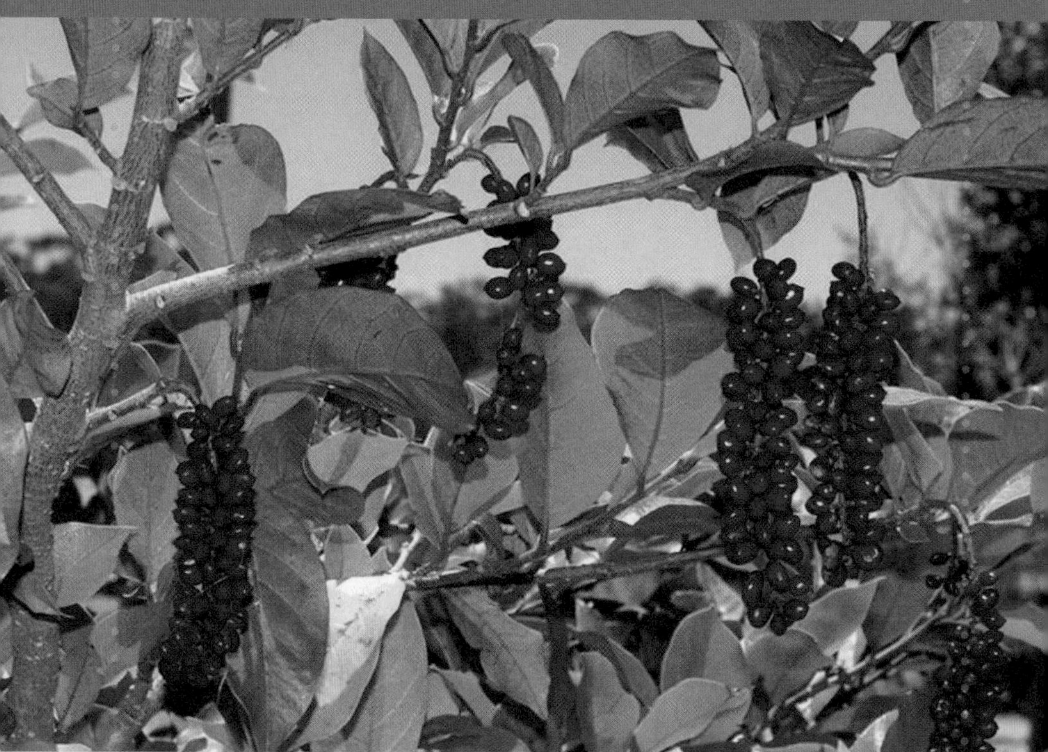

Scientific Name *Antidesma ghaesembilla* Gaertn.

Common Names Yangu, Black Currant Tree.

Aboriginal Names Marnda (Wunambal, Gaambera) (Karadada et al., 2011), Goowarroorlji, Kuwaarrurlji, Berenggarrji, Perengkarrji (Gija) (Purdie et al., 2018 Wightman, 2003), Nguji (Jaru) (Wightman, 2003), Yaangu minya, Wiliwa ninya (Kwini) (Cheinmora et al., 2017; Crawford, 1982).

Field Notes Yangu grows as a shrub or tree to 10 m in height. It has ovate, alternate leaves and small, yellow-green flowers, about 1 mm in diameter that are present on long spikes between August and December. Its fruit are globose berries around 5 mm in diameter that are full of seeds. Yangu occurs in alluvial and basalt soils near swamps and watercourses, and in sandstone gorges across the top end from the Kimberley region in Western Australia to the Northern Territory and the Cape York Peninsula in Queensland. It also occurs

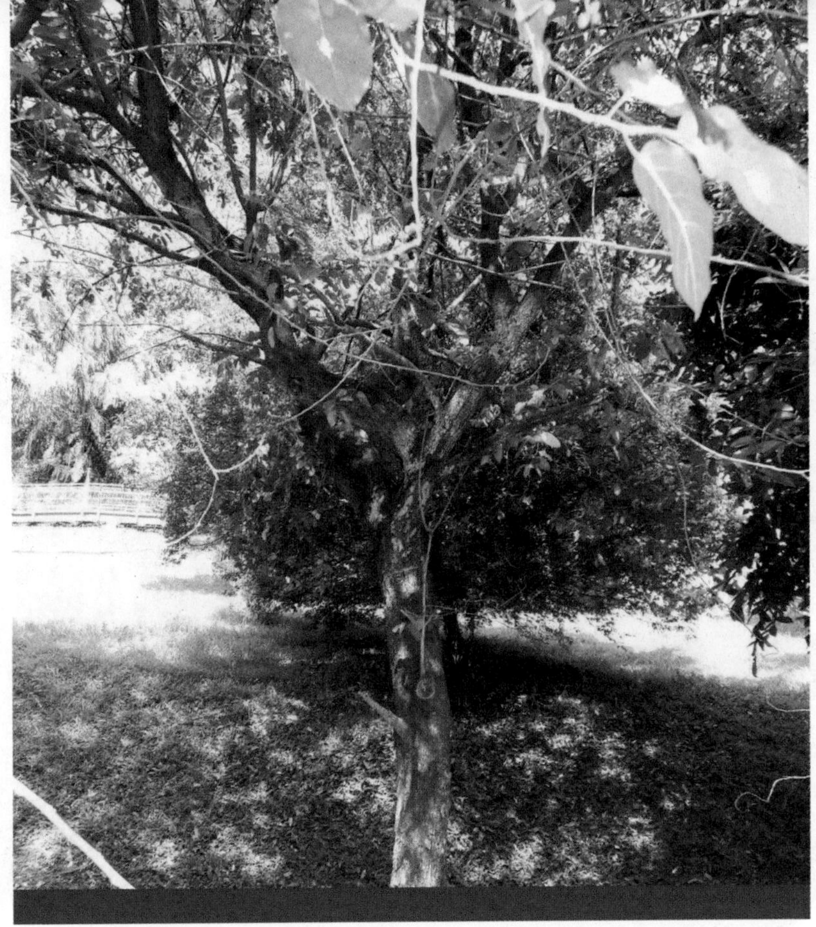

in southern China, on the Indian subcontinent, in Cambodia, Indonesia, Laos, Malaysia, Myanmar, New Guinea, the Philippines, Thailand and Vietnam (ALA, 2022; Fern, 2021; WAH, 2022).

Medicinal Uses The leaves of Yangu trees were crushed and used as a poultice to treat headaches, scurf (flakes on the surface of the skin), abdominal swelling and fever (Fern, 2021). In Far North Queensland, the leaves are mashed with leaves of a paperbark (Melaleuca species), boiled and applied as a poultice to areas of arthritic and rheumatic pain (Edwards, 2005).

Other Uses Yangu trees have small, edible fruit that turn deep red to black when ripe. They are mainly eaten raw by children as a snack. The fruit are available from mid-November to February (Cheinmora et al., 2017; Crawford, 1982; Isaacs, 1987; Jackes, 2010; Karadada et al., 2011; Purdie et al., 2018; Vigilante et al., 2013; Wightman, 2003).

Yellow Boxwood

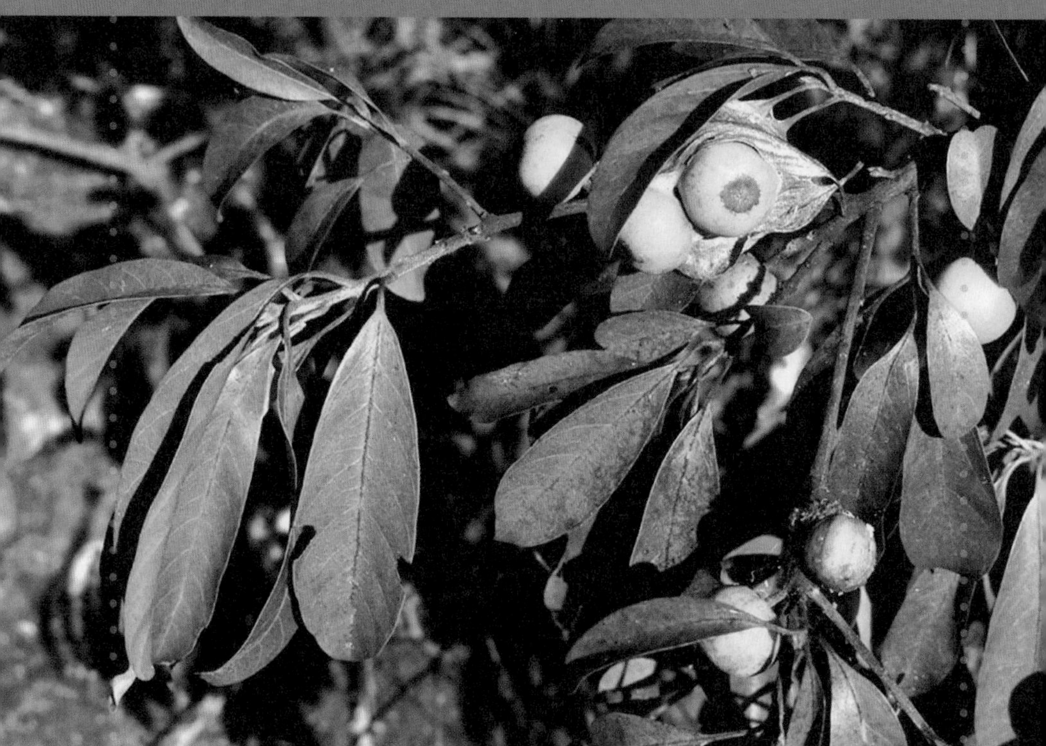

Scientific Name *Planchonella arnhemica* (Benth.) P.Royen, previously known as *Planchonella pohlmaniana* (F.Muell.) Dubard (misapplied).

Common Names Yellow Boxwood, Black Apple, Engraver's Wood, Queensland Yellow Box, Pohlmann's Jungle Plum, Beleam, Arlian, Northern Yellow Boxwood.

Aboriginal Name Mangarr winya (Kwini) (Cheinmora, et al., 2017; Crawford, 1982).

Field Notes Yellow Boxwood grows as a large shrub or tree up to 8 m in height. It has greyish brown, scaly bark that exudes a milky juice when cut, and simple, green and glossy oblanceolate leaves that are up to 130 mm long. Its small, insignificant, creamy-white flowers grow in clusters of up to 12 in the leaf forks. Its globular fruit are green or black and roughly 30 mm in diameter containing five brown, glossy seeds. Yellow Boxwood is usually found in dry

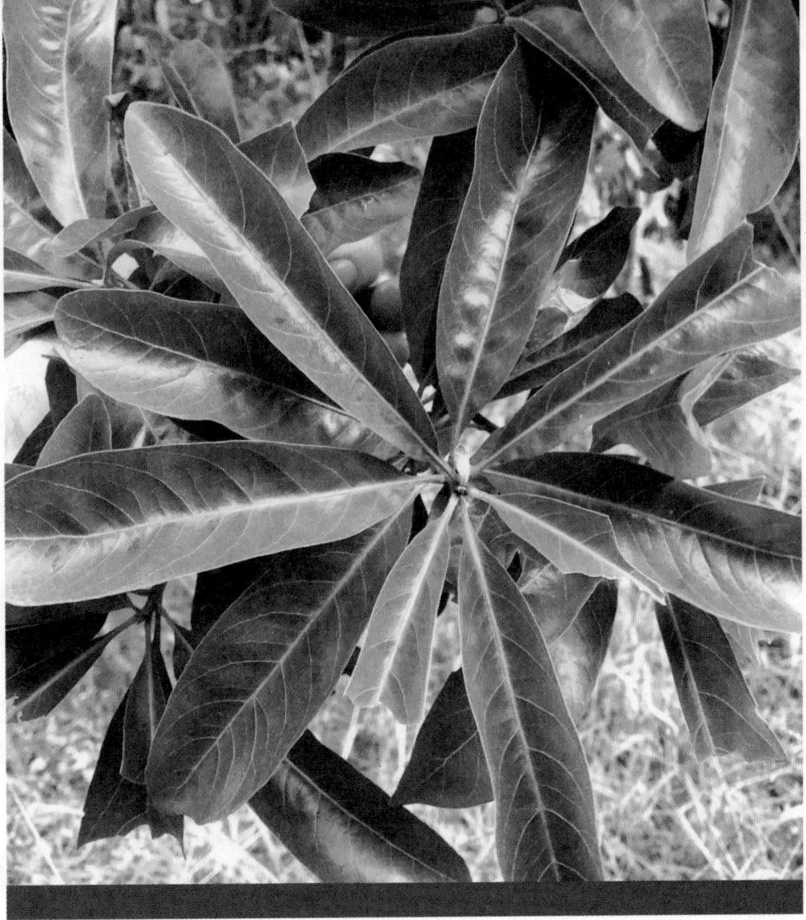

rainforests or on outcrops and rocky ridges in the Kimberley region of Western Australia, the far north of the Northern Territory, the Cape York Peninsula and down the east coast of Queensland as far south as the border with New South Wales (ALA, 2022; Lassak & McCarthy, 2001; SMIP, 2022; WAH, 2022).

Medicinal Uses Infusions or decoctions of the twigs and leaves of Yellow Boxwood were used as an antiseptic wash to bathe wounds and sores. Poultices of crushed leaves and twigs were applied to boils and carbuncles to ripen them and help draw them out (Cock, 2011; Lassak & McCarthy, 2001; Low, 1990).

Other Uses The fruit and seeds of Yellow Boxwood are edible. The seeds were eaten either raw or roasted. The fruit are available from mid-November to February (Bindon, 2014; Cheinmora, et al., 2017; Crawford, 1982; Cribb & Cribb, 1981; Fox & Garde, 2018; Isaacs, 1987; Vigilante et al., 2013).

Yellow Buttons

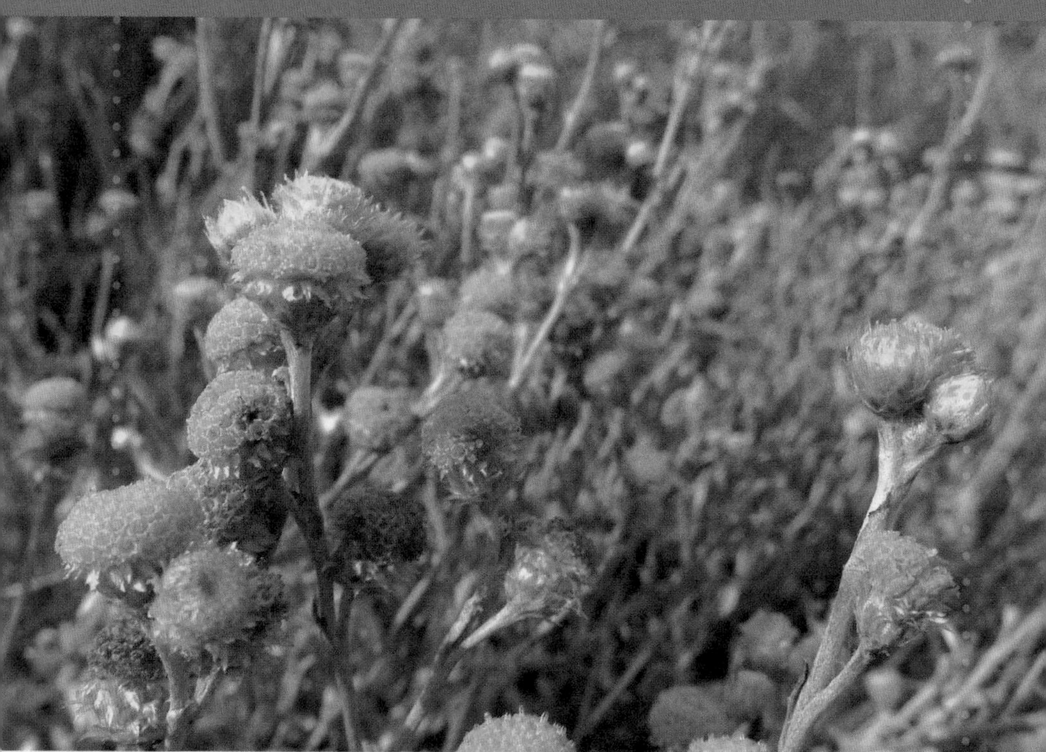

Scientific Name *Chrysocephalum apiculatum* (Labill.) Steetz, previously known as *Helichrysum apiculatum* (Labill.) DC.

Common Names Yellow Buttons, Common Everlasting Flower.

Field Notes Yellow Buttons is an erect perennial herb that branches near the base and grows to around 800 mm in height. Its silver to grey leaves vary in shape from linear-lanceolate, narrow obovate to spathulate, are tapered at both ends and up to 60 mm long and 25 mm wide. Its bright yellow flower heads appear in clusters at the ends of the stems, mainly during summer and autumn, but have also been seen at other times of the year. Its fruit are narrowly oblong-obovoid achenes that are four-angled and slightly compressed and glabrous. Yellow Buttons occurs in a variety of habitats in the Pilbara and Kimberly regions of Western Australia, as well as the drier parts of the state, and in all the other states and territories, including Tasmania (ALA, 2022; ANPSA, 2021; Lassak & McCarthy, 2001; WAH, 2022).

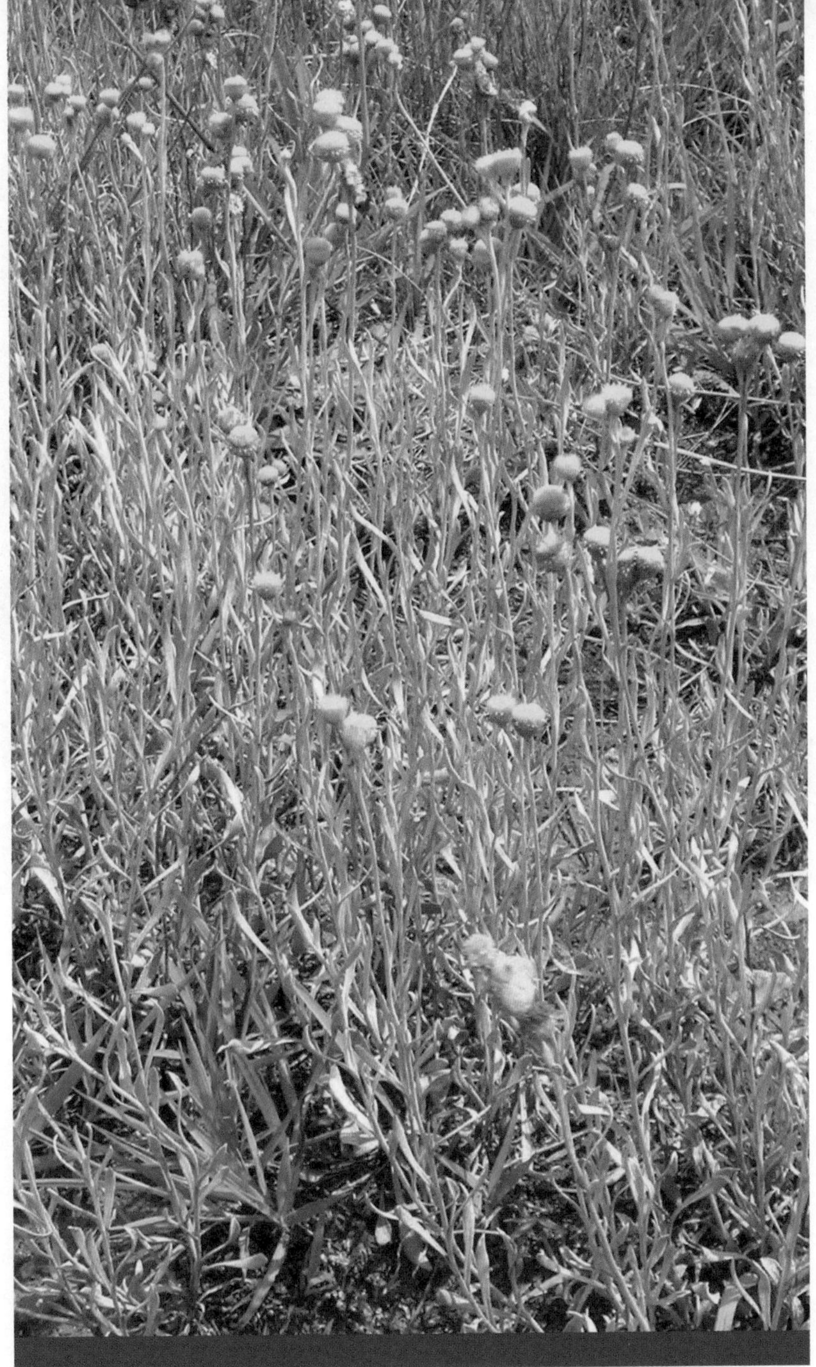

Medicinal Uses Decoctions of the Yellow Buttons plant were taken internally as a vermifuge to expel intestinal parasites (Fern, 2021; Lassak & McCarthy, 2001; Low, 1990).

Yellow Mangrove

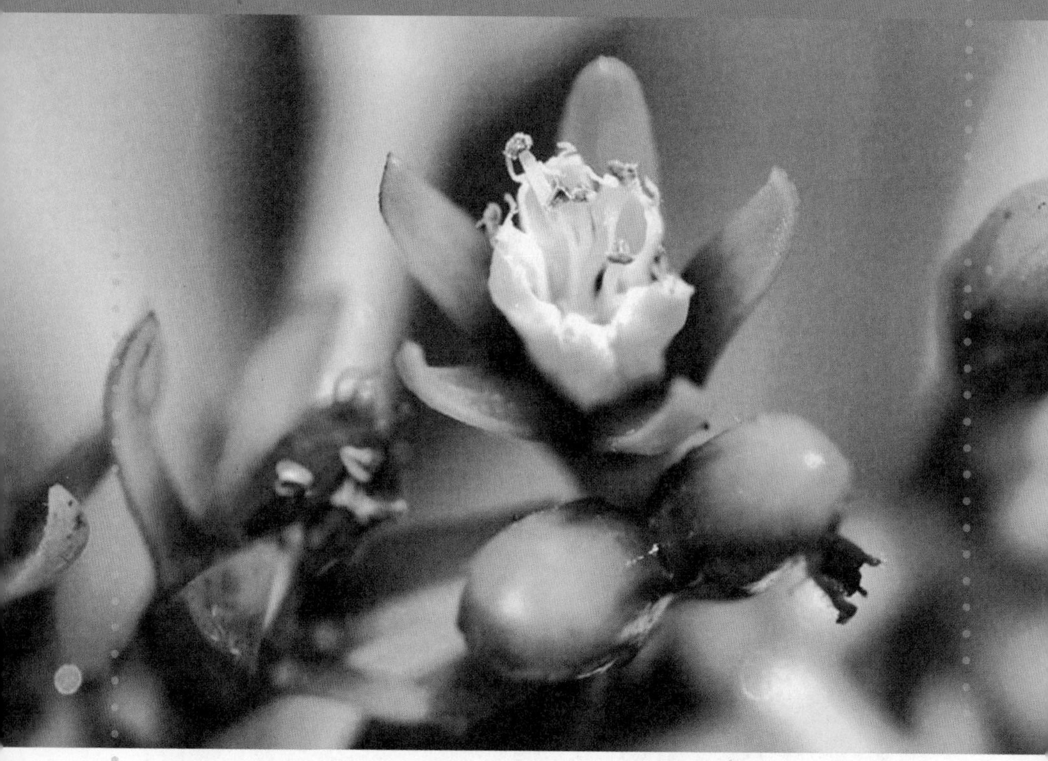

Scientific Name *Ceriops australis* (C.T.White) Ballment, T.J.Sm. & J.A.Stoddart.

Common Names Yellow Mangrove, Smooth-fruited Yellow Mangrove.

Aboriginal Names Goorril (Bardi) (Paddy et al., 1993), Jarrgarla (Wunambal, Gaambera) (Karadada et al., 2011), Darrngarla ninya (Kwini) (Cheinmora et al., 2017).

Field Notes Yellow Mangrove grows as a shrub or small tree up to 10 m in height with short, stocky flanged buttresses. Its obovate to obovate-elliptic leaves are a glossy, yellowish-green in colour and up to 100 mm long and 40 mm wide. Its yellowish-green to orange-red flowers that have creamy white petals form in a dense cluster of two to ten flowers that are around 50 mm long. Its fruit are inverted, pear-shaped drupes about 10 mm or so in length. Yellow Mangrove occurs in inner and drier mangrove stands, usually on the borders

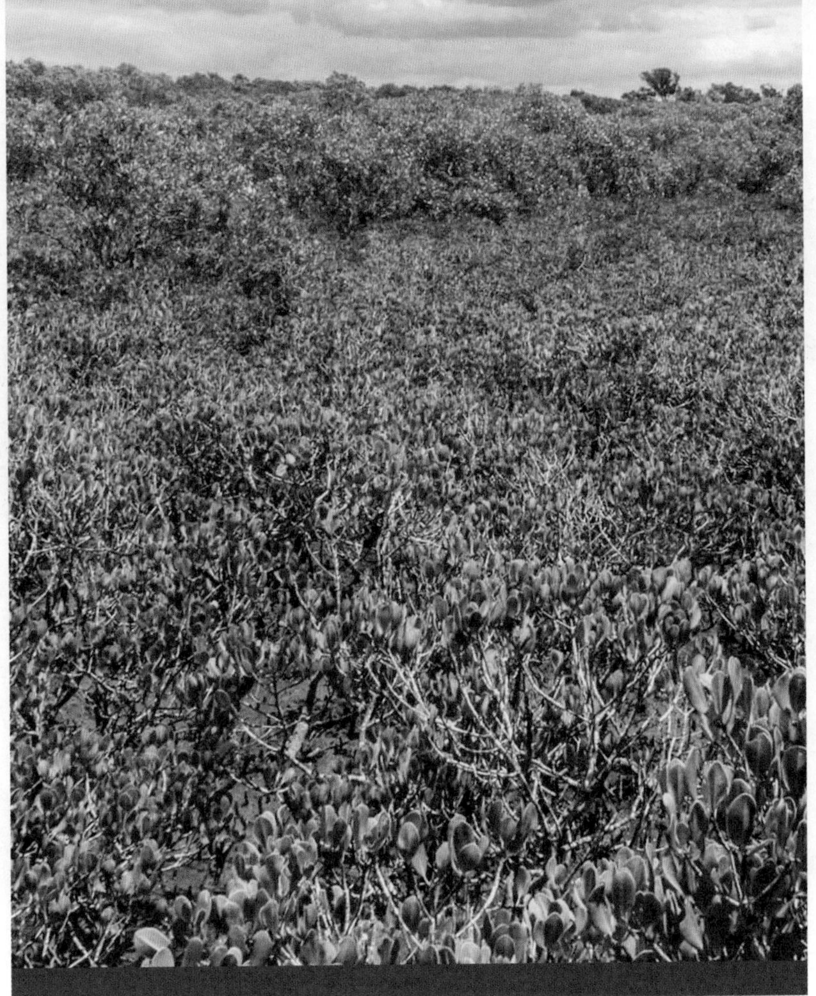

of saltpans and on the landward borders of other mangroves, often forming dense shrublands, around the coast of northern Australia from Exmouth in Western Australia to Moreton Bay in Queensland (ALA, 2022; SMIP, 2022).

Medicinal Uses Infusions of the inner red bark of Yellow Mangrove were used as a wash to treat skin disorders. The wood was burnt and the ashes were used for a similar purpose. Apparently, *Ceriops australis* and *Ceriops tagal* were considered to be the same species until they were shown to be genetically different. *Ceriops tagal* is used in a similar way in other parts of the north including the Tiwi Islands (ALA, 2022; SMIP, 2022).

Other Uses The outer bark of Yellow Mangrove has been used as a dye and for tanning (ALA, 2022).

Yijarda

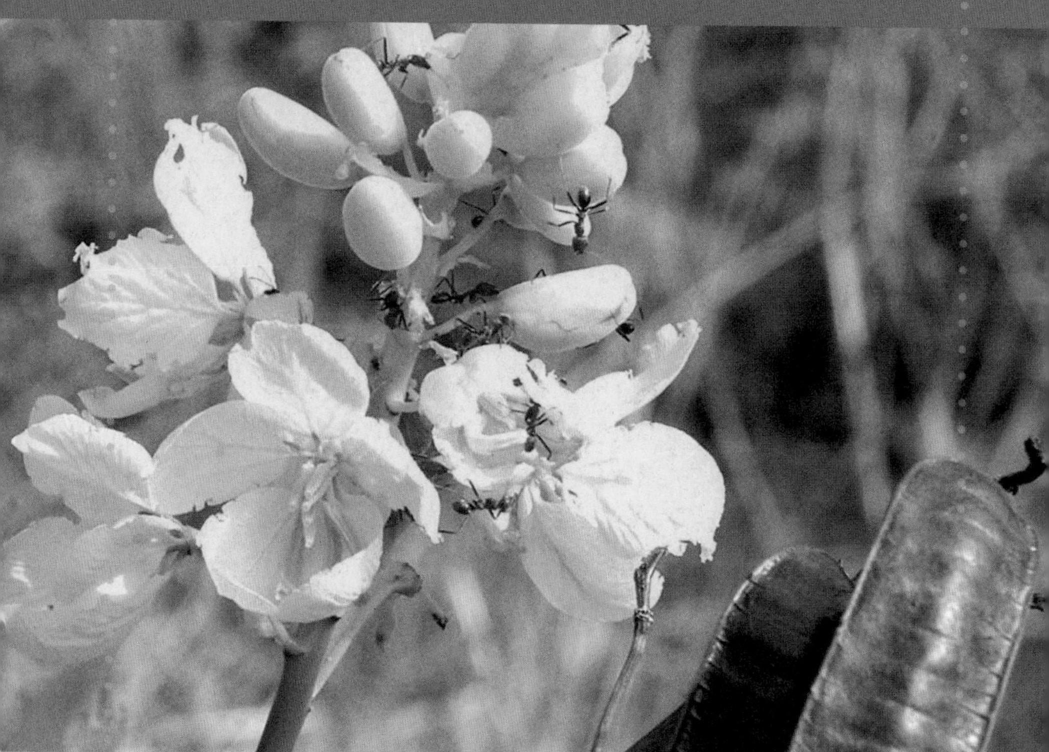

Scientific Name *Senna magnifolia* (F.Muell.) Randell.

Common Name Yijarda.

Aboriginal Names Yijarda, Ganbirrganbirr (Jaru) (Wightman, 2003).

Field Notes Yijarda is an erect, spreading, glabrous shrub that grows up to 4 m in height. Its ovate leaf blades are opposite on the stems and up to 50 mm long and 30 mm wide. Its yellow, buttercup-like flowers are present between March and August. Its fruit or seed pods are long, straight, flat and up to 70 mm long by 15 mm wide. Yijarda occurs in skeletal, gravelly soils, red sand and clay on limestone outcrops, stony ridges and quartzite hills in the Kimberley region of Western Australia and north-east Queensland (ALA, 2022; WAH, 2022).

Medicinal Uses Decoctions of the leaves were used as an antiseptic wash to bathe skin sores and wounds to aid the healing process (Wightman, 2003).

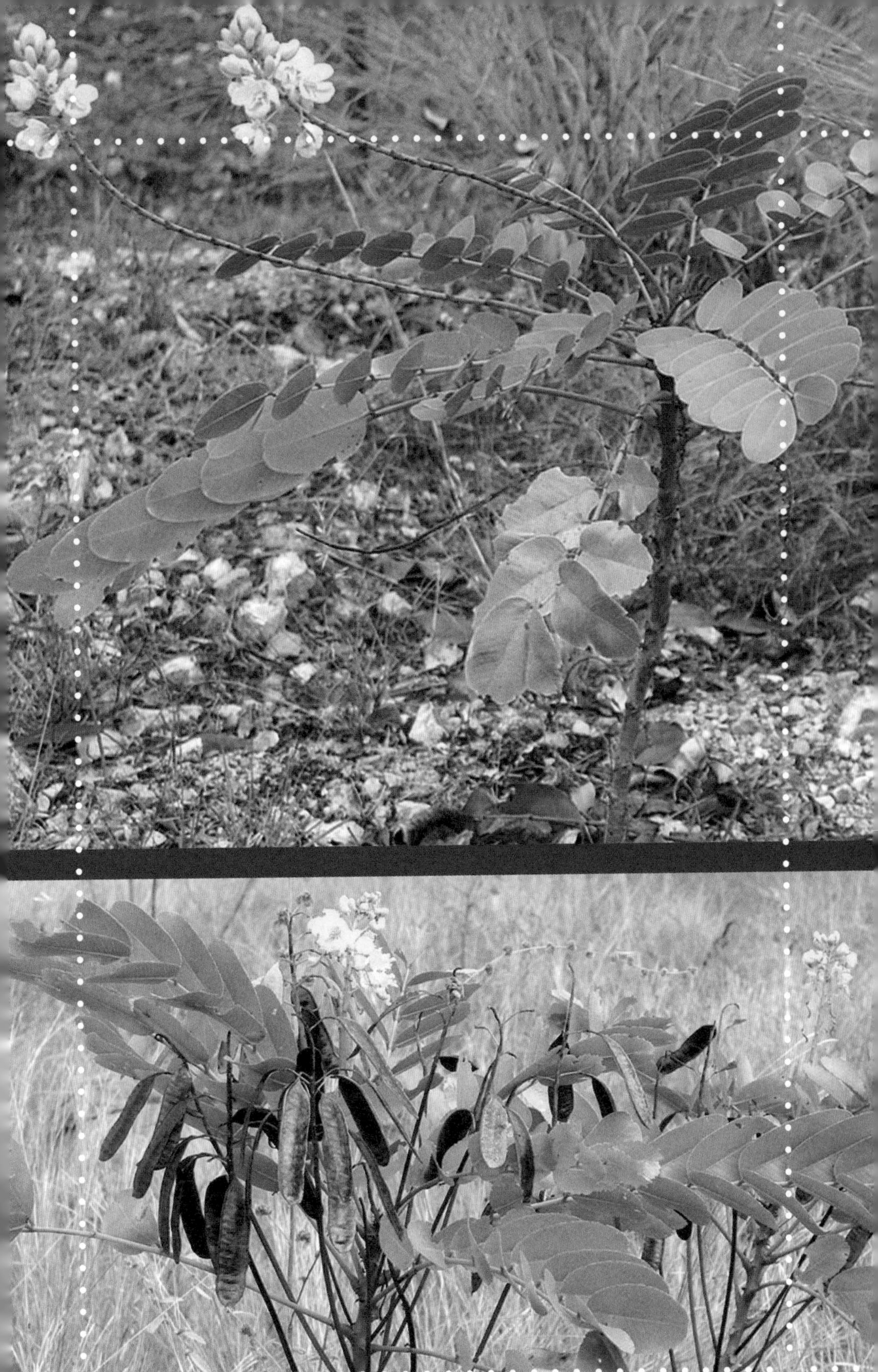

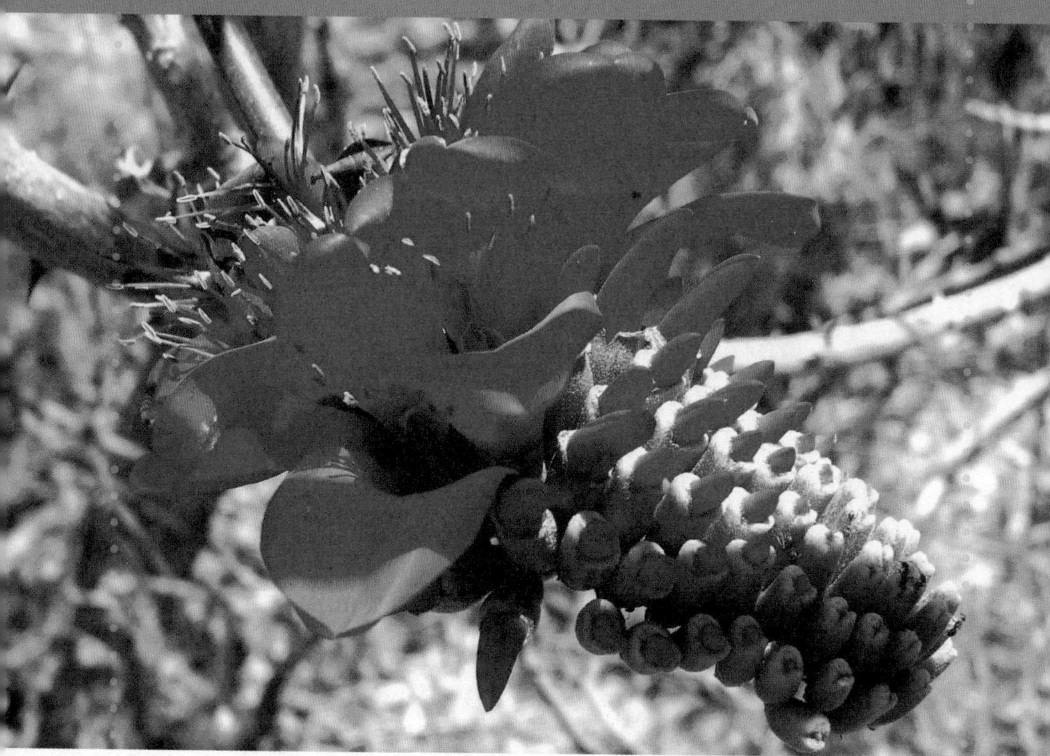

Scientific Name *Erythrina vespertilio* Benth.

Common Names Yulbah, Bat's Wing Coral Tree, Batwing Coral Tree, Corkwood, Cork Tree, Grey Corkwood, Red Bean Tree, Heilaman Tree.

Aboriginal Names Ngawaleng (Miriwoong) (Leonard et al., 2013), Gandiwali (Bunuba) (Oscar et al., 2019), Gandiwal (Wunambal, Gaambera) (Karadada et al., 2011), Garndiwarlel, Karntiwarlel (Gija) (Purdie et al., 2018), Jirndiwili (Gooniyandi) (Dilkes-Hall et al., 2019), Ranyi (the plants with prickles), Yinindi (the plants without prickles) (Jaru) (Wightman, 2003), Yarnkal minya (Kwini) (Cheinmora et al., 2017; Crawford, 1982), Kumpupanu, Marlayi (Kukatja) (Valiquette, 1993), Marlayi, Yinirnti (Ngardi) (Cataldi, 2004), Yinirnti (Walpiri) (Northern Tanami IPA, 2015), Jurnpu (Karajarri) (Moss et al., 2021).

Field Notes Yulbah is a deciduous tree that grows up to 15 m in height. Its bark is greyish-brown and uneven. Its branches and branchlets, and usually its leaf stalks, are very thorny. Its leaves have three lobes with the outer lobes curling to resemble bat wings. Its scarlet to orange-red flowers are pendulous, and around 30–40 mm long. Flowering is between May and November. Yulbah occurs in sand, clay and loam over basalt or limestone in gorges and alongside rivers and creeks in the Pilbara and Kimberley regions of Western Australia, the Northern Territory, Queensland and New South Wales, where its range extends down the east coast to around Port Macquarie (ALA, 2022; ANPSA, 2022; Lassak & McCarthy, 2001; WAH, 2022).

Medicinal Uses Decoctions of the leaves of Yulbah were taken internally as a sedative. Infusions of the bast, or fibre, from the inner bark of the tree and bark were applied externally to sore eyes due to conjunctivitis and to the head for headaches (Cheinmora et al., 2017; Cock, 2011; Crawford, 1982; Isaacs, 1987; Lassak & McCarthy, 2001; Reid, 1986).

Other Uses Some Aboriginal groups ate the fibrous roots of the young Yulbah trees. They are stripped of the bark then roasted in hot ashes before eating (Fox & Garde, 2018; Hiddins, 2001; Isaacs, 1987; Purdie et al., 2018; Wightman, 2003; Williams, 2010). The timber from Yulbah trees was used to make throwing sticks and shields (Cheinmora et al., 2017; Fern, 2021; Reid, 1986). The seeds were used to make necklaces and body ornaments (Cheinmora et al., 2017; Fern, 2021). The straight twigs from this tree were good for making fire by the 'traditional drilling method' (Purdie et al., 2018).

Glossary of Terms Used by Herbalists

Not all the terms listed below have been used in this book, but for carrying out investigation of traditional herbal medicine, it helps to have knowledge of the terms used by herbalists.

Anodyne Relieves mild pain.

Anthelmintic A medicine that expels worms.

Antibilious Acts on the bile, relieving biliousness.

Anti-emetic Stops vomiting.

Antilithic Prevents the formation of stones in the urinary organs.

Antiperiodic Preventing regular recurrences.

Antirheumatic Relieves or cures rheumatism.

Antiscorbutic Cures or prevents scurvy.

Antiseptic A medicine that prevents putrefaction.

Antispasmodic Relieves or prevents spasms.

Aperient Gently laxative without purging.

Aperitive Stimulates the appetite for food.

Aromatic A stimulant, spicy, anti-griping.

Astringent Causes contraction and arrests discharges.

Carminative Expels wind from the bowels.

Cathartic Evacuates the bowels (a purgative).

Cholagogue Increases the flow of bile into the intestine.

Decoction A method of extracting dissolved oils, volatile organic compounds and other chemical substances by mashing herbal or plant material, which may include stems, roots, bark and rhizomes, and then boiling them in water.

Demulcent Soothing, relieves inflammation, especially for skin and mucous membranes.

Deobstruent Removes obstructions.

Depurative Purifies the blood.

Diaphoretic Produces perspiration.

Discutient Dissolves and heals tumours.

Diuretic Increases the secretion and flow of urine.

Emetic Produces vomiting.

Emmenagogue Promotes menstruation.

Emollient Softens and soothes inflamed parts when locally applied.

Esculent Edible.

Expectorant Facilitates expulsion of mucus or phlegm from the lungs and throat.

Febrifuge Abates and reduces fevers.

Hepatic Pertaining to the liver.

Infusion A method of extracting desired chemical compounds or flavours from plants by steeping them in a solvent such as water, oil or alcohol.

Laxative Promotes bowel action.

Lithotriptic Dissolves calculi (stones) in the urinary system.

Nauseant Produces vomiting.

Nervine Acts specifically on the nervous system, stops nervous excitement, tonic.

Parturient Induces and promotes labour at childbirth.

Pectoral A remedy for chest afflictions.

Refrigerant Cooling.

Resolvent Dissolves boils, tumours and other inflammations.

Rubefacient Increases circulation and produces red skin.

Sedative Quiets nerve action and promotes sleep.

Steep To soak an item in liquid such as water or alcohol.

Stomachic Excites the action of the stomach, has the effect of strengthening it and relieving indigestion.

Styptic Arrests haemorrhage from cuts.

Sudorific Produces profuse perspiration.

Tonic A remedy which is invigorating, strengthening and toning.

Vermifuge Expels worms from the intestines.

List of Images

102-3 Caustic Weed, photos by Dr Neil Blair
104-5 Cedar Mangrove, photos by Ria Tan
106 Centipede Fern, photo by Lauren Gutierrez
107 Centipede Fern, photo by Russell Cumming
108-9 Chaff Flower, photo by Lauren Gutierrez
110-11 Chain Fruit, photos by Russell Cumming
112 Chinese Salacia, photo by Cerlin Ng
113 Chinese Salacia, photo by Russell Cumming
114-15 Climbing Deeringia, photos by Lauren Gutierrez
116 Climbing Fern, photo by Russell Cumming
117 Climbing Fern, photo by Wibowo Djatmiko
118-19 Climbing Maiden Hair, photos by Lauren Gutierrez
120 Clubleaf Wattle, photo by Mark Marathon
121 Clubleaf Wattle, photo by Russell Cumming
122 Clump Yellow Pea Bush, photo by Mark Marathon
123 Clump Yellow Pea Bush, photo by Steve & Alison Pearson
124 Coast Roly-poly, photo by Russell Cumming
125 Coast Roly-poly, photo by Harry Rose
126 Coastal Caper, photo by Craig Nieminski
127 Coastal Caper, photo by Bill & Mark Bell
128 Coastal Jack Bean, photo by Sam Fraser-Smith
129 Coastal Jack Bean, photo by Bob Peterson
130 Cockroach Bush, photo by Bill & Mark Bell
131 Cockroach Bush, photo by Nathan Johnson
132-33 Coffee Bush, photos by Russell Cumming
134-35 Comet Grass, photos by Russell Cumming
136 Common Hakea, photo by Craig Nieminski
137 Common Hakea, photo by Mark Marathon
138 Conkerberry, photo by Northwestplants
140-41 Conkerberry, photos by Mark Marathon
142 Coolibah Mistletoe, photo by Russell Cumming
143 Coolibah Mistletoe, photo by North Queensland Plants
144 Cordia Tree, photo by Russell Cumming
145 Cordia Tree, photo by Steve & Alison Pearson
146 Crab's Eye (flowers), photo by Forest & Kim Starr
146 Crab's Eye (seed pod), photo byVinayaraj
148 Crocodile Tree, photo by Tom Harley
149 Crocodile Tree, photo by earth.com
151 Croton, photo by CSIRO
152 Cucumis, photo by Ranjithsiji
153 Cucumis, photo by Mark Marathon
154-55 Currant Bush, photos by Russell Cumming
156-57 Cuthbertson's Wattle, photos by Mark Marathon
158 Daly River Satinash, photo by Craig Nieminski
159 Daly River Satinash (fruit), photo by Cerlin Ng
159 Daly River Satinash (habit), photo by Doreen Massey
160 Damson Plum, photo by Russell Cumming
161 Damson Plum, photo by Forrest & Kim Starr
162 Desert Cassia, photo by Julie Burgher
163 Desert Cassia, photo by Forest & Kim Starr
164 Desert Oak, photo by Terry Feuerborn
165 Desert Oak, photo by Kevin Trotman
166-67 Desert Spurge, photos by Russell Cumming
168 Djabaru, photo by Craig Nieminski
169 Djabaru, photo by Russell Cumming
170 Dog's Balls, photos by Russell Cumming
172 Dogwood, photo by Jacopo Werther
173 Dogwood, photo by Russell Cumming
174 Dogwood Hakea, photo by Russell Cumming
175 Dogwood Hakea, photo by Steve & Alison Pearson
176 Droopy Leaf, photo by Dinesh Valke
177 Droopy Leaf, photo by Siddarth Machado
178-79 Dumara Bush, photos by Roger Fryer & Jill Newland
180-81 Emu Apple, photos by Craig Nieminski
182 Entire-Leaf Wild Grape, photo by Craig Nieminski
183 Entire-Leaf Wild Grape, photo by Cerlin Ng
189 Coolabah, photo by Stan Shebs
189 Darwin Box, photo by Craig Nieminski

192 River Gum, photo by CSIRO
193 Kimberley White Gum, photo by Dean Nicolle
193 Snappy Gum, photo by Dean Nicolle
194 False Cedar, photo by Russell Cumming
195 False Cedar, photographer unknown
196 Fibrebark-Melaleuca nervosa-flowers, photo by Ian Sutton
197-98 Fibrebark, photo by Russell Cumming
198 Fitzroy Wattle, photo by Russell Cumming
199 Fitzroy Wattle, photo by Mark Marathon
200 Flannel bush, photo by Bill & Mark Bell
201 Flannel Bush, photo by Leif Stridvall
202-3 Flinders River Poison, photos by Bill & Mark Bell
204 Forked Mistletoe, photo by Craig Nieminski
205 Forked Mistletoe, photo by Russell Cumming
206 Fragrant Opilia, photo by Craig Nieminski
207 Fragrant Opilia - Opilia amentacea - foliage & flowers, photo by Russell Cumming
208 Freshwater Mangrove, photo by Cerlin Ng
208 Freshwater Mangrove, photo by Dinesh Valke
210-22 Frogsmouth, photos by Annmarie Wise-Green
212 Gadji, photo by Reuben C. J. Lim
213 Gadji, photo by Mark Marathon
214-16 Gandungai, photo by Forest & Kim Starr
216 Ganmanggu (tubers), photo by William Haun
218 Garuga, photo by Russell Cumming
219 Garuga, photo by Wendy Cutler
220-21 Gawar, photo by Steve & Alison Pearson
222 Gidgee, photo by Arthur Chapman
223 Gidgee, photo by Mark Marathon
224 Goat's Foot Vine, photo by Colin Meurk
225 Goat's Foot Vine, photo by sclereid0309
226 Gobin, photo by Andrew Price
228-29 Golden Beard Grass, photos by Russell Cumming
230 Goolyi Bush, photo by Mauro Halpern
231 Goolyi Bush, photo by Leonora Enking
232 Gooramurra, photo by Steve & Alison Pearson
233 Gooramurra, photo by Ethel Aardvark
234 Great Morinda, photo by Forest & Kim Starr
236 Green Birdflower, photo by Freya Thomas
237 Green Birdflower, photo by Bill & Mark Bell
238 Green Crumbweed, photo by Russell Cumming
240 Green Tree Ant, photo by Jordan Dean
242 Grey-leaf Heliotrope, photo by Ragnhild & Neil Crawford
243 Grey-leaf Heliotrope, photo by J.M.Garg
244 Gubinge, photo by Craig Nieminski
245 Gubinge, photo by Louise Beames
246 Gummy Spinifex, photo by Russell Cumming
247 Gummy Spinifex, photo by Kevin Matthews
248-49 Guttapercha Tree, photos by Margaret Donald
250 Hairy Lolly Bush, photo by Craig Nieminski
251 Hairy Lolly Bush, photo by John Tann
252 Hard Cascarilla, photo courtesy of CSIRO
253 Hard Cascarilla, photos by Russell Cumming
254-55 Harpoon Bud, photos by Russell Cumming
256 Helicopter Tree, photo by Mark Marathon
258 Honey sugarbag, photo by Waltja Tjutangku Palyapayi Aboriginal Corporation
260-61 Hopbush, photo by North Queensland Plants
262 Hopbush, photo by Arthur Chapman
263 Hopbush, photo by Steve & Alison Pearson
264 Ironwood, photo by Russell Cumming
266 Jalkay, photos by Russell Cumming
269 Java Brucei, photo by Steve & Alison Pearson
268 Java Brucei, photo by Reuben C. J. Lim
270-71 Jersey Cudweed, photos by Harry Rose
272 Jigal Tree, photo by Steve & Alison Pearson
274 Joolal, photo by Steve & Alison Pearson
276 Kankulang, photo by Craig Nieminski
277 Kankulang, photo by Margaret Donald
278 Kapok Bush, photos by Joe Stephens

279 Kapok Bush, photo by Margaret Donald
280 Kapok Mangrove, photo by Russell Cumming
281 Kapok Mangrove, photographer unknown
282-83 Karnbor, photo by Craig Nieminski
284-85 Kimberley Heather, photos by Geoff Whalan
286 Kunai Grass, photo by John Tann
287 Kunai Grass, photo by Harry Rose
288 Laba, photo by CSIRO
289 Laba, photo by Evan Davies
290 Lather Leaf, photo by David Eickhoff
291 Lather Leaf, photo by Forest & Kim Starr
292-93 Lawyer Vine, photos by John Tann
294 Leafy Nine Awn, photo by Craig Nieminski
295 Leafy Nine Awn, photo by Mark Marathon
296 Leichardt Pine, photo by Steve & Alison Pearson
296 Leichardt Pine, photo by Russell Cumming
299-301 Lemon Grass, photos by Arthur Chapman
300 Lemon-scented Grass, photo by Maura Thoenes
302-3 Lemonwood, photos by Steve & Alison Pearson
304 Little Gooseberry Tree, photo by Cerlin Ng
305 Little Gooseberry Tree, photo by Russell Cumming
306 Lollybush, photo by Adrienne Markey
306 Lollybush, photo by Ethel Aardvark
308 Lotus, photo by Paul Barker Hemings
309 Lotus, photo by Douglas Sprott
309 Lotus, photo by Hans Hillewaert
310 Love Vine, photo by David Eickhoff
311 Love Vine, photo by Scot Nelson
313 Love Vine, photo by CSIRO
314115 Maangga, photographer unknown
316-17 Magabala, photos by the CSIRO
318 Malaiino (fruit), photo by William Milliken
318 Malaiino (leaves), photo by Li Chieh Pan
319 Malaiino, photo by R. Purdie, ANBG
320 Malara, photo by Louise Beames
321 Malara, photo by Tom Harley
321 Malara, photo by Steve & Alison Pearson
322 Mamukata, photo by Craig Nieminski
323 Mamukata, photo by russell Cumming
324-27 Mangaloo, photos by Craig Nieminski
328 Maroon Bush, photo by Bruce Skinner
329 Maroon Bush, photo by Russell Dahms
329 Maroon Bush (fruit), photographer unknown
330-31 Marsh Stemodia, photographer unknown
332 Milky Mangrove, photo by John McPherson
333 Milky Mangrove, photo by Russell Cumming
333 Milky Mangrove, photo by Steve & Alison Pearson
334 Mimosa Bush, photo by Forest & Kim Starr
334 Mimosa Bush, photo by Margaret Donald
336 Mistletoe, photo by Tony Van Kampen
337 Mistletoe, photo by Pete Woodall
338-39 Moonia, photos by Kevin Thiele
340 Musk Basil, photo by Mark Marathon
341 Musk Basil, photo by Dinesh Valke
342-43 Myrtle Mangrove, photo by Russell Cumming
344 Namana, photo by Kevin Theile
345 Namana, photo by Mark Marathon
346 Native Apple, photographer unknown
347 Native Apple, photo by Craig Nieminski
348-49 Native Bryony, photos by Dinesh Valke
350-51 Native Coleus, photos by Russell Cumming
352 Native Cowpea, photo by Craig Nieminski
353 Native Cow Pea, photo by Dinesh Valke
354-55 Native Fig, photos by Forest & Kim Starr
356 Native Fuchsia, photo by Julie Burgher
356 Native Fuchsia, photo by Arthur Chapman
357 Native Fuchsia, photo by Geoff Derrin
358 Native Hibiscus, photos by Forest & Kim Starr
360 Native Lasiandra, photo by Bahamut Chao

361 Native Lasiandra, photo by Graham Carpenter
362 Native Myrtle, photo by Russell Cumming
363 Native Myrtle, photo by Margaret Donald
363 Native Myrtle, photo by Arthur Chapman
364-64 Native Plumbago, photos by Forest & Kim Starr
366 Native Poplar, photo by Mark Marathon
367 Native Poplar, photo by Steven & Alison Pearson
368-69 Native Rosella, photos by Dinesh Valke
370 Native Walnut, photo by Craig Nieminski
371 Native Walnut, photo by Steve & Alison Pearson
371 Native Walnut (habit), photo by Bill & Mark Bell
372-73 Needleleaf Wattle, photos by Russell Cumming
374 Ngurubi, photo by Natalie Tapson
375 Ngurubi, photo by Ian McMaster
376-77 Nine-leaved Indigo, photos by Russell Cumming
378 Nodding Swamp Orchid, photo by Vinayaraj V R
379 Nodding Swamp Orchid, photo by 57Andrew
380-81 Nonda, photos by Russell Cumming
382 North Coast Wattle, photo by Russell Cumming
383 North Coast Wattle, photos by Mark Marathon
384-85 Northern Cane Grass, photos by Russell Cumming
386 Northern Cottonwood, photo by Russell Cumming
388 Northern Kurrajong, photos by Brian Kane
390 Northern Sandalwood, photo by Russell Cumming
392 Northern Star Wattle, photo by Louise Beames
393 Northern Star Wattle, photo by Adrienne Markey
394-95 Oakleaf Fern, photos by Russell Cumming
396-97 Old World Forked Fern, photos by Forest & kim Starr
398-99 Onion Lily, photos by North Queensland Plants
400 Orange Jasmine, photo by Forest and Kim Starr
401 Orange Jasmine, photo by Dinesh Valke
402 Orange Spade Flower, photo by Mark Marathon
403 Orange Spade Flower, photo by Craig Nieminski
404 Pagurda, photo by Nathan Johnson
405 Pagurda, photo by Mark Marathon
406-7 Papawitilpa, photos by Arthur Chapman
408 Pemphis, photo by Arthur Chapman
409 Pemphis, photo by Ria Tan
410 Pied Piper Bush, photo by Andrew Steward
411 Pied Piper Bush, photo by Bev Stockwell and Sally Danen
412 Pink River Apple, photo by Craig Nieminski
413 Pink River Apple, photo by Louise Beames
414-15 Pink Star Flower, photos by North Queensland Plants
416-17 Pirrungu, photos by Russell Cumming
418 Pituri, photo by Kevin Thiele
419 Pituri, photo by Arthur Chapman
420 Pornupan, photo by Ton Rulkens
421 Pornupan, photo by Ria Tan
422 Poverty Bush, photo by Ian McMaster
423 Poverty Bush, photo by Craig Nieminski
424 Puffballs, photo by Lenny Worthington
425 Puffball, photo by Martin Jambon
426 Puncture Vine, photo by Forest & Kim Starr
427 Puncture Vine, photo by David Eickhoff
428 Purslane, photos by Russ Kleinman
430 Quinine Bush (fruit), photo by Steve & Alison Pearson
430 Quinine Bush (flower buds), photo by Craig Nieminski
431 Quinine Bush (habit), photo by Russell Cumming
432 Quinine Tree, photos by Craig Nieminski
433 Quinine Tree, photo by Margaret Donald
434 Rag Weed, photo by Ann Peach
435 Rag Weed, photo by Steve Doyle
436 Ranji, photo by Tom Harley
437 Ranji, photo by Figs of Australia
438 Ranji Bush, photographer unknown
439 Ranji Bush, photo by Bill & Mark Bell
440 Red Ash, photo by Margaret Donald
441 Red Ash, photo by Tony Rodd
442-43 Red Bush Apple, photos by Craig Nieminski

445 Red Bush Apple, photo by Robert Webster
447-48 Red Fungus, photos by Arthur Chapman
448 Red Root, photo by Craig Nieminski
450 Redfruit Kurrajong, photo by Tatiana Gerus
450 Redfruit Kurrajong (fruit), photo by Steve & Alison Pearson
451 Redfruit Kurrajong, photo by Russell Cumming
452 Rhynchosia, photographer unknown
453 Rhynchosia (vine), photo by Russell Cumming
453 Rhynchosia (flowers), photo by Mark Marathon
454-55 River Fig, photos by Tony Rodd
455 River Fig (habit), photo by Margaret Donald
456 River Mangrove, photo by Craig Nieminski
457 River Mangrove, photo by John Tann
457 River Mangrove, photo by Russell Cumming
458 River Teatree, photo by Ian Sutton
459 River Teatree, photo by Mark Marathon
460-61 Rock Grevillea, photos by Joe Stephens
461 Rock Grevillea (fruit), photo by Craig Nieminski
462 Salt Wattle, photo by Tom Harley
463 Salt Wattle, photographer unknown
464 Saltwater Paperbark, photo by Murray Fagg
465 Saltwater Paperbark (foliage & flowers), photo by Louise Beames
465 Saltwater Paperbark (habit), photo by Russell Cumming
466-67 Sand Palm, photos by J. Brew
468 Sandhill Wattle, photo by Craig Nieminski
469 Sandhill Wattle, photo by Mark Marathon
471 Sandpaper Fig, photo by Margaret Donald
470 Sandpaper Fig, photo by Russell Cumming
472 Sandpaper Fig, photo by Craig Nieminski
473 Sandpaper Fig, photo by Louise Beames
474 Saw-edged Spurge, photo by Craig Nieminski
475 Saw-edged Spurge, photo by Russell Cumming
476 Scarlet Bloodroot, photo by Arthur Chapman
477 Scarlet Bloodroot, photo by Russell Cumming
478-79 Scent Grass, photos by John Horsfall
480-81 Scraggy Wattle, photos by Russell Cumming
481 Scraggy Wattle, photo by Arthur Chapman
482-83 Scrambling Clerodendrum, photos by Forest & Kim Starr
484 Screwpine, photo by Craig Nieminski
485 Screwpine, photo by Matthew Stevens
487 Screwpine, photo by Russell Cumming
487 Screwpine (habit), photo by Margaret Donald
488 Scurvy grass, photo by Bill & Mark Bell
489 Scurvy grass, photo by Russell Cumming
490 Scurvy Weed, photo by Joe Stephens
491 Scurvy Weed, photo by iNaturalist
492 Sea Purslane, photo by Anita Gould
493 Sea Purslane, photos by Forest & Kim Starr
494 Signal Mistletoe, photo by Craig Nieminski
495 Signal Mistletoe, photo by Margaret Donald
495 Signal Mistletoe, photo by Margaret Donald
496-97 Silky Grevillea, photo by Russell Cumming
497 Silky Grevillea (shrub in flower), photo by Dinesh Valke
498 Silky Heads, photo by John Tann
499 Silky Heads, photo by Russell Cumming
500 Silky Oilgrass, photo by Arthur Chapman
501 Silky Oilgrass, photo by Mark Marathon
502 Silver Cadjeput (flowers), photo by Tom Harley
502 Silver Cadjeput (tree in habit), photo by Margaret Donald
503 Silver Cadjeput, photo by Russell Cumming
504 Sleepy Morning, photo by Forest and Kim Starr
505 Sleepy Morning, photo by Forest and Kim Starr
506-7 Smartweed, photos by Russell Cumming
508 Smelly Bush, photo by Mark Marathon
509 Smelly Bush, photo by Russell Cumming
510 Snakevine, photo by Craig Nieminski
512 Spike Rush, photo by Nadiah Manjato
513 Spike Rush, photo by John Winder

514-15 Spinifex, photo by Craig Nieminski
516 Split Jack, photo by Steve & Alison Pearson
517 Split Jack, photos by Mark Marathon
518-19 Spotted-leaved Red Mangrove, photos by Russell Cumming
520-21 Spreading Sneezewood, photos by Neil Blair
522 Stem-fruit Fig (fruit), photo by Russell Cumming
522 Stem-fruit Fig (habit), photo by Scott Zona
523 Stem-fruit Fig, photo by Vinayaraj V R
524-25 Sticky Hopbush, photo by Forest and Kim Starr
526 Stiffleaf Sedge, photo by John Tann
527 Stiffleaf Sedge, photo by Mark Marathon
528 Stinking Passionflower, photo by Leon Brooks
530 Stinkweed, photo by Adrienne Markey
531 Stinkweed, photo by Laurinda Timmins
532 Strychnine Bush, photo by Craig Nieminski
533 Strychnine Bush (fruit), photo by Russell Cumming
533 Strychnine Bush (habit), photo by Joe Stephens
534-35 Supplejack, photos by Steve & Alison Pearson
536 Swamp Crinum, photo by Craig Nieminski
537 Swamp Crinum, photo by Brenda Jarratt
538-39 Swamp Morning Glory, photos by Forest & Kim Starr
539 Swamp Morning Glory (plants ready for market), photo by Eric in SF
540-41 Swamp Tea Tree, photos by Mahmud Yussop
542 Tamarind, photo by Mauricio Mercadante
543 Tamarind, photos by Forest & Kim Starr
544-45 Taro, photos by Forest & Kim Starr
546 Tarvine, photo by Jackie Miles
547 Tarvine, photo by Aaron Bean
548-49 Three-leaved Cayratia, photos by Dinesh Valke
550 Tickweed, photo by Jeevan Jose
551 Tickweed, photographer unknown
552 Timon Tree, photo by Craig Nieminski
553 Timon Tree, photo by Mark Marathon
554-55 Tree Orchid, photos by Craig Nieminski
556 Trefoil Rattlepod, photo by Craig Nieminski
557 Trefoil Rattlepod, photo by Russell Cumming
558 Tropical Reed, photo by Tony Rodd
559 Tropical Reed, photo by Show Ryu
560 Tropical Speedwell,, photo by Craig Nieminski
561 Tropical Speedwell, photo by Russell Cumming
562 Turpentine Wattle, photo by Mark Marathon
564 Umbrella Bush, photographer Russell Cumming
565 Umbrella Bush, photo by J. Stanley
566 Vitex, photo by Craig Nieminski
567 Vitex, photographer unknown
568 Walara, photo by Russell Cumming
568 Walara (fruit), photo by Tony Rodd
569 Walara, photo by Steve & Alison Pearson
570 Warty Fuchsia Bush, photo by Natalie Tapson
571 Warty Fuchsia Bush, photo by Geoff Derrin
572-73 Weeping Denhamia, photos by Craig Nieminski
574-75 Weeping Pittosporum, photos by John Tan
576-77 Weeping Tea-tree, photos by Tony Rodd
578 Whipstick Wattle, photo by Craig Nieminski
579 Whipstick Wattle, photo by Russell Cumming
580-81 White Apple, photo by Russell Cumming
581 White Apple (habit), photo by North Queensland Plants
582 White Berry Bush, photo by Brian Kane
583 White Berry Bush, photo by Bernard Dupont
584 White Cheeswood, photo by Craig Nieminski
585 White Cheeswood, photo by Tom Harley
586 White Cypress Pine, photo by Margaret Donald
588 White Dragon Tree, photo by Steve & Alison Pearson
590 White Grevillea, photo by Russell Cumming
591 White Grevillea, photo by Tatiana Gerus
592 White Mangrove, photo by Ria Tan
592 White Mangrove (habit), photo by Brian Kane
593 White Mangrove, photo by Ton Rulkens

594 White Mangrove (fruit), photo by Brian Kane
594 White Mangrove, photo by Ton Rulkens
595 White Mangrove (flower), photo by Craig Nieminski
595 White Mangrove (foliage), photo by Dinesh Valke
596 White Nymph Water Lily, photo by Gail Hampshire
597 White Nymph Water Lily, photo by Joe Stephens
598 White Turkeybush, photo by Craig Nieminski
599 White Turkeybush, photo by Northern Australian Plants
600 White Wild Musk Mallow, photo by Gail Hampshire
601 White Wild Musk Mallow, photo by Russell Cumming
602-3 Wickham's Wattle, photo by Arthur Chapman
604 Wild Gardenia, photo by Craig Nieminsk
605 Wild Gardenia, photo by Russell Cumming
606 Wild Mango, photo by Craig Nieminski
607 Wild Mango (flower), photo by Joe Stephens
607 Wild Mango (fruit), photo by Craig Nieminski
609 Wild Melon, photo by Russell Cumming
610 Wild Nutmeg, photo by Craig Nieminski
611 Wild Nutmeg, photo by Territory Native plants
612 Wild Orange, photo by Craig Nieminski
614 Wild Parsnip, photo by Craig Nieminsk
615 Wild Parsnip, photo by Roger Fryer and Jill Newland
616 Wild Peach, photo by Craig Nieminski
617 Wild Peach, photo by Mark Marathon
618-19 Wild Pear, photos by Craig Nieminski
622-23 Wild Plum, photos by Russell Cumming
624 Witchweed, photo by Craig Nieminski
625 Witchweed, photo by Adrienne Markey
625 Witchweed, photo by Roger Fryer and Jill Newland
626 Witinti, photo by Bill & Mark Bell
627 Witinti, photo by Ian Sutton
628 Yangu, photo by Russell Cumming
629 Yangu, photo by Reuben Lim
630 Yellow Boxwood, photo by Russell Cumming
631 Yellow Boxwood, photo by Greg Tasney
632 Yellow Buttons, photo by John Tann
633 Yellow Buttons, photo by Harry Rose
634 Yellow Mangrove, photo by Craig Nieminski
635 Yellow Mangrove, photo by John Robert McPherson
636-37 Yijarda, photos by Russell Cumming
638 Yulbah, photo by Bill & Mark Bell

Allen. M. (2019). *To Your Health*. www.pressreader.com/australia/gourmet-traveller-australia/20190318/281578061975299 .

Arrawarra Culture. (n.d.). *Fact Sheet 15: Bush Medicine*. www.arrawarraculture.com.au/fact_sheets/pdfs/15_Medicine.pdf

Atlas of Living Australia (ALA). (2022). www.ala.org.au/

AusGrass2. (2022). *Grasses of Australia*. www.AusGrass2.myspecies.info/

Austin, P., Nathan, D. (1998). *Kamilaroi/Gamilaraay Web Dictionary*. www.dnathan.com/language/gamilaraay/dictionary/

Australian Bushfoods. (2022). www.ausbushfoods.com

Australian National Botanic Gardens. (2000). *Aboriginal Bush Medicine*. www.anbg.gov.au/gardens/education/programs/pdfs/aboriginal-bush-medicines.pdf

Australian National Botanic Gardens (ANBG). (2022). www.anbg.gov.au/index.html

Australian Native Edible & Medicinal Seed Service. (n.d.). www.rarefruitblog.files.wordpress.com/2016/06/australiannativeedible.pdf

Australian Native Plants Society (Australia) (ANPSA). (2022). www.anpsa.org.au

Australian Plants Society SA Region. (2022). www.australianplantssa.asn.au

Australian Plants Online (2022). www.australianplantsonline.com.au/ .

Australian Seed. (2022). www.australianseed.com

Australian Tropical Rainforest Plants (ATRP). (2020). https://apps.lucidcentral.org/rainforest/text/intro/index.html

Bailey, F. (1881). Medicinal Plants of Queensland. *The Proceedings of the Linnean Society of New South Wales*. Vol 5. Sydney: F.W. White.

Bancroft, K. (n.d.). *Monitoring Mangroves*. www.library.dbca.wa.gov.au/static/Journals/080052/080052-35.010.pdf (document no longer available).

Barker, R. (1991). *A Checklist of Native Plants Reportedly Edible*. www.anpsa.org.au/foodplantsSG/checklist1991.pdf

Barney, G., Cann, C., Carrington, B., Juli, M., Nodea, N., Nyadbi, L., Peters, R., Purdie, S., Thomas, M., Kofod, F., Leonard, S. (2013). *Jadagen, Warnkan, Barnden: Changing Climate in Gija Country*. Kununurra: Warmun Art Centre.

Bates, D. (1985). *Native Tribes of Western Australia*. Canberra: National Library of Australia.

Benjamin, A., Manickam, V. (2007). Medicinal pteridophytes from the Western Ghats. *Indian Journal of Traditional Knowledge*. 6: 611-618.

Bennett, D., Leung, G., Wang, E., Ma, S., Lo, B., McElwee, K., Cheng, K. (2015). Ratite Oils Promote Keratinocyte Cell Growth and Inhibit Leukocyte Activation. *Poultry Science*. 94(9): 2288-96.

Bindon, P. (1996). *Useful Bush Plants*. Perth: Western Australian Museum.

Bindon, P. (2014). *Backyard Bush Tucker*. Yass: Anthony J MacQuillan.

Bininj Kunwok. (2022). www.bininjkunwok.org.au

Biodiversity India. (2022). *India Biodiversity Portal*. www.indiabiodiversity.org/

Bowman, M., King, D., Reu, S., Fisher, R. (2000). *Common Grasses of Central*

Australia. Land & Water Resources Research & Development Corporation. www.southwestnrm.org.au/sites/default/files/uploads/ihub/central-australian-grasses.pdf (this document is no longer available).

Brand-Miller, J., Holt, S. (1998). Australian Aboriginal Plant Foods: a Consideration of Their Nutritional Composition and Health Implications. *Nutrition Research.* 11: 5-23.

Brisbane Rainforest Action & Information Network (BRAIN). (2022). www.brisrain.org.au/default.asp

Bureau of Meteorology. (2014). *Indigenous Weather Knowledge, Wardaman Calendar: Wujerrijin - dry season.* www.bom.gov.au/iwk/wardaman/wujerrijin.shtml

Bush Heritage Australia. (n.d.). *Bunuba*. https://www.bushheritage.org.au/places-we-protect/western-australia/bunuba

Bush Heritage Australia. (2019). Food for thought. In *December Newsletter*. www.bushheritage.org.au/newsletters/2020/summer/food-for-thought

BushcraftOz. (2022). *The Australian Bushcraft Forum*. www.bushcraftoz.com/

Cairns to Cape Tribulation. (2016). *Swamp Crinum: Crinum uniflorum*. www.cairnstocape.com.au/florafauna/Crinum-uniflorum/84

Calvert, G. (2016). *Wetland Plants of the Wet Tropics*. https://www.wettropicsplan.org.au/wp-content/uploads/2020/11/Wetland-Plants-of-the-Wet-Tropics-FINAL-WEB-compressed-b.pdf

Calvert, G. (2018). *Bush Tucker of the Wet Tropics*. https://www.wettropics.gov.au/rainforest_explorer/Resources/Documents/factsheets/bushTuckerOfTheWetTropics.pdf

Cancilla, D., Wingfield, B. (2017). *Ethnobotanical and Ethnozoological Values Desktop Assessment - Eliwana Project*. www.fmgl.com.au/docs/default-source/approval-publications/eliwana-iron-ore-mine-project-environmental-review-document/appendix-22-ethnobotanical-and-ethnozoological-values-ecoscape-2018.pdf

Cataldi, L. (2004). *A Dictionary of Ngardi*. https://ses.library.usyd.edu.au/bitstream/handle/2123/21407/110322%20-%20Final%20Master%20Compressed.pdf?sequence=3

Cheinmora, D., Charles, A., Karadada, T., Waina, B., Nylerin, F., Waina, L., Punchi, M., Chalarimeri, A., Unghango, D., Saunders, T., Sefton, M., Vigilante, T., Wightman, G. (2017). *Belaa Plants and Animals: Biocultural Knowledge of the Kwini People of The Far North Kimberley, Australia.* Wyndham: Balangarra Aboriginal Corporation.

Children's Health Queensland. (2019). *Milky mangrove* (*Excoecaria agallocha*). www.childrens.health.qld.gov.au/poisonous-plant-milky-mangrove-excoecaria-agallocha/

Cicada Woman Tours. (2013). *Plants Used by Aboriginal People*. www.cicadawoman.weebly.com/uploads/8/7/3/4/8734418/plants_used_by_aboriginal_people_april_2013.pdf

City of Darwin. (2013). *Creating Habitat for Darwin Gardens*. www.darwin.nt.gov.au/sites/default/files/publications/attachments/crting_habitat_for_darwin_gardens_web_version_june2013_2mb.pdf

City of Townsville (n.d.). *Green Tree Ants: Oecophylla smaragdina*. www.soe-townsville.org/greentreeants/index.html

Clarke, P. (1987). Aboriginal Uses of Plants as Medicines, Narcotics and Poisons in Southern South Australia. *Journal of the Anthropological Society of South Australia*. 25(5).

Clarke, P. (2007). *Aboriginal People and Their Plants*. Kenthurst NSW: Rosenberg Publishing.

Clarke, P. (2008). Aboriginal healing practices and Australian bush medicine. *Journal of the Anthropological Society of South Australia*. 33: 3-38

Clendon, M., Lalbanda, P., Peters, A., Utemorrah, D. (2000). *A Provisional Worrorra Dictionary*. Halls Creek: Kimbrley Language Resource Centre.

Cock, I. (2011). *Medicinal and Aromatic Plants – Australia*. www.researchgate.net/publication/264424689_Medicinal_and_aromatic_plants_-_Australia

Coppin, P. (2008). *Nyoongar Food Plant Species*. www.petercoppin.com/factsheets/edible/nyoongar.pdf

Crawford, I. (1982). Traditional Aboriginal Plant Resources in the Kalumburu Area: Aspects in Ethno-economics. *Records of the Western Australian Museum*, supplement 15. www.museum.wa.gov.au/sites/default/files/1.Crawford.pdf

Cribb, A., Cribb, J. (1981). *Wild Medicine in Australia.* Sydney: Fontana-Collins.

Customary Medicinal Knowledgebase (CMKB) (2019). Database of native plants. www.biolinfo.org/cmkb_dev/cmkb/web

Dann, D. (2003). *Waranygu: Digging for Food*. Geraldton: Yamatji Language Centre.

Darwin City Council. (n.d.). *Darwin EM Native Vegetation Book*. www.harvestcorner.org.au/site/assets/files/1023/darwin_native_vegetation_book_06v2.pdf

De Angeles, D. (2005). *Aboriginal Use Plants of the Greater Melbourne Area*. https://www.maribyrnong.vic.gov.au/files/assets/public/aboriginal-plant-use-of-the-greater-melbourne-area.pdf

Deegan, B., Sturt, B., Ryder, D., Butcher, M., Brumby, S., Long, G., Nagarra Badngarri, N., Lannigan, J., Blythe, J., Wightman, G. (2010). *Jaru Plants and Animals: Aboriginal Flora and Fauna Knowledge from the South-east Kimberley and Western Top End, North Australia*. Halls Creek: Kimberley Language Resource Centre.

Department of Agriculture and Fisheries. (2022). www.daf.qld.gov.au

Department of Primary Industries. (2022). www.dpi.nsw.gov.au

Department of Primary Industries and Regional Development. (2022). www.agric.wa.gov.au

Devanesen, D. (2000). *Traditional Aboriginal Medicine Practice in the Northern Territory*. www.digitallibrary.health.nt.gov.au/prodjspui/bitstream/10137/2703/1/Reading_TraditionalAboriginalMedicinePracticeInTheNorthernTerritory.pdf

Dilkes-Hall, I., Maloney, T., Davis, J., Malo, H., Cherel, E., Street, M., Cherrabun, W., Cherel, B. (2019). Understanding Archaeobotany through

Ethnobotany: an Exampla from Gooniyandi Country, Northwest, Western Australia. *Journal of the Anthropological Society of South Australia*.

Dobbs, R., Davies, C., Pettit, N., Pusey, B., Walker, M., Tingle, F. (2015). *Nyul Nyul Freshwater Management and Monitoring Plan*. Darwin: Charles Darwin University

Dollin, A. Dollin, L. (2021). Aussie Bee. www.aussiebee.com.au/index.html

Edwards, S. (2005). *Medical Ethnobotany of Wik, Wik-Way and Kugu peoples of Cape York Peninsula, Australia: an Integrated Collaborative Approach to Understanding Traditional Phytotherapeutic Knowledge and its Applications*. www.discovery.ucl.ac.uk/id/eprint/10105289/1/10105153.pdf/

eFlora.SA. (2022). *Electronic Flora of South Australia*. www.flora.sa.gov.au.

El Questro. (n.d.). *El Questro Top 20 Plants*. https://www.elquestro.com.au/_/media/parks/elquestro/pdfs/elq2014---kimberley-top-20-plants2125.pdf?la=en

Ens, E., Walsh, F., Clarke, P. (2017). *Aboriginal People and Australia's Vegetation: Past and Current Interactions*. www.researchgate.net/publication/317350497_Aboriginal_people_and_Australia's_vegetation_Past_and_current_interactions

Environs Kimberley. (n.d.). *Monsoon (vine) thickets on coastal sand dunes of Dampier Peninsula*. www.dpaw.wa.gov.au/images/documents/plants-animals/tecs/Monsoon-vine-thickets-Dampier-Peninsula.pdf

Environs Kimberley. (2016). eK News: Bulletin of Environs Kimberley – Issue 77 / April.

Eulo, P. (n.d.). *Budjiti Traditional Use of Plants on Naree Station*. www.bushheritage.org.au/getmedia/dd8f5a68-2dd8-4ed0-a61c-354bea63c525/Budjiti-booklet

Ewart, A., Davies, O. (1917). *The Flora of the Northern Territory*. Melbourne: McCarron, Bird & Co.

Fern, K. (2021). *Useful Tropical Plants*. https://tropical.theferns.info

Ferns of Western Australia. (2022). https://fernswa.myspecies.info/

Flavel, M. (2018). *Traditional Diet of the Kiwirrkurra Community Living in the Gibson Desert: Chemical Composition and Functional Characterisation of Identified Foods*. http://arrow.latrobe.edu.au:8080/vital/access/manager/Repository/latrobe:42830

Flora of Australia Online. (2022). https://profiles.ala.org.au/opus/foa

FloraNT. (2022). eflora.nt.gov.au/home

Flowers of India. (2022). www.flowersofindia.net

Foulkes, P. (n.d.). *Kimberley Plants*. www.wkfl.asn.au/nature/cam.htm

Fox, G., Garde, M. (2018). An-me Arri-ngun. *The Food We Eat: Traditional Plant Foods of the Kundjeyhmi People of Kakadu National Park*. Jabiru: Gundjeihmi Aboriginal Corporation.

Fruitipedia. (2022). www.fruitipedia.com.

Glasby, M. (2018). *A Survival Guide*. www.wanowandthen.com/EBooks/survival.pdf

Global Biodiversity Information Facility (GBIF). (2022). www.gbif.org

Gott, B. (2010). *Aboriginal Plants in the Grounds of Monash University*. https://www.monash.edu/__data/assets/pdf_file/0004/542119/Guide-to-the-Aboriginal-Garden-Clayton-Campus.pdf

Grier, N. (n.d.). *Rowes Bay Wetlands Learnscape*. www.creektocoral.org/learnscapes/rowesbay/plants.htm

Grossmann, K. (n.d.). *How to Use Emu Oil: Aboriginal superfood*. www.radiantlifecatalog.com/blog/bid/71172/how-to-use-emu-oil-aboriginal-superfood

Guse, D. (2005). Our Home Our Country: A Case Study of Law, Land, and Indigenous Cultural Heritage in the Northern Territory, Australia. www.ris.cdu.edu.au/ws/portalfiles/portal/23681592/Thesis_CDU_6490_Guse_D.pdf

Hansen, V., Horsfall, J. (2016). *Noongar Bush Medicine: Medicinal Plants of the South-west of Western Australia*. Crawley: UWA Publishing.

Health Benefits Times. (2020). *Health Benefits of Orange Jasmine*. www.healthbenefitstimes.com/orange-jasmine/

Herbal Medicine Research Centre (2002). *Compendium of medicinal plants used in Malaysia, vol. 2*. Kuala Lumpur: Institute for Medical Research, Kuala Lumpur, Malaysia.

Herbalistics. (2022). https://herbalistics.com.au/product/duboisia-hopwoodii-pituri-seed/

Herbiguide. (2022). www.herbiguide.com.au

Hiddins, L. (2001). *Bush Tucker Field Guide*. Ringwood: Penguin Books.

Inner Path Herbal Materia Medica. (2019). www.innerpath.com.au/matmed/0HerbsIndex.htm

Isaacs, J. (1987). *Bush Food: Aboriginal Food and Herbal Medicine*. Sydney: Ure Smith Press.

Jackes, B. (2010). *Plants of Magnetic Island*. https://researchonline.jcu.edu.au/18043/1/Plants_of_Magnetic_Island.pdf

James Cook University. (2022). www.jcu.edu.au

Jones, D., (1996). *The Status and Management of Colubrina asiatica (Latherleaf) in Everglades National Park*. Florida: South Florida Natural Resources Center, Everglades National Park, Homestead.

Kakadu National Park. (2016). *Turkey Bush*. www.parksaustralia.gov.au/kakadu/discover/nature/plants/turkey-bush/

Kamenev, M. (2011). *Top 10 Aboriginal Bush Medicines*. www.australiangeographic.com.au/topics/history-culture/2011/02/top-10-aboriginal-bush-medicines/

Kane, B. (2022). *Bush Trees, Medicines and Fruit of Broome*. www.wkfl.asn.au/nature/bushfruits.html

Kapitany, A. (2020). *Edible Succulent Plants*. www.australiansucculents.com/edible-succulents

Karadada, J., Karadada, L., Goonack, W., Mangolamara, G., Bunjuck, W., Karadada, L., Djanghara, B., Mangolamara, S., Oobagooma, J., Charles, A., Williams, D., Karadada, R., Saunders, T. Wightman, G. (2011). *Uunguu*

Plants and Animals: Aboriginal Biological Knowledge from Wunambul Gaambera Country in the North-west Kimberley, Australia. Wyndham: Wunambal Gaambera Aboriginal Corporation.

Kaur, M., Nitika. (2015). Review on Sea Purslane. *Journal of Pharmacognosy and Phytochemistry*. 3(5): 22-24.

Kemarre, A. (2019). *Bush Medicine*. www.utopialaneart.com.au/pages/bush-medicine-exhibition

Kenneally, K. (2018). Kimberley Tropical Monsoon Rainforests of Western Australia: Perspectives on Biological Diversity. *Journal of the Botanical Research Institute of Texas* 12(1): 149–228.

Kenneally, K., Choules Edinger, D., Willing, T. (1996). *Broome and Beyond: Plants and People of the Dampier Peninsula, Kimberley, Western Australia*. Como, WA: Department of Conservation and Land Management.

Khan, K., Khan, M., Ahmad, M., Mazari, P., Hussain, I., Ali, B., Fazal, H., Khan, I. (2011). Ethno-medicinal Species of genus Ficus L. Used to Treat Diabetes in Pakistan. *Journal of Applied Pharmaceutical Science*. 6: 209-211.

Kimberley Specialists. (2020). www.kimberleyspecialists.com/farwayrbio.htm

Kumar, S., Malhotra, R., Kumar, D. (2010). *Euphorbia hirta*: Its Chemistry, Traditional and Medicinal Uses, and Pharmacological Activities. *Pharmacognosy Review*. 4(7): 58–61.

Lake, M. (2015). *Australian Rainforest Woods: Characteristics, Uses and Identification*. Clayton South: CSIRO Publishing.

Land for Wildlife. (n.d.). *Bush Foods: Grasses.* www.wildlife.lowecol.com.au/wp-content/uploads/sites/25/Bush-Foods.pdf

Lands, M. (1997). Mayi: *Some Bush Fruits of the West Kimberley*. Broome: Magabala Books.

Lassak, E. and T. McCarthy. (2008). *Australian Medicinal Plants*. Sydney: Reid New Holland.

Lee, G. (2003). *Mangroves in the Northern Territory*. Department of Infrastructure, Planning and Environment, Darwin.

Leonard, S., Kofod, F., Olawsky, K. (2013), *Miriwoong Seasonal Calendar*. Kununurra: Mirima Dawang Woorlab-gerring.

Leonard S., Mackenzie, J., Kofod, F., Parsons, M., Langton, M., Russ, P., Ormond-Parker, L., Smith, K., Smith, M. (2013). *Indigenous Climate Change Adaptation in the Kimberley Region of North-Western Australia. Learning from the past, Adapting in the Future: Identifying Pathways to Successful Adaptation in Indigenous Communities*. National Climate Change Adaptation Research Facility, Gold Coast. https://nccarf.edu.au/indigenous-climate-change-adaptation-kimberley-region-north-western-australia-learning/

Lepp, H. (2012). *Aboriginal Use of Fungi.* www.anbg.gov.au/fungi/aboriginal.html

Lindsay, L. (1997). *Capricornia Cuisine: Bush Tucker in Central Queensland.* www.anpsa.org.au/APOL5/mar97-2.html

Lindsay, L. (Ed). (2004). Association of Societies for Growing Australian Plants. *Newsletter Number 47*. June.

Lister, P., Holford, P., Haigh, T., Morrison, D.A. (1996). *Acacia in Australia: Ethnobotany and potential food crop*. pp. 228-236. In J. Janick (ed.), *Progress in New Crops*. Alexandria, VA: ASHS Press.

Low, T. (1990). *Bush Medicine: A Pharmacopoeia of Natural Remedies*. North Ryde: Collins Angus & Robertson.

Low, T. (1991). *Wild Food Plants of Australia*. North Ryde: Collins Angus & Robertson.

Macquarie University. (2020). *Smilax australis R. Br.* www.biolinfo.org/cmkb_dev/cmkb/web/index.php/plantspecies/356

Maiden, J. (1889). *Useful Native Plants*. Sydney: Turner & Henderson.

Mader, G. (2007). The Good Oil. *Journal of the Australian Academy of the History of Pharmacy*. 3(33): 6-7.

Mangroves Australia. (2022). *Indigenous Uses of Mangroves*. www.mangrove-saustralia.wordpress.com/2021/01/20/indigenous-uses-of-mangroves/

Manjari, G., Saran, S., Rao, A., Devipriya, S. (2017). Phytochemical Screening of Aglaia elaeagnoidea and their Efficacy on antioxidant and Antimicrobial Growth. *International Journal of Ayurveda and Pharma Research*. 5(2). http://ijaprs.com/index.php/ijapr/article/view/469

Martin, S. (2014). *Bush Tukka Guide*. Richmond: Explore Australia Publishing.

Mary River Catchment Coordinating Committee. (MRCCC). (n.d.). *A Guide to Some Edible/Useful (Mostly) Local Species.* www.mrccc.org.au/wp-content/uploads/2013/10/Edible-and-useful-native-plants.pdf

Maslin, B., Van Leeuwen, S. Reid, J. (2010). *Wattles of the Pilbara*. www.world-widewattle.com/speciesgallery/descriptions/pilbara/html/default.htm

McConnell, K., O'Connor, S. (1997). 40,000 Year Record of Food Plants in the Southern Kimberley Ranges, Western Australia. *Australian Archaeology*, 45(1): 20-31.

McConvell, P., Saunders, T., Spronck, S. (2013). *Linguistic Prehistory of the Australian Boab.* Selected Papers from the 44th Conference of the Australian Linguistic Society.

McDonald, E. (1988). *Wildflowers of the Pilbara*. Brisbane: Boolarong Publications.

McGregor, W. (n.d.). *Region: The Kimberley*. www.hum.au.dk/ling/research/Kimberley%20languages%20map.htm (this link is no longer active)

McMahon, G. (2006). *Bushtucker in the Top End*. www.dpir.nt.gov.au/__data/assets/pdf_file/0020/228008/ff15_bushtucker_in_top_end.pdf

McNiven, J., Hitchcock, G. (eds) (2015). Goemulgaw Lagal: Natural and Cultural Histories of the Island of Mabuyag, Torres Strait. *Memoirs of the Queensland Museum: Culture.* 8 (1). http://hdl.handle.net/1885/71687

Medical Plants in Singapore. (2019). *Hibiscus tiliaceus*. www.medicinalplants insingapore.wikifoundry.com/page/Hibiscus+tiliaceus

Michie, M. (1993). *The Use of Mangroves by Aborigines in Northern Australia*. Channel Island Field Study Centre Occasional Paper, No. 5.

Milgin, A., J. Watson & L. Thompson. (2009). *Bush Tucker and Bush Medicine of the Nyikina*. Port Melbourne: Pearson.

Mirima Dawang Woorlab-gerring, (2021). *Miriwoong Language App*.

Moore, A. (2008). *Water Chestnuts*. www.permaculturenews.org/2008/11/29/water-chestnuts/

Morse, J. (2005). *Bush Resources: Opportunities for Aboriginal Enterprise in Central Australia.* www.nintione.com.au/resource/DKCRC-Report-02-Bush-Foods.pdf

Native Plants Queensland – Townsville Branch. (2020). www.npqtownsville.org.au

Native Tastes of Australia. (2022). *Bush Remedies*. www.tasteaustralia.biz/bushfood/bush-remedies/

Nguyen, D. (1993). *Medicinal Plants of Vietnam, Cambodia, and Laos*. Santa Monica, CA: Nguyen Van Duong.

Noosa's Native Plants. (2022). www.noosasnativeplants.com.au

Northern Agricultural Catchments Council (NACC). (2022). *Coastal Plant Pocket Guide*. Phone App.

Northern Tanami IPA. (2015). *Northern Tanami Indigenous Protected Area Plan of Management*. https://www.clc.org.au/wp-content/uploads/2021/04/Northern-Tanami-IPA-Plan-of-Management.pdf

Northern Territory Department of Health. (1981 & 1983). Traditional Aboriginal Medicines Project: Newsletters No. 2 & 3.

Northern Territory Parks and Wildlife Commission. (n.d.). Cassia Hill Self-Guided Walk (Information Sheet). www.nt.gov.au/__data/assets/pdf_file/0008/804725/cassia-hill-self-guided-walk.pdf

NSW Government Local Land Services. (n.d.). *Shrubs*. www.archive.lls.nsw.gov.au/__data/assets/pdf_file/0003/495840/archive-shrubs.pdf (this link is no longer active).

NSW Government Office of the Environment & Heritage. (2020). *Lemon-scented Grass – Profile*. www.environment.nsw.gov.au/threatenedspecie-sapp/profile.aspx?id=10267

Nutrition Security. (2020). *Wild Edible Plants*. www.wildedibles.teriin.org/index.php?album=Wild-edibles (This website is no longer available).

Nyinkka Nyunyu Art and Culture Centre. (n.d.). *Mayi: Bush Tucker Recipes*. https://wumpurrarni-kari.libraries.wsu.edu/digital-heritage/mayi-bush-tucker-recipes

Olive Pink Botanic Garden. (2010). *Medicinal & Bush Food Plants*. www.opbg.com.au/wp-content/uploads/2010/03/Medicinal-and-Bushfood-plants.pdf (this document is no longer available as the website is no longer offering it for download).

Olive Pink Botanic Garden. (2013). Silver Cassia. www.opbg.com.au/thegardens/factfiles/silver-cassia/

Oscar, M., Chungal, D., Hoad, S., Bedford, P., Aitken, M., Reynolds, S., Miller, J. (2019). *Yarrangi Thangani Lundu, Mayi Yani-U: Bunuba Trees and Bush Foods*. Fitzroy Crossing: Environs Kimberley, Broome and Bunuba Dawangarri Aboriginal Corporation.

Outback Joe (2018). *Green Ants*. www.outbackjoe.com/macho-divertissement/bush-tucker-plants-and-animals/green-ants/

Oz Native Plants. (2022). www.oznativeplants.com

Packer, J., Brouwer, N., Harrington, D., Gaikwad, J., Heron, R., Yaegl Community Elders, Ranganathan, S., Vemulpad, S., Jamie, J. (2012). An Ethnobotanical Study of Medicinal Plants Used by the Yaegl Aboriginal Community in Northern New South Wales, Australia. *Journal of Ethnopharmacology*, 139(1): 244-255.

Paddy, E., Paddy, S., Smith, M. (1993). *Boonyja Bardag Gorna: All Trees are Good for Something*. Perth: WA Museum.

Palm Pedia. (2015). www.palmpedia.net

Pearn, J. (2004). *Medical Ethnobotany of Australia: Past and Present*. Paper presented to the Linnean Society, London, 30 September. Transcript published by University of Queensland. espace.library.uq.edu.au/eserv.php?pid=UQ:10307&dsID=jp_meia_ls_04.pdf

Peile, A. (1997). *Body and Soul: An Aboriginal View*. Perth: Hesperian Press.

Philippine Medicinal Plants. (2015). *Dilang-butiki: Creeping dentella*. www.stuartxchange.com/Dilang-butiki.html

Philippine Medicinal Plants. (2015). *Katil: Chinese Bush Carrot*. www.stuartx-change.org/Katil.html

Pl@ntUse. (2022). www.uses.plantnet-project.org/en/Main_Page

PlantNET. (2022). The NSW Plant Information Network System. Royal Botanic Gardens and Domain Trust, Sydney. https://plantnet.rbgsyd.nsw.gov.au

Plants for a Future (PFAF). (2022). www.pfaf.org

Plants of the World Online. (2021). www.plantsoftheworldonline.org

Preedy, V., Watson, R., Patel, V. (2011). *Nuts and Seeds in Health and Disease Prevention*. New York: Elsevier Inc.

Purdie, S., Patrick, P., Nyadbi, L., Thomas, P., Fletcher, D., Barrett, G., Ramsey, M., Watbi, D., Martin, M., Thomas, M., Thomas, M., Widalji, P., Kofod, F., Thomas, S., Mung Mung, P., Peters, R., Blythe, J., Wightman, G. (2018). *Gija Plants and Animals: Aboriginal Flora and Fauna Knowledge from the East Kimberley, North Australia*. Batchelor; Palmerston: Northern Territory Government - Department of Environment and Natural Resources

Queensland Bushfoods Association. (2022). *Edible Species*. www.ausbush-foods.com/bushfoodsonline/reports/Plants/edible species.xls

Rare Fruit Council of Australia (RFCA). (1993). *Bush Foods – An Annotated List: Fruit and Seeds Eaten by Aboriginal People in Northern Australia*. www.rfcarchives.org.au/Next/Fruit/AusNative/AnnotatedBushfoods7-93.htm

Readford, H. (2011). Pisolithus sp. www.bushcraftoz.com/threads/pisolithus-sp.7264/

Reid, E. (1986), *The Records of Western Australian Plants Used by Aboriginals as Medicinal Agents*. Bentley: WAIT School of Pharmacy.

Richards, E., Hudson, J. (2012). *Interactive Walmajarri–English Dictionary: with English–Walmajarri finderlist.* http://ausil.org/Dictionary/Walmajarri/Index-en.htm

Rippey, E., Rowland, B. (1995). *Plants of the Perth Coast and Islands*. Perth: University of Western Australia Press.

Roebuck Bay Working Group. (n.d.). *Coastal Gardens: A Planting Guide for Broome on the Dampier Peninsula*. www.roebuckbay.org.au/pdfs/coastal-gardens-web-version.pdf

Save Our Waterways Now. (n.d.). www.saveourwaterwaysnow.com.au

Searle, S. (2020). *Traditional Uses of Australian Acacias*. www.wattleday.asn.au/about-wattles/aboriginal-and-torres-strait-islander-knowledge-and-culture/practical-uses

Sindhuja, R., Rajendran, A., Jayanthi, P., Binu-Thomas, Sivalingam, R. (2012). Traditional Phytomedicines in Kinathukadavu Hills in Southern Western Ghats of Coimbatore. *International Journal of Applied BioResearch*. 9: 1-7.

Slockee, C. (2019). *Plant Profile – Cottonwood*. www.abc.net.au/gardening/factsheets/plant-profile---cottonwood/11708398

Smith, M., Kalotas, C. (1985). Bardi Plants: an Annotated List of Plants and Their Use by the Bardi Aborigines of Dampierland, in North-western Australia. *Records of the Western Australian Museum*. 12 (3): 317-359.

Smith, N. (1991). Ethnobotanical Field Notes from the Northern Territory, Australia. *Journal of the Adelaide Botanical Gardens*. 14(1): 1-65.

Smith, P., Smith, J. (2009). Flora and Fauna Impact Assessment Proposed Nyikina Cultural Centre, Derby, West Kimberley (report to Nyikina Incorporated). www.researchgate.net/publication/340827962_Flora_and_Fauna_Impact_Assessment_Proposed_Nyikina_Cultural_Centre_Derby_West_Kimberley_report_to_Nyikina_Incorporated

Society for Kimberley Indigenous Plants and Animals (SKIPA). (2022). *A Blog About Kimberley Indigenous Plants and Animals*. www.skipas.wordpress.com/

Some Magnetic Island Plants (SMIP). (2022). www.somemagneticislandplants.com.au.

Spearritt, G. (2016). *Plants of Duggan Park, Toowoomba*. www.amarooeec.eq.edu.au/Supportandresources/Formsanddocuments/Documents/plants-of-duggan-park.pdf

Steptoe, D. Passananti, J. (2012). *Bush Medicine: Aboriginal Remedies for Common Ills*. www.australiangeographic.com.au/topics/history-culture/2012/05/bush-medicine-aboriginal-remedies-for-common-ills/

Subhan, N. (2016). *Phytochemical and Pharmacological Investigations of Australian Acacia: An Ethnomedicine-guided Bioprospective Approach*. www.researchoutput.csu.edu.au/ws/portalfiles/portal/92489962/Subhan_Nusrat_thesis.pdf

Sujatha, S., B. Renuga. (2014). Integrated Imminent Wide Scientific Potential from Tropical Weedy Medicinal Plant of Tephrosia Purpurea (Linn.) Pers. An overview. *World Journal of Pharmaceutical Research*. 3 (4): 119-137.

Sustainable Gardening Australia. (2020). *Some Useful Bushfoods*. www.sgaonline.org.au/bushfoods-info/

Territory Native Plants. (2022). www.territorynativeplants.com.au

Thomson, S. (2018). *Plants as Medicine*. www.abc.net.au/gardening/factsheets/plants-as-medicine/10152430

Tiwi Land Council. (2001). *Tiwi Plants & Animals: Aboriginal Flora and Fauna Knowledge from Bathurst and Melville Islands, Northern Australia*. www.tiwilandcouncil.com/documents/Uploads/Tiwi%20plants%20and%20animals%20booklr.pdf

Top End Native Plants Society. (2020). *Recommended Top End Native Plants for Landscaping*. www.topendnativeplants.org.au/

Trails WA. (n.d.). *Ngurin Bush Tucker Trail, Roebourne*. www.karratha.wa.gov.au/Ngurin-Bush-Tucker-Trail

Tuckerbush. (2020). *Edible Australian Tucker Bush*. www.tuckerbush.com.au/

Tungmunnithum, D., Pinthong, D., Hano, C. (2018). Flavonoids from *Nelumbo nucifera* Gaertn., a Medicinal Plant: Uses in Traditional Medicine, Phytochemistry and Pharmacological Activities. *Medicines*. 5(4): 127.

Uddin, K., Juraimi, A., Hossain, S., Un Nahar, A., Ali, E., Rahman, M. M. (2014). Purslane Weed (Portulaca oleracea): a Prospective Plant Source of Nutrition, Omega-3 Fatty Acid, and Antioxidant Attributes. *Scientific World Journal*. 2014. https://doi.org/10.1155/2014/951019

Uluru-Kata Tjuta National Park. (n.d.). www.parksaustralia.gov.au/uluru/

Valiquette, H. (ed.) (1993). *A Basic Kukatja to English Dictionary*. Wirrimanu: Luurnpa Catholic School.

Venkatesh, S., Reddy, Y., Ramesh, M., Swamy, M., Mahadevan, N., Suresh, B. (2008). Pharmacognostical Studies on Dodonaea viscosa Leaves. *African Journal of Pharmacy and Pharmacology*. 2(4): 83-88.

VicFlora. (2022). https://vicflora.rbg.vic.gov.au

Vigilante, T., Toohey, J., Gorring, A., Blundell, V., Saunders, T., Mangolamara, S., George, K., Oobagooma, J., Waina, M., Morgan, K., Doohan, K. (2013). Island Country: Aboriginal Connections, Values and Knowledge of the Western Australian Kimberley Islands in the Context of an Island Biological Survey. *Records of the Western Australian Museum*, supplement 81. www.museum.wa.gov.au/sites/default/files/WAM_Supp81_Internals%20pp145-181.pdf

Webb, L. (1959). The Use of Plant Medicines and Poisons by Australian Aborigines. *Mankind*. 7: 137-146.

Western Australian Herbarium (WAH) (2022). *FloraBase–the Western Australian Flora. Department of Biodiversity, Conservation and Attractions*. https://florabase.dpaw.wa.gov.au

Western Australia Now and Then. (2022). *Aboriginal Medicine*. www.wanowandthen.com/Aboriginal-Medicine.html

Wheaton, T. (ed.) (1994). *Plants of the Northern Australian Rangelands*. Darwin: Department of Lands, Housing and Local Government.

Wheatstone Project. (n.d.). *A Field Guide to the Native Flora of the Onslow Region*. https://australia.chevron.com/-/media/australia/publications/documents/nature-book-onslow-flora.pdf

White, V., White, G. (n.d.). *Peanut Tree Sterculia quadrifida*. www.witjutigrub.

com.au/index.php/info-sheets/17-peanut-tree-sterculia-quadrifida

Whitehouse, M., Turner, A., Davis, C., Roberts, M. (1998). Emu Oil (s): a Source of Non-toxic Transdermal Anti-inflammatory Agents in Aboriginal Medicine. *Inflammopharmacology*. 6(1): 1-8.

Wightman, G. (2003). *Plants and Animals of Kija and Jaru Country: Aboriginal Knowledge Conservation and Ethnobiological Research in the upper Ord Catchment, Western Australia.* Land & Water Australia.

Wightman, G. (2017). *Climbers and Vines of Mangarrayi* Country. Katherine: DNRETAS, Diwurruwurr-Kija Aboriginal Corporation.

Wild. (2020). *10 Aboriginal Medicine Plants and Their Uses*. www.wild.com.au/features/koori-aboriginal-medicine-plants/

Williams A., Sides, T. (2008). *Wiradjuri Plant Use in the Murrumbidgee Catchment*. https://catalogue.nla.gov.au/Record/4585882

Williams, C. (2010). *Medicinal Plants in Australia Volume 1: Bush Pharmacy*. Kenthurst NSW: Rosenberg Publishing.

Williams, C. (2011). *Medicinal Plants in Australia Volume 2: Gums, Resins, Tannin and Essential Oils.* Kenthurst NSW: Rosenberg Publishing.

Williams, C. (2012). *Medicinal Plants in Australia Volume 3: Plants, Potions and Poisons*. Kenthurst NSW: Rosenberg Publishing.

Williams, C. (2013). *Medicinal Plants in Australia Volume 4: An Antipodean Apothecary*. Kenthurst NSW: Rosenberg Publishing.

Williams, C. (2020). *Bush Remedies*. Dural: Rosenberg Publishing.

Williams, L. (2020). *Medicine Country – The Kimberley*. www.goldenbayiridology.com/2020/11/03/medicine-country-the-kimberley-western-australia-by-lisa-williams/

Willing, T. (2014). *Tukujana Nganyjurrukura Ngurra: Literature Review for Terrestrial & Marine Environments on Karajarri Land and Sea Country.* https://d3r4tb575cotg3.cloudfront.net/static/Karajarri%20Literature%20Review_2014.pdf

Wilson, D., Scott-Virtue, L., Kohen, J. (n.d.). *Food Plants*. www.kimberleyspecialists.com/farwayrbio.htm

Wiynjorrotj, P., Flora, S., Daybilama Brown, N., Jatbula, P., Galmur, J., Katherine, M., Merlin, F., Wightman, G. (2005). *Jawoyn Plants and Animals*. Darwin: Northern Territory Government.

Woodall, G., Moule M., Eckersley P., Boxshall B., Puglisi, B. (2010). *New Root Vegetables for the Native Food Industry: Promising Selections from South Western Australia's Tuberous Flora*. www.aff.org.au/wp-content/uploads/RIRDC_09-161.pdf

World Wide Wattle. (2022). www.worldwidewattle.com/

Yamatji Marpla Aboriginal Corporation (YMAC). (2016). *Traditional Ecological Knowledge of Nyangumarta Warrarn Indigenous Protected Area*. www.ymac.org.au/wp-content/uploads/2013/05/899-Ethno-booklet.pdf

Young, L,, Vitenbergs, A. (2007). *Lola Young: Medicine Woman & Teacher*. Fremantle: Fremantle Arts Centre Press.

Young, R., Jackett, N., Graff, J. (2012). *Report to the Kimberley Land Council*

Aboriginal Corporation & Native Title Claim Group. www.epa.wa.gov.au/sites/default/files/PER_documentation/Ecologia%202012%20Thunderbird%20Cultural%20Heritage%20Flora%20and%20Fauna%20Assessment_0.pdf

Yunupinu, B., Yunupinu-Marika, L., Marika, D., Marika, B., Marika, B., Marika, R., Wightman, G. (1995). Rirratjunu Ethnobotany: Aboriginal Plant Use from Yirrkala, Arnhem Land, Australia. *Northern Territory Botanical Bulletin*. 21: 57.

Zhou Y.X., Xin H.L., Rahman K., Wang S.J., Peng C., Zhang H. (2015). Portulaca oleracea L.: A review of Phytochemistry and Pharmacological Effects. *Biomed Research International*. 2015. https://doi.org/10.1155/2015/925631

Index